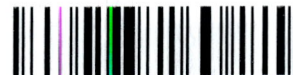

Additional Reviewer's Comments for:

"12 Lead ECG Interpretation in Acute Coronary Syndrome with Case Studies ..... the Cardiac Catheterization Lab" :

"Sir William Osler, Physician-in-Chief and Professor of Medicine for Johns Hopkins Hospital proclaimed, 'He who studies medicine without books sails an uncharted sea, but he who studies medicine without patients does not go to sea at all.' His wisdom, expressed nearly a century ago, could not ring truer in today's practice of medicine. An effective tool for educating today's physicians is the employment of case studies which combine both elements of Sir Osler's quote: academic literature and practical experience. This textbook provides both, and I highly recommend it for all residents and fellows in emergency medicine and cardiology."

Matthew Glover, MD, FACP, FACC
- Interventional Cardiologist
St. Joseph's Hospital
Tampa, Florida

"This outstanding book follows the patient from the field (EMS) to the ER to the cath lab, one of the few of its kind. Use of Cath Lab Case Studies provides a new and valuable perspective to learning 12 Lead ECG interpretation. I strongly recommend it for all health care providers who deal with cardiac patients."

Charles Sand, MD, FACEP, FACP
- Medical Director, Bayflite
- Medical Director, Hillsborough County Fire Rescue
- Past President, American Heart Association, Florida and Puerto Rico Affiliate
- Emergency Department Physician, St. Josephs' Hospital
Tampa, Florida

"ECG's are one of the few sophisticated diagnostic tests widely available to paramedics. This book arms paramedics with the tools to make the accurate and sophisticated assessments which are the foundation of exceptional patient care."

Mike Taigman
- Author, "Taigman's Advanced Cardiology in Plain English"
- Emergency Medical Services Educator and Conference Speaker and Lifelong Student
Sacramento, California

"I cannot imagine a critical care nurse who would not benefit from utilizing this book. A combination of highlighting essential information, lots of graphic images and providing review questions facilitates rapid, effective learning."

Walter Page Young, RN, BSN, CEN
- Education Specialist, Clinical Education
St. Joseph's Hospital
Tampa, Florida

"This book provides a valuable tool for nurses who desire to strengthen their ECG knowledge. I highly recommend it to all nurses who care for patients with Acute Coronary Syndrome."

Caroline "Nikki" Campbell, RN, MSN, CMSRN
- Education Specialist, Clinical Education
St. Joseph's Hospital
Tampa, Florida

ON THE COVER: mid-right photograph: Wendy Wiesler, RN and Humberto Coto, MD, perform PTCA on CODE STEMI patient. lower right photograph: Wendy Tracy with daughter Brooke visit Wayne Ruppert, Sr at York Hospital in York, PA

The CATH LAB SERIES Presents:

12 LEAD ECG INTERPRETATION

IN

ACUTE CORONARY SYNDROME

With CASE STUDIES
from the

CARDIAC CATHETERIZATION LAB

By: Wayne Ruppert, CVT

Medical Editors: Humberto Coto, MD, FACP, FACC
Matthew Glover, MD, FACC
Xavier Prida, MD, FACC
Charles Sand, MD, FACEP, FACP

TARGET AUDIENCE:

This book is intended for medical professionals whom are competent in basic single lead ECG rhythm strip analysis, and desire to learn the basic concepts of 12 lead ECG interpretation, and to identify 12 lead ECG patterns associated with Acute Coronary Syndrome (ACS). It is not intended to teach "basic single-lead rhythm strip analysis."

ISBN: 978-0-9829172-1-3
Library of Congress Control Number: 2010935678

TriGen Publishing
23110 SR 54 #221
Lutz, FL 33549

Email: editor@TriGenPress.com

ABOUT THE AUTHOR:

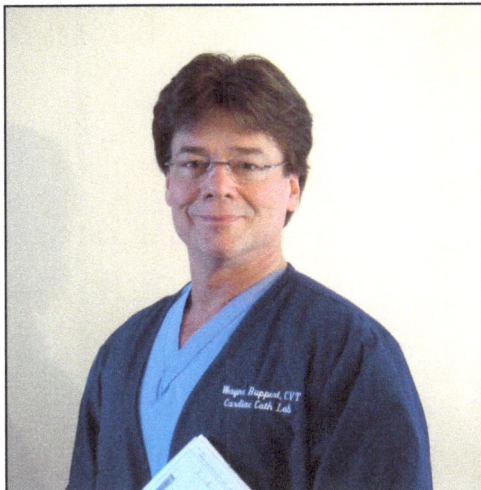

Wayne Ruppert is an Interventional Cardiovascular Technologist and Electrophysiology Technologist for the St. Joseph's Hospitals in Lutz and Tampa, Florida. Mr. Ruppert has logged over 10,000 cardiac catheterizations and electrophysiology studies since 1996. He has taught 12 Lead ECG Interpretation at St. Joseph's since 1997 and at York Hospital in York, PA since 2000.

In 1982, Mr. Ruppert learned the art of 12 Lead ECG Interpretation under the direction of the late Dr. Henry J.L. Marriott.

Mr. Ruppert is an accomplished national conference speaker, and has taught at multiple national conferences since 1989. He is certified as an Instructor in ACLS, PALS, and BCLS.

He began his career with the paramedic response squad operated by York Hospital in 1980, in York, PA. He has served as an EMT and Paramedic Instructor in Pennsylvania and Florida, and Field Training Officer / Director of Education for the Pinellas County, Florida EMS system. From 1991 to 1993, he served as the National Director of Quality Improvement for a publicly traded private ambulance company, where he developed, implemented and coordinated quality improvement and continuing education programs for 14 operations nationwide.

He is also a certified law enforcement officer, and serves as a Reserve Deputy for the Pasco County, Florida, Sheriff's Office.

He resides in Florida with his wife and two children. One adult son, Jeremy, resides in Texas.

ABOUT THE MEDICAL EDITORS:

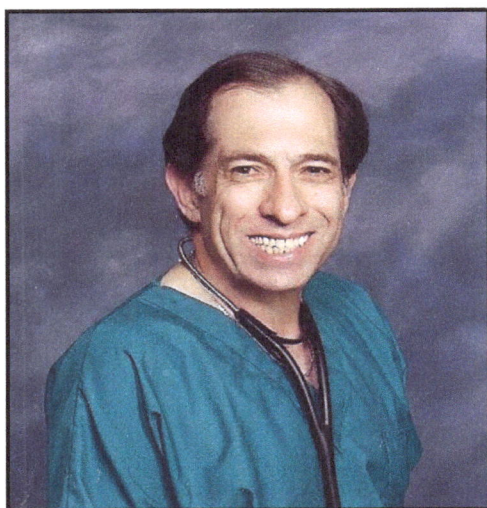

Humberto Coto, MD, FACP, FACC is board certified in Cardiovascular Medicine, Interventional Cardiology and Internal Medicine.

Dr. Coto received his undergraduate degree from Boise State College in 1972 and his Medical Degree from the Autonomous University of Guadalajara in 1976. He completed his internal medicine residency at East Tennessee State University. After completing his cardiology fellowship at University of Louisville School of Medicine, Louisville, Kentucky, he remained at University of Louisville as Co-Director of Interventional Cardiology and Assistant Professor of Cardiology.

He currently serves as the Chief of Cardiology at the St. Joseph's Hospital Heart Institute, and has served on the medical staff at the St. Joseph's Hospital Heart Institute as an Interventional Cardiologist since 1995.

Dr. Coto served as an Assistant Clinical Professor of Medicine for the University of South Florida between 1991 and 1996. He is also the past President of the Hillsborough County Medical Society.

In addition to his medical pursuits, Dr. Coto serves the Hillsborough County Sheriff's Office as a volunteer officer and Field Training Officer, and has logged hundreds of hours on patrol in his community.

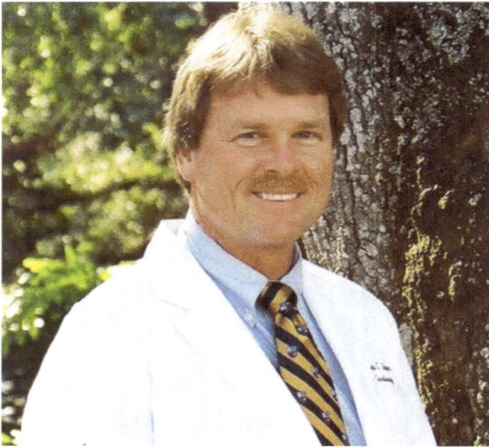

Matthew A. Glover, MD, FACC, FACP is board certified in Cardiovascular Medicine, Interventional Cardiology and Internal Medicine.

Dr. Glover received his undergraduate degree from University of Florida, and his Medical Degree from the University of South Florida in 1975. He completed his medical residency at the University of California – San Francisco, and cardiology fellowship at the Naval Regional Medical Center in San Diego, California
.

He has served on the medical staff at the St. Joseph's Hospital Heart Institute as an Interventional Cardiologist since 1982.

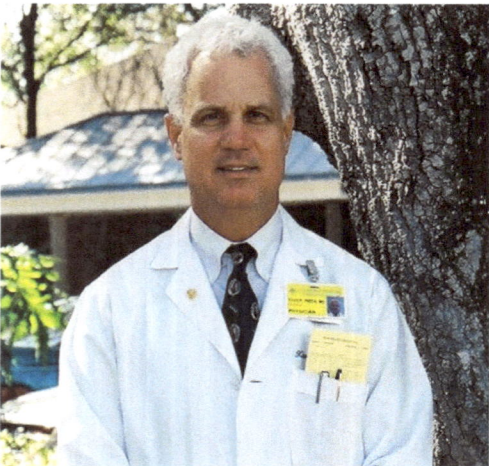

Xavier E. Prida, MD, FACC, FACP is board certified in Cardiovascular Medicine, Interventional Cardiology and Internal Medicine.

Dr. Prida received his undergraduate degree from University of Florida, and his Medical Degree from the University of Miami in 1980. He completed his medical residency at Cornell University Medical Center in New York, and his cardiology fellowship at Shands Hospital at the University of Florida, Gainesville, Florida

He has served on the medical staff at the St. Joseph's Hospital Heart Institute as an Interventional Cardiologist since 1987.

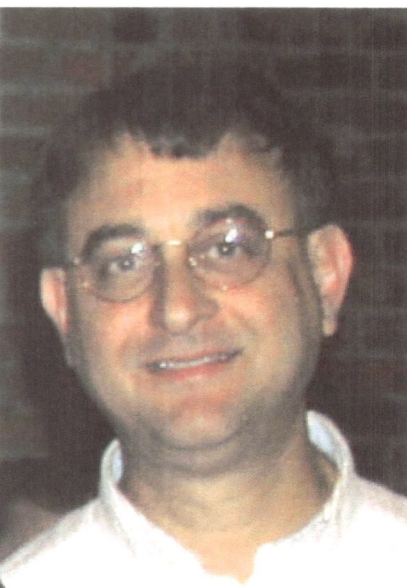

Charles Sand, MD, FACEP, FACP is board certified in Emergency Medicine by the American College of Emergency Physicians, and in Internal Medicine.

Dr. Sand received his undergraduate degree from the University of Florida, and his Medical Degree from the University of Miami School of Medicine in 1985. He completed his internal medicine residency at the Emory University Affiliated Hospitals in 1988, and his emergency medicine residency at the University of Florida Health Science Center in Jacksonville, Florida .

He has served on the medical staff at the St. Joseph's Hospital as an Emergency Physician since 1993.

Dr. Sand has served as the American Heart Association as the Florida-Puerto Rico AHA affiliate president and past National ACLS Florida representative. He participates in community, state, and national education and committee work on heart disease and stroke, and has served on and chaired a number of EMS and FCEP committees.

THE AUTHOR'S PERSONAL PAGE:

THIS BOOK IS DEDICATED to the *passion* that led most of us to seek careers in medicine: -- *the passion to save the life of a fellow human being.* It fuels our need for excellence, and motivates us to seek every opportunity to hone our lifesaving skills. The *knowledge* contained in this book has directly assisted my medical colleagues and I with saving the lives of several people, some of whose case studies are presented in this book. I wish to pass along this knowledge to other health care professionals, with hope that many more will be saved in the future.

"There is no greater reward in medicine than watching someone you helped resuscitate leaving the hospital, surrounded by their family."

Early in my career, I learned to appreciate the value of the 12 Lead ECG as a tool to discover life-threatening conditions. Shortly before the above photograph was taken, I attended my first 12 Lead ECG Workshop—conducted by the late **Dr. Henry J. L. Marriott**—in Lancaster, PA, in June of 1982. Weeks later, I used the Physiocontrol LifePak 5 monitor in this photograph to discover a patient's anterior wall MI by "walking" the single positive lead across the patient's chest. This knowledge greatly enhanced my ability to discover life-threatening conditions, and in several cases, made a significant difference in patient outcome.

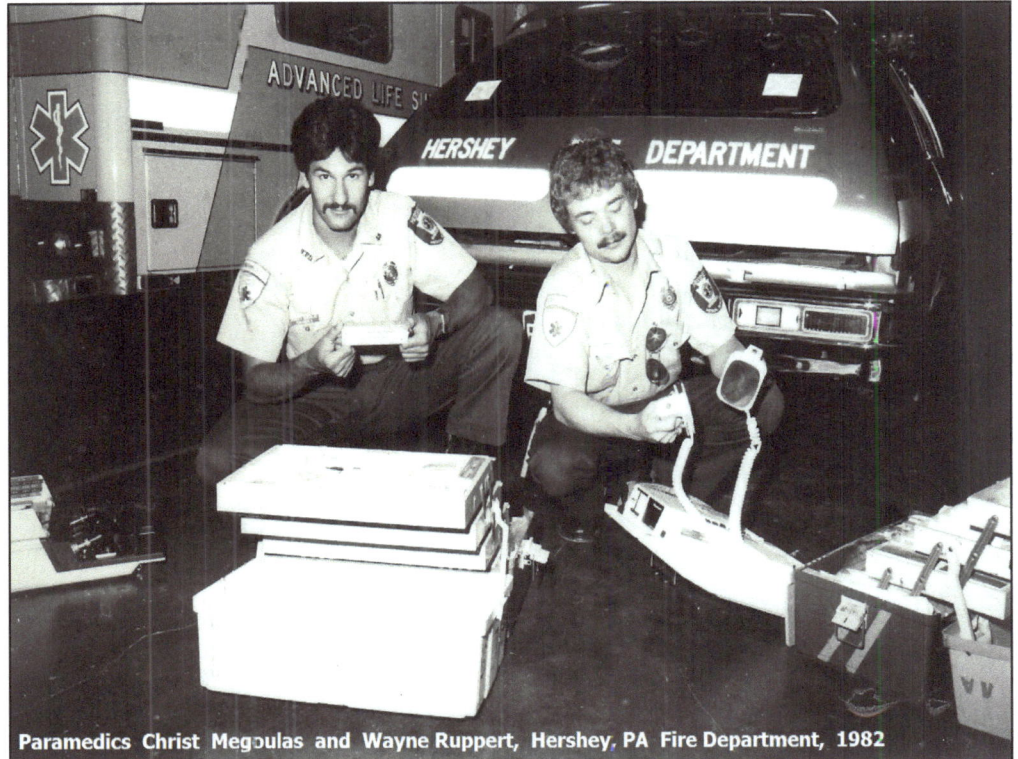

Paramedics Christ Megoulas and Wayne Ruppert, Hershey, PA Fire Department, 1982

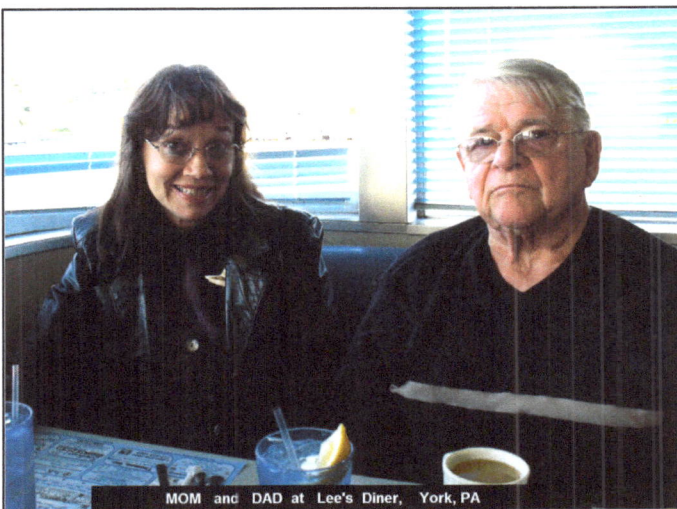

MOM and DAD at Lee's Diner, York, PA

SPECIAL THANKS TO MY PARENTS, WAYNE AND GAIL RUPPERT, FOR PROVIDING ME WITH THE GIFT OF LIFE, AND FOR THEIR ENDLESS LOVE AND GUIDANCE, WHICH HAS TAUGHT ME HOW TO MAKE THE BEST OF THAT GIFT!

A Tribute to Dr. Henry J.L. Marriott
June 10, 1917 – August 31, 2007

I credit world renowned cardiologist **Dr. Henry J. L. "Barney" Marriott** as being *"the man who taught the world to read ECGs."* When I told him this in 2007, at the age of 90, he laughed and humbly replied, "you give me far too much credit." In addition to teaching thousands of physicians and nurses across the globe to read ECGs, Dr. Marriott is the man who taught me to read ECGs in 1982.

After completing his medical education at Oxford University as a Rhodes Scholar in 1943, he served his residency St Mary's Hospital in London.

At St. Mary's, he cared for injured and dying British soldiers returning from the frontlines of World War II. In 1944 he served in the Penicillin Research Unit under Sir Alexander Fleming, who discovered Penicillin. Dr. Marriott had the unique opportunity to successfully treat some of the first cases of bacterial endocarditis with penicillin.

In 1948, while serving as Assistant Professor of Medicine at Johns Hopkins University and Hospital in Baltimore, MD, he was asked to teach ECG interpretation to fourth year medical students. This marked the beginning of over six decades of

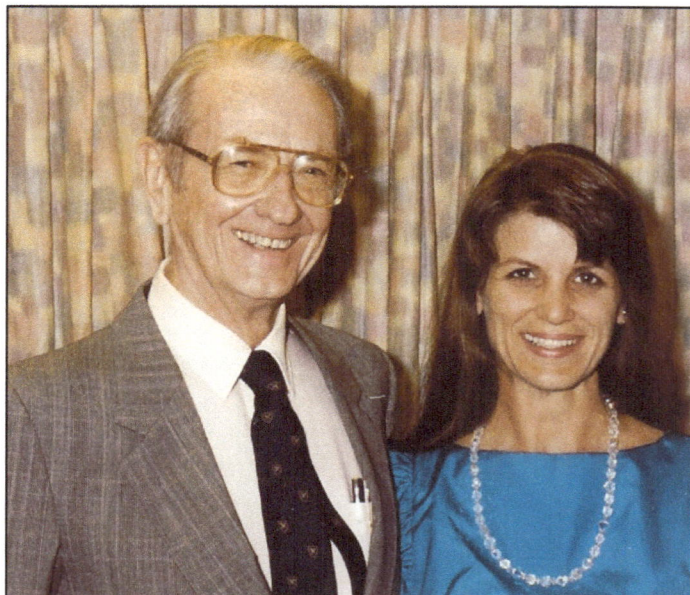

Dr. Henry J. L. Marriott and Jonni Cooper, PhD. Photo taken on the QE 2, while enroute to Austria via England, for a meeting of physicians.

achievement in cardiology research, writing, and education. To date, his contributions to medicine and humanity remain equaled by few, and second to none.

In 1952, he wrote "Medical Milestones," a book for laymen, which was published by Williams and Wilkens of Baltimore. With a forward written by Sir Alexander Fleming, the book became an instant best-seller, and made him a household name with physicians and the public alike.

In 1954, he wrote "Practical Electrocardiography," the book which has defined the standard and served as the base for nearly every ECG book written since. Over the next thirty four years, he published seven more editions of this book, until it was picked up by Galen Wagner, MD, FACC, Director of the Duke Medical School Clinical Research Study Program and the Editor of The *Journal of Electrocardiography*. Dr. Wagner has eloquently blended the most recent discoveries learned in the Electrophysiology Lab with the teachings of Dr. Marriott; a truly unbeatable combination that continues to make "Marriott's Practical Electrocardiography" requisite reading for every cardiac-care clinician world-wide.

From 1946 until his passing in 2007, Dr. Marriott taught the art of Electrocardiography to *thousands* of physicians, nurses, and other medical professionals at universities, hospitals, and conventions worldwide.

I had the distinct honor to attend Marriott ECG workshops in 1982 and in 1994. The conference in 1994, held at a convention center in Clearwater Beach, Florida, was attended by several hundred medical professionals, some whom had traveled around the world for the opportunity to hear him speak. At that time, I was developing a 12 lead ECG curriculum for field paramedics. I wanted Dr. Marriott's feedback on my ideas, so he invited me to join him and Dr. Jonni Cooper for lunch. I was astounded that the internationally renowned cardiologist had noticed me, let alone offered for me to join him for lunch. – I could not believe my good fortune! During our lunch meeting, he listened intently as I explained my ideas, and then provided several insightful and relevant suggestions.

And once again, on a mid-summers day in 2007, I had the honor of being present with Dr. Marriott as he, at the age of 90, taught ECG interpretation to nurses and monitor techs at the 5 North nurses station at St. Joseph's Hospital in Tampa, Florida. On this day, he was clad in a patient's gown, his body ravaged by the disease consuming it, but his mind as young and sharp as the day he stepped forth from the polished halls of Oxford University to "change the world" nearly 70 years prior. This proved to be his last ECG class – for he passed away shortly thereafter, in the arms of his research and teaching partner, Dr. Jonni Cooper.

The mission of Barney Marriott lives on, being carried out by Dr. Jonni Cooper and the staff of the Marriott Heart Foundation and the American College of Cardiovascular Nurses (ACCN) in Riverview, Florida.   www.marriottheart.org

TABLE of CONTENTS:

CASE STUDIES of ACUTE CORONARY SYNDROME:

STEMI CASE STUDIES

NSTEMI CASE STUDIES

UNSTABLE ANGINA CASE STUDIES:

BRUGADA SYNDROME and other STEMI MIMICS:

MEDICAL ABBREVIATIONS USED IN THIS BOOK:

ABCs	airway, breathing, and circulation
ACLS	Advanced Cardiac Life Support
ACS	acute coronary syndrome
ADP(s)	accelerated diagnostic protocol(s)
AF	atrial fibrillation
AHA	American Heart Association
ALS	advanced life support (prehospital care)
AMI	acute myocardial infarction
ASA	aspirin
ASHD	arteriosclerotic heart disease, atherosclerotic heart disease
AV	atrio-ventricular
aVF	augmented voltage foot (left leg ECG lead)
aVL	augmented voltage left (ECG lead)
aVR	augmented voltage right (ECG lead)
BBB	bundle branch block
BMP	basic metabolic panel
BP	blood pressure
CABG	coronary artery bypass graft(s)
CAD	coronary artery disease
CAOx4	conscious, alert, oriented to person, place, time and event
CBC	complete blood count
CHF	congestive heart failure
CK	creatine kinase (cardiac marker)
CK-MB	creatine kinase - MB isoenzyme (cardiac marker)
COPD	chronic obstructive pulmonary disease
CPK	phosphocreatine kinase (cardiac marker)
CRP	c-reactive protein (cardiac inflammation marker)
CX, CIRC.	circumflex
DES	drug-eluting stent
DIAG	diagonal
DIB	difficulty in breathing
ECG	electrocardiogram (usually refers to single lead or telemetry)
ED/ER	emergency department / room
EF	ejection fraction
ECG, EKG	electrocardiogram (ECG), electrokardiogramm (German for ECG)
EMS	emergency medical services
EP	electrophysiology
EST	exercise stress test
FACC	Fellow of the American College of Cardiology
FACEP	Fellow of the American College of Emergency Physicians
FACIM	Fellow American College of Internal Medicine
FACP	Fellow of the American College of Physicians
HDL	high density lipoprotein
HR	heart rate
IABP	intr-aortic balloon pump
ICD	internal (implanted) cardiac defibrillator
IWMI	inferior wall myocardial infarction
JACC	Journal of American College of Cariology
K+	potassium
LA	left atrium
LAD	left anterior descending (artery)
LAFB	left anterior fascicular block
LAH	left atrial hypertrophy

LBB	left bundle branch
LBBB	left bundle branch block
LDL	low density lipoprotein
LMCA	left main coronary artery
LPFB	left posterior fascicular block
LV	left ventricle
LVEF	left ventricular ejection fraction
LVH	left ventricular hypertrophy
LQTS	long QT syndrome
MCL	modified chest lead
MG++	magnesium
MI	myocardial infarction
mm	millimeters
MONA	morphine, oxygen, nitroglycerin, aspirin
MSEC	milliseconds
MV	mitral valve
NEJM	New England Journal of Medicine
NIH	National Institutes of Health
NL	normal
NSTEMI	non-ST segment elevation myocardial infarction
02 SAT	oxygen saturation
OM	obtuse marginal (artery)
P	pulse
PCI	percutaneous coronary intervention
PDA	posterior descendiing artery
PLV	posterior lateral vessel(s)
PMHx	past medical history
PTCA	percutaneous transluminal coronary angioplasty
PVC	premature ventricular contraction
R	respirations / respiratory rate
RA	right atrium
RAH	right atrial hypertrophy
RBB	right bundle branch
RBBB	right bundle branch block
RCA	right coronary artery
RV	right ventricle
RVH	right ventricular hypertrophy
RVMI	right ventricular myocardial infarction
SA	sino-atrial
SA NODE	sino-atrial node, sinus node
SACS	Simple Acute Coronary Syndrome (Score)
SAO2	oxygen saturation
SOB	shortness of breath
STAT	from Latin word *statim*, meaning. "immediately"
STEMI	ST segment elevation myocardial infarction
SVT	supra-ventricular tachycardia (narrow complex)
UA	unstable angina
VF	ventricular fibrillation
V-FIB	ventricular fibrillation
VLDL	very low density lipoprotein
VT, V-TACH	ventricualr tachycardia
V-TACH	ventricular tachycardia
WBC	white blood cell(s)
WNL	within nomal limits
WPW, W-P-W	Wolff-Parkinson-White Syndrome

HOW TO USE THIS BOOK:

☞   If you wish to expediently master the essential concepts in this book:

- READ the sentences that are highlighted in this color.
- STUDY all graphic images and photographs.
- CORRECTLY ANSWER the REVIEW QUESTIONS at the end of each section.   If you are not sure of the correct answer, the page where the information in the question originate is noted in parentheses. Turn to the page indicated and review the material.
- *Adherence to the above recommended practice will optimize your successful mastery of this material.*

A note from the author before you get started:

This work has evolved from a PowerPoint handout that I created for my 12 Lead ECG workshops, which I have been conducting since 1997. It encompasses everything I have learned from veteran medical practitioners (my mentors), books, medical journals, and from my own practical experience in the prehospital environment, emergency department, and from assisting with over 10,000 cardiac catheterizations and electrophysiology studies, spanning from 1978 to the current time.

Suffice to say, although this book represents *the best I that I have to offer* at the current time, I have no doubt that there are folks who will read this book, and will have thoughts they would like to share.   From those of you who take the time to read my work, I appreciate your feedback, whether it's complimentary or "constructive."   You can correspond with me at:

wayne@ECGTraining.org

ROLE OF THE ECG IN PATIENT EVALUATION:

Like everything else in medicine, science and technological advancements are evoking changes in the way we use the multi-lead ECG.

In the 1950s and 60s, the 12 Lead ECG was a primary diagnostic tool in cardiology. Early pioneers of that era, such as Wenckebach, Wilson, Katz, Marriott and others taught us how to diagnose ischemia, infarction, necrosis, hypertrophy, and a host of other cardiac disorders through interpretation of the ECG.

With today's advancements in the fields of diagnostic imaging, echocardiography, cardiac catheterization and electrophysiology, we have diagnostic tools that overshadow the ECG in sensitivity and specificity. As such, we have learned that many traditional ECG diagnoses are often inaccurate and unreliable.

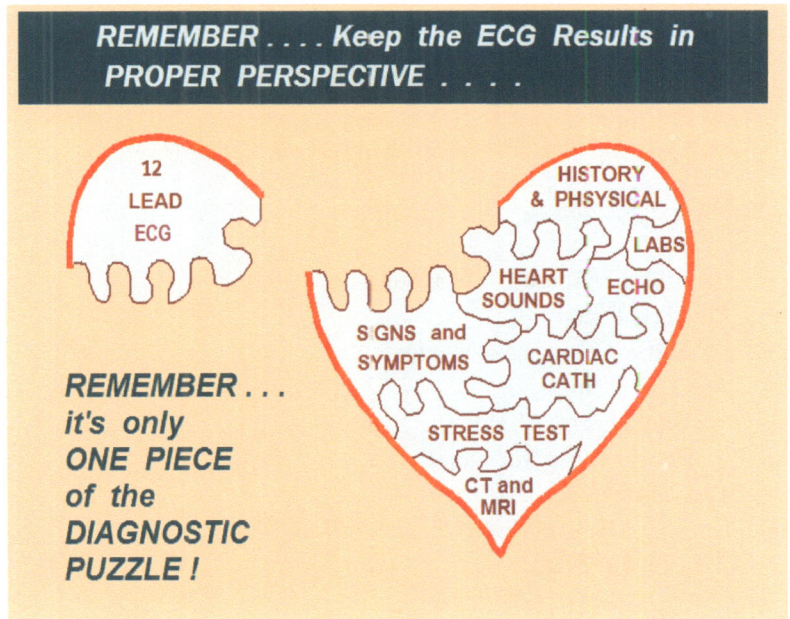

REMEMBER . . . . Keep the ECG Results in PROPER PERSPECTIVE . . . .

REMEMBER . . . it's only ONE PIECE of the DIAGNOSTIC PUZZLE !

In the emergency setting, acute myocardial infarction can be missed when the ECG lacks typical S-T segment elevation. Wide QRS tachycardias—which can be ventricular tachycardia, bypass-tract tachycardia with antedromic conduction (W-P-W), or SVT with aberrancy—are frequently misdiagnosed, and in some cases impossible to differentiate on the 12 Lead ECG. Patients who have severe coronary artery blockages – even some suffering acute myocardial infarction – may present with perfectly normal 12 lead ECGs.

DESPITE ALL OF OUR TECHNOLOGICAL ADVANCES IN DIAGNOSTIC CARDIOLOGY.....

THE 12 LEAD ECG IS THE QUICKEST AND MOST COST-EFFICIENT FRONT-LINE TRIAGE TOOL THAT WE HAVE TODAY.

When the ECG is taken at face value, without consideration of the patient's assessment findings and risk factor profile—or worse, the ECG machine's computer-derived diagnosis is accepted without question—the outcome may be catastrophic.

Despite our technological advances in diagnostic cardiology and the ECGs propensity for error, the 12 lead ECG is undisputedly one of the most expedient and cost-efficient front-line triage tools we have today. Per the American Heart Association, *obtaining a 12 Lead ECG within ten minutes upon arrival at the emergency department* is part of the "golden standard" of care when dealing with suspected MI patients.

In dealing with other life-threatening conditions such as symptomatic bradycardias, wide complex tachycardias, Torsades de Pointes, myocarditis, critical electrolyte imbalances and cardiac ischemia, the 12 Lead ECG often provides us with a "key piece of the diagnostic puzzle," aiding us in selecting and executing the appropriate treatment modality in a timely manner.

In the non-acute setting, obtaining a 12 Lead ECG as part of a comprehensive routine exam is a necessary practice to help identify the presence of "silent killers," such as *Wolff-Parkinson-White, Long Q-T* and *Brugada Syndromes*. In addition, ischemia and chamber hypertrophy can often be detected on the resting 12 Lead ECG. In cases where the ECG is normal and all disease processes are ruled out, the "normal ECG" serves as an invaluable "baseline" ECG at a future date, when the patient returns with suspicious symptoms.

The ECGs *greatest strength* is its usefulness as a tool to assist us with diagnosing life-threatening conditions. When used properly, it can help us to save lives. ***Conversely, its greatest weakness is its notable lack of sensitivity and specificity,*** which can lead to misdiagnosis, improper treatment, and catastrophic outcomes.

Simply stated, *we cannot **rely solely on the ECG to provide us with the patient's diagnosis.*** In order to ***maximize diagnostic accuracy*** while concurrently *minimizing diagnostic error,* we must rely on other indicators which will compensate for the ECGs' *lack of sensitivity and specificity*.

During a suspected cardiac patient's *initial assessment*, the following parameters must be assessed:

- Primary Complaint / Symptoms
- Physical Exam:
- ABCs / Shock Assessment
- ECG monitoring
- Vital signs / SAO2
- Heart / Lung Sounds
- 12 Lead ECG
- Cardiac Markers / other Pertinent Lab Results
- Risk Factor Profile

Our goal is *to collect the above data within thirty minutes of patient arrival*. With the advent of point-of-care testing for cardiac markers, we find this goal is reasonably attained. One of American Heart Association's defined clinical standards is for Health Care Providers (including EMS services) to "obtain and interpret a 12 lead ECG on all suspected cardiac patients within *ten minutes of arrival.*" With the above information at hand, most life-threatening conditions—such as ACS or lethal dysrhythmias—can usually be ruled out.

For patients who don't meet obvious STEMI / NSTEMI criteria, a process for evaluating possible Unstable Angina (UA) and low risk chest pain patients, called *"accelerated diagnostic protocols"* (ADPs), are employed. ADPs utilize serial ECGs and cardiac markers in combination with other diagnostic testing, such as cardiac echo, stress testing and CT coronary angiography to definitively rule out ACS and other abnormal cardiac conditions. (ADPs are presented in more detail on pages 158 – 162).

"The ST-SEGMENT-ELEVATION MYOCARDIAL INFARCTION (STEMI) CHAIN of SURVIVAL" and the ROLE of the 12 LEAD ECG

The metaphor "STEMI CHAIN of SURVIVAL" was originally coined by Dr. Joseph P. Ornato in an editorial featured in the American Heart Association's **Circulation** journal in 2007.[1] This insightful article describes the need for our communities to develop a nationwide standard for the initial management of STEMI. Dr. Ornato compares his vision for development of a nationwide "STEMI ALERT" program to that which was initiated over 25 years ago by the American College of Surgeons Committee on Trauma which spurred our nation to develop one of the finest and most effective trauma care systems in the world.

The four main components, or "links" in the "STEMI Chain of Survival" are featured below. In his editorial, Dr. Ornato addresses specific issues and opportunities for improvement within each of the four links:

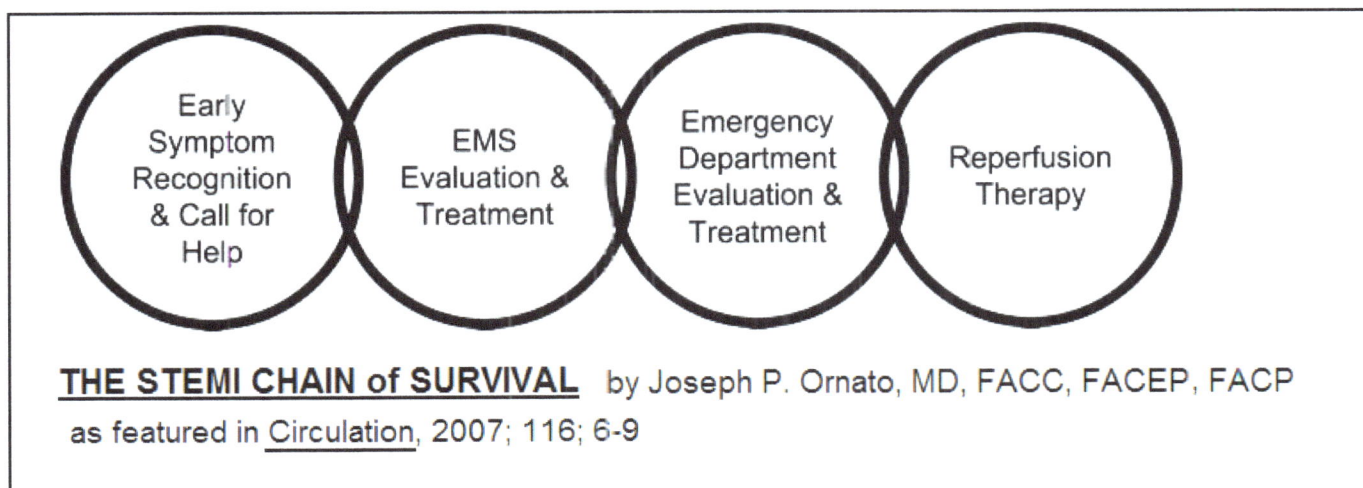

Early Symptom Recognition & Call for Help

EMS Evaluation & Treatment

Emergency Department Evaluation & Treatment

Reperfusion Therapy

THE STEMI CHAIN of SURVIVAL by Joseph P. Ornato, MD, FACC, FACEP, FACP

as featured in Circulation, 2007; 116; 6-9

After viewing Dr. Ornato's "STEMI Chain of Survival," the first thought that comes to mind is that the old saying, "a chain is as strong as its weakest link" holds true here. It is obvious that if any of the above links fail, our STEMI patient's outcome may be disastrous.

The strength of the second link (EMS care) and third link (hospital ER care) are largely dependent upon the capabilities of EMS and ED staff to quickly obtain and correctly interpret a 12 lead ECG.

Two of the issues which need to be addressed with respect to the prehospital care link is that many EMS systems still are not 12 lead ECG capable, and many paramedic education curriculums still regard 12 lead ECG interpretation as an *enhanced* versus a *core* skill competency.

Within the realm of the hospital, basic 12 lead ECG training is still not part of the nursing curriculum. A majority of the nurses I have interacted with in my career have been trained in single-lead rhythm strip anaylsis, but have not been educated to interpret a 12 lead ECG. Although the *primary responsibility* for "formally diagnosing" STEMI obviously rests on the shoulders of physicians, it is essential that the other health care professionals whom interact with the patient – in many cases before the patients see a physician – be able to quickly identify ST segment elevation and other indicators of Acute Coronary Syndrome (ACS) on the 12 lead ECG. This early identification expedites the patient's progression through earlier phases of care. In some communities, it's the EMS provider's interpretation of the 12 Lead ECG that gets patients transported to hospitals with aggressive reperfusion programs, and activates cardiac cath lab response teams. In the ED, it is frequently one of the nursing staff who identifies ST segment elevation on an ECG, and brings it to the attention of a physician.

This book is dedicated to building and strengthening the 12 Lead ECG interpretation skills of EMS and ED team members, and thereby helping to reinforce the middle two links in the STEMI Chain of Survival..

---

[1] Ornato, Joseph P, Circulation 2007;116;6-9

A dedicated *AMI and STROKE ALERT TEAM:* One Hospital's Model Approach to Decreasing Door-to-Reperfusion Times in the "STEMI Chain of Survival:"

If the bulk of this book is dedicated to "strengthening the 2nd and 3rd links in the STEMI Chain of Survival," then the information presented on this single page could aid hospitals in reinforcing the last two links: *Emergency Department Evaluation and Treatment*, and *Reperfusion Therapy*.

The AMI and STROKE ALERT TEAM at St. Josephs' Hospital in Tampa, Florida is comprised of a small group of highly trained and skilled nurses who are on call within the hospital 24 hours per day, 7 days per week. The AMI Team is activated either by the hospital's MedCom staff (who receive advanced notification from EMS of the arrival of a Cardiac Alert patient), or by ED team members when a suspected AMI patient arrives at the Triage Desk.

AMI Team nurses are chosen from the ranks of veteran nurses with critical care backgrounds, are ACLS and NIH Stroke Score certified, and have been trained by the author of this book in 12 Lead ECG interpretation.

AMI Team nurses are familiar with the clinical and administrative protocols utilized by the ED and cardiac cath lab for treating STEMI patients.

In the ED, AMI Team nurses assist ED staff with patient evaluation, initial preparation for cardiac catheterization, obtaining consent for cardiac catheterization, and transport of the patient to the cardiac catheterization suite.

When patients are transferred to St. Joseph's from non-PCI capable hospitals, they serve as the clinical liaison between nursing staff at the sending facility and the cardiac cath lab staff at St. Joseph's.

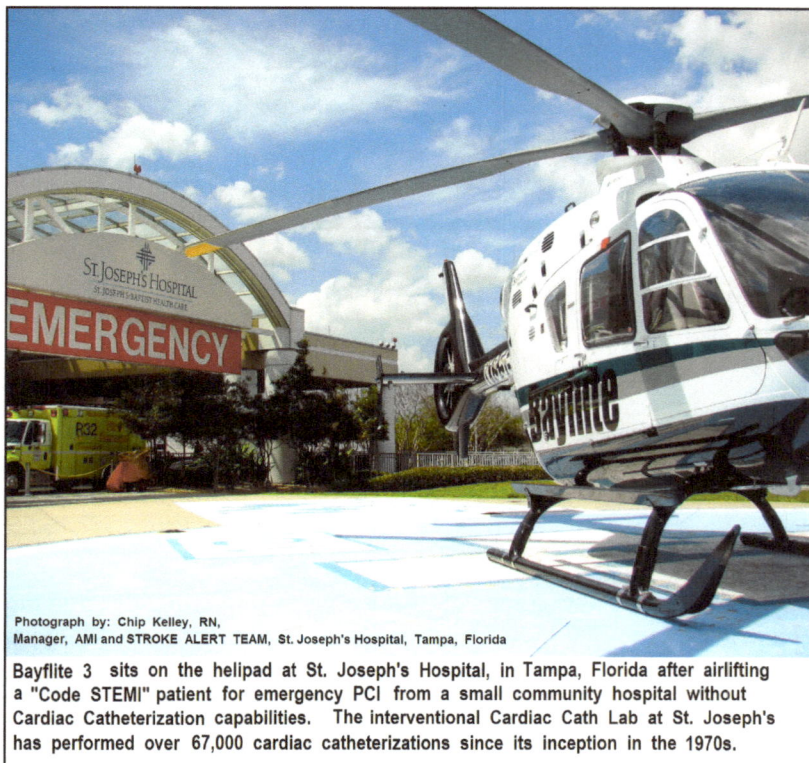

Photograph by: Chip Kelley, RN, Manager, AMI and STROKE ALERT TEAM, St. Joseph's Hospital, Tampa, Florida

Bayflite 3 sits on the helipad at St. Joseph's Hospital, in Tampa, Florida after airlifting a "Code STEMI" patient for emergency PCI from a small community hospital without Cardiac Catheterization capabilities. The interventional Cardiac Cath Lab at St. Joseph's has performed over 67,000 cardiac catheterizations since its inception in the 1970s.

Since 2005, AMI Team nurses have been facilitating every step of the way from the moment a patient is diagnosed with STEMI until the patient's arrival in the cardiac catheterization lab. There's no doubt they've played an instrumental role in keeping the hospital's door-to-reperfusion times well below the 'gold standard' of 90 minutes.

Two additional "strong links" in Tampa's "STEMI Chain of Survival" are St. Joseph Hospital's Cardiac Catheterization Lab, and the region's two primary 911 Advanced Life Support EMS services: Tampa Fire Rescue, and Hillsborough County Fire Rescue.

The Cardiac Catheterization Lab has been serving the citizens of Tampa, Florida for over 30 years. Currently, the Heart Institute at St. Joseph's Hospital maintains a full-service, interventional cardiac catheterization program, providing 24 hour per day, 7 day per week service to STEMI patients. In addition to adult cardiac catheterization services, the Heart Institute operates two electrophysiology (EP) labs, and maintains both pediatric interventional cardiac catheterization and electrophysiology programs.

Regarding the area's EMS providers, both Tampa Fire Rescue and Hillsborough County Fire Rescue provide advanced life support (ALS) level services that are trained and equipped to provide 12 Lead ECG interpretation. When suspected AMI patients are encountered in the field, they contact St. Joseph's MedCom center, who initiates the Cardiac Alert process.

For more information about St. Joseph's AMI and Stroke Alert program, contact team manager Chip Kelley, RN at: chip.kelley@baycare.org

Patient Management is the act of coordinating and overseeing all aspects of *patient evaluation, diagnosis, and treatment.* In the "big picture" of patient management, the 12 LEAD ECG often provides a *key piece of the diagnostic puzzle,* aiding us in rapidly diagnosing potentially life-threatening disorders.

The main focus of this book is teaching clinicians to assimilate the data obtained from the 12 LEAD ECG with *other pertinent assessment information* in order to intelligently determine the next appropriate step(s) to be taken in the continuum of providing patient care.

There are three major objectives we must meet in order to accomplish this. We must educate medical professionals to routinely:

1. **Collect and analyze data from *multiple sources* to maximize accuracy in diagnosing potentially life-threatening cardiac disorders.** Due to problems with *sensitivity* and *specificity*, the ECG frequently provides misleading diagnostic information. Therefore we can not rely solely on the ECG to make accurate diagnostic decisions. We must assimilate data from the patient's *verbal history, physical exam, lab tests,* and *risk factor profile* – in conjunction with the ECG – in order to provide a maximum level of diagnostic accuracy.

2. **Recognize abnormal ECG patterns which are consistent with specific cardiac disorders.** Through the use of actual case studies, we review pertinent ECG abnormalities and pathophysiologies which are associated with Acute Coronary Syndrome. Every case study is followed through the Cardiac Catheterization and/or Electrophysiology (EP) Labs, where the true diagnosis is obtained. With this information, we *validate* or *re-qualify traditional ECG diagnoses, provide case summaries* and *highlight key teaching points.*

3. **Use an Algorithmic approach to patient evaluation.** Algorithms facilitate *accuracy, speed,* and *consistency* in the assessment and treatment of abnormal medical conditions. They provide *structure and organization to complex, dynamic scenarios, keep our minds focused on appropriate priorities,* and *channel our actions to be consistent with accepted diagnostic and therapeutic practices.*

☞ A medical team leader's *patient management skills* are of equal importance to patient outcome as are the skills of *patient assessment* and *treatment.* Patient management is the "putting it all together" aspect of patient care. Requisites for successful patient management include:
- *Knowledge of which diagnostic modalities and therapeutic interventions are necessary,*
- The *ability to prioritize the appropriate order of events*
- The ability to accept input from other team members and integrate appropriate suggestions into the care plan
- The ability to effectively coordinate the actions of team members
- the *ability to rapidly make changes "mid-stream," when the patient's condition changes.*

The Primary Patient Management Algorithm shown on the next page serves as the "central nervous system" for coordinating all patient care activities described in this book, in chronological order, which include:

- *patient evaluation,*
- *clinical decision making*
- *implementation of therapeutic interventions*

We suggest you become familiar with this algorithm, as it serves as the "main blueprint" for this curriculum, as well as Book 2 and Book 3 of this series (listed at bottom of algorithm, next page).

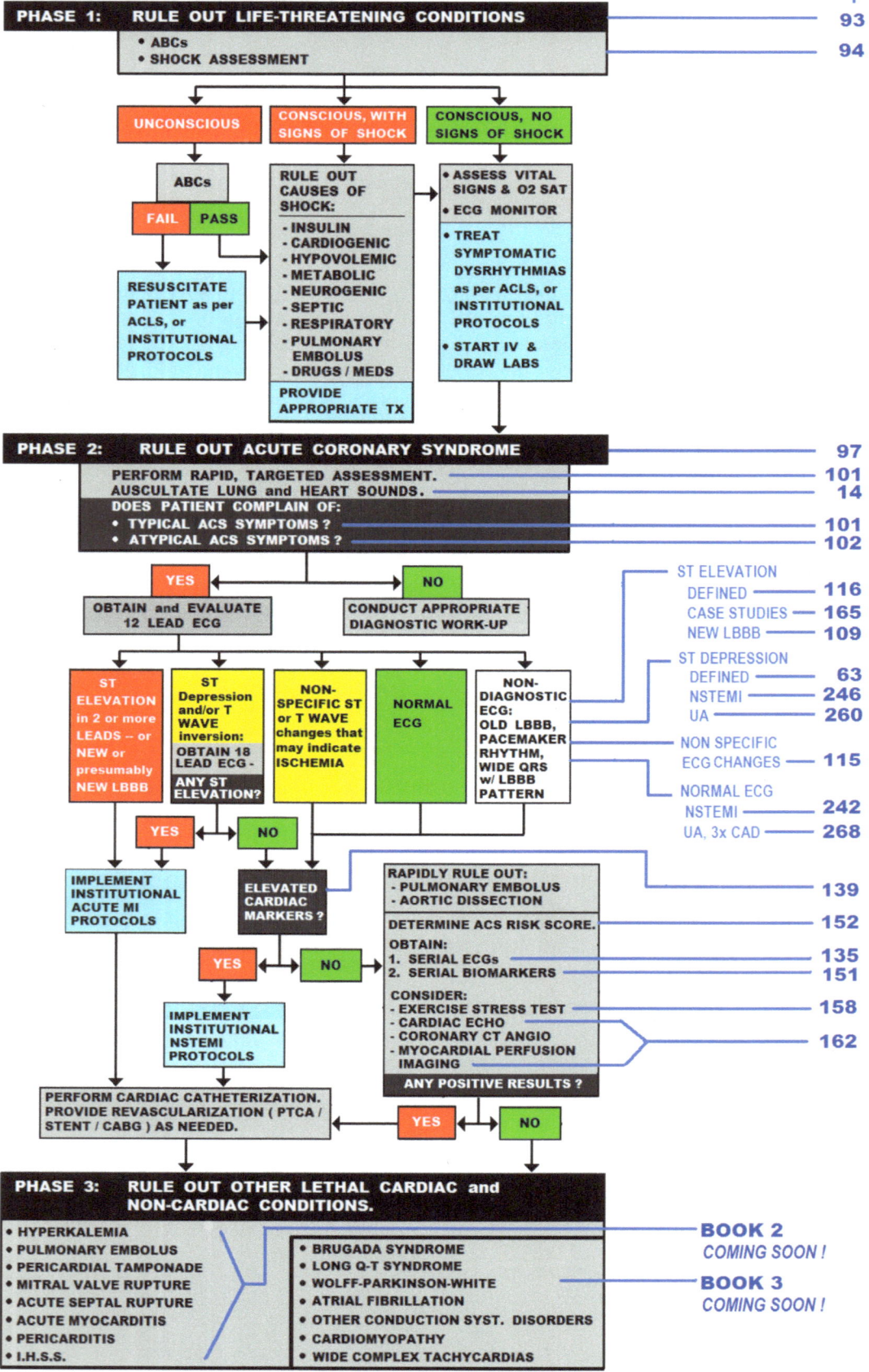

PRIMARY CARDIAC PATIENT MANAGEMENT ALGORITHM

PAGE REFERENCE:

PHASE 1: RULE OUT LIFE-THREATENING CONDITIONS — 93

- ABCs
- SHOCK ASSESSMENT — 94

UNCONSCIOUS

CONSCIOUS, WITH SIGNS OF SHOCK

CONSCIOUS, NO SIGNS OF SHOCK

ABCs → FAIL / PASS

RESUSCITATE PATIENT as per ACLS, or INSTITUTIONAL PROTOCOLS

RULE OUT CAUSES OF SHOCK:
- INSULIN
- CARDIOGENIC
- HYPOVOLEMIC
- METABOLIC
- NEUROGENIC
- SEPTIC
- RESPIRATORY
- PULMONARY EMBOLUS
- DRUGS / MEDS

PROVIDE APPROPRIATE TX

- ASSESS VITAL SIGNS & O2 SAT
- ECG MONITOR
- TREAT SYMPTOMATIC DYSRHYTHMIAS as per ACLS, or INSTITUTIONAL PROTOCOLS
- START IV & DRAW LABS

PHASE 2: RULE OUT ACUTE CORONARY SYNDROME — 97

PERFORM RAPID, TARGETED ASSESSMENT. — 101
AUSCULTATE LUNG and HEART SOUNDS. — 14
DOES PATIENT COMPLAIN OF:
- TYPICAL ACS SYMPTOMS ? — 101
- ATYPICAL ACS SYMPTOMS ? — 102

YES → **OBTAIN and EVALUATE 12 LEAD ECG**

NO → **CONDUCT APPROPRIATE DIAGNOSTIC WORK-UP**

ST ELEVATION in 2 or more LEADS -- or NEW or presumably NEW LBBB

ST Depression and/or T WAVE inversion: OBTAIN 18 LEAD ECG - ANY ST ELEVATION?

NON-SPECIFIC ST or T WAVE changes that may indicate ISCHEMIA

NORMAL ECG

NON-DIAGNOSTIC ECG: OLD LBBB, PACEMAKER RHYTHM, WIDE QRS w/ LBBB PATTERN

ST ELEVATION
- DEFINED — 116
- CASE STUDIES — 165
- NEW LBBB — 109

ST DEPRESSION
- DEFINED — 63
- NSTEMI — 246
- UA — 260

NON SPECIFIC
- ECG CHANGES — 115

NORMAL ECG
- NSTEMI — 242
- UA, 3x CAD — 268

YES / **NO**

IMPLEMENT INSTITUTIONAL ACUTE MI PROTOCOLS

ELEVATED CARDIAC MARKERS ?

RAPIDLY RULE OUT:
- PULMONARY EMBOLUS
- AORTIC DISSECTION — 139

DETERMINE ACS RISK SCORE. — 152

OBTAIN:
1. SERIAL ECGs — 135
2. SERIAL BIOMARKERS — 151

CONSIDER:
- EXERCISE STRESS TEST — 158
- CARDIAC ECHO
- CORONARY CT ANGIO
- MYOCARDIAL PERFUSION IMAGING — 162

ANY POSITIVE RESULTS ?

YES / **NO**

IMPLEMENT INSTITUTIONAL NSTEMI PROTOCOLS

PERFORM CARDIAC CATHETERIZATION. PROVIDE REVASCULARIZATION (PTCA / STENT / CABG) AS NEEDED.

YES / **NO**

PHASE 3: RULE OUT OTHER LETHAL CARDIAC and NON-CARDIAC CONDITIONS.

- HYPERKALEMIA
- PULMONARY EMBOLUS
- PERICARDIAL TAMPONADE
- MITRAL VALVE RUPTURE
- ACUTE SEPTAL RUPTURE
- ACUTE MYOCARDITIS
- PERICARDITIS
- I.H.S.S.

- BRUGADA SYNDROME
- LONG Q-T SYNDROME
- WOLFF-PARKINSON-WHITE
- ATRIAL FIBRILLATION
- OTHER CONDUCTION SYST. DISORDERS
- CARDIOMYOPATHY
- WIDE COMPLEX TACHYCARDIAS

BOOK 2 *COMING SOON !*

BOOK 3 *COMING SOON !*

I. Review of Essential Cardiac A & P

As is true with the rest of the human body, we can classify the three main types of cells found in the heart as belonging to one of the following groups:

- **Myocardial** (muscle tissue): cells which contract when electrically stimulated and do the "work" associated with pumping blood throughout the body.
- **Structural** (connective tissue): cells which make up the "structures of the heart," such as the heart valves, chordae tendineae, the disc-shaped "skeleton of the heart," and cardiac blood vessels. Basically, any cells which do not contract or conduct electricity are classified as structural cells.
- **Electrical** (nerve tissue): cells which initiate and or conduct electrical currents, such as the sinus and AV nodes, bundle branches, and purkinje fibers.

MYOCARDIUM - AT THE CELLULAR LEVEL:

MYOCARDIAL CELLS AT REST have POSITIVELY charged IONS on the OUTSIDE of the membrane, and NEGATIVELY charged IONS on the INSIDE

Ca++ Na+ Ca++ Na+ Ca++

Cl- Cl- K+ Cl- K+ Cl- K+ Cl-

Ca++ Na+ Ca++ Na+ Ca++

zzzZZ

At rest, myocardial cells are POSITIVELY charged on the outside, and NEGATIVELY charged on the inside. The image to the left depicts a myocardial cell at rest.

The action that normally results in CARDIAC MUSCLE CELL CONTRACTION is known as *depolarization.* During depolarization, there is an "exchange of ions" which causes a normal cardiac muscle cell to contract.

In a normal functioning heart, depolarization of a cardiac muscle cell is triggered by the depolarization of a neighboring cell. The initial "wave of depolarization" is generated by the sinus node, which distributes the wave of depolarization throughout the heart via the heart's electrical conduction system. When everything is working properly, the wave of depolarizing cells causes the heart to contract—and pump blood: the atria pump blood to the ventricles, "packing them full of blood," and the ventricles pump blood to the lungs and the rest of the body.

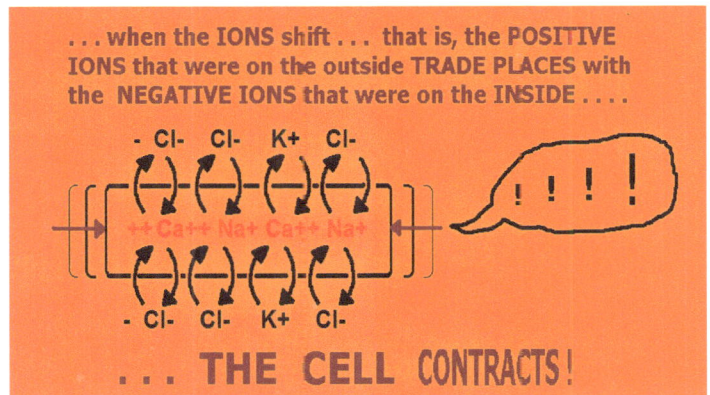

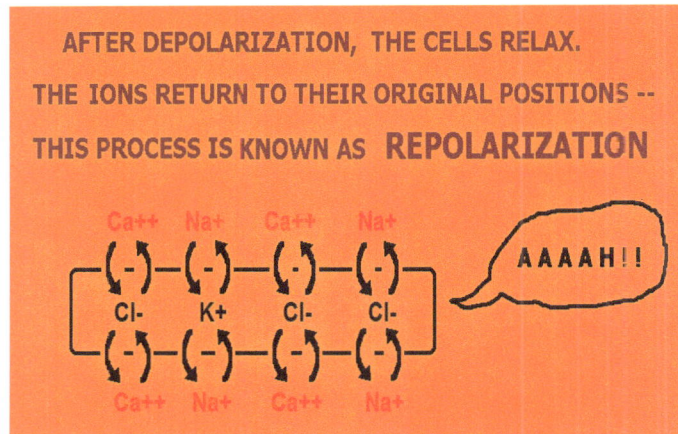

. . . when the IONS shift . . . that is, the POSITIVE IONS that were on the outside TRADE PLACES with the NEGATIVE IONS that were on the INSIDE . . . .

- Cl- Cl- K+ Cl-

++ Ca++ Na+ Ca++ Na+

- Cl- Cl- K+ Cl-

! ! ! !

. . . THE CELL CONTRACTS!

AFTER DEPOLARIZATION, THE CELLS RELAX.

THE IONS RETURN TO THEIR ORIGINAL POSITIONS --

THIS PROCESS IS KNOWN AS REPOLARIZATION

Ca++ Na+ Ca++ Na+

(-)—(-)—(-)—(-)

Cl- K+ Cl- Cl-

(-)—(-)—(-)—(-)

Ca++ Na+ Ca++ Na+

AAAAH!!

After a cell has depolarized (and contracted), the process of *repolarization* begins. During repolarization, the cell relaxes to its original elongated shape, and the ions shift to their original positions: positively charge ions return to the exterior of the cell, and negatively charged ions return to the interior of the cell.

From the beginning of *depolarization* until the end of *repolarization,* the myocardial cell is considered to be "refractory." During the *refractory period,* cardiac cells cannot be *depolarized again*—the repolarization process must be completed before another depolarization can occur.

CARDIAC CELL ACTION POTENTIAL:

> ☞ NOTE: You *do not* need to understand the phases of action potential in order to effectively read and interpret an ECG. Understanding action potential does, however, make it easier to understand more complicated processes such as the pacemaker function of the SA and AV nodes, escape pacemaker mechanisms, ectopic foci, and reentry.

Action potential describes the cell's *trans-membrane potential*. In simpler terms, it describes the capacity to generate and/or conduct electrical current within a single cell. All *cardiac muscle cells* and *electrical system cells* have action potential.

After *cardiac muscle* and *electrical cells* have completed repolarization, they enter a *resting state*, known as PHASE 4 of the Action Potential. In this resting state, cell interiors have a slightly negative charge, which measures between – 80mA and – 90mA.

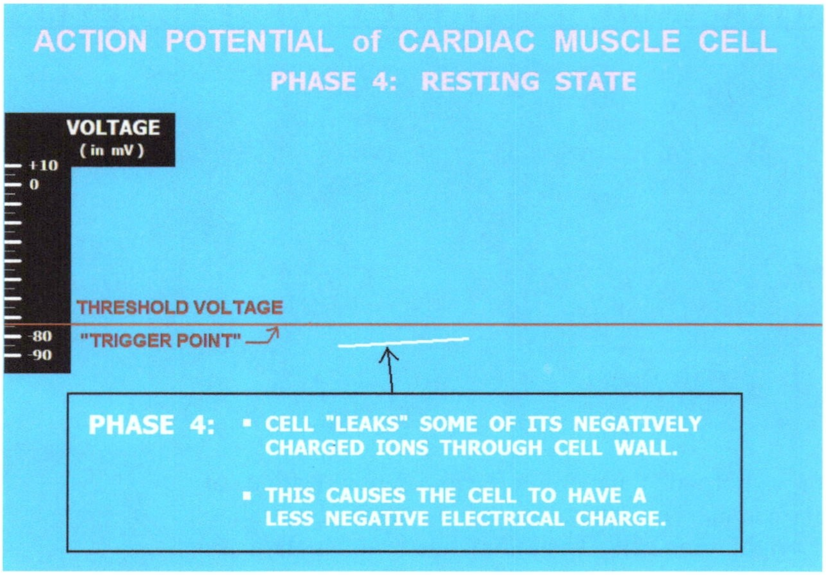

During phase 4 of the Action Potential, cardiac muscle and electrical system cells are "recharged" and "ready to go."

During phase 4, cells "leak out" some of their negatively charged ions. This causes the cell's overall electrical charge to become slightly less negative, as indicated in the above diagram.

ACTION POTENTIAL of CARDIAC MUSCLE CELL
PHASE 4: RESTING STATE

VOLTAGE (in mV)

THRESHOLD VOLTAGE
"TRIGGER POINT"

PHASE 4:
- CELL "LEAKS" SOME OF ITS NEGATIVELY CHARGED IONS THROUGH CELL WALL.
- THIS CAUSES THE CELL TO HAVE A LESS NEGATIVE ELECTRICAL CHARGE.

One of two events trigger the cell to depolarize (and enter phase 0):

1. A neighboring cell will depolarize, which triggers this cell to depolarize:

In a normally functioning heart, the SA node depolarizes first. This causes cells immediately surrounding the SA node to depolarize. This *wave of depolarization* spreads rapidly, cell-to-cell, throughout the heart via the cardiac electrical system and into muscle tissue, where the wave of depolarization causes muscle cell contraction.

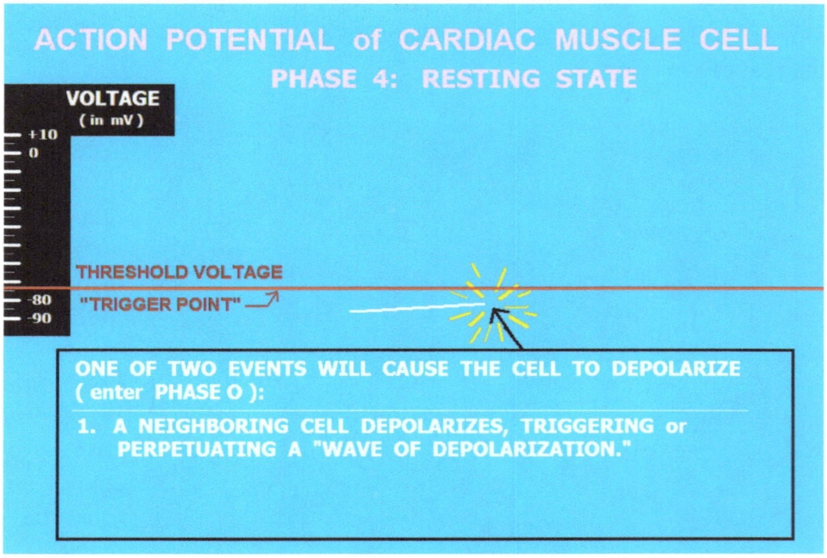

---OR---

ACTION POTENTIAL of CARDIAC MUSCLE CELL
PHASE 4: RESTING STATE

VOLTAGE (in mV)

THRESHOLD VOLTAGE
"TRIGGER POINT"

ONE OF TWO EVENTS WILL CAUSE THE CELL TO DEPOLARIZE (enter PHASE O):
1. A NEIGHBORING CELL DEPOLARIZES, TRIGGERING or PERPETUATING A "WAVE OF DEPOLARIZATION."

2. Through the trait of *automaticity*, the cell will self-depolarize.

If depolarization is not initiated by a neighboring cell, eventually the cell may leak out enough of its own *negatively charged ions* to reach the *threshold voltage*, or its "trigger point," causing it to self-depolarize. This is known as *automaticity*, and outside of the body's nervous system, this trait is unique to the heart. At the moment the cell *begins to depolarize*, we say it is now entering PHASE 0.

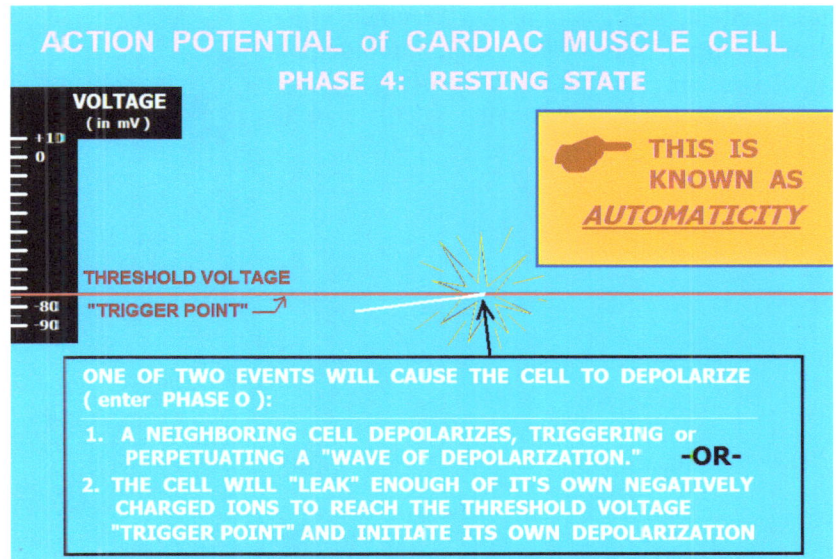

ACTION POTENTIAL of CARDIAC MUSCLE CELL
PHASE 4: RESTING STATE

VOLTAGE (in mV)

THIS IS KNOWN AS *AUTOMATICITY*

THRESHOLD VOLTAGE
"TRIGGER POINT"

ONE OF TWO EVENTS WILL CAUSE THE CELL TO DEPOLARIZE (enter PHASE 0):
1. A NEIGHBORING CELL DEPOLARIZES, TRIGGERING or PERPETUATING A "WAVE OF DEPOLARIZATION." **-OR-**
2. THE CELL WILL "LEAK" ENOUGH OF IT'S OWN NEGATIVELY CHARGED IONS TO REACH THE THRESHOLD VOLTAGE "TRIGGER POINT" AND INITIATE ITS OWN DEPOLARIZATION

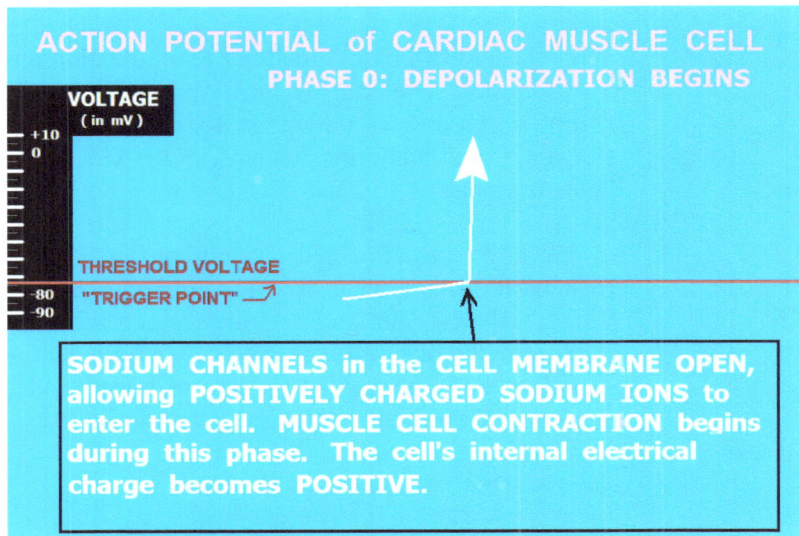

ACTION POTENTIAL of CARDIAC MUSCLE CELL
PHASE 0: DEPOLARIZATION BEGINS

VOLTAGE (in mV)

THRESHOLD VOLTAGE
"TRIGGER POINT"

SODIUM CHANNELS in the CELL MEMBRANE OPEN, allowing POSITIVELY CHARGED SODIUM IONS to enter the cell. MUSCLE CELL CONTRACTION begins during this phase. The cell's internal electrical charge becomes POSITIVE.

DURING PHASE 0, sodium channels in the cell wall open, allowing sodium ions to rapidly enter the cell. This rapid influx of positively charged sodium ions changes the cell's internal electrical charge from negative to positive. Cardiac muscle cells begin to contract during this phase.

Just as quickly as sodium entered the cell, it makes a hasty retreat, which defines PHASE 1 of the action potential . . . and at the same moment when sodium ions are getting pumped back out of the cell, the *calcium channels* open, and the *slower but steady* calcium ions enter the cell. This serves to keep the cell positively charged.

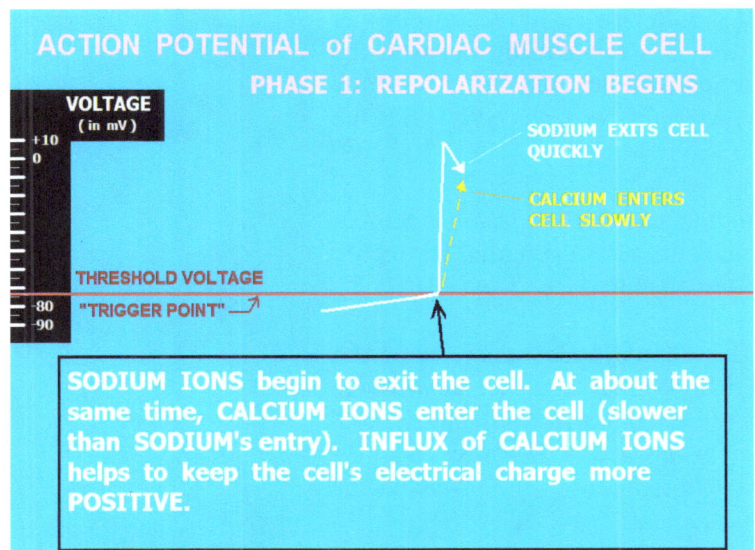

ACTION POTENTIAL of CARDIAC MUSCLE CELL
PHASE 1: REPOLARIZATION BEGINS

VOLTAGE (in mV)

SODIUM EXITS CELL QUICKLY

CALCIUM ENTERS CELL SLOWLY

THRESHOLD VOLTAGE
"TRIGGER POINT"

SODIUM IONS begin to exit the cell. At about the same time, CALCIUM IONS enter the cell (slower than SODIUM's entry). INFLUX of CALCIUM IONS helps to keep the cell's electrical charge more POSITIVE.

DURING PHASE 2, sodium ions finish their hasty retreat, and calcium ions complete their slow entry into the cell, prolonging repolarization, and thereby *prolonging the refractory period* of the cell. (This trait is unique to cardiac cells).

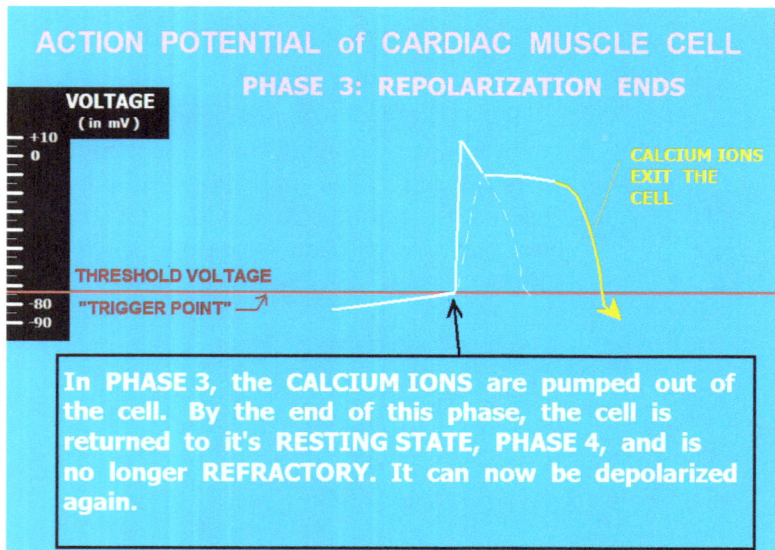

ACTION POTENTIAL of CARDIAC MUSCLE CELL
PHASE 2: REPOLARIZATION

VOLTAGE (in mV)
+10
0

CALCIUM FINISHES ITS SLOW ENTRY INTO CELL

SODIUM FINISHES ITS EXIT FROM CELL

THRESHOLD VOLTAGE
"TRIGGER POINT"
-80
-90

REPOLARIZATION is prolonged by the slow-moving CALCIUM IONS, which continue moving into the cell. By the end of PHASE 2, the SODIUM IONS have returned to their original positions, outside the cell.

ACTION POTENTIAL of CARDIAC MUSCLE CELL
PHASE 3: REPOLARIZATION ENDS

VOLTAGE (in mV)
+10
0

CALCIUM IONS EXIT THE CELL

THRESHOLD VOLTAGE
"TRIGGER POINT"
-80
-90

In PHASE 3, the CALCIUM IONS are pumped out of the cell. By the end of this phase, the cell is returned to it's RESTING STATE, PHASE 4, and is no longer REFRACTORY. It can now be depolarized again.

IN PHASE 3, the calcium ions exit the cell.

By the end of phase 3, cellular repolarization has occurred. The cell is no longer considered refractory, and is now able to be depolarized again. And this brings us back to PHASE 4, the resting stage.

We have just finished describing the Action Potential of a typical cardiac ventricular muscle cell. If you were able to follow along with this process, the rest of this section on action potential will be easy, and will help you to understand a great deal more about how the heart works.

It should now be of no surprise that there is a relationship between the action potential of *cardiac ventricular muscle cells* and the ECG.

In the case of *ventricular muscle cells*, the action potential is roughly equivalent to the *Q-T interval*.

This should make sense, since the QRS complex signifies *ventricular muscle depolarization*, and the *S-T segment* and *T wave* signify *repolarization of ventricular muscle*.

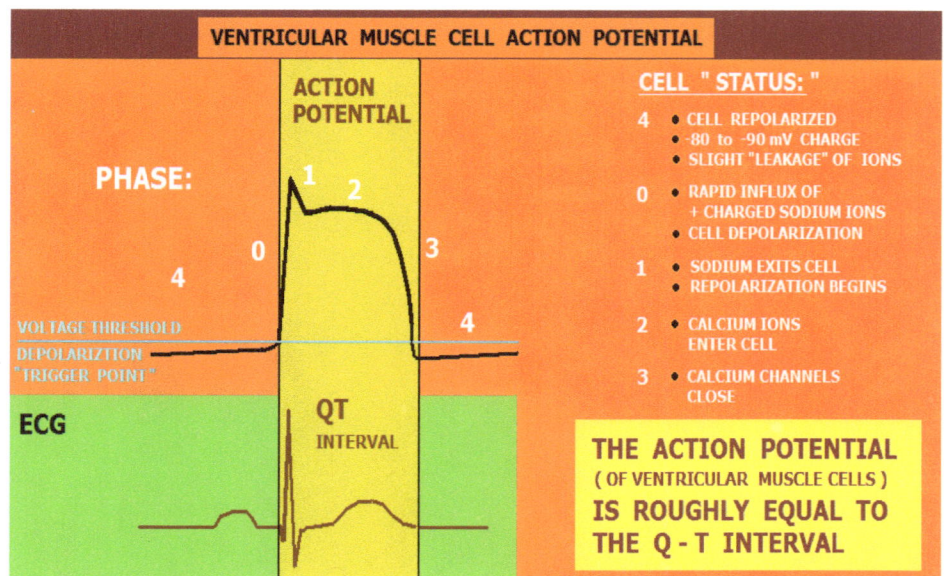

VENTRICULAR MUSCLE CELL ACTION POTENTIAL

ACTION POTENTIAL

PHASE:

1
2
0
3
4
4

VOLTAGE THRESHOLD
DEPOLARIZTION
"TRIGGER POINT"

ECG

QT INTERVAL

CELL " STATUS: "

4 • CELL REPOLARIZED
• -80 to -90 mV CHARGE
• SLIGHT "LEAKAGE" OF IONS

0 • RAPID INFLUX OF + CHARGED SODIUM IONS
• CELL DEPOLARIZATION

1 • SODIUM EXITS CELL
• REPOLARIZATION BEGINS

2 • CALCIUM IONS ENTER CELL

3 • CALCIUM CHANNELS CLOSE

THE ACTION POTENTIAL
(OF VENTRICULAR MUSCLE CELLS)
IS ROUGHLY EQUAL TO
THE Q - T INTERVAL

Next, we will look at the *action potentials* of several different types of heart cells. We'll start with *pacemaker cells*. That is, cells that make up the SA and AV NODES.

Because pacemaker cells don't have fast sodium channels, and calcium channels let ions in *slowly*, the *speed of cellular depolarization* is *slow*, and therefore, so is the *spread* of the *wave of depolarization* to other cells within the SA and AV NODES. *Being slow and steady are desired traits of pacemaker cells.*

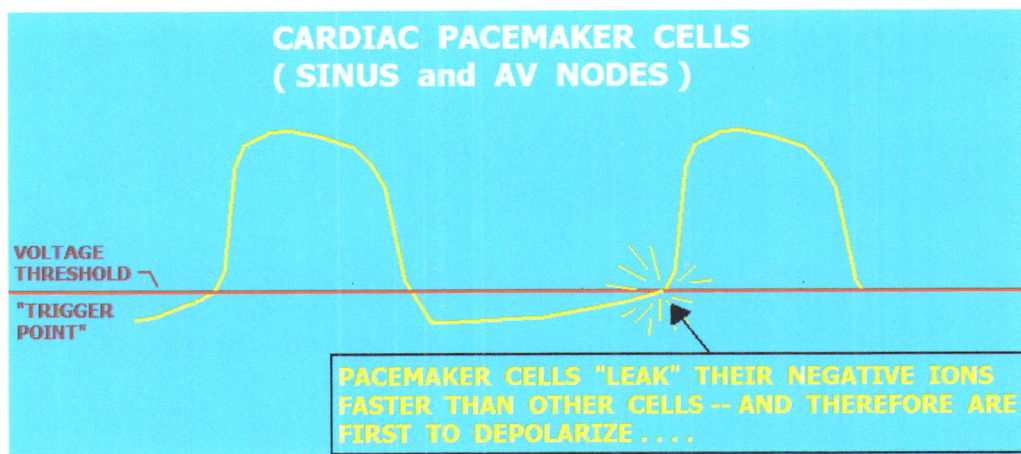

While pacemaker cells depolarize slowly, they are the fastest to "leak out" negative ions during PHASE 4, which causes them to reach the voltage threshold faster than any other cardiac cells. In the normal functioning heart, the cells of the SA NODE leak ions at the fastest rate, causing them to depolarize first. Of course when this happens, the wave of depolarization spreads throughout the heart's electrical system, causing atrial depolarization, AV node depolarization and finally, ventricular depolarization. In simpler terms, depolarization of the SA node triggers the entire heartbeat!

What determines inherent rates of pacemaker cells is how fast they leak ions in PHASE 4 and reach the voltage threshold, the "trigger point" for depolarization.

The image to the right illustrates how the different rates of leakage of potassium ions during PHASE 4 results in the different "intrinsic pacemaker rates."

So if you ever wondered why a sinus rate was 60 – 100, and an AV nodal rate was 40 – 60, this is why!

For some unlucky folks, their purkinje cells do not leak enough

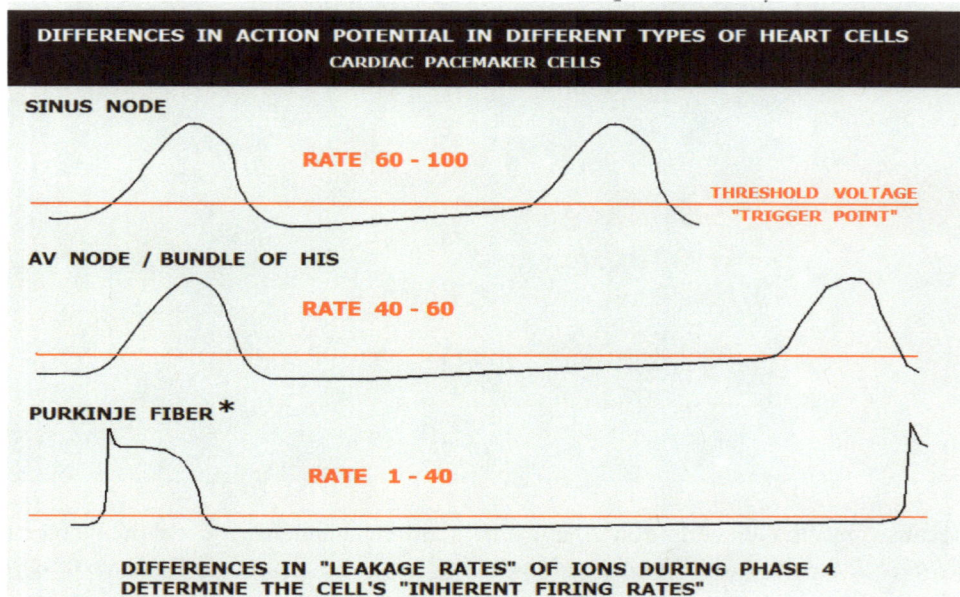

DIFFERENCES IN ACTION POTENTIAL IN DIFFERENT TYPES OF HEART CELLS
CARDIAC PACEMAKER CELLS

SINUS NODE

RATE 60 - 100

THRESHOLD VOLTAGE "TRIGGER POINT"

AV NODE / BUNDLE OF HIS

RATE 40 - 60

PURKINJE FIBER *

RATE 1 - 40

DIFFERENCES IN "LEAKAGE RATES" OF IONS DURING PHASE 4 DETERMINE THE CELL'S "INHERENT FIRING RATES"

ions to reach the *threshold potential*. When these individuals suffer from any condition which causes complete heart block, they have no ventricular escape rhythm; their resulting ECG rhythm is *ventricular standstill* or *asystole*. They need STAT CPR and cardiac pacing to survive.

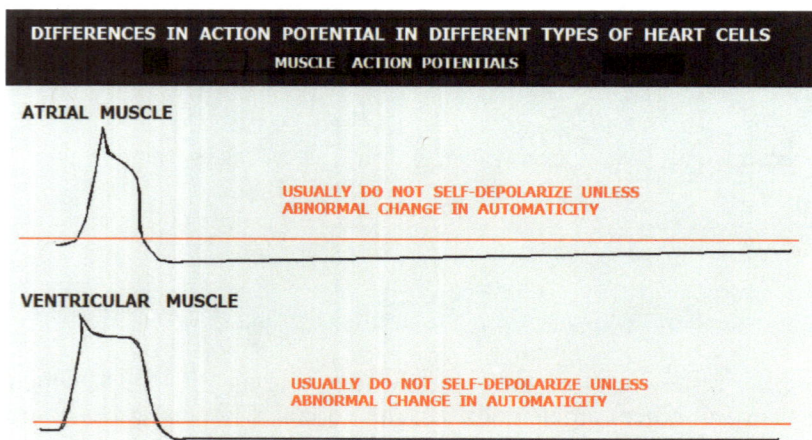

DIFFERENCES IN ACTION POTENTIAL IN DIFFERENT TYPES OF HEART CELLS
MUSCLE ACTION POTENTIALS

ATRIAL MUSCLE

USUALLY DO NOT SELF-DEPOLARIZE UNLESS ABNORMAL CHANGE IN AUTOMATICITY

VENTRICULAR MUSCLE

USUALLY DO NOT SELF-DEPOLARIZE UNLESS ABNORMAL CHANGE IN AUTOMATICITY

Unlike pacemaker cells, cardiac muscle cells have very little or no leakage of ions during PHASE 4, which explains why muscle cells generally don't serve as a pacemaker.

Also, note that the action potential of *atrial muscle* is slimmer than the action potential of ventricular *muscle*. *The narrower the action potential, the shorter the refractory period—which in this case means ATRIAL MUSCLE can handle a faster rate heart rate than VENTRICULAR MUSCLE—that is, before you start seeing problems, such as* fibrillation. .

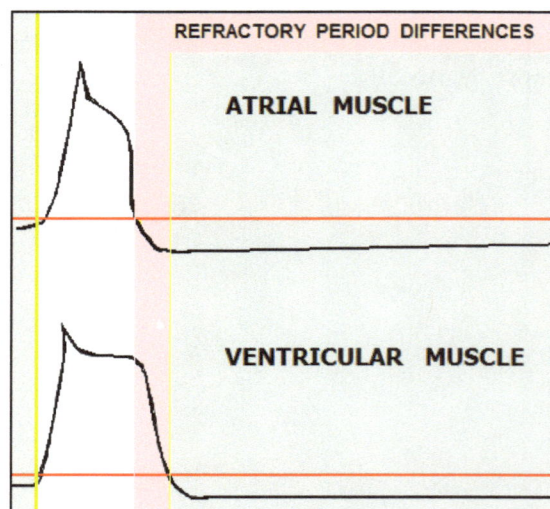

REFRACTORY PERIOD DIFFERENCES

ATRIAL MUSCLE

VENTRICULAR MUSCLE

THE STRUCTURE OF THE HEART:

The heart is comprised of four chambers: two atria, whose primary job is to "pack the ventricles full of blood," and two ventricles, whose primary job is to pump blood to the lungs and the rest of the body.

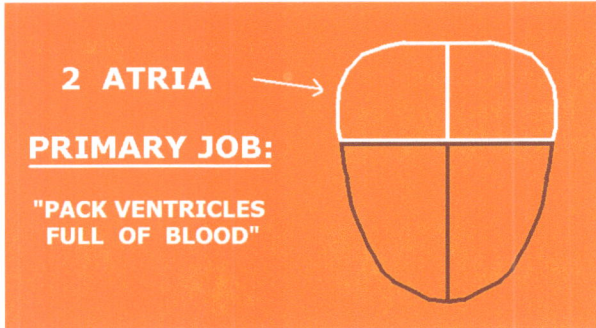

2 ATRIA

PRIMARY JOB:

"PACK VENTRICLES FULL OF BLOOD"

When functioning properly, the atrial kick contributes approximately 10-20% of the total cardiac output. When the atria don't function properly, as in atrial fibrillation, the ventricles may compensate by increasing heart rate and stroke volume.

2 VENTRICLES

PRIMARY JOB:

"PUMP BLOOD TO THE LUNGS AND THE REST OF THE BODY"

Because people can live without their atria contracting, our main concern during cardiac emergencies is, "what is the ventricular rate," and "how well are the ventricles are contracting?" These two factors play a major role in determining the patient's hemodynamic stability.

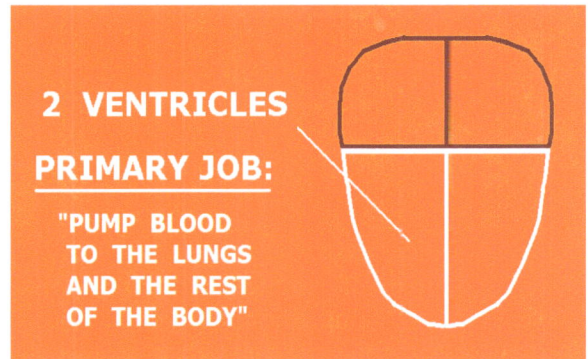

THE CHAMBER MOST IMPORTANT TO KEEPING THE PATIENT ALIVE

(and the ONLY one you can't live without)

IS THE

LEFT VENTRICLE

WHICH IS OFTEN REFERRED TO AS THE PUMP.

Regarding heart rate, I become concerned about hemodynamic compromise when my patient's resting ventricular heart rate is below 50 or above 150. These numbers are not etched in stone, nor do they apply to everyone. Each person's age, cardiovascular status, and overall physical condition determine at what heart rates they become hemodynamically unstable.

Pressures in the heart chambers vary, as the next two diagrams will illustrate. In the normal heart, ventricular pressures are greater than atrial pressures. Pressures on the left side of the heart are normally greater than those on the right side. Normal LV systolic pressures range from 90 – 140mmhg, while the normal RV systolic pressures range is 17 – 32mmhg.

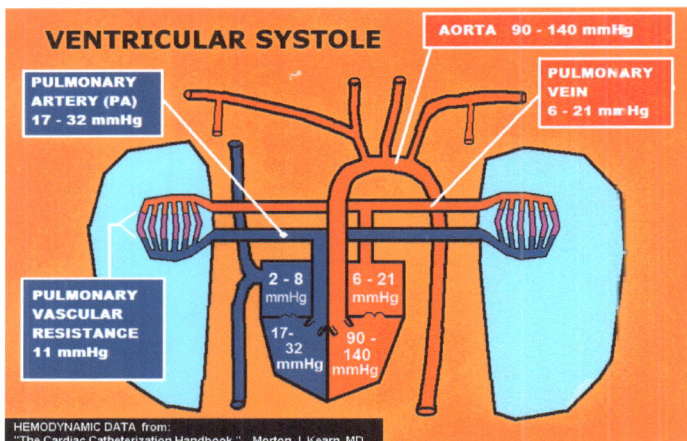

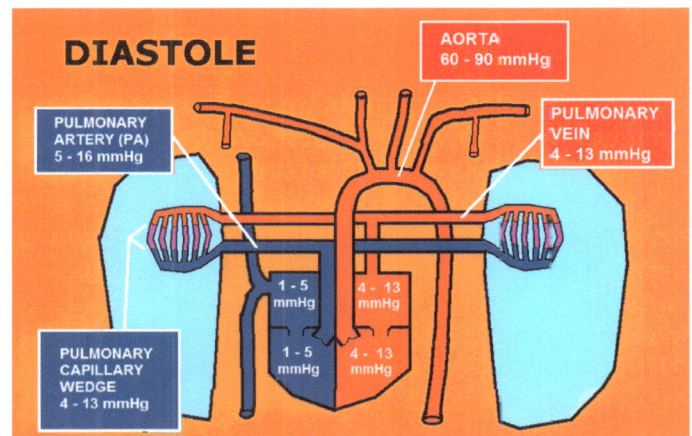

VENTRICULAR SYSTOLE

- AORTA 90 - 140 mmHg
- PULMONARY ARTERY (PA) 17 - 32 mmHg
- PULMONARY VEIN 6 - 21 mmHg
- PULMONARY VASCULAR RESISTANCE 11 mmHg
- 2 - 8 mmHg
- 6 - 21 mmHg
- 17 - 32 mmHg
- 90 - 140 mmHg

HEMODYNAMIC DATA from: "The Cardiac Catheterization Handbook," Morton J. Kearn, MD

DIASTOLE

- AORTA 60 - 90 mmHg
- PULMONARY ARTERY (PA) 5 - 16 mmHg
- PULMONARY VEIN 4 - 13 mmHg
- PULMONARY CAPILLARY WEDGE 4 - 13 mmHg
- 1 - 5 mmHg
- 4 - 13 mmHg
- 1 - 5 mmHg
- 4 - 13 mmHg

HEART VALVES and BASIC HEART SOUND ASSESSMENT:

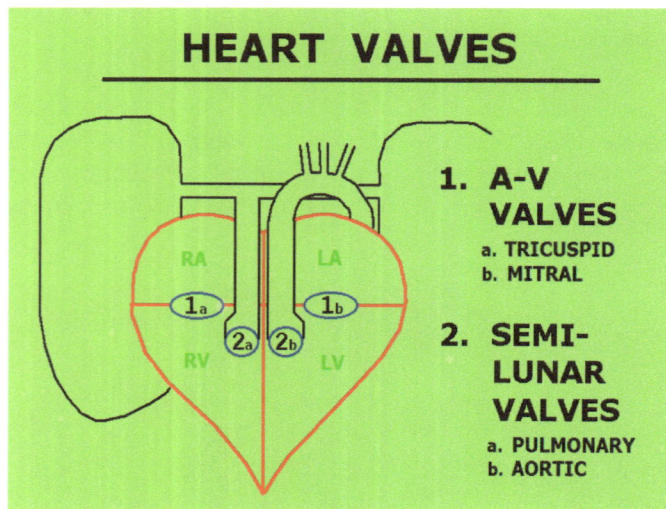

HEART VALVES

1. **A-V VALVES**
   a. TRICUSPID
   b. MITRAL

2. **SEMI-LUNAR VALVES**
   a. PULMONARY
   b. AORTIC

The chambers of the heart are separated by valves, which keep blood moving in one direction and prevent *backflow*.

There are two atrio-ventricular valves (abbreviated "AV valves") which separate the atria from the ventricles, and two semi-lunar valves, which are located in the outflow tract of each ventricle.

At the beginning of ventricular systole, pressure in the ventricles rise, forcing the mitral and tricuspid valves to close. Closure of the AV valves prevents the backflow of blood into the atria. Concurrently, the aortic and pulmonary valves open, allowing blood to be pumped to the lungs and to the rest of the body.

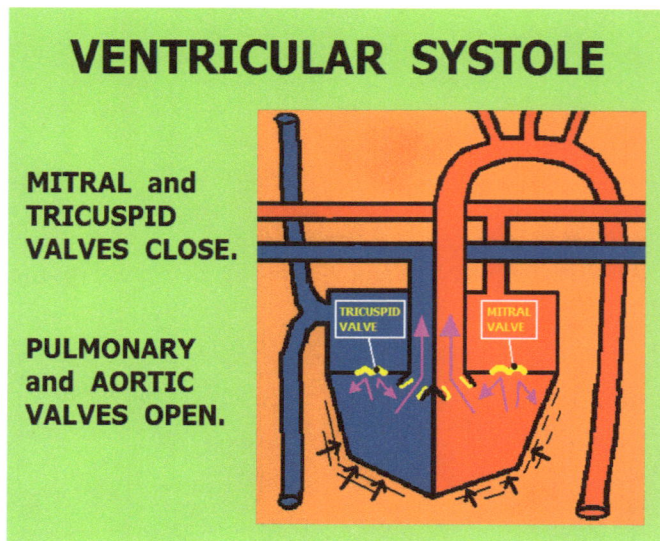

VENTRICULAR SYSTOLE

MITRAL and TRICUSPID VALVES CLOSE.

PULMONARY and AORTIC VALVES OPEN.

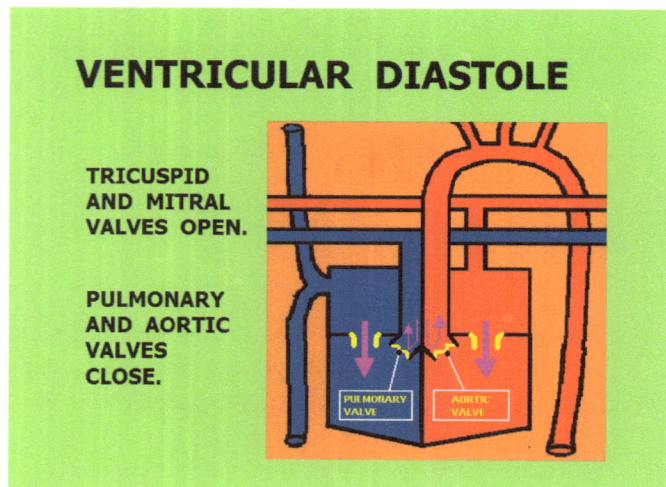

VENTRICULAR DIASTOLE

TRICUSPID AND MITRAL VALVES OPEN.

PULMONARY AND AORTIC VALVES CLOSE.

After ventricular systole is complete, the ventricles relax. Pressure drops in the ventricular chambers. When ventricular pressure drops below pressures in the pulmonary artery and aorta, the pulmonary and aortic valves close. This prevents blood in the pulmonary artery and aorta from "dropping backwards" into the ventricles.

The leaflets of the AV valves are secured to the base of the ventricles by the chordae tendineae and the papillary muscles. During ventricular systole, these structures extend to hold the AV valves in the closed position. The papillary muscles are dependent upon adequate myocardial tissue perfusion to maintain their integrity and function properly. Therefore in cases of extensive myocardial infarction, the papillary muscles can tear, resulting in ACUTE MITRAL VALVE RUPTURE. This is usually seen 7 – 10 days post-extensive MI.

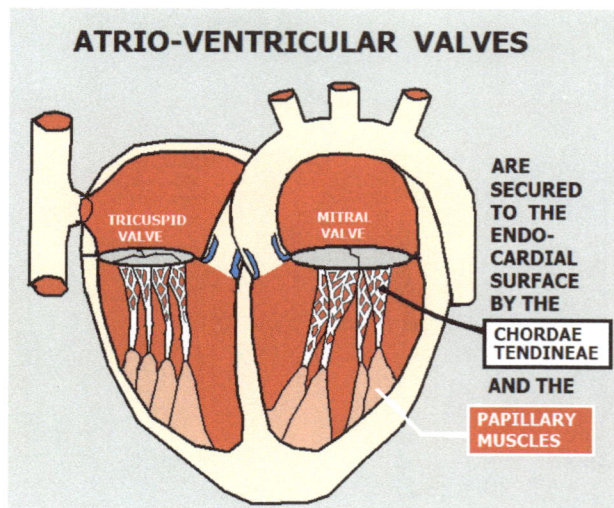

ATRIO-VENTRICULAR VALVES

TRICUSPID VALVE

MITRAL VALVE

ARE SECURED TO THE ENDO-CARDIAL SURFACE BY THE CHORDAE TENDINEAE AND THE PAPILLARY MUSCLES

THE SEMILUNAR VALVES

PULMONARY VALVE

AORTIC VALVE

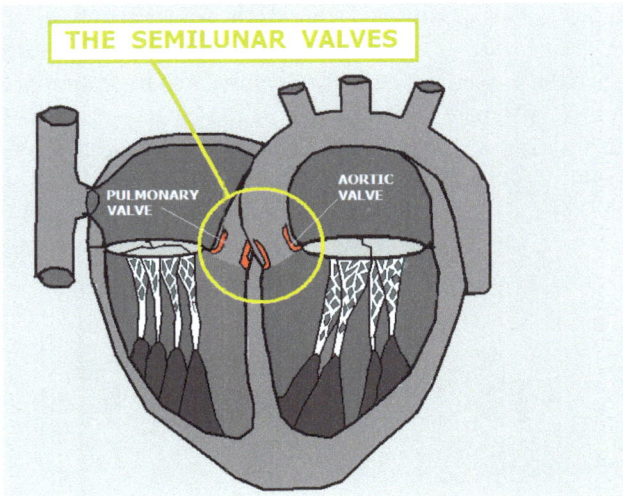

The semi-lunar valves (aortic and pulmonary) are comprised of connective tissue. They are not secured with muscle tissue and therefore are usually not vulnerable to damage from myocardial infarction.

BASIC HEART SOUNDS ASSESSMENT: is an important component of the initial cardiovascular assessment. Your ability to pick up on abnormal heart sounds may be the first indicator that a life-threatening condition exists, such as in cases of *acute papillary muscle tear* resulting in *mitral valve failure.* Specific heart sound abnormalities often go hand-in-hand with the conditions listed in the diagram to the right.

VERY **BASIC HEART SOUNDS ASSESSMENT**

ABNORMAL EKG CHANGES THAT MAY PRESENT WITH ABNORMAL HEART SOUNDS:

- ACUTE MI
- CHAMBER HYPERTROPHY
- RECENT MI (NECROSIS)
- PERICARDITIS

BASIC HEART SOUNDS COVERED:

❑ **Normal Heart Sounds**

❑ **Murmurs**
  - systolic
  - diastolic

❑ **Friction Rubs**

SCOTT DAVIDSON, RN auscultating heart sounds at St. Joseph's Hospital Heart Institute Tampa, FL

We review the heart sounds you see listed with the picture to the left. Our goal is to provide you with a basic introduction to heart sounds assessment, since this subject is not often covered in nursing and paramedical programs. If you've had little or no exposure to heart sounds assessment prior to reading this book, we urge you to get your hands on a good *heart sounds assessment CD,* or download an auditory file of such. When I "Googled" abnormal heart sounds, pages of available resources popped up, including several university-based sources. This is one subject where *listening to actual examples* is far superior to *reading descriptions* of these sounds in a textbook. None-the-less, we will do our best to offer accurate *descriptions* of each. One final piece of advice is to listen to as many heart sounds as possible. Listen to your own. Listen to family members. When I was learning, I even listened to my dog's heart sounds, a very sweet and mild-mannered Labrador retriever

It helps to have a stethoscope with a bell-shaped head, like the one shown in the picture to the right. The bell-shape is better for picking up low tones, such heart sounds. Of course if you only have a diaphragm type stethoscope that will probably do just fine in most situations.

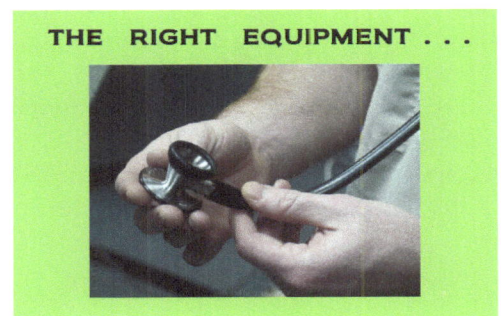

THE RIGHT EQUIPMENT . . .

TYPICAL STETHOSCOPE POSITIONS FOR HEART SOUNDS ASSESSMENT

First, note that positions 1 through 4 are identical to where ECG leads V1 through V4 are located. Positions 1 and 1b are used to hear the tricuspid and pulmonary velves. Positions 2, 3, and 4 are used to assess sounds of the mitral and aortic valves. Position 5, located under the right clavicle, is used to isolate sounds made by the aortic valve – soundwaves of heart sounds are carried by liquid (blood), which flows from the aorta into the subclavian arteries.

Normal heart sounds, known as "S1" and "S2," are generated by the closing of heart valves during the cardiac cycle.

We often say that the heart sounds of a normal heartbeat sounds like "Lub-Dup ……Lub-Dup…….Lub Dup."

HEART SOUNDS ASSESSMENT

HEART SOUNDS ARE GENERATED BY THE SOUND OF THE HEART VALVES <u>CLOSING</u>.

THERE ARE TWO NORMAL HEART SOUNDS, KNOWN AS: <u>S-1</u> and <u>S-2</u>

WE OFTEN DESCRIBE THESE HEART SOUNDS AS "LUB - DUP"

HEART SOUNDS ASSESSMENT

S1 is heard at the BEGINNING of VENTRICULAR SYSTOLE.

IT IS MADE BY THE SOUND OF THE MITRAL and TRICUSPID VALVES CLOSING

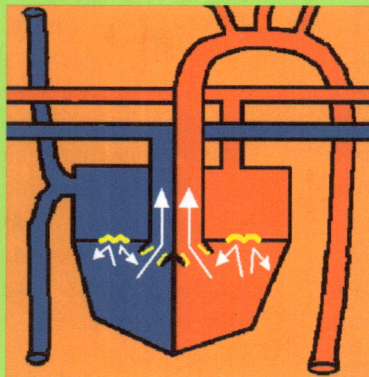

S1 is the first normal heart sound, the "Lub" of "<u>Lub</u>-Dup," and is caused by the sounds of the atrio-ventricular (A-V) valves "slamming shut," at the beginning of ventricular systole. As the ventricles begin to contract, the Tricuspid and Mitral valves are pushed shut, which prevents blood from being "ejected retrograde" into the right and left atria. During this phase, blood is being pumped through the open pulmonary and aortic valves.

HEART SOUNDS ASSESSMENT

S2 OCCURS AT THE BEGINNING OF DIASTOLE.

IT IS THE SOUND OF THE PULMONARY AND AORTIC VALVES CLOSING.

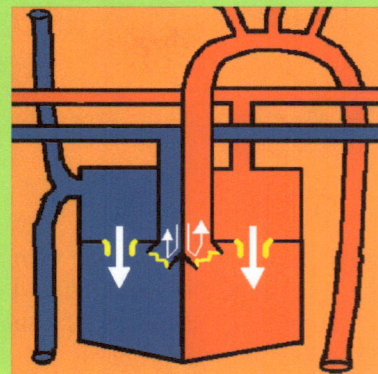

At the end of ventricular systole, the ventricles begin to relax. As relaxation occurs, intra-ventricular pressure drops rapidly. When the intraventricular pressure falls below the pressure in the pulmonary and systemic circulation, the semi-lunar valves (pulmonary and aortic valves) close. The closing of these valves causes the second heart sound, S2, to be heard. S2 is the "Dup" of "Lub-<u>Dup</u>…. Lub-<u>Dup</u>."

Normal heart sounds are crisp, clear, and produce a well-defined, tympanic "Lub-Dup . . . Lub-Dup . . . Lub- Dup" sound.

When a heart valve leaks, you can often detect the leakage with a stethoscope. It typically makes a "swishing" sound, known as a *murmur*. Valve leakage can result from:

- Congenital disorders
- Stretching of a heart chamber associated with hypertrophy
- Leaflets that don't overlap properly (incompetent valve)
- Damage from infections (rheumatic fever, endocarditis)
- Rupture of papillary muscles
- Rupture of ventricular septum

When there is a very small leak, the murmur may be hard to detect. Many such murmurs are considered benign, and are monitored by the patient's physician over the course of years. When a physician detects a change in the patient's murmur, an echocardiogram and/or right-sided cardiac catheterization is most likely indicated. Of course, any time a new murmur is detected, it should be evaluated by a physician as soon as possible.

CAUSE OF SYSTOLIC (S1) MURMUR

- **DAMAGE TO MITRAL and/or TRICUSPID VALVE(s)**

- **CAUSES REGURGITATION**

☞ **SOUNDS LIKE:**

"SWISH - DUP . . . SWISH - DUP . . ."

When a murmur is heard during S1 (ventricular systole), it results from either tricuspid or mitral valve leakage. In most cases, the *mitral valve* is most prone to leakage, due to the higher pressures associated with the left ventricle. (Normal left ventricular systolic pressures are 90 – 140 mm/hg, as opposed to the lower pressure of the right ventricle, which is normally 17 – 32 mm/hg systolic).

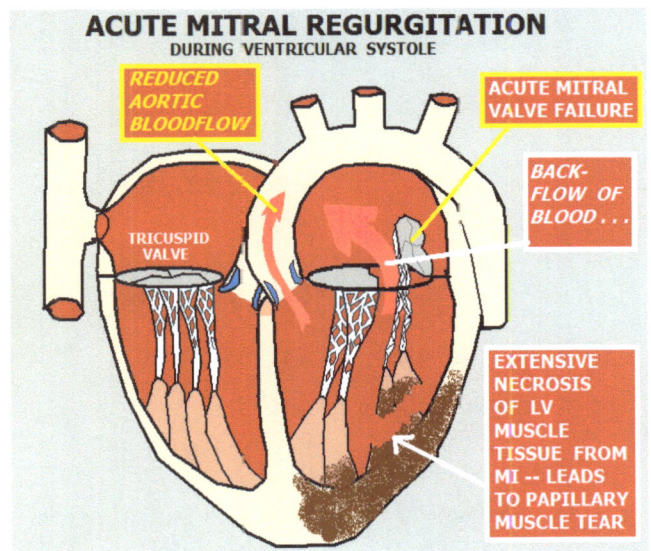

When a new S1 (systolic) murmur is detected during or after an acute MI, ACUTE MITRAL VALVE RUPTURE should be considered. Patients suffering from this disorder are often in shock, with hypotension and pulmonary edema. This condition is often an urgent, life-threatening condition. Acute mitral valve rupture usually is found in cases of acute / recent (7 – 10 days) post extensive, transmural MI.

ACUTE MITRAL REGURGITATION
DURING VENTRICULAR SYSTOLE

REDUCED AORTIC BLOODFLOW

ACUTE MITRAL VALVE FAILURE

BACK-FLOW OF BLOOD . . .

TRICUSPID VALVE

EXTENSIVE NECROSIS OF LV MUSCLE TISSUE FROM MI -- LEADS TO PAPILLARY MUSCLE TEAR

CAUSE OF DIASTOLIC (S2) MURMUR

- **DAMAGE TO AORTIC and/or PULMONIC VALVE(s)**

- **CAUSES REGURGITATION**

☞ **SOUNDS LIKE:**

"LUB - SWISH . . . LUB - SWISH . . ."

When the murmur is heard during S2, it is commonly referred to as a "diastolic murmur," because S2 marks the beginning of diastole. Of course, the presence of an S2 murmur is usually the result of leakage of the pulmonary or aortic (semi-lunar) valves. Just like with S1 murmurs, S2 murmurs usually result from failure of the valve on the left side of the heart (in this case, the *aortic valve*) due to the higher left-sided pressures.

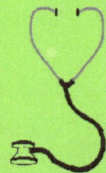

Friction rubs, described in the above diagrams, are most commonly associated with *acute pericarditis*. As you will see in our acute MI and pericarditis case studies, the ECGs in both conditions can be identical – acute pericarditis can sometimes present with S-T elevation in one region of the heart, which is more consistent with an acute MI. Since friction rubs can be heard with pericarditis and acute MI, it is not a good idea to rely solely on the presence or absence of a friction rub to differentiate between the two conditions.

The table below provides a summary of basic emergency heart sounds assessment:

- RAPID EMERGENCY HEART SOUNDS ASSESSMENT -

HEART SOUND	INDICATIVE OF:	ETIOLOGY	SUSPECTED ECG CHANGES / NOTES
• NEW S-1 (SYSTOLIC) MURMUR	• MITRAL VALVE REGURGITATION	• ACUTE RUPTURE OF PAPILLARY MUSCLE	• OFTEN SEEN 2-10 DAYS POST EXTENSIVE MI. often seen with INFERIOR-POSTERIOR MI.
	• L→R VENTRICLE SHUNTING	• VENTRICULAR-SEPTAL RUPTURE	• ACUTE ANTERIOR-SEPTAL WALL MI, NEW BUNDLE BRANCH BLOCKS / NEW HIGH GRADE (2° / 3° HEART BLOCK)
• PRVIOUSLY DIAGNOSED S1 MURMUR	• CHRONIC MITRAL or TRICUSPID VALVE REGURG.	• MITRAL or TRICUSPID INCOMPETENCE	• corresponding ATRIAL / VENTRICULAR HYPERTROPHY ; PULMONARY HYPERTENSION
• NEW S-2 (DIASTOLIC) MURMUR	• AORTIC REGURGITATION	• ACUTE AORTIC VALVE FAILURE	• OFTEN SECONDARY TO: ACUTE AORTIC DISSECTION, ENDOCARDITIS, DECELERATION TRAUMA
• PREVIOUSLY DIAGNOSED S2 MURMUR	• CHRONIC AORTIC or PULMONARY VALVE REGURG.	• AORTIC or PULM. VALVE INCOMPTETENCE	• Hx of: CONGENITAL CARDIAC PROB., RHEUMATIC DISEASE, PROGRESSIVE CALCIFICATIONS (elderly), ASHD.
• FRICTION RUB	• PERICARDITIS	• INFECTIOUS PROCESSES	• PERICARDITIS FINDINGS
	• ACUTE MYOCARDITIS		• MYOCARDITIS FINDINGS
		• ACUTE / RECENT MI	• ACUTE / EVOLVING MI EKG CHANGES

THE CORONARY ARTERIES

If you work in any area where you're likely to encounter acute MI patients, it is in your best interest—and that of your patients—for you to learn the common anatomy of the coronary arteries.

By learning the two most common arterial anatomic configurations—which together account for approximately 90% of the population—you will be able to anticipate and prepare for complications that may arise as you care for acute MI patients.

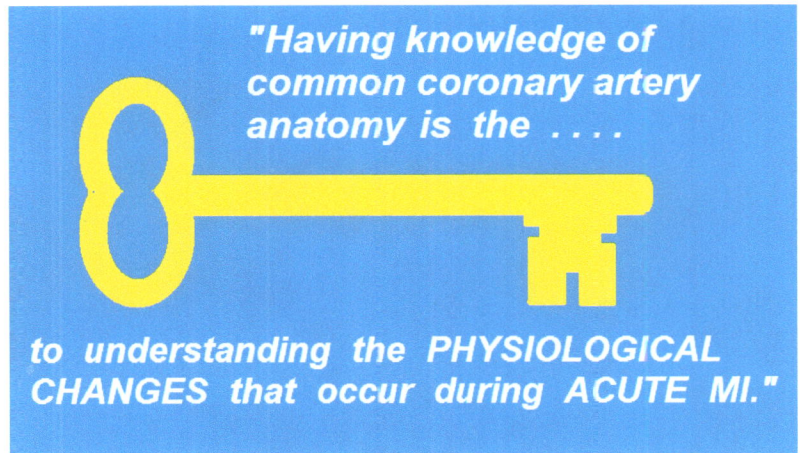

"Having knowledge of common coronary artery anatomy is the . . . .

to understanding the PHYSIOLOGICAL CHANGES that occur during ACUTE MI."

The process for applying this knowledge begins once you've obtained a "positive" ECG for a patient whom you suspect is suffering from Acute Coronary Syndrome, or ACS:

FIRST, INTERPRET THE ECG, THEN. . .

- ⚬➡ IDENTIFY THE AREA OF THE HEART AFFECTED BY THE MI
- ⚬➡ RECALL THE ARTERY WHICH SERVES THAT REGION . . .
- ⚬➡ RECALL OTHER STRUCTURES SERVED BY THAT ARTERY . . .
- ⚬➡ ANTICIPATE FAILURE OF THOSE STRUCTURES . . .
- ⚬➡ INTERVENE APPROPRIATELY !

If you don't already know how to identity an acute MI on an ECG, no problem; we'll cover that later. Right now, we'll focus on the coronary artery anatomy.

The coronary arteries originate in the ascending aorta, superior to the aortic valve. With rare exception, there are two main arteries: the right coronary artery (RCA) and the left main coronary artery (LMCA).

We further subdivide the left main coronary artery into its two branches, the *left anterior descending artery* (LAD) and the *circumflex artery* (CX).

For all practical purposes, we say that most people have THREE main coronary arteries:

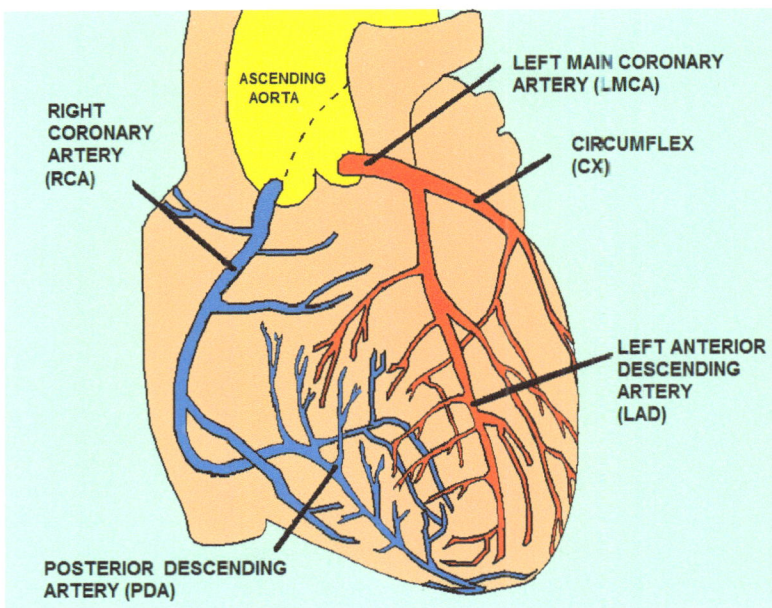

RIGHT CORONARY ARTERY (RCA)
LEFT ANTERIOR DESCENDING ARTERY (LAD)
CIRCUMFLEX ARTERY (CX)

The diagram seen to the left depicts how approximately 75 - 80% of the population's coronary arteries are anatomically configured. This anatomy is referred to as a "common right-dominant system." The term "right dominant" implies that the distal RCA gives rise to the *posterior descending artery* (PDA), which supplies blood to the inferior wall of the left ventricle. The second most common arterial configuration is the "left dominant" system, (10-15% population) where the circumflex artery gives rise to the PDA, which supplies the inferior wall.

ASCENDING AORTA

LEFT MAIN CORONARY ARTERY (LMCA)

RIGHT CORONARY ARTERY (RCA)

CIRCUMFLEX (CX)

LEFT ANTERIOR DESCENDING ARTERY (LAD)

POSTERIOR DESCENDING ARTERY (PDA)

COMMON RIGHT DOMINANT SYSTEMS (75 – 80 % population)

RIGHT CORONARY ARTERY (RCA):

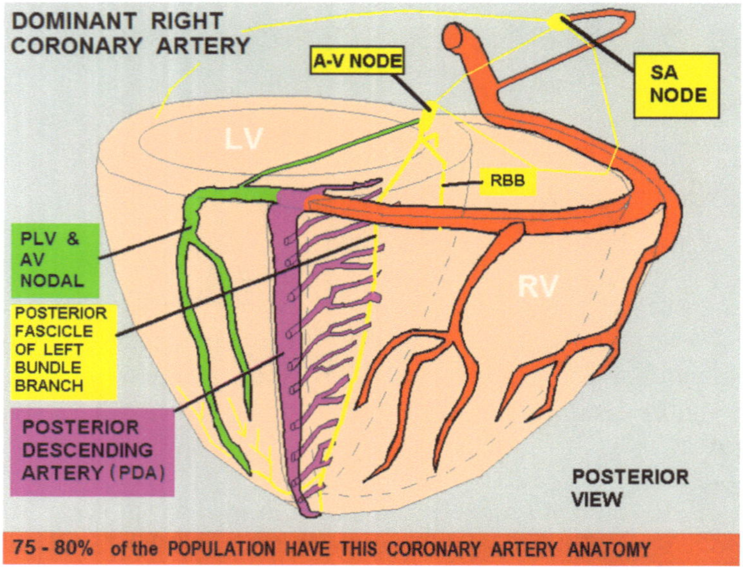

The image to the left is a posterior view of the ventricles and the RCA (shown in red). The RCA feeds the *sinus node and *right ventricle*. The PDA (purple) arises from the RCA and rests over the posterior intra-ventricular septum. The PDA perfuses the back 1/3 of the intra-ventricular septum and the inferior wall of the left ventricle. The PLVs (posterior lateral vessels) (green), supply blood to approximately ½ of the posterior wall of the left ventricle, *and the AV node.*

The diagram below shows a cutaway view of the right and left ventricles, and portrays the arterial distributions shared by 75 – 80% of the population whom have a ***dominant right coronary artery***.

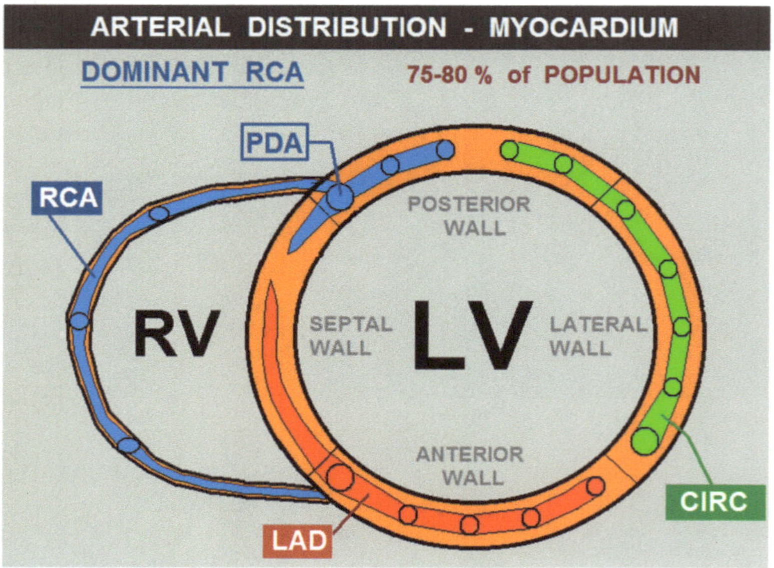

In patients with dominant RCA systems, the RCA (shown in blue) feeds *100% of the right ventricle* and approximately 15 – 25% of the left ventricle. The Circumflex distribution (green) supplies approximately 30% of the left ventricle (LV) muscle mass, and the LAD supplies approximately 45%. Note that in this majority subset of the population, the POSTERIOR WALL is perfused dually by the distal RCA and Circumflex arteries.

ECG leads II, III, and aVF view the region of myocardium supplied blood by a dominant RCA, which is the inferior wall of the left ventricle. Leads V1 – V3 will show reciprocal ST depression in cases of acute posterior wall MI.

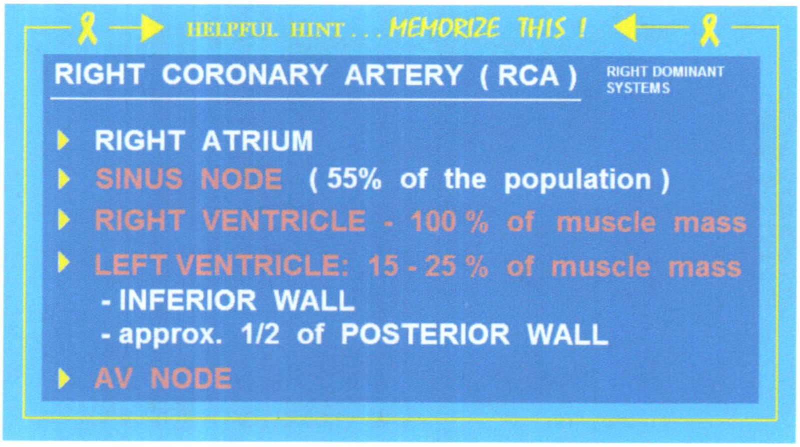

To the left is a list of structures served by a dominant RCA. Since approximately 75 – 80% of the population have this arterial configuration, you can see why there is such a high incidence of SINUS BRADYCARDIA, AV NODAL BLOCKS (1st, 2nd, and 3rd degree heart blocks), and RIGHT VENTRICULAR INFARCTION in cases of ACUTE INFERIOR WALL STEMI. This knowledge will greatly enhance your ability to treat and anticipate complications when caring for patients with inferior wall MI.

---

* The sinus node artery arises from the RCA in approximately 55% of the population, and the mid-circumflex (CX) artery in the remaining 45% of the population. The origin of the SA nodal branch has no relationship to whether the RCA or the CX is dominant.

LEFT MAIN CORONARY ARTERY (LMCA):

The ostium of the Left Main Coronary Artery (LMCA) is located just above the aortic valve in the ascending aorta. It is typically a short (2-10mm) artery. The LMCA, (red) supplies blood to the LAD (purple) and Circumflex (green).

In 75 – 80% of the population (those with a dominant right coronary artery), the LMCA supplies blood to approximately 75% of the left ventricle, as shown by the cut-away view of the heart below.

In RCA dominant patients, the LMCA supplies blood to the ANTERIOR, SEPTAL and LATERAL regions of the left ventricle, and to approximately ½ of the POSTERIOR wall.
.

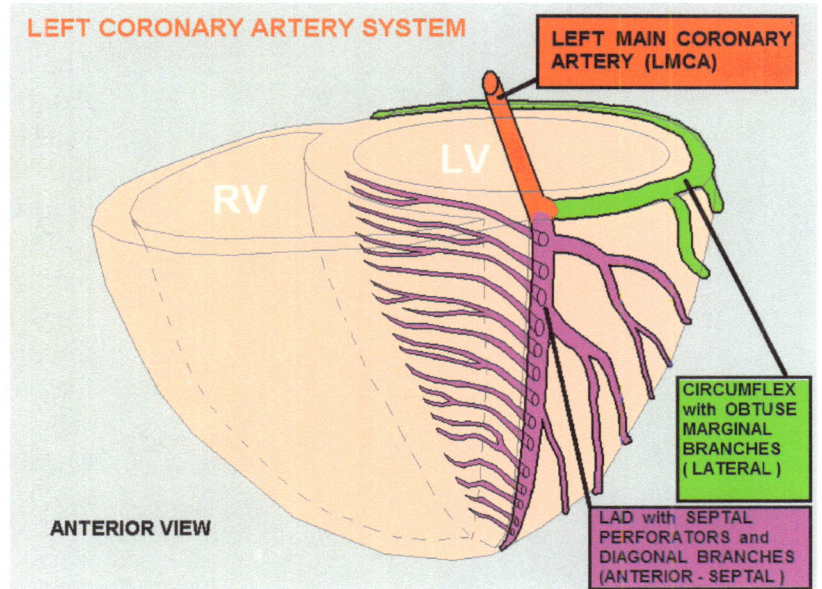

LEFT CORONARY ARTERY SYSTEM

LEFT MAIN CORONARY ARTERY (LMCA)

CIRCUMFLEX with OBTUSE MARGINAL BRANCHES (LATERAL)

LAD with SEPTAL PERFORATORS and DIAGONAL BRANCHES (ANTERIOR - SEPTAL)

ANTERIOR VIEW

cutaway view of the
LEFT MAIN CORONARY ARTERY (LMCA)

☞ **SUPPLIES APPROXIMATELY 75% OF LV MUSCLE MASS**

RIGHT DOMINANT SYSTEM

POSTERIOR WALL

RV SEPTAL WALL LV LATERAL WALL

CIRCUMFLEX (CX) ARTERY

ANTERIOR WALL

RIGHT CORONARY ARTERY (RCA)

LEFT MAIN CORONARY ARTERY (LMCA)

LEFT ANTERIOR DESCENDING (LAD) ARTERY (below LMCA)

A total obstruction of the Left Main Coronary Artery is almost always fatal, with rare exceptions:

- patients who develop the total occlusion when in extremely close proximity to a hospital providing aggressive PTCA and/or thrombolytic therapy, and
- patients who have developed collateral circulation from the RCA.

ECG leads which view LMCA territory include: I, aVR, aVL, V1 – V6.

(This leaves only II, III, and aVF – the inferior wall – which is supplied blood by the RCA in 75-80% of the population).

⚡ → HELPFUL HINT ... *MEMORIZE THIS !* ← ⚡

LEFT MAIN CORONARY ARTERY (LMCA) RIGHT DOMINANT SYSTEM

▶ **LEFT ANTERIOR DESCENDING ARTERY (LAD)**
  BUNDLE BRANCHES
  BUNDLE OF HIS
  ANTERIOR / SEPTAL WALL ———————— 35 - 45%
▶ **CIRCUMFLEX ARTERY (CX)**
  SINUS NODE (45% POPULATION)
  LATERAL WALL ———————————— 20 - 30%
💣 TOTAL LV MUSCLE MASS ———————— 55 - 75%

LEFT ANTERIOR DESCENDING ARTERY (LAD):

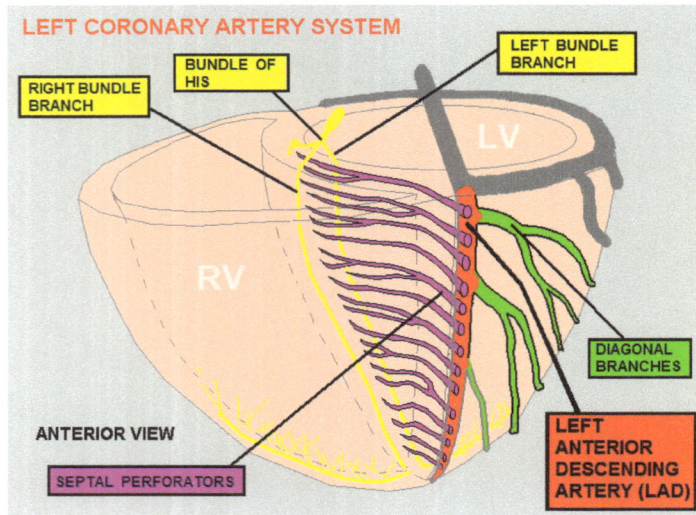

The LAD (red) arises from the Left Main Coronary Artery, and terminates at the apex of the left ventricle. The LAD supplies blood to the *anterior wall* of the left ventricle via multiple *diagonal* branches (shown in green) and to 2/3 of the *septal wall* via multiple *septal perforators* (shown in purple). The total LV muscle mass supplied by the LAD is approximately 45%. The *Bundle of His*, the *anterior fascicle* of the *left bundle branch* and the *right bundle branch* are located within the septum, and receive their blood supply from the septal perforator arteries, which originate from the LAD.

The image to the right highlights (purple) the amount LV muscle mass which received its blood supply from the LAD. A total blockage of the LAD usually results in an ANTERIOR-SEPTAL WALL MI.

ECG leads V1 – V4 view the region of myocardium supplied by the LAD. Leads V1 and V2 also "see" the intr-ventricular septum.

Occasionally the LAD's distribution will extend into the lateral wall, where in cases of STEMI, result in leads V5 and/or V6 showing ST segment elevation.

In less than 5% of the population, the LAD will extend around the apex of the heart and supply the inferior wall ("transapical" LAD).

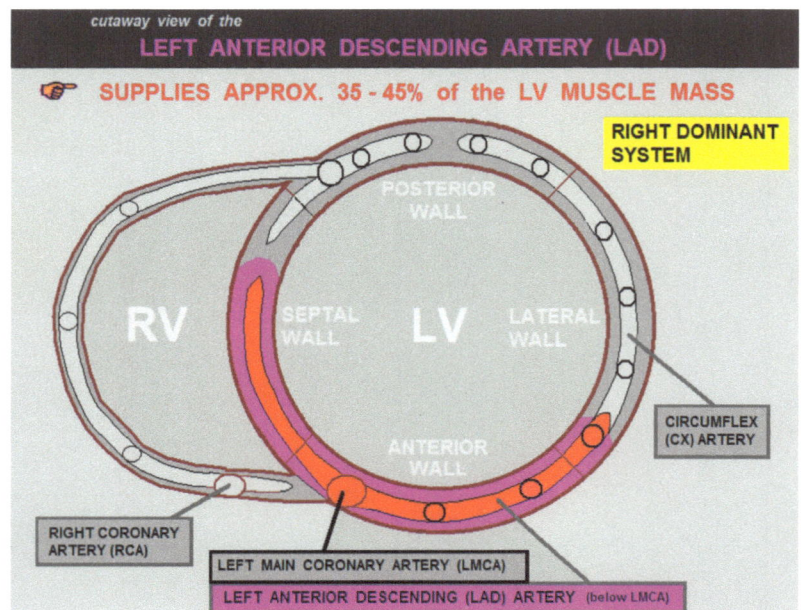

ACUTE ANTERIOR-SEPTAL MI frequently results in severe cardiogenic shock from pump failure and CHF with pulmonary edema. Damage to the *Bundle of His* and *Bundle Branches* may disrupt conduction of electrical impulses from the atria to the ventricles and result in severe heart blocks (2nd degree type II, and 3rd degree heart block) with slow, wide QRS complex (idioventricular) escape rhythms.

22

CIRCUMFLEX ARTERY (CX):

LEFT CORONARY ARTERY SYSTEM

CIRCUMFLEX ARTERY (CX)

LV

RV

OBTUSE MARGINAL (OM) BRANCHES

ANTERIOR VIEW

In right dominant systems, the circumflex artery (shown in red) is usually small, its territory limited to the *left atrium, lateral wall* and up to ½ of the *posterior wall* of the left ventricle, and in 45% of the population, the *sinus node*.

The CX supplies blood to the lateral wall via several *obtuse marginal* (OM) branches, (shown in purple).

ECG leads I, aVL, V5 and V6 view the lateral wall, supplied by the circumflex artery.

In right-dominant systems, the circumflex artery supplies blood to approximately 20 – 30% of the *left ventricle* muscle mass.

Occlusion of a non-dominant circumflex artery typically results in an infarction of the ***lateral wall*** of the left ventricle.

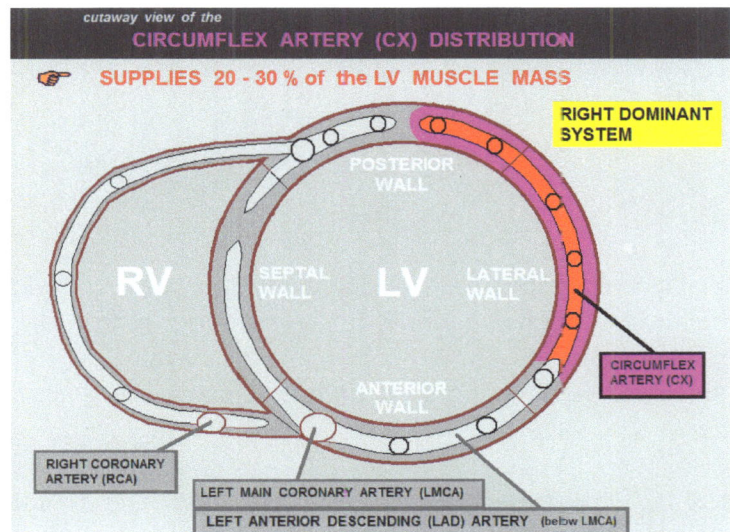

cutaway view of the
CIRCUMFLEX ARTERY (CX) DISTRIBUTION

☞ SUPPLIES 20 - 30 % of the LV MUSCLE MASS

RIGHT DOMINANT SYSTEM

POSTERIOR WALL

RV

SEPTAL WALL

LV

LATERAL WALL

CIRCUMFLEX ARTERY (CX)

ANTERIOR WALL

RIGHT CORONARY ARTERY (RCA)

LEFT MAIN CORONARY ARTERY (LMCA)

LEFT ANTERIOR DESCENDING (LAD) ARTERY (below LMCA)

⟶ HELPFUL HINT . . . *MEMORIZE THIS !* ⟵

CIRCUMFLEX ARTERY (CX)   RIGHT DOMINANT SYSTEMS

▸ **LEFT ATRIUM**
▸ **SINUS NODE (45% of the population)**
▸ **LEFT VENTRICLE: 20 - 30 % of muscle mass**
  - LATERAL WALL
  - up to 1/2 of POSTERIOR WALL

COMMON LEFT DOMINANT SYSTEMS:

<mark>The second most common coronary arterial configuration is the left dominant system, which accounts for approximately 10 - 15% of the population.</mark>

What differentiates a *right-dominant system* from a *left-dominant system* is: ***"which coronary artery feeds the inferior wall: the Right Coronary Artery or the Left Circumflex?"*** In a right-dominant system, the RCA gives rise to the posterior descending artery and posterior lateral vessels. In a left-dominant system, the circumflex artery gives rise to the posterior descending artery and posterior lateral vessels.

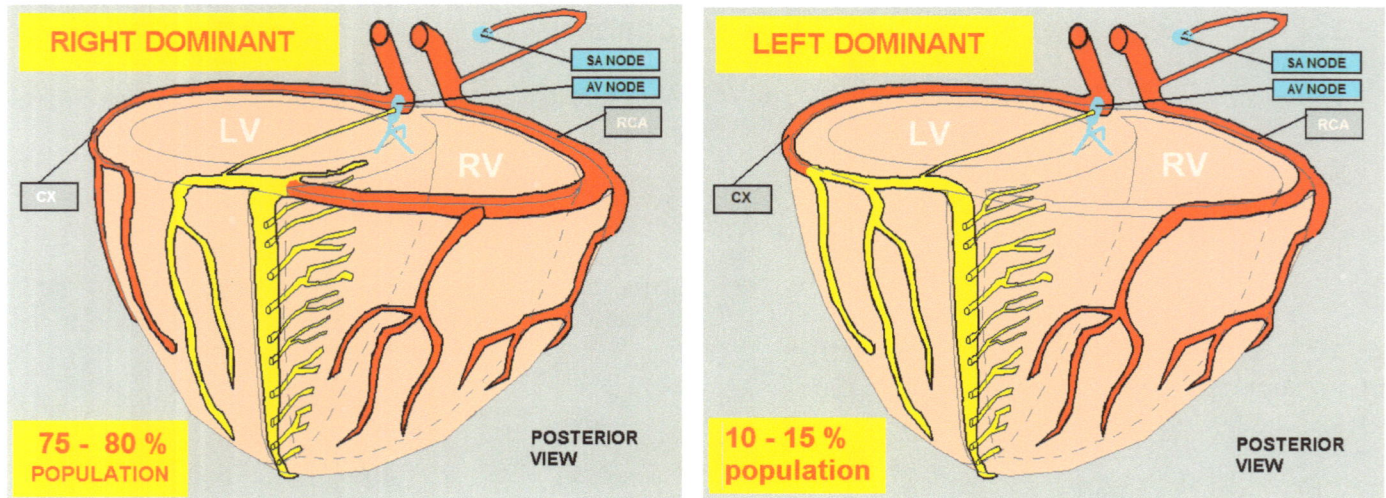

The above diagrams illustrate the difference between right and left dominant systems. While this anatomic variance appears to be minor, it plays a major role in the event of acute MI. <mark>When a person with a right-dominant system has an occlusion of their circumflex artery, the area of infarct usually effects 20-30 percent of their LV muscle mass—usually not enough to cause profound cardiogenic shock. In contrast, when patients who have *left dominant system*s obstruct their circumflex artery, the area of infarct can effect up to 55% of their LV muscle mass—the LATERAL, POSTERIOR, and INFERIOR WALLS—enough to cause profound cardiogenic shock, with high incidence of complications and mortality.</mark> The diagrams below illustrate the differences in the amount of LV muscle mass supplied by a non-dominant circumflex (below left) and a dominant circumflex artery (below right). In both images, the circumflex distribution is shown in green:

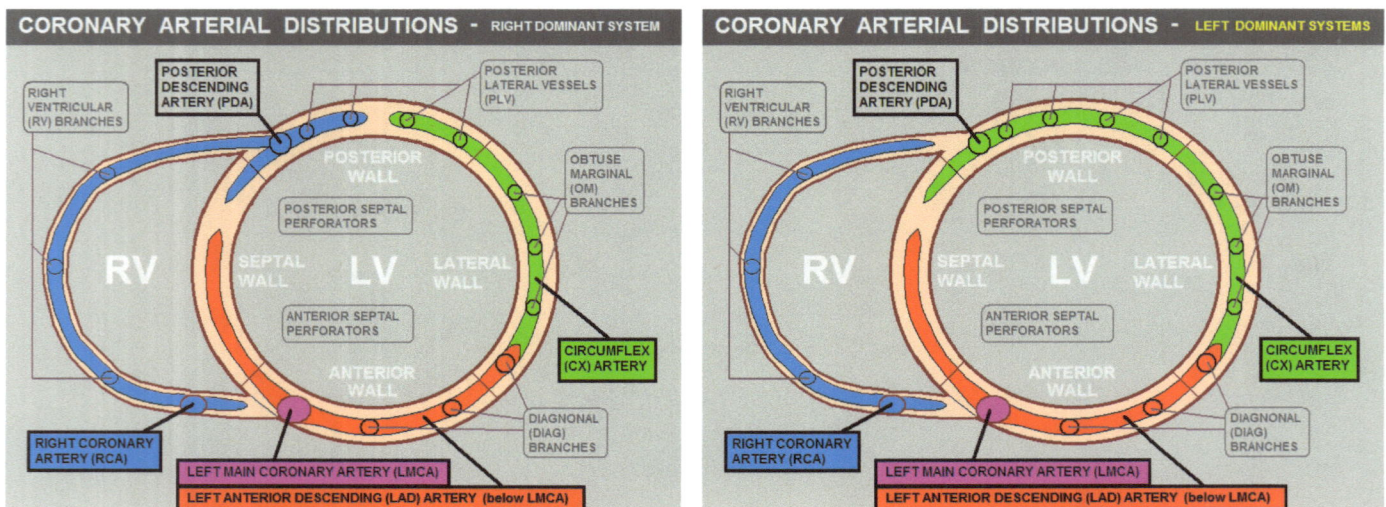

The table below lists the main differences in the structures served by *dominant right* and *dominant left* systems:

RIGHT DOMINANT SYSTEMS 75 - 80% of the POPULATION	LEFT DOMINANT SYSTEMS 10 - 15% of the POPULATION

R C A
 • RIGHT ATRIUM
 • SINUS NODE
 • RIGHT VENTRICLE (55% pop.)
 • LEFT VENTRICLE MUSCLE MASS --- 15 - 25
  - INFERIOR WALL
  - 1/2 POSTERIOR WALL
 • AV NODE
	• RIGHT ATRIUM
	 • SINUS NODE
	 • RIGHT VENTRICLE (55% pop.)
	 • LEFT VENTRICLE MUSCLE MASS --15 - 25%
	  - INFERIOR WALL
	  - 1/2 POSTERIOR WALL
	 • AV NODE

C X
 • LEFT ATRIUM
 • SINUS NODE (45% of pop.)
 • LEFT VENTRICLE MUSCLE MASS -- 20 - 30%
  - LATERAL WALL
  - 1/2 POSTERIOR WALL
	• LEFT ATRIUM
	 • SINUS NODE (45% of pop.)
	 • LEFT VENTRICLE MUSCLE MASS --20 - 30%
	  - LATERAL WALL
	  - 1/2 POSTERIOR WALL

AMOUNT OF LV SUPPLIED BY RCA: 15 - 25% AMOUNT OF LV SUPPLIED BY CX: 20 - 30%	AMOUNT OF LV SUPPLIED BY RCA: 0% *AMOUNT OF LV SUPPLIED BY CX: 35 - 55%*

When a patient with a non-dominant circumflex artery suffers occlusion of the left main coronary artery, 55-75% of their LV muscle mass is affected.

When a patient with a dominant circumflex artery suffers occlustion of the left main coronary artery, nearly 100% of their LV muscle mass is affected. In either scenario, MI caused by occlusion of the left main coronary artery carries a very high mortality rate.

ANGIOGRAPHY of DOMINANT RIGHT and DOMINANT LEFT CORONARY ARTERIES:

The images below are from two patients with relatively disease-free coronary arteries. Patient 1 has a DOMINANT RIGHT SYSTEM, where the RCA supplies blood to the inferior and approximately ½ of the posterior wall.

Note the differences in territorial distributions between PATIENT 1 and PATIENT 2:

PATIENT 1: RIGHT (RCA) DOMINANT CORONARY ARTERIAL VASCULATURE (75 -80% of POPULATION):

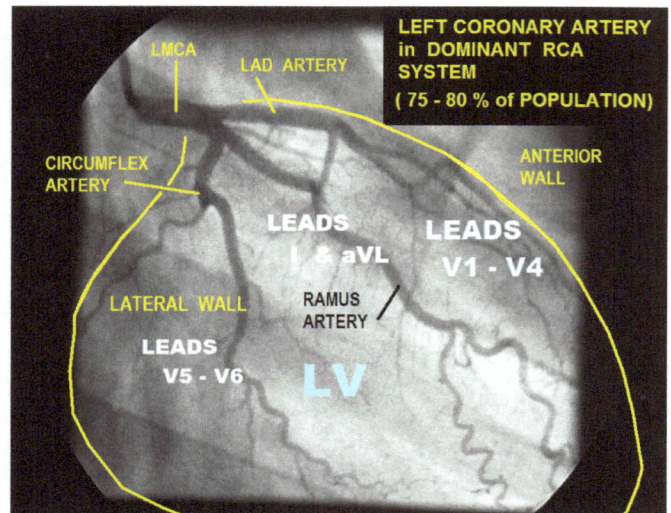

If PATIENT 1 were to suffer acute obstruction of his RCA, ECG leads II, III, and aVF would most likely exhibit ST segment elevation. If he were to incur occlusion of his circumflex artery, most likely leads V5 and V6 would show ST segment elevation.

PATIENT 2: LEFT (CX) DOMINANT CORONARY ARTERIAL VASCULATURE (10-15% POPULATION):

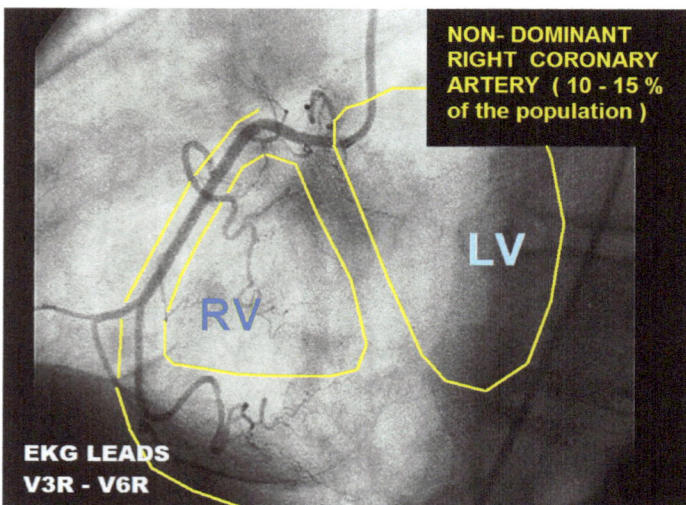

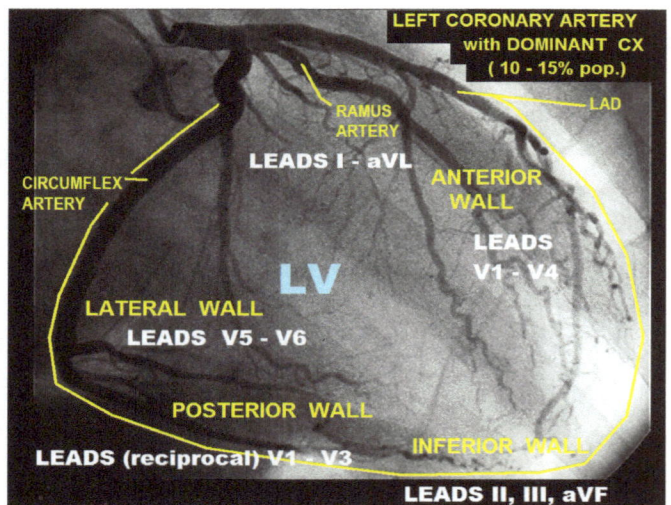

If PATIENT 2 were to incur obstruction of his RCA, the 12 Lead ECG most likely would not show ANY ST segment elevation. In most cases, only a RIGHT SIDED or 18 LEAD ECG, which display lead s V3R – V6R (right precordial leads) would show ST elevation. If he were to obstruct his circumflex artery, ECG leads V5, V6, II, III, and aVF would show ST elevation, and leads V1 – V3 would show RECIPROCAL ST Segment DEPRESSION.

LESS COMMON CORONARY ARTERY ANATOMICAL VARIATIONS:

In this section, we present variations in coronary artery anatomy that make up between 10 – 15% of the population. Since these anatomical variations are less common than the "standard right and left dominant systems," it is not imperative that you memorize them; just be aware that they exist – so when you see an MI presenting on an ECG that "just doesn't make sense," your patient may have one of these less-common coronary arterial variations.

In this book, we don't go into great detail discussing each variation. In the ECG conference series that use this textbook, we provide actual coronary angiography, taken during cardiac catheterization, which show each anatomical variation.

As you can see, most of these variations involve the blood supply to the INFERIOR and POSTERIOR wall of the left ventricle. These variations account for why patients presenting with INFERIOR WALL MI can present with so many varying degrees of hemodynamic stability. In the Acute Coronary Syndrome / STEMI section of this book, we present actual case studies of INFERIOR WALL MI in patients with each of these variations.

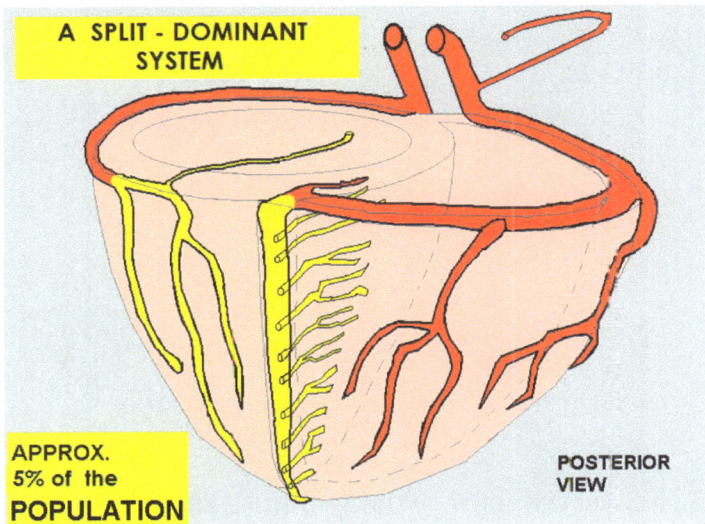

A SPLIT - DOMINANT SYSTEM

APPROX. 5% of the POPULATION

POSTERIOR VIEW

In patients with a split-dominant system, the RCA supplies the inferior wall of the left ventricle, and the circumflex supplies most of the posterior wall and the AV node.

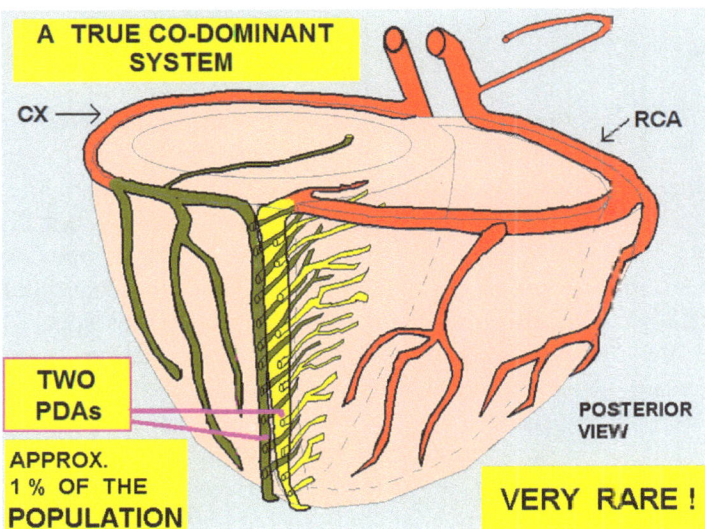

A TRUE CO-DOMINANT SYSTEM

CX →

← RCA

TWO PDAs

APPROX. 1 % OF THE POPULATION

POSTERIOR VIEW

VERY RARE !

Patients with a true co-dominant system have two posterior descending arteries, both which are visible during coronary angiography. Of significant note, my father has this anatomical variation. He experienced INFERIOR WALL MI from occlusion of his RCA. Because his inferior wall is perfused dually by the RCA and Circumflex branches, he suffered NO measurable decrease in his left ventricular ejection fraction (LVEF). It was measured at 60% before and after the MI. (NORMAL LVEF range is 55 – 70%)

EXTREME RIGHT DOMINANT

LV

RV

APPROX. 5 - 10 % POPULATION

POSTERIOR VIEW

In patients with this anatomical variation, their entire POSTERIOR WALL is fed by the right coronary artery. So when these folks are unfortunate enough to have a blockage in their RCA, they usually present with INFERIOR-POSTERIOR WALL MI. In our live case study, our patient presented with profound cardiogenic shock, which is typical for inferior-posterior wall MI.

In the less than 5% of the population who have a trans-apical LAD, when they incur a blockage in their LAD, they will present with ANTERIOR-SEPTAL-INFERIOR WALL MI – and their ECGs often show ST elevation in the anterior leads (V1-V4), along with ST elevation in the inferior leads (II, III, and aVF). This type of clinical ECG presentation is so rare that it has been known to confuse clinicians, causing them to misdiagnose the patient with ACUTE PERICARDITIS.

If you are aware that the LAD does indeed feed the INFERIOR WALL in a very small slice of our population, you will not be caught "off-guard" when a patient arrives in your ED with ANTERIOR-SEPTAL-INFERIOR WALL STEMI, such as the patient in Case Study 10, on page 226.

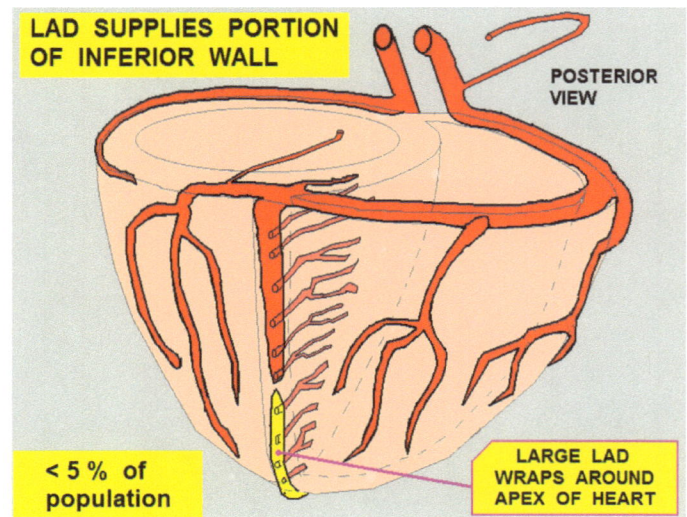

LAD SUPPLIES PORTION OF INFERIOR WALL

POSTERIOR VIEW

< 5 % of population

LARGE LAD WRAPS AROUND APEX OF HEART

Because the "culprit artery" is the LAD, there is usually a significant amount of LV involvement, with accompanying cardiogenic shock, pump failure, pulmonary edema, and in our case study, multiple episodes of spontaneous ventricular fibrillation (V-Fib) requiring multiple defibrillations and an Amiodarone infusion.

ANOMALOUS CORONARY ARTERY VARIATIONS:

Although "anomalous" refers to "irregular" or "abnormal," in the context of coronary arteries, the term often refers to patients whom have a single coronary artery that supplies the entire myocardium. In the three cases I've seen in the cath lab spanning over 12 years, the ostium originated in the right coronary sinus of the aortic root. The anomalous branch originated from the proximal segment of an otherwise normal-appearing RCA. The anomalous branch traversed the epicardial surface between the aorta and pulmonary artery and gave rise to the LAD and Circumflex branches. All three patients found their way to the cath lab after experiencing syncope of unknown etiology, and were free of cardiovascular disease. There is a well documented relationship between patients with this specific anomaly – where an anomalous artery is "sandwiched" between the aortic and pulmonary trunks – and sudden death, which is most likely attributed to compromised blood flow when the anomalous branch is compressed during physical exertion. All three patients underwent successful surgical correction. Other common abnormalities include patients whose left circumflex branch or LAD originates off of the RCA. All told, over 20 abnormal variations in coronary artery anatomy have been described in medical literature. A majority of the patients with coronary arterial anomalies are asymptomatic and unaware of their anatomical difference. The relevancy of this with respect to your ECG evaluation skills is that when you attempt to read the ECG of a patient with an undiagnosed coronary artery anomaly whom is experiencing ACS, the ECG may not resemble anything you've seen in the books!

THE CARDIAC ELECTRICAL SYSTEM:

The electrical system of the heart is comprised of *nodes, bundles*, and *fascicles*. The main difference between heart muscle cells and electrical system cells is that electrical system cells have *automaticity* – the capability of initiating their own depolarization. Additionally, electrical cells conduct waves of depolarization much faster than muscle cells.

The diagram below illustrates the basic components of the cardiac electrical system, and indicates the coronary artery that usually supplies blood to each component:

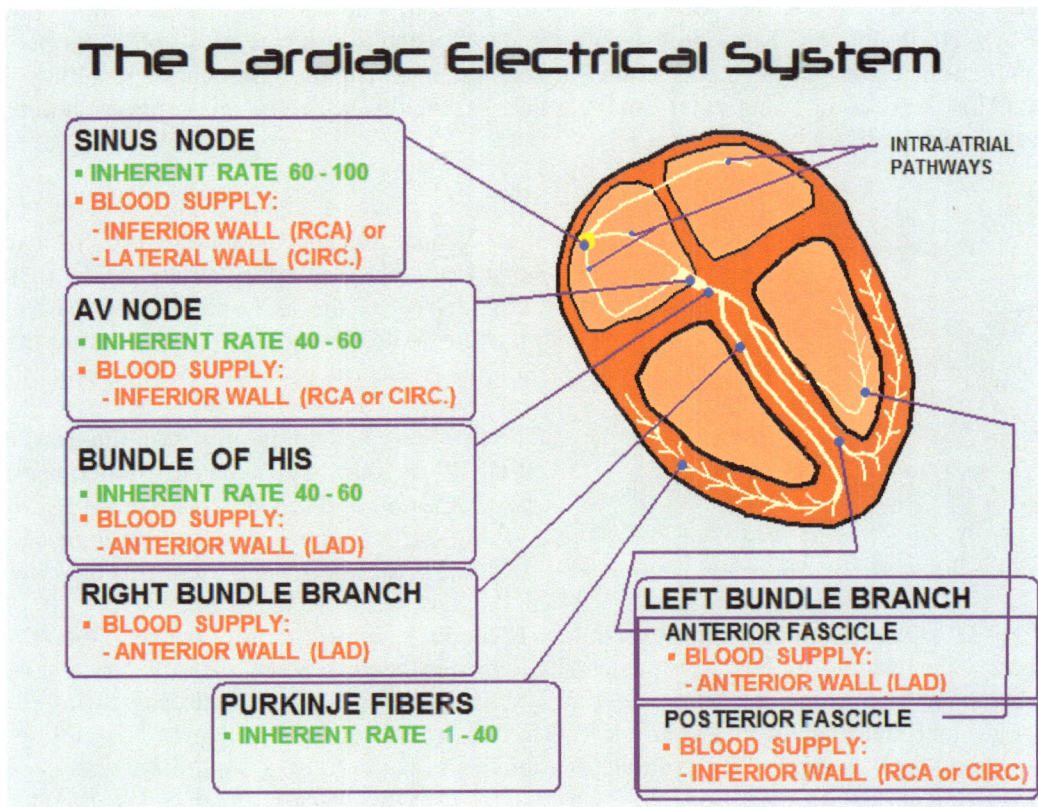

The Cardiac Electrical System

SINUS NODE
- INHERENT RATE 60 - 100
- BLOOD SUPPLY:
  - INFERIOR WALL (RCA) or
  - LATERAL WALL (CIRC.)

AV NODE
- INHERENT RATE 40 - 60
- BLOOD SUPPLY:
  - INFERIOR WALL (RCA or CIRC.)

BUNDLE OF HIS
- INHERENT RATE 40 - 60
- BLOOD SUPPLY:
  - ANTERIOR WALL (LAD)

RIGHT BUNDLE BRANCH
- BLOOD SUPPLY:
  - ANTERIOR WALL (LAD)

PURKINJE FIBERS
- INHERENT RATE 1 - 40

INTRA-ATRIAL PATHWAYS

LEFT BUNDLE BRANCH
ANTERIOR FASCICLE
- BLOOD SUPPLY:
  - ANTERIOR WALL (LAD)
POSTERIOR FASCICLE
- BLOOD SUPPLY:
  - INFERIOR WALL (RCA or CIRC)

The Sinus (SA) Node is located in the high right atrium. It is the primary pacemaker in normal hearts. It has the fastest *leakage rate of negative ions* during PHASE 4 of the Action Potential, and therefore is the first area of the heart to depolarize. The sinus node's inherent depolarization rate is 60 – 100 beats per minute. The SA node is sensitive to sympathetic and parasympathetic innervation, meaning it responds to many changes in the body, such as exercise, stress, hypoxia, hypovolemia (increases in heart rate), stimulants (such as caffeine) and drugs, both of the *legal, therapeutic* kind, and the illegal kind (cocaine, PCP, etc).

Intra-atrial Pathways carry the wave of depolarization throughout the atria.

On the ECG, depolarization of the atria is recorded as a *P wave*. In the normal heart, the P wave is the first recorded waveform on the ECG, and represents atrial depolarization.

Once atrial depolarization is complete and a P wave has been recorded on the ECG, the wave of depolarization arrives at the AV Node.

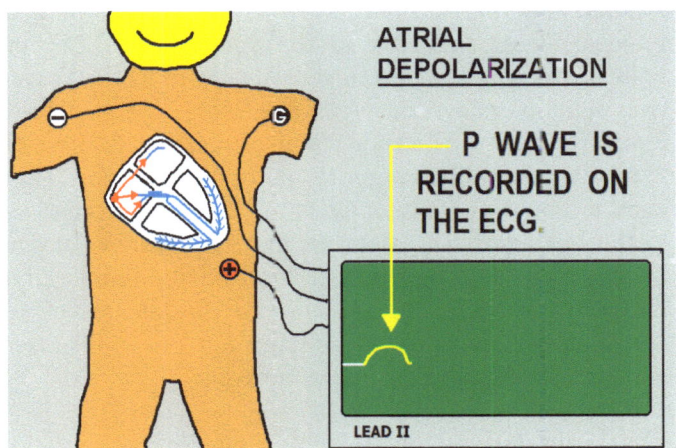

ATRIAL DEPOLARIZATION

P WAVE IS RECORDED ON THE ECG

LEAD II

The AV Node is located in the region of the lower right atrium.   Its job is two-fold:

1)   the AV Node acts like a rate filter – it slows the wave of depolarization, so that it takes approximately $1/10^{th}$ of a second for the impulse to traverse the AV node. This allows time for blood to get pumped from the atria to the ventricles. If there were no AV nodal delay, the atria would be squeezing blood into the ventricles at about the same time the ventricles would be contracting, and result in the "atria fighting against the force of the ventricles." When patients are in *atrial fibrillation*, hundreds of fibrillatory impulses bombard the AV node per minute. The AV node filters out many of the erratic fibrillatory impulses, and usually keeps the ventricular response rate under control.

2) the AV Nodes serves as a "back-up" pacemaker. In the event that no wave of depolarization comes down from the atria to the AV Node, the AV Node will depolarize itself, usually at a rate of 40-60 beats per minute—with subsequent conduction down through the Bundle of His and Bundle Branches, resulting in ventricular depolarization. This results in "junctional bradycardia" — usually with enough cardiac output to sustain the patient's hemodynamic stability.

THE P-R SEGMENT

ELECTRICAL ACTIVITY
DURING P-R SEGMENT:

- Depolarization wave in A-V node

- Atrial Repolarization

.10 SECOND
ISOELECTRIC PAUSE

LEAD II

While the wave of depolarization is being "held up" within the AV node for approximately $1/10^{th}$ of a second, there is no measurable electrical activity being picked up on the skin surface by the ECG electrodes. Therefore, the ECG machine writes an isoelectric line during this period. We call this isoelectric pause the *P-R segment*.

The two activities going on within the heart during the P-R SEGMENT that we need to remember is *AV nodal depolarization* and *atrial repolarization. We examine the P-R SEGMENT for signs of abnormal atrial repolarization, such as in cases of acute pericarditis and atrial infarction.*

The Bundle of His is located just below the AV Node.   It conducts current rapidly between the AV Node and the Bundle Branches. The Bundle of His is capable of pacing the heart. When the AV Node fails to propagate impulses from the atria, such as in cases of conduction system disorders like Lev's disease, or inferior wall MI, the Bundle of His may take over pacing the ventricles. Rhythms paced by the Bundle of His closely resemble AV Nodal rhythms: rate 40-60, narrow QRS complexes (unless the patient has a *bundle branch block*). When AV nodal conduction is intact, you may see inverted P waves after the QRS, usually in the S-T segment. When there is AV nodal block, such as is often seen with INFERIOR WALL MI, you may see complete heart block: normal appearing P waves that have no relationship to the narrow QRS complexes, with a rate of 40 – 60 beats per minute. This rhythm is sometimes referred to as "A-V disassociation. The Bundle of His usually gets its blood supply from the Left Anterior Descending (LAD) artery.

The Bundle Branches are located within the intraventricular septum, and are the main "electrical conduits" which carry impulses from the atria to the ventricles. The bundle branches originate at the distal Bundle of His. There are two main bundles; the *right bundle branch* and the *left bundle branch*.   The right bundle branch (RBB) conducts the wave of depolarization to the right ventricle. The left bundle branch (LBB) conducts the wave of depolarization to the left ventricle. Because the left ventricle has more muscle mass than the right, the left bundle branch divides into two fascicles: the *left anterior fascicle,* which feeds the anterior left ventricle and the *left posterior fascicle,* which feeds the left posterior ventricle.

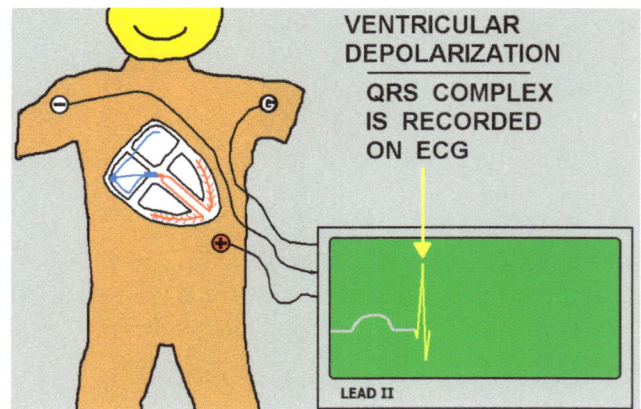

VENTRICULAR DEPOLARIZATION

QRS COMPLEX
IS RECORDED
ON ECG

LEAD II

The *right bundle branch* and *anterior fascicle* of the left bundle branch are located in the *anterior* intraventricular septum, and receive their blood supply from the left anterior descending (LAD) artery.

A total blockage of the proximal LAD artery usually results in an extensive ANTERIOR-SEPTAL WALL MI. Septal infarctions can damage the bundle branches and result in high grade (2nd / 3rd degree) heart block.

The *posterior fascicle* of the left bundle branch is located in the posterior intraventricular septum, and receives its blood supply from the posterior descending artery (PDA). The PDA branches off from the RCA in 75 – 80% of the population and the circumflex artery in 15 – 20%.

The Purkinje Fibers receive the wave of depolarization from the bundle branches and disburse it throughout the ventricles, causing depolarization and contraction of ventricular muscle. The electrical cells of the purkinje network are capable of Automaticity if no wave of depolarization is received from the bundle branches above. The purkinje fibers intrinsic rate is 1 – 40 beats per minute.

After ventricular depolarization, comes ventricular repolarization. This is seen on the ECG as the S-T segment and T wave.

One important concept to remember is if another electrical stimulus—such as an electrical shock or PVC—is introduced to a mass of cardiac tissue during repolarization, it may result in dys-synchrony of the normal cardiac cycle. In the ventricles, this may result in in Torsades de Pointes, or ventricular fibrillation.

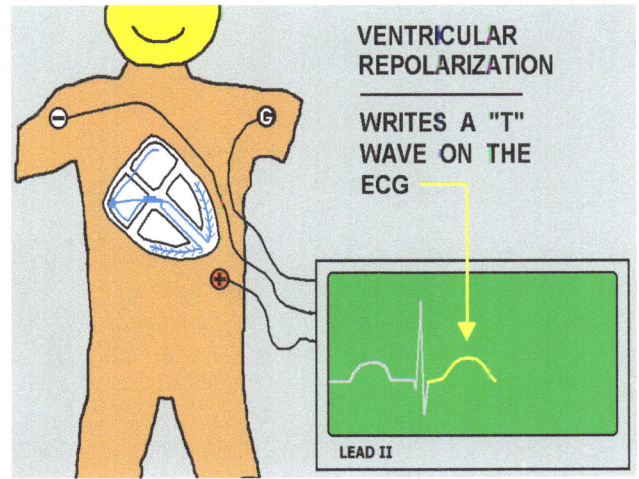

VENTRICULAR REPOLARIZATION

WRITES A "T" WAVE ON THE ECG

LEAD II

During the T-WAVE, we say that that VENTRICULAR REPOLARIZATION is occurring.

PEAK of T WAVE

T wave

QRS

ELECTRICAL STIMULUS TO VENTRICLES during this phase MAY result in TORSADES, V-FIB, and / or V-TACH.

ELECTRICAL STIMULUS TO VENTRICLES during this phase is VERY LIKELY to result in TORSADES, V-FIB, and / or V-TACH.

As a general rule, I think of the phase beginning at the end of the QRS complex to the tip of the T wave as the "absolute refractory period," and the tip of the T wave to the end of the T wave as the "relative refractory period."

To demonstrate how predictably the heart responds to being "electrically stimulated" during the absolute refractory period, we make our patients go into cardiac arrest every time we implant an internal defibrillator (ICD) — that's where we give the ICD a "test run"— to make sure it works, before we send the patient home!!

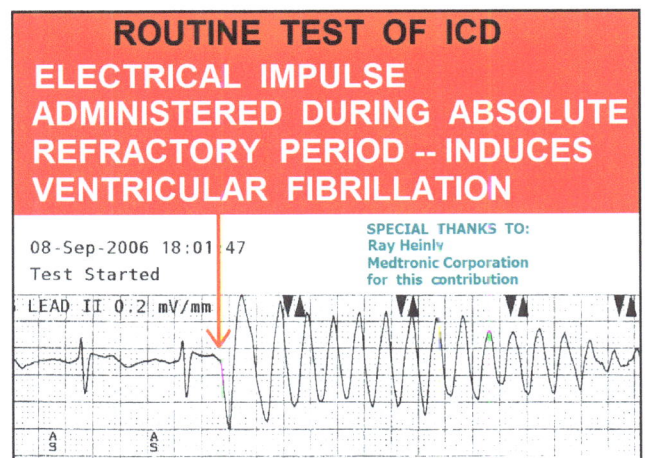

ROUTINE TEST OF ICD

ELECTRICAL IMPULSE ADMINISTERED DURING ABSOLUTE REFRACTORY PERIOD -- INDUCES VENTRICULAR FIBRILLATION

08-Sep-2006 18:01 47
Test Started

LEAD II 0.2 mV/mm

SPECIAL THANKS TO: Ray Heinly Medtronic Corporation for this contribution

31

NORMAL INTRINSIC HEART RATES:

The table seen to the right depicts normal rates for the heart's common pacemaker sites. Knowing these normal ranges may help you with identifying a patient's heart rhythm.

Multiple factors affect automaticity, such as the presence of certain medications, toxins, the body's temperature, Ph, blood gases, electrolytes and more. When automaticity is affected by any of these factors, heart rates may deviate from normal values.

NORMAL INTRINSIC RATES:

SA NODE:	60 - 100
AV NODE:	40 - 60
VENTRICLES:	1 - 40

THE SKELETON OF THE HEART

An important structure that often gets overlooked in traditional cardiac A & P programs is the "skeleton of the heart," which is a disc-shaped structure, made of connective tissue which separates the atria from the ventricles.

There are five openings in the skeleton of the heart, as seen in the diagram to the right: one for each of the four heart valves (*tricuspid, mitral, pulmonary* and *aortic)*, and one for the *Bundle of His.*

This gasket-like structure functions like an "electrical insulator" – it prevents electrical impulses from traveling between the atria and ventricles, except for current traversing the Bundle of His.

If the skeleton of the heart did not exist, every impulse of atrial depolarization reaching the bottom of the atria would flow directly into the ventricle beneath it, resulting in immediate ventricular depolarization. There would be no $1/10^{th}$ of a second AV Nodal delay. The atria

and ventricles would contract at nearly the same time. The sequence of ventricular contraction would be nearly opposite that of normal, causing a drop in cardiac output. If there were no skeleton of the heart to electrically insulate the atria from the ventricles, many patients who went into atrial fibrillation would quickly deteriorate into ventricular fibrillation.

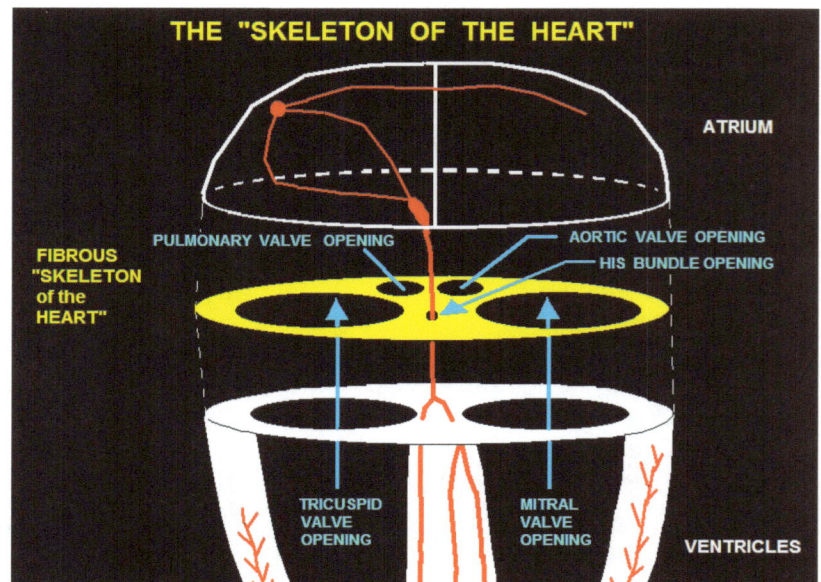

Occasionally people have an abnormal opening in the skeleton of their heart, resulting in current "leakage" between the atria and ventricles. This opening is known as a *bypass tract.* Some bypass tracts only conduct current *antegrade* (from the atria to the ventricles), and other bypass tracts only conduct *retrograde* (from the ventricles to the atria.). Some bypass tracts are capable of conducting current in both directions.

In cases where current is conducted antegrade (from the atria to the ventricles) through a bypass tract, ventricular muscle cells beneath the bypass tract depolarize early, resulting in a shortened P-R interval, and abnormally wide QRS complexes with *delta waves.* When this occurs, we say there is *pre-excitation. This phenomenon is known as the WOLFF-PARKINSON-WHITE SYNDROME.*

☞ REVIEW QUESTIONS:

REINFORCE YOUR KNOWLEDGE OF ESSENTIAL CONCEPTS:
(questions originate from highlighted text and graphic images)

Role of the ECG and Essential Cardiac Anatomy and Physiology

1. (p.1) Your patient is suffering from Acute Myocardial Infarction due to a sudden total obstruction of his Circumflex Artery. He has chest pain, and his Cardiac Markers are elevated. However his 12 Lead ECG shows no ST elevation or depression, and is "completely normal" in all aspects. This "false negative ECG" is an example of:
   a. Poor technique being used to record the 12 Lead ECG
   b. The lack of sensitivity, which is one of the ECGs inherent flaws
   c. The nursing staff waited too long to obtain the ECG, and missed the MI
   d. The patient refused to cooperate, and falsified his ECG results

2. (p. 1) Your patient's ECG shows sinus rhythm, narrow QRS complexes, and ST segment depression in leads V1 through V4. Some possible causes of this abnormality include: *anterior wall ischemia, acute posterior wall myocardial infarction*, and *non-Q wave myocardial infarction of the anterior wall*. The fact that your patient's ECG abnormality can mean several different diagnoses is an example of lack of specificity, which is one of the ECGs inherent flaws:
   a. True
   b. False

3. (p. 1) Clinicians should always accept the ECG computer-derived diagnosis as being correct.
   a. True
   b. False

4. (p. 1) When patients present with symptoms which are suspicious for Acute Coronary Syndrome, the American Heart Association recommends that a 12 Lead ECG be obtained and interpreted within the first _____ of the patient's arrival.
   a. 2 minutes
   b. 10 minutes
   c. 30 minutes
   d. 60 minutes

5. (p. 14) Necrosis to the papillary muscles, such as which results from extensive myocardial infarction, can lead to _____, often within 7 – 10 days post-MI.
   a. cardiac arrest
   b. acute renal failure
   c. bacterial endocarditis
   d. acute mitral valve regurgitation

6. (p. 20) When referring to the coronary arteries, 75-80% of the population is right dominant. Being *right dominant* means:
   a. the right coronary artery gives rise to the posterior descending artery which supplies blood to the inferior wall of the left ventricle.
   b. the patient is right-handed
   c. the patient's right ventricle pumps blood directly into the aorta and the systemic circulation
   d. the right ventricle is enlarged, resulting in ST depression with inverted, asymmetrical T waves in leads V1 and V2.

7. (p. 20) When a dominant Right Coronary Artery is blocked, *Inferior Wall MI* usually results, and can be accompanied by *right ventricular MI*, *sinus bradycardia*, and *AV nodal blocks* (1st, 2nd, and 3rd degree heart blocks).
   a. True
   b. False

8. (p. 21) The left main coronary artery supplies blood to most of the left ventricle. Total occlusion of the left main coronary artery is often fatal.
   a. True
   b. False

9. (p. 22) The left anterior descending artery supplies blood to the _____ - _____ walls of the left ventricle.
   a. inferior-lateral
   b. basilar-septal
   c. inferior-posterior
   d. anterior-septal

10. (p. 22) Total occlusion of the left anterior descending artery often results in _____ and _____.
    a. acute renal failure, hyperkalemia
    b. cardiogenic shock, pulmonary edema
    c. sinus bradycardia, postural hypotension
    d. 1st degree heart block, atrial fibrillation

11. (p. 23) The sinus node receives it blood supply from the circumflex artery in _____% of the population.
    a. 10
    b. 45
    c. 75
    d. 100

12. (p. 24) In patients who are left dominant, their _____ gives rise to the posterior descending artery, which supplies inferior wall of the left ventricle.
    a. circumflex artery
    b. left main coronary artery
    c. left anterior descending artery
    d. right coronary artery

13. (p. 24) In patients who are left dominant, their circumflex artery supplies the _____, _____, and _____ walls of the left ventricle, which comprises up to approximately _____ % of the left ventricle.
    a. anterior, septal, inferior -- 75%
    b. anterior, inferior, posterior – 35%
    c. apical, septal, atrial – 100%
    d. inferior, posterior, lateral – 55%

14. (p. 28) There is a very small percentage of the population whose coronary artery anatomy is very unusual, such as patients who have a single artery that supplies the entire myocardium. It is important to be aware of this because:
    a. when such patients experience ACS, their ECGs may look very different from what you're used to seeing
    b. you can refer the patient to the Guinness Book of World Records
    c. you can add the ECG -- minus patient identification data – to your collection of abnormal ECGs to astound and impress your co-workers with
    d. when you see the confusing ECG, you can shove it back into the patient's chart, hand it off to a co-worker, and say, "I'm overdue for my lunch break. Please cover for me."

II. Basic 12 Lead ECG Concepts

ECG PAPER:

ECG PAPER - THE VERTICAL AXIS:

- SMALL BOXES = 1mm SQUARES

- THE VERTICAL AXIS REPRESENTS AMPLITIUDE (VOLTAGE)

- IN VERTICAL DIRECTION, THERE ARE 5 SMALL BOXES IN EACH LARGE (5mm) BOX

- 1 mv CALIBRATION SPIKE = 10 mm

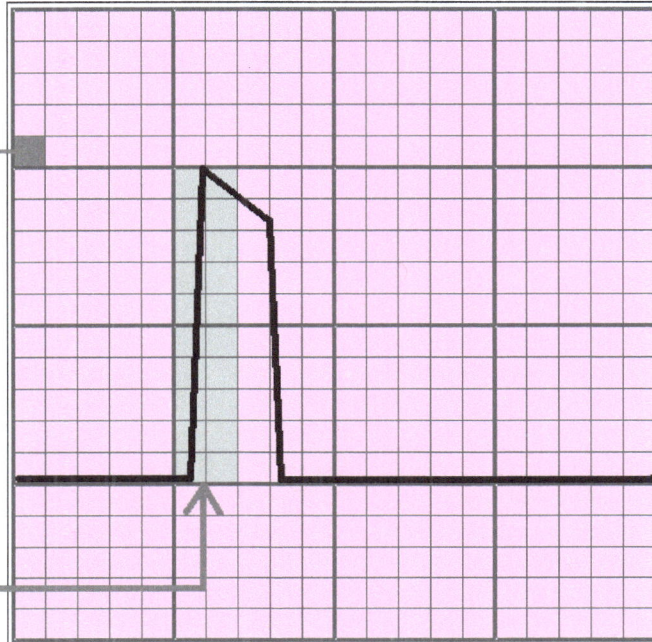

ECG PAPER - THE HORIZONTAL AXIS:

THE HORIZONTAL AXIS REPRESENTS TIME . . .

STANDARD SPEED FOR RECORDING ADULT EKGs = 25 mm / SECOND

EACH 1mm BOX = .04 SECONDS, or 40 MILLISECONDS (40 ms)

5 SMALL BOXES = .20 SECONDS, or 200 MILLISECONDS (200 ms)

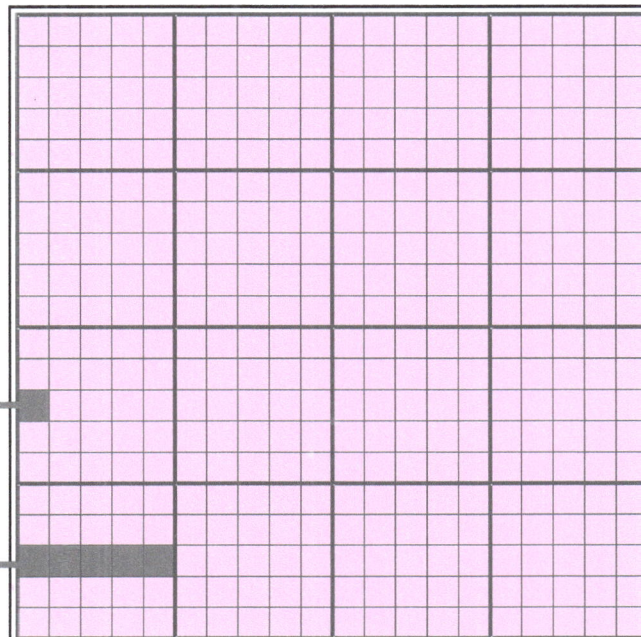

THE ECG MACHINE:

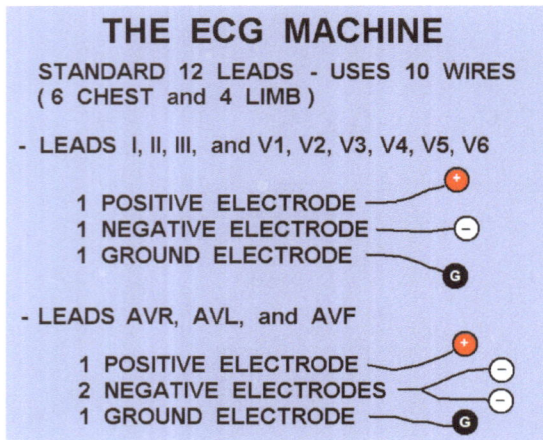

THE ECG MACHINE
STANDARD 12 LEADS - USES 10 WIRES
(6 CHEST and 4 LIMB)

- LEADS I, II, III, and V1, V2, V3, V4, V5, V6

    1 POSITIVE ELECTRODE ⊕
    1 NEGATIVE ELECTRODE ⊖
    1 GROUND ELECTRODE ⏺G

- LEADS AVR, AVL, and AVF

    1 POSITIVE ELECTRODE ⊕
    2 NEGATIVE ELECTRODES ⊖ ⊖
    1 GROUND ELECTRODE ⏺G

For nine of 12 leads, the ECG machine uses three lead wires each, as seen in the diagram to the left. These leads are I, II, III and V1 through V6. In case you didn't know, the "V" designation (as in V1 through V6) stands for "vector." How's that for a nice piece of ECG trivia?

The augmented voltage leads (AVR, AVL, and AVF) utilize four lead wires each.

It is not all that important for you to know which position all of the wires are in for each lead. What IS important is that you know *where the POSITIVE electrode is located* for each lead. I found the best way to understand the 12 lead ECG is to imagine that the positive electrode is an "EYE." The eye (positive electrode) is the electrode that "sees" movement of the heart's electrical currents.

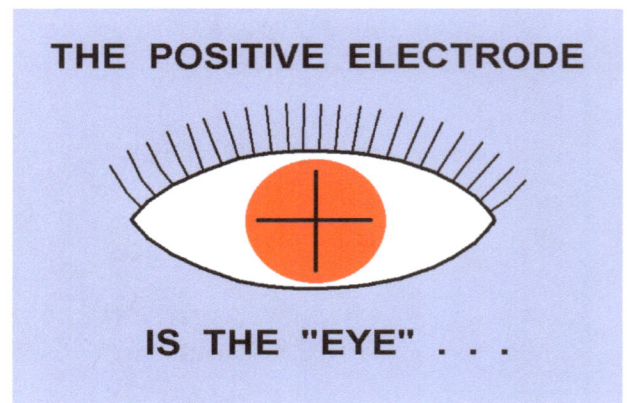

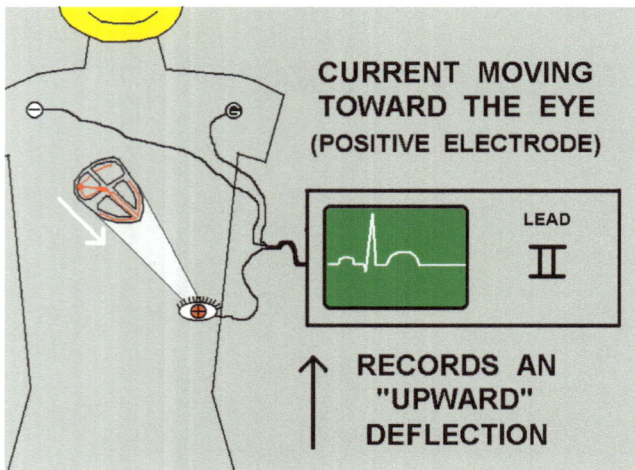

THE POSITIVE ELECTRODE

IS THE "EYE" . . .

CURRENT MOVING TOWARD THE EYE
(POSITIVE ELECTRODE)

LEAD **II**

↑ RECORDS AN "UPWARD" DEFLECTION

For example, the positive electrode in limb lead II is located on the patient's left leg. (We sometimes "cheat" when hooking patients up for telemetry monitoring and place the left leg leads on the lower left abdomen, as seen in our example to the left). In this case, the "eye" (positive electrode) is "seeing" current moving toward it during the normal cardiac cycle. Whenever current moves *toward* a positive electrode, the ECG machine records a *positive* deflection.

Conversely, whenever current moves *away from* the positive electrode, the ECG machine records a *negative* waveform, as seen in the example to the right. In LEAD AVR, the positive electrode is on the patient's *right arm*. Therefore, most current is moving *away from* the positive electrode, which makes most of the recorded heartbeat of lead AVR *negative*.

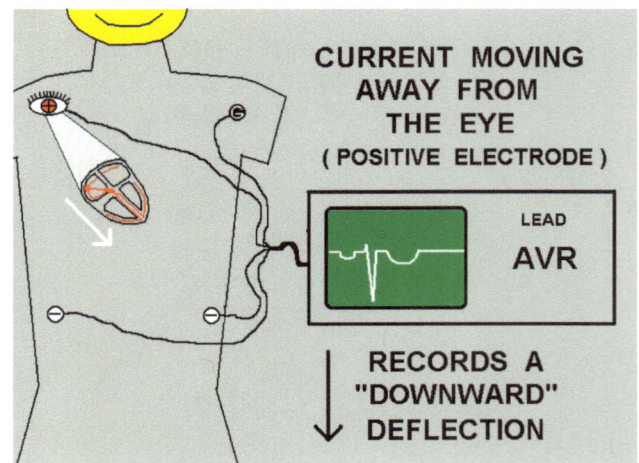

CURRENT MOVING AWAY FROM THE EYE
(POSITIVE ELECTRODE)

LEAD **AVR**

↓ RECORDS A "DOWNWARD" DEFLECTION

THE 12 LEAD ECG:

The standard 12 lead ECG machine utilizes ten wires to obtain the ECG tracing. Four leads are placed on the patient's extremities, and six leads are placed on the patient's chest.

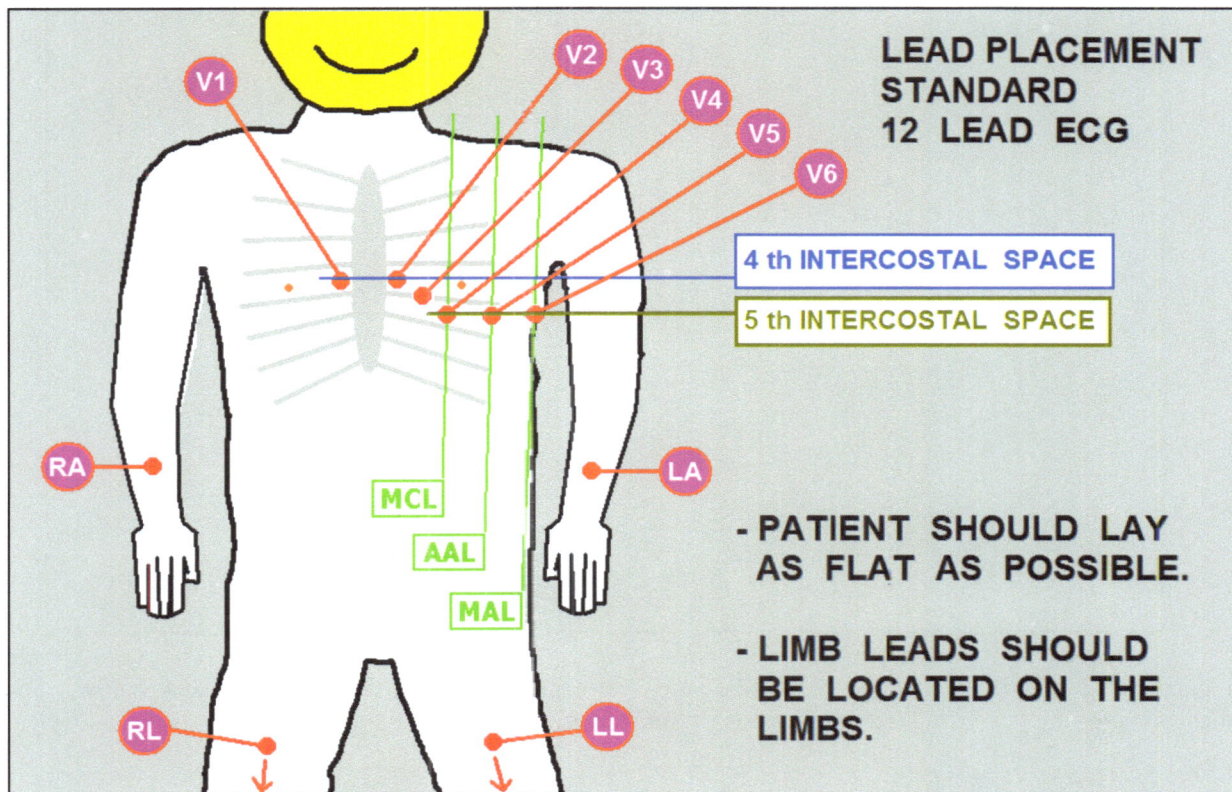

First, have the patient lay flat, if possible. When the patient is unable to lay flat, such as in cases of CHF, you may be able to get the patient in a reverse-trendelenberg position. I have found that improper patient positioning, such as when a patient is "doubled over," can result in false abnormal S-T segments, which become "normal" when the patient lays flat.

The four limb leads should be placed on the limbs, as distally as possible. I find you get less muscular artifact if the leads are placed over a bony prominence, such as over the tibia (shin bones) in the legs, and the forearms, as shown in the above diagram.

Lead V1 is placed at the fourth intercostal space just to the right of the patient's sternum. The landmark to quickly find the 4th intercostal space (with most patients) is the nipple line. Just remember....for some unfortunate folks, gravity has not been too kind, so you may discover their nipple line is located at the level of their patella, so just be careful! ☺ Lead V2 is located at the 4th intercostal space to the left of the sternum. The standard way to find V3 is to first find V4, then place V3 directly in the middle between V2 and V4. To find V4, go where the 5th intercostal space and the mid-clavicular line intersect. V5 is located on the same horizontal plane as V4, at the anterior axillary line. V6 is located on the same horizontal plane as V4 and V5, at the point where the mid-axillary line intersects. To be technically correct, do not follow the contour of the ribs when positioning V5 and V6—you should remain on the same horizontal plane as V4.

A standard 12 lead ECG looks like this:

38 yr	Vent. rate	64	BPM	Normal sinus rhythm
Male	PR interval	130	ms	Normal ECG
	QRS duration	96	ms	No previous ECGs available
Room:ER	QT/QTc	396/408	ms	
	P-R-T axes	40 11 61		

D.O.S.:

I aVR V1 V4

II aVL V2 V5

III aVF V3 V6

In the standard 12 lead ECG, you get "3 second snips" of each lead, which is laid out as seen below. Some ECG machines also provide you with three continuous rhythm strips, as seen in our example of the author's ECG:

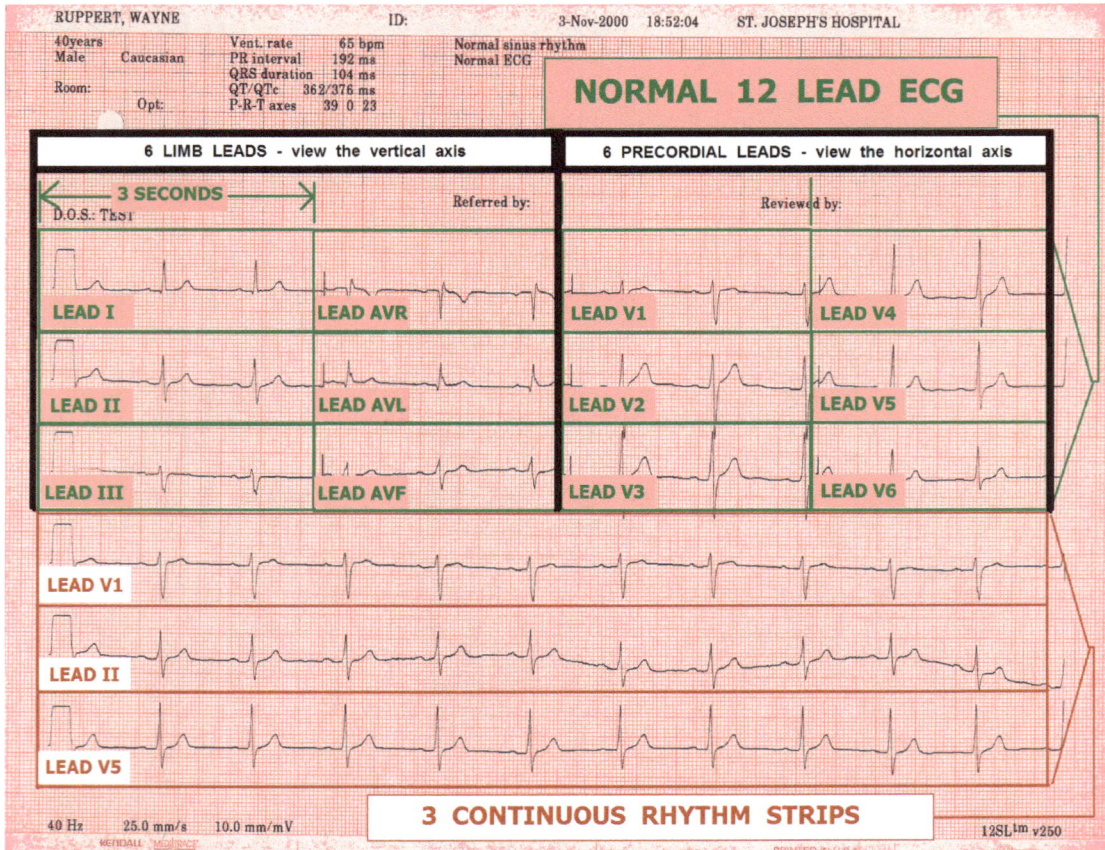

RUPPERT, WAYNE   ID: 3-Nov-2000 18:52:04   ST. JOSEPH'S HOSPITAL

40years		Vent. rate	65 bpm	Normal sinus rhythm
Male	Caucasian	PR interval	192 ms	Normal ECG
		QRS duration	104 ms	
Room:		QT/QTc	362/376 ms	
	Opt:	P-R-T axes	39 0 23	

NORMAL 12 LEAD ECG

6 LIMB LEADS - view the vertical axis   6 PRECORDIAL LEADS - view the horizontal axis

← 3 SECONDS →   Referred by: Reviewed by:

D.O.S.: TEST

LEAD I   LEAD AVR   LEAD V1   LEAD V4

LEAD II   LEAD AVL   LEAD V2   LEAD V5

LEAD III   LEAD AVF   LEAD V3   LEAD V6

LEAD V1

LEAD II

LEAD V5

3 CONTINUOUS RHYTHM STRIPS

40 Hz   25.0 mm/s   10.0 mm/mV   12SL^lm v250

38

Now we're going to look at how the 12 lead ECG machine "sees" each area of the heart. When I teach 12 lead ECG classes, I tell my students to image a "crystal-clear" human body made of glass. The only thing inside of it is a heart, located in it's normal position within the thoracic cavity. Then, dip the glass model in liquid chocolate—like the kind you get at Dairy Queen. Once the chocolate has dried, scratch away little peep-holes where the positive electrodes of a 12 lead ECG are normally positioned. Now, our model should look like the one in the picture to the right:

To understand what part of the heart each lead of the ECG sees, simply imagine yourself peeping through the peepholes in this model. For example, to see what lead V1 sees, peep through the hole labeled "V1." In doing so, you will see the front surface of the heart, commonly known as the *anterior wall* of the left ventricle.

	AREAS VIEWED by 12 LEAD ECG	+	TYPICAL CORONARY ARTERIAL DISTRIBUTION
AVR	BASILAR SEPTAL	→	1st SEPTAL PERFORATOR
AVL, I	LATERAL ANTERIOR	→	1st DIAGONAL or RAMUS or 1st OBTUSE MARGINAL
V1, V2	ANTERIOR	→	LEFT ANTERIOR DESCENDING
	SEPTAL	→	LEFT ANTERIOR DESCENDING
	POSTERIOR (recip.)	→	POSTERIOR LATERAL VESSELS
V3, V4	ANTERIOR	→	LEFT ANTERIOR DESCENDING
V5, V6	LATERAL	→	CIRCUMFLEX
II, III, AVF	INFERIOR	→	RIGHT CORONARY ARTERY or CIRCUMFLEX

Next, we'll break the 12 lead ECG down into groups of leads that view each region of the heart:

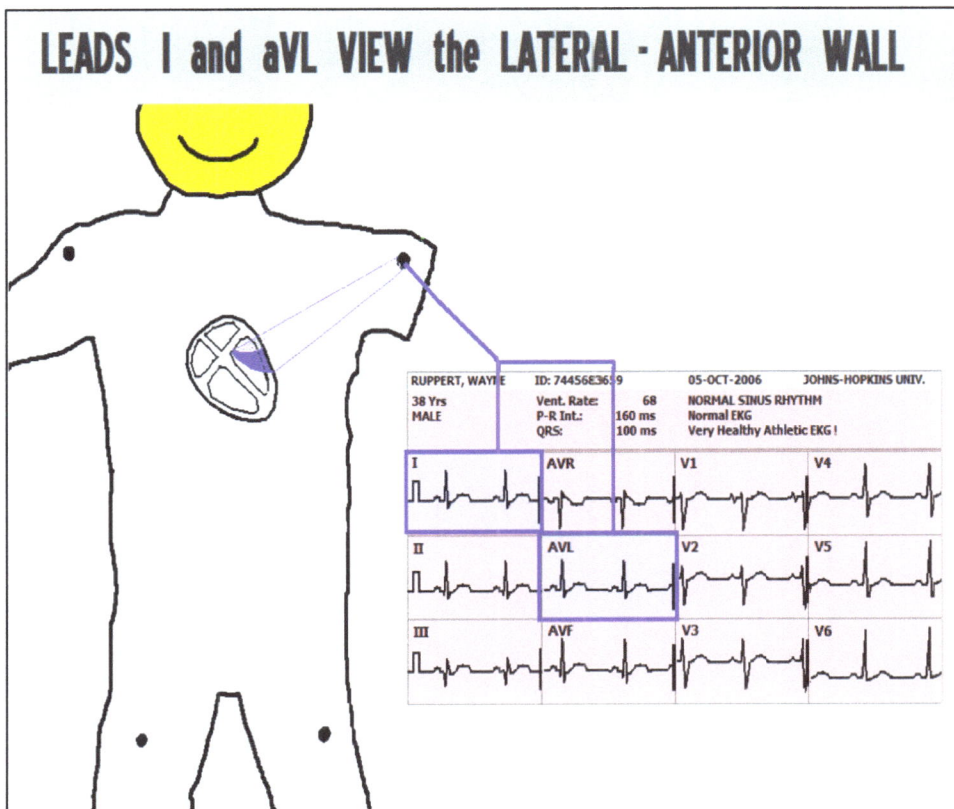

LEADS I and aVL VIEW the LATERAL - ANTERIOR WALL

Traditional ECG curricula state that leads I and AVL, located on the left shoulder, view the *lateral wall* of the left ventricle. To be more accurate, we say Leads I and aVL view the superior anterior-lateral aspect of the left ventricle. Thinking of it in this manner will help us to identify the specific coronary artery involved in acute MI, or the "culprit artery," and also helps to identify where along the course of the artery – proximal or distal – the lesion is located. For example, if Leads I and aVL are elevated along with V1 – V4 (anterior wall MI), the blockage is usually in the proximal LAD. If Leads I and aVL are elevated along with V5 and V6 (lateral wall MI), the blockage will likely be in the proximal circumflex artery.

In the next three images, note that the "area of infarction" (shaded in brown) is the same region of myocardium in each of the three hearts. However, the origin of the blocked artery is different. In the image to the right, the blocked artery originates from the circumflex artery. In the image below, the blocked artery has its own origin off of the Left Main Coronary Artery; it is not part of the LAD, nor is it part of the circumflex. When this artery has its own takeoff from the LMCA, we call it a "Ramus Artery." In the bottom right image, the blocked artery originates off of the LAD. Right now, we want you to see that the region viewed by leads I and aVL can originate from an artery that branches off of the *circumflex* or *left anterior descending artery*, or from a *ramus artery* off of the LMCA.

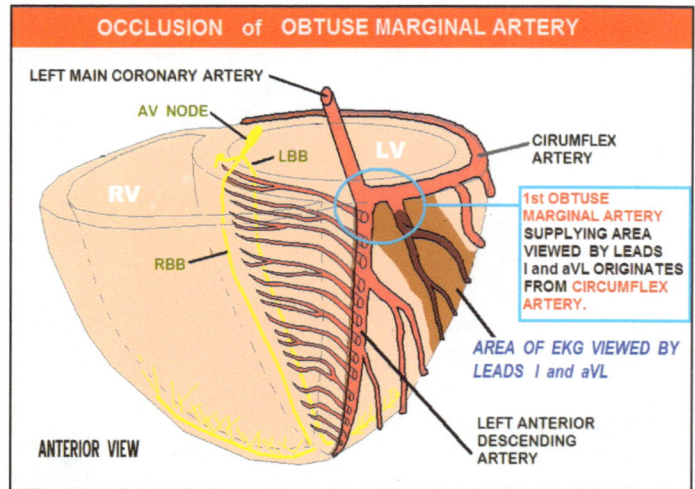

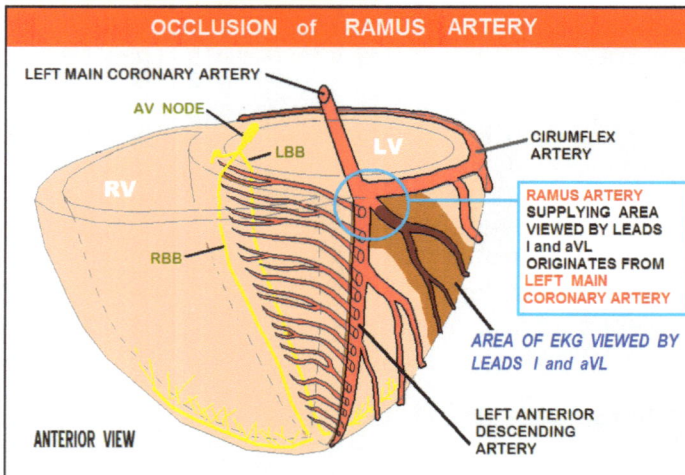

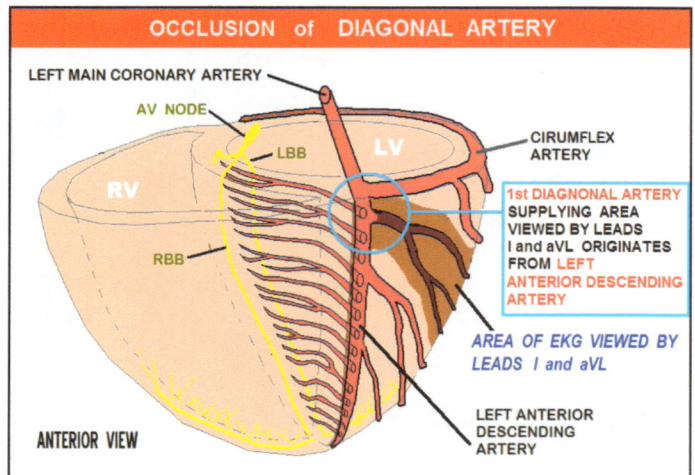

OCCLUSION of OBTUSE MARGINAL ARTERY

LEFT MAIN CORONARY ARTERY
AV NODE
LBB
RBB
RV
LV
CIRUMFLEX ARTERY
1st OBTUSE MARGINAL ARTERY SUPPLYING AREA VIEWED BY LEADS I and aVL ORIGINATES FROM CIRCUMFLEX ARTERY.
AREA OF EKG VIEWED BY LEADS I and aVL
LEFT ANTERIOR DESCENDING ARTERY
ANTERIOR VIEW

OCCLUSION of RAMUS ARTERY

LEFT MAIN CORONARY ARTERY
AV NODE
LBB
RBB
RV
LV
CIRUMFLEX ARTERY
RAMUS ARTERY SUPPLYING AREA VIEWED BY LEADS I and aVL ORIGINATES FROM LEFT MAIN CORONARY ARTERY
AREA OF EKG VIEWED BY LEADS I and aVL
LEFT ANTERIOR DESCENDING ARTERY
ANTERIOR VIEW

OCCLUSION of DIAGONAL ARTERY

LEFT MAIN CORONARY ARTERY
AV NODE
LBB
RBB
RV
LV
CIRUMFLEX ARTERY
1st DIAGNONAL ARTERY SUPPLYING AREA VIEWED BY LEADS I and aVL ORIGINATES FROM LEFT ANTERIOR DESCENDING ARTERY
AREA OF EKG VIEWED BY LEADS I and aVL
LEFT ANTERIOR DESCENDING ARTERY
ANTERIOR VIEW

Leads II, III, and aVF view the INFERIOR WALL of the LEFT VENTRICLE.

LEADS II, III, and aVF VIEW
INFERIOR WALL of the LEFT VENTRICLE

RUPPERT, WAYNE   ID: 7445683659   05-OCT-2006   JOHNS-HOPKINS UNIV.
38 Yrs   Vent. Rate: 68   NORMAL SINUS RHYTHM
MALE   P-R Int.: 160 ms   Normal EKG
QRS: 100 ms   Very Healthy Athletic EKG !
I   AVR   V1   V4
II   AVL   V2   V5
III   AVF   V3   V6

FED by the RCA (75 - 80 % pop) or the CIRCUMFLEX (10 - 15 %)

Leads II, III, and aVF utilize the lead wire on the left lower leg as the positive electrode. Therefore, leads II, III, and aVF all view the bottom of the heart, or the INFERIOR WALL of the left ventricle.

Remember that the inferior wall receives its blood supply from the RIGHT CORONARY ARTERY in 75 – 80% of the population. In 10 – 15% of the population, the inferior wall gets its blood supply from the CIRCUMFLEX ARTERY.

In the remaining 5 – 15% of the population, the inferior wall gets its blood supply from a combination of the RCA and Circumflex arteries or from a "trans-apical LAD" in 1% of the population.

Leads V1 - V4 view the ANTERIOR and SEPTAL WALL of the LEFT VENTRICLE.

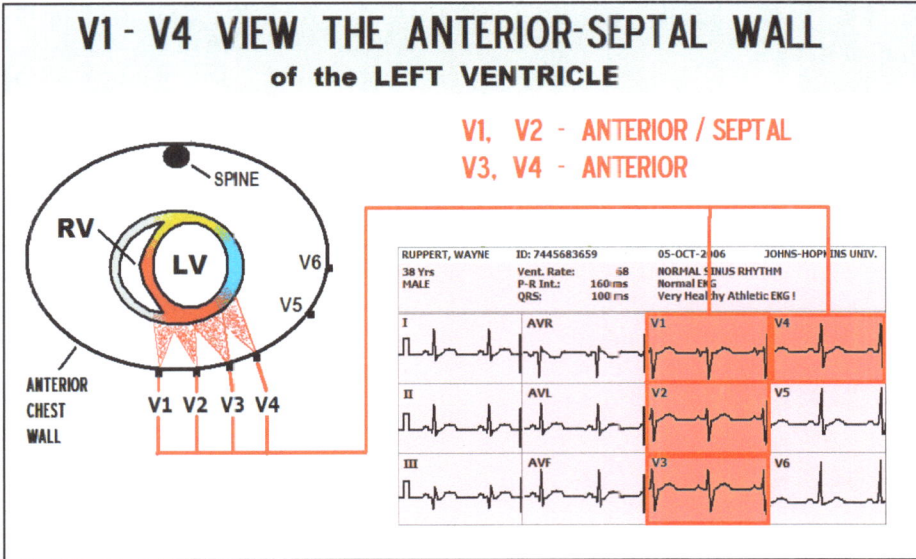

V1 - V4 VIEW THE ANTERIOR-SEPTAL WALL of the LEFT VENTRICLE

V1, V2 - ANTERIOR / SEPTAL
V3, V4 - ANTERIOR

SPINE
RV
LV
V6
V5
ANTERIOR CHEST WALL
V1 V2 V3 V4

RUPPERT, WAYNE   ID: 7445683659   05-OCT-2006   JOHNS-HOPKINS UNIV.
38 Yrs   Vent. Rate: 68   NORMAL SINUS RHYTHM
MALE   P-R Int.:   160 ms   Normal EKG
QRS: 100 ms   Very Healthy Athletic EKG !

In this cutaway anatomical view of a patient's chest wall with the heart inside the chest cavity, you can see the relationship of ECG leads V1 – V4 to the patient's heart. Leads V1 – V4 view the ANTERIOR wall of the left ventricle. Leads V1 and V2 also see the intraventricular septum.

Recall from the CARDIAC A&P chapter, the anterior wall is fed by the LEFT ANTERIOR DESCENDING ARTERY. In cases of ANTERIOR WALL MI, suspect that the LAD is the "culprit" artery.

ALSO, Leads V1 – V3 view the POSTERIOR WALL of the LEFT VENTRICLE via reciprocal changes.

In the STANDARD 12 LEAD ECG, there are no leads that directly view the POSTERIOR WALL.

Therefore when you're evaluating the ECG of a patient in which you see ST segment elevation in the INFERIOR LEADS (II, III, and aVF), and you also notice ST SEGMENT DEPRESSION in leads V1 – V3, you should suspect that POSTERIOR WALL MI is also present. Remember, there is a high incidence of *posterior involvement* in cases of *inferior wall STEMI* because the same artery that feeds the inferior wall usually also feeds part – or all – of the posterior wall.

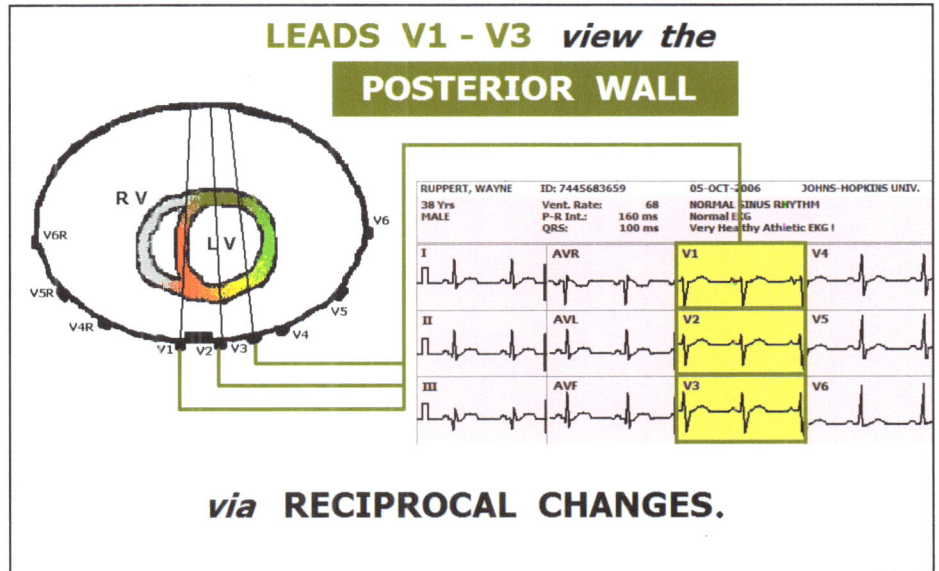

LEADS V1 - V3 view the POSTERIOR WALL

via RECIPROCAL CHANGES.

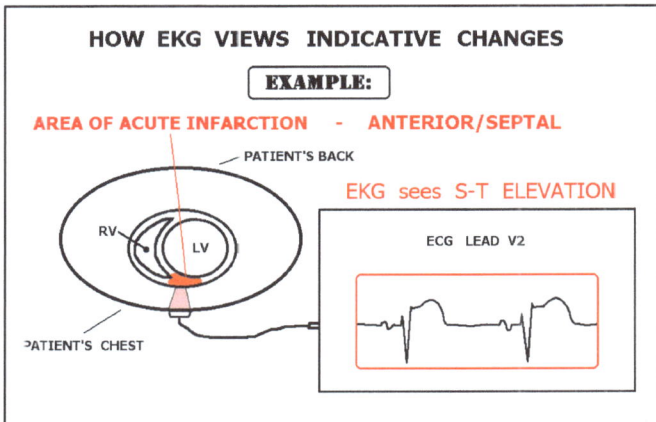

HOW EKG VIEWS INDICATIVE CHANGES

EXAMPLE:

AREA OF ACUTE INFARCTION - ANTERIOR/SEPTAL

PATIENT'S BACK

EKG sees S-T ELEVATION

ECG LEAD V2

RV   LV

PATIENT'S CHEST

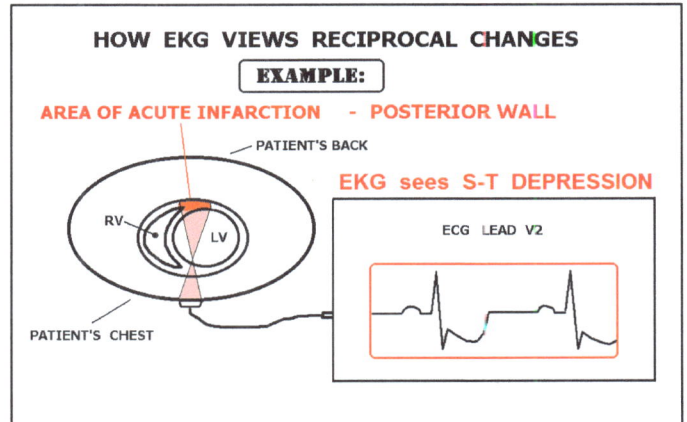

HOW EKG VIEWS RECIPROCAL CHANGES

EXAMPLE:

AREA OF ACUTE INFARCTION - POSTERIOR WALL

PATIENT'S BACK

EKG sees S-T DEPRESSION

ECG LEAD V2

RV   LV

PATIENT'S CHEST

V5 - V6 VIEW THE LATERAL WALL
of the LEFT VENTRICLE

Leads V5 and V6 view the LATERAL WALL, which is commonly fed by the CIRCUMFLEX ARTERY.

In cases of ANTERIOR WALL MI, ST elevation in V5 and possibly V6 is sometimes noted. This results when the LAD territory extends into the lateral wall. *Patient's hearts don't always "read the book," so they may present a little differently than how its traditionally presented in a textbook!*

LEAD aVR has been traditionally ignored by many clinicians who read ECGs. We have learned Lead aVR can supply us with critical information. Lead aVR views the BASILAR SEPTUM, and usually receives its blood supply from the first large septal perforator which arises from the proximal left anterior descending artery. In STEMI, ST segment elevation in aVR is associated with occlusion of the proximal LAD, above the takeoff of the first septal perforator, and may also indicate occlusion of the Left Main Coronary Artery (LMCA). Elevation of aVR is usually associated with extensive anterior-septal MI. In cases of ischemia without AMI, ST segment elevation in lead aVR has been associated with severe triple-vessel disease, and/or obstructive lesions of the Left Main Coronary Artery.

Now when you view each lead of the 12 Lead ECG, you should think of:
- THE REGION OF THE HEART VIEWED BY EACH LEAD
- THE CORONARY ARTERY THAT COMMONLY SUPPLIES THAT REGION

As previously stated, <mark>the standard 12 lead ECG has two significant blind spots: the posterior wall of the left ventricle, which is viewed only by reciprocal changes in the anterior leads, and the right ventricle, which is not viewed by indicative or reciprocal leads, as illustrated below:</mark>

CHEST LEADS V1 - V6
WHAT EACH LEAD "SEES" . . .

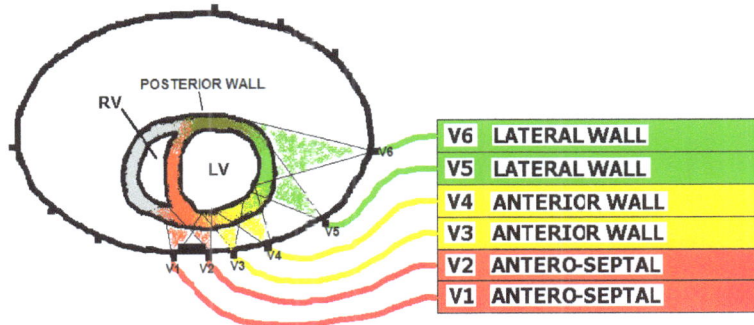

<mark>The 18 lead ECG provides six more leads: 3 that view the right ventricle, and 3 that view the posterior wall.</mark> Leads V4R, V5R, and V6R are located in the same anatomical position as V4, V5, and V6, only on the right side of the patient's chest. These leads, of course, view the right ventricle. Leads V7, V8 and V9 are located at the same horizontal plane as V6, on the patient's back, between V6 and the spine. These leads directly view the posterior wall. When combined with the standard six chest leads, the myocardium is covered fairly well, as seen in the illustration below:

CHEST LEADS V1 - V6 *PLUS* V4R, V5R, V6R, and V7, V8, V9
WHAT EACH LEAD "SEES" . . .

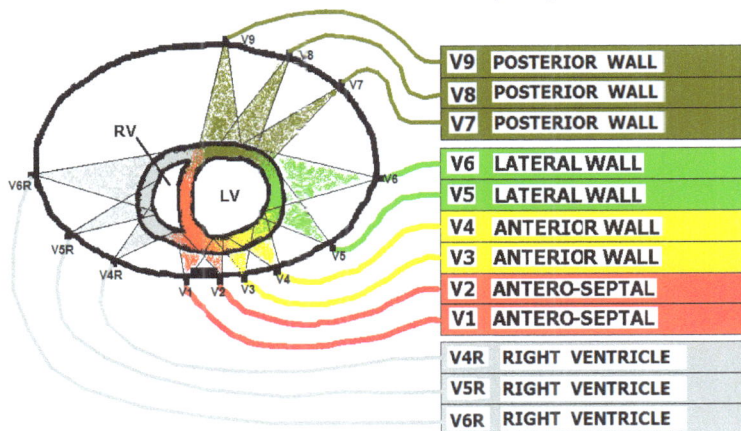

It would be an appropriate evolution of electrocardiography if the 18 lead ECG became the industry standard. Until then, there is a viable option that is immediately available to all medical practitioners who desire to see 18 leads: *first, obtain your 12 lead ECG, then reposition the six chest leads to view the posterior wall and the right ventricle.* That is, three leads on the patient's back, and three leads on the right side of the chest, as seen in the diagrams on the next page:

HOW TO REPOSITION 6 CHEST LEADS to OBTAIN 3 R VENTRICLE and 3 POSTERIOR LEADS

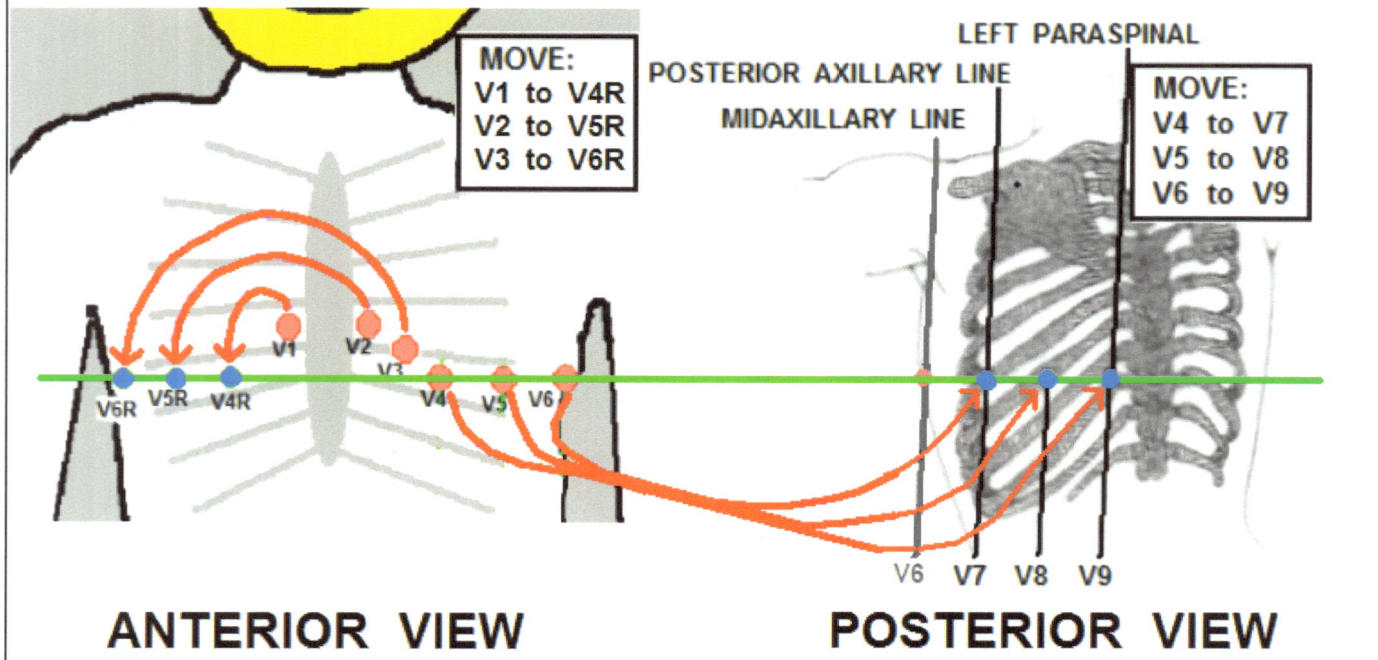

MOVE:
V1 to V4R
V2 to V5R
V3 to V6R

LEFT PARASPINAL
POSTERIOR AXILLARY LINE
MIDAXILLARY LINE

MOVE:
V4 to V7
V5 to V8
V6 to V9

V6R V5R V4R   V1 V2 V3   V4 V5 V6

V6 V7 V8 V9

ANTERIOR VIEW   **POSTERIOR VIEW**

The image above is presented with written permission and compliments from Jonni Cooper, PhD, RN, of the Marriott Heart Foundation, and author of the superb textbook, "ECG Essentials."

LEAD PLACEMENT V4R, V5R, V6R

V1 V2 V3 V4

V4R
V5R
V6R

PAL PARASPINAL LINE SPINE

1/2 BETWEEN V7 & V9

V6 V6 HORIZONTAL PLANE

V7 V8 V9

Special thanks to Antonio Mejia, RN, our "model" for the above 18 Lead ECG lead placement photos. Antonio is an extremely competent and pleasant co-worker in the Cath Lab, and is a talented cartoonist. One day I expect to see Antonio's cartoons in the comic section of the Sunday News each week. Thanks, Antonio!

The advantage of the 18 lead ECG is that it provides better sensitivity and specificity in diagnosing ischemia, acute MI, and necrosis. In terms of sensitivity, the standard 12 lead ECG of a patient suffering from an *acute right ventricular MI* could look normal, with no S-T segment elevation or depression. However an 18 lead ECG of the same patient would show S-T segment elevation in V4R – V6R.

The ECG shown below is that of Antonio Mejia, our "model" featured on the previous page. At the current time, Antonio is in his thirties, and is in excellent health.

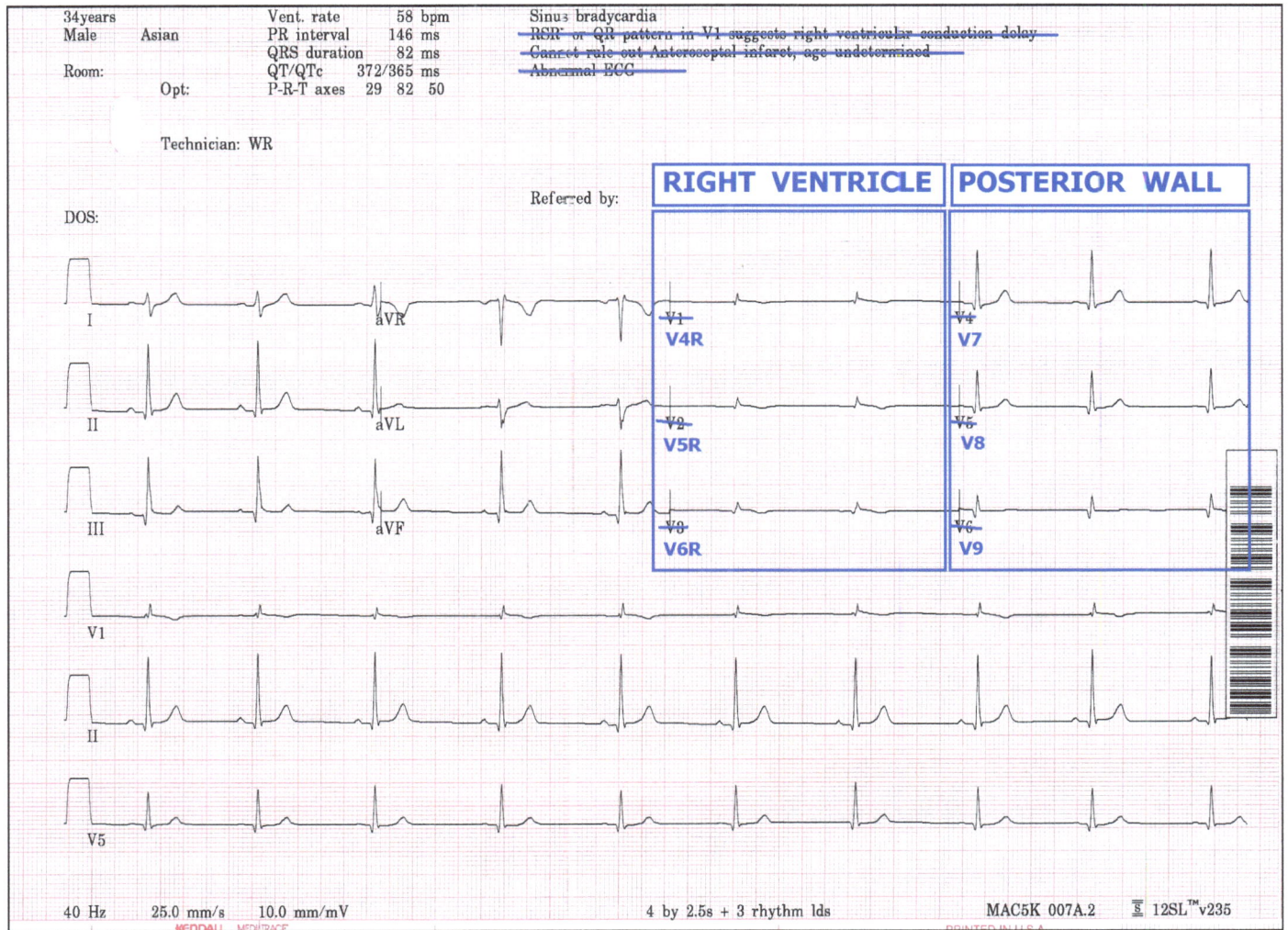

The 18 Lead ECG is obtained by relocating Leads V1 – V3 to the V4R – V6R positions, and V4 – V6 should be relocated to the V7 – V9 positions. Note the low amplitude QRS complexes in the right ventricular leads. I have observed the low amplitude QRS finding in healthy people, no doubt resulting from the smaller muscle mass of the right ventricle. Also of note are the qR patterns seen in V4R – V6R. The posterior leads, V7 – V9, are consistent in size and deflection to that of other left ventricular leads.

Also note we had to strike lines through the computer's diagnosis. When you reposition leads outside of their usual 12 lead positions, the computer doesn't know you've done this. Therefore any complexes that don't match what is "normal" for the standard 12 lead will be diagnosed as an abnormality. Also, you should correctly indicate which leads you have modified, as we have done in the above example.

One major benefit in using the 18 lead ECG is its improved specificity in diagnosing abnormalities. For example, the 12 lead ECG of a patient suffering from acute posterior wall MI will show S-T segment depression in leads V1 – V3. The problem with this finding is that the discovery of depressed S-T segments in V1 – V3 can indicate other possible diagnoses, such as *anterior wall ischemia*, and acute *anterior non-Q wave MI*. If you obtain an 18 lead ECG on a patient suffering from acute posterior wall MI, the patient's S-T segment elevation in leads V7, V8, and/or V9 provides a more specific diagnosis of posterior wall MI.

The tables below displays some important data from research conducted by [2]Wung, et. al from the University of Arizona:

WHY DO WE OBTAIN AN 18 LEAD ECG ?
☞ **STANDARD 12 LEAD DOES NOT "DIRECTLY VIEW" POSTERIOR WALL and RIGHT VENTRICLE.**
THE 18 LEAD ECG PROVIDES:
❑ **IMPROVED SPECIFICITY in diagnosis of acute POSTERIOR WALL MI**
❑ **IMPROVED SENSITIVITY in diagnosis of RIGHT VENTRICULAR MI**
❑ **IMPROVED SPECIFICITY in IDENTIFICATION of CULRIT ARTERY**

INTERPRETATION OF 18 LEAD ECG:
❑ S-T ↑ V3R - V5R = RV MI
❑ S-T ↑ V7 - V9 = POSTERIOR MI
❑ *S-T ↓ V3R - V5R +   S-T ↑ V7 - V9 = CIRCUMFLEX OCCLUSION
❑ *S-T ↑ V3R - V5R +   S-T ↓ V7 - V9 = RCA OCCLUSION

As you can see from the data provided by Dr. Wung's study, there is improved specificity in identification of the culprit artery during acute MI (RCA vs. Circumflex). This information could shave several minutes from a patient's door – to -- reperfusion time in the Cath Lab!

I have also found that using leads V4r, V5r, and V6r adequately displays ST elevation in cases of right ventricular MI.

Indications for obtaining an 18 lead ECG is anytime there is S-T elevation in leads II, III, and /or AVF, and/or any time there is ST depression in anterior leads V1 - V4. [3]

Use of the 18 lead ECG provides an 8% increase in sensitivity for acute MI over that of the standard 12 lead ECG.[4]

---

[2] S Wung et al, Journal of Electrocardiography, vol 39, Issue 3, 275-281
[3] AHA/ACC/HRS Scientific Statement: Recommendations for the Standardization and Interpretation of the Electrocardiogram, Circulation, 2007, vol 115 pp-1306 - 1324
[4] Amsterdam, E. et al, "AHA Scientific Statement for Testing of Low-Risk Patients Presenting to the Emergency Department With Chest Pain" - Circulation 2010;122:756-776:

ASSESSMENT of ECG WAVEFORMS and INTERVALS:

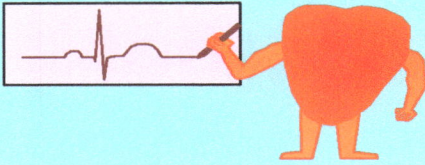

PUTTING IT ALL ON PAPER . . .

WAVEFORMS and INTERVALS . . .

☞ NOTE: All measurements in this book are in reference to ECGs recorded at the standard adult speed (25mm/sec), and standard amplitude (1mV = 10mm), unless specified otherwise.

THE P WAVE

- SHOULD BE AN UPRIGHT, CONVEX-SHAPED DOME IN ALL LEADS EXCEPT AVR and V1
- SHOULD BE LESS THAN .2 mv (2 mm) HIGH
- SHOULD BE LESS THAN 100 ms (2.5mm) LONG

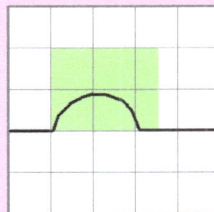

IN LEAD AVR: SHOULD BE INVERTED

IN LEAD V1, MAY BE:
- POSITIVE
- OR BI-PHASIC

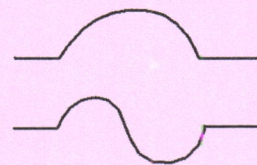

ATRIAL HYPERTROPHY.

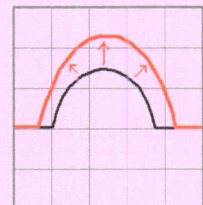

When P waves are taller than 2mm and/or longer than 2.5mm, there is ATRIAL HYPERTROPHY; one or both atria are enlarged.

USE LEAD II to begin your evaluation for ATRIAL HYPERTROPHY. P waves that are *too tall* (higher than 2mm) favor *right atrial hypertrophy*. P waves that are *too long* (longer than 2.5mm) favor *left atrial hypertrophy*.

When the P WAVE is

TOO LARGE

We think of

ATRIAL HYPERTROPHY

THE P WAVE

LEAD V1

- WHEN THE P WAVE IS BI-PHASIC IN V1, IT DISPLAYS BOTH R and L ATRIAL DEPOLARIZATION

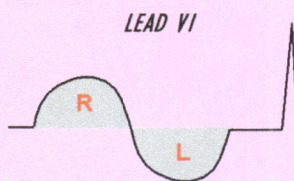

If you discover that P waves are too large in Lead II, then go to Lead V1 to determine which atrium is enlarged. The P wave in Lead V1 is often biphasic, as show in the image to the left.

The images at the top of the next page illustrate the P wave in Right Atrial Hypertrophy (top left image), and Left Atrial Hypertrophy (top right image).

RIGHT ATRIAL ENLARGEMENT

P-WAVE IN V1

In LEAD V1, the POSITIVE DEFLECTION of the P WAVE will be LARGER, or MORE DOMINANT.

LEFT ATRIAL ENLARGEMENT

P-WAVE IN V1

In LEAD V1, the NEGATIVE DEFLECTION of the P WAVE will be LARGER, or MORE DOMINANT.

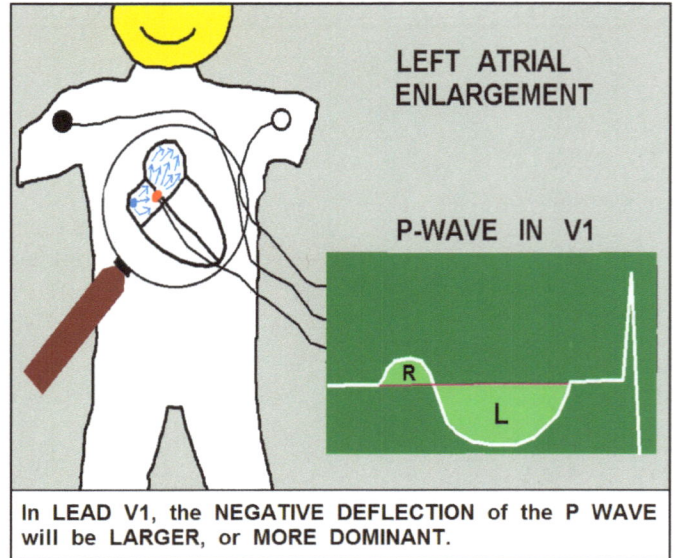

THE P-R SEGMENT:

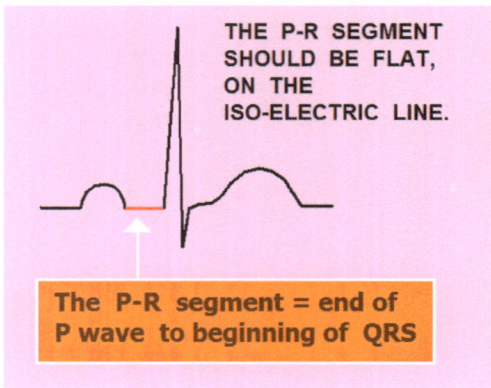

THE P-R SEGMENT SHOULD BE FLAT, ON THE ISO-ELECTRIC LINE.

The P-R segment = end of P wave to beginning of QRS

The *P-R segment* is usually depicted on the ECG as a *pause* between the P wave and the QRS complex. It is normally isoelectric.

When the P-R segment is elevated or depressed, consider *acute pericarditis* and *atrial infarction.*

.

In *acute pericarditis*, P-R segment depression is most pronounced in Lead II, and P-R segment elevation is most pronounced in lead AVR. *Atrial infarction* is sometimes seen in cases of acute inferior wall MI and acute lateral wall MI.

The DELTA WAVES of WOLFF-PARKINSON-WHITE SYNDROME (WPW)

are seen on the EGGs of patients with NON- CONCEALED forms of WPW, and result from the *premature depolarization of ventricular muscle* located beneath an ACCESSORY BYPASS TRACT.

Cause:

1. P-R INTERVAL TOO SHORT (< 120 ms.)
2. QRS DURATION TOO LONG (> 120 ms.)

☞ Think of ACCESSORY BYPASS TRACTS as *ABNORMAL GAPS* in the CONNECTIVE TISSUE FRAMEWORK that separates -- and *ELECTRICALLY INSULATES --* the ATRIA from the VENTRICLES. *SEE page 32, "The SKELETON of the HEART "* for *more information.*

THE P-R INTERVAL:

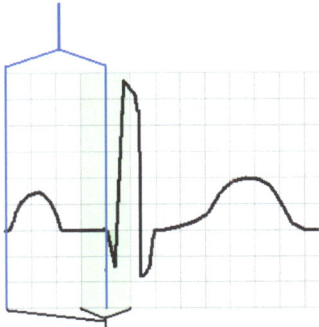

NORMAL DURATION
120 - 200 ms

The P-R interval is measured from the beginning of the P wave to the beginning of the QRS complex, as indicated by the blue lines in the diagram to the left.

The normal P-R interval should not be shorter than 120ms or longer than 200ms. (3-5mm on adult ECG – 25mm/sec).

The P-R Interval measurement should always be CONSISTENT from one beat to the next.

In cases where the P-R interval is too short, consider the following possible causes:

- ECTOPIC ATRIAL ACTIVITY - P wave axis may be abnormal (inverted in leads where normally upright)
- PRE-EXCITIATION (W-P-W) - look for *delta waves* and *wide QRS complexes.*
- JUNCTIONAL BEATS - P waves inverted in most leads, heart rate may be in junctional range (40-60). In rhythms originating in the Bundle of His region, P waves may be inverted and found after the QRS, in the S-T segment.

P - R INTERVAL TOO SHORT . . .
LESS THAN 120 mSEC

THINK:

- ECTOPIC ATRIAL ACTIVITY
- PRE-EXCITATION (WPW)
- JUNCTIONAL BEATS / RHYTHM
  (P WAVES NEARLY ON TOP OF QRS,
  POSSIBLY INVERTED)

P - R INTERVAL TOO LONG
GREATER THAN 200 mSEC

THINK:

- HEART BLOCK

When the P-R interval is too long (greater than 200ms) think of Heart Block. If the only abnormality is a prolonged P-R Interval, you're looking at first degree heart block. If there is more than one P wave for each QRS, and/or the P-R interval varies with each QRS, then you're looking at a 2nd or 3rd degree heart block.

When the P-R interval varies from one beat to the next, the underlying rhythm is most likely 2nd degree type I heart block (Wenckebach), or 3rd degree (complete) heart block.

CLUE: When P-R intervals vary, but the R-R interval is regular, with no "skipped beats," think *3rd degree heart block.* When the RR interval is irregular, (such as when QRS complexes have been dropped), think *Wenckebach.*

P - R INTERVAL INCONSISTENT
(VARIES FROM BEAT TO BEAT)

THINK:

- 2° TYPE 1 HEART BLOCK
  (WENCKEBACH)

- 3° HEART BLOCK
  (COMPLETE HEART BLOCK)

THE QRS COMPLEX:

Normal QRS complexes may be negative, positive, or biphasic, depending on which lead you're looking at. First, we'll break down the QRS complex, like the one seen to the right: a *Q wave* is present when the first deflection of the QRS is negative. An *R wave* is the first positive waveform, whether or not a Q wave is present. An *S wave* is any negative deflection following an R wave.

THE QRS COMPLEX

- MAY CONSIST OF ONE OR SEVERAL DEFLECTIONS, as indicated below:

If the first deflection is NEGATIVE, it is known as the " Q WAVE. "

The first POSITIVE deflection is known as the " R WAVE. "

If there is a NEGATIVE deflection after the R WAVE, it is known as the " S WAVE. "

- HERE ARE SOME COMMON VARIATIONS OF QRS COMPLEXES:

qR   RS   R   Rsr'   Qr

QS   qRSr'   qR   rS   Rr'

To the left are several variations of QRS complexes, along with their technically correct designators. We refer to all of them as "QRS" complexes, but technically speaking, the only "true QRS" is the one in the illustration above: it has a Q, an R, and an S wave.

Next, we'll look at some basic rules concerning QRS complexes.

QRS WIDTH (Duration):

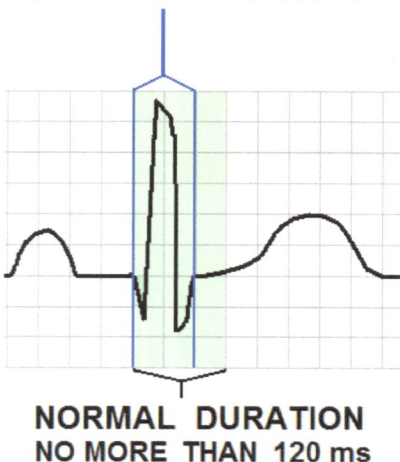

The QRS complex should not be wider than 120ms, (3mm on ECGs recorded at the standard adult speed of 25mm/sec).

NORMAL DURATION
NO MORE THAN 120 ms

QRS COMPLEX TOO WIDE
(WIDER THAN 120 ms)

THINK:

- BUNDLE BRANCH BLOCK
- VENTRICULAR COMPEX (ES)
- PACED RHYTHM
- L VENTRICULAR HYPERTROPHY
- ELECTROLYTE IMBAL. (↑K+ ↓Ca++)
- DELTA WAVE (PRE-EXCITATION)

When the QRS is wider than normal, it can indicate several possible disorders, as shown in the image to the right:

QRS HEIGHT (Amplitude):

QRS AMPLITUDE

is influenced by:

- age
- physical fitness
- body size
- conduction system disorders
- chamber hypertrophy

The vertical size of QRS complexes are a reflection of current, or *amplitude*. Many variables effect QRS height, and are listed in the table to the right. Conditions that effect generation and conduction of current within the heart, and the amount of impedance between the heart and ECG electrodes all have an effect on vertical QRS size.

Use the patient's *overall QRS amplitude* as a guideline for when to consider obtaining additional diagnostic testing for hypertrophy (such as an *echocardiogram* and/or *right sided cardiac catheterization*). To calculate the *Overall QRS Amplitude,* add the height of the tallest R wave to the depth of the deepest S wave (in millimeters). If the total exceeds 30mm, we consider the possibility of *Ventricular Hypertrophy.*

TOTAL QRS AMPLITUDE

is measured by finding the TALLEST POSITIVE DEFLECTION (R WAVE) and the DEEPEST NEGATIVE DEFLECTION (S WAVE) on the 12 LEAD EKG and ADDING THE VALUES TOGETHER

QRS AMPLITUDE

MAXIMUM NORMAL VALUES are difficult to define due to differences in PATIENT AGE, BODY SIZE, and FITNESS.

HOWEVER A GENERAL VALUE GUIDELINE IS: 3.0 mV (30 mm on normally calibrated EKG)

This guideline, like many other ECG diagnoses, *lacks desirable sensitivity and specificity*—for example, in the early stages of *Right Ventricular Hypertrophy* (RVH), the only ECG changes may be changes in axis, as seen in limb lead I and lead V1, and reversal of R wave progression in the precordial leads, *with the patient's total QRS amplitude remaining less than 30mm.*

☞ If any doubt exists as to whether there is ventricular hypertrophy, additional diagnostic testing, such as obtaining an echocardiogram, should be considered.

The ECG below illustrates how to determine the OVERALL QRS AMPLITUDE:

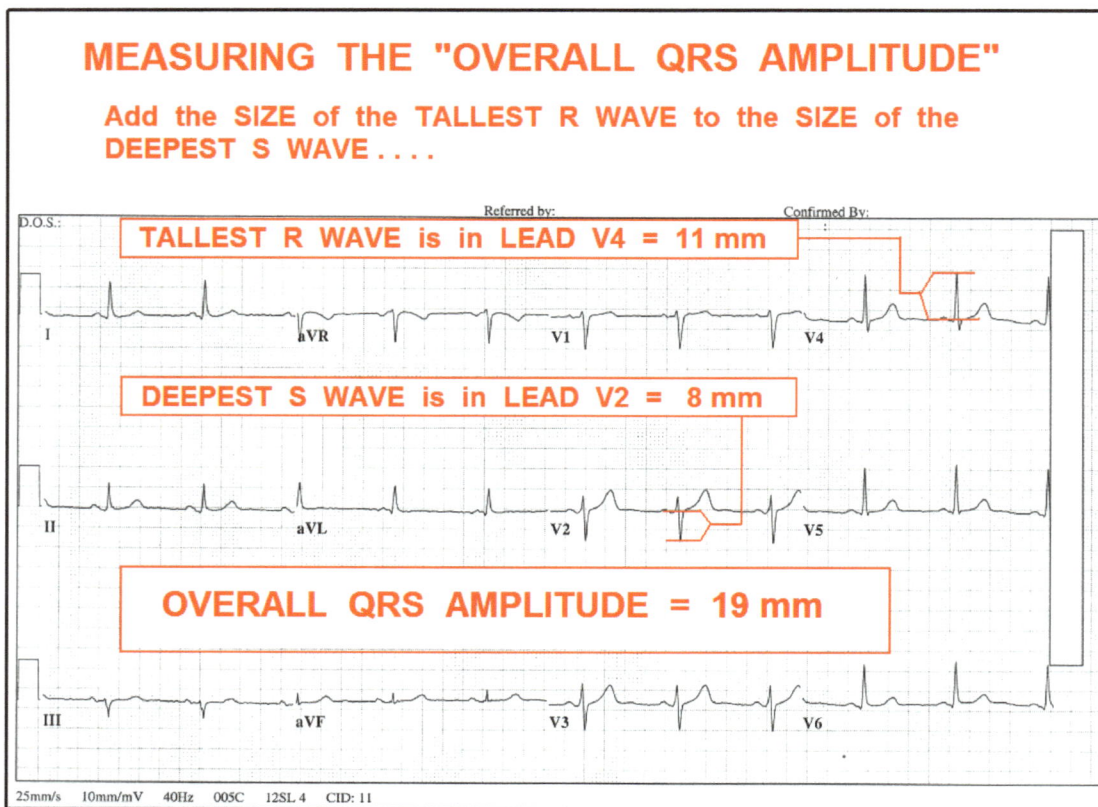

MEASURING THE "OVERALL QRS AMPLITUDE"

Add the SIZE of the TALLEST R WAVE to the SIZE of the DEEPEST S WAVE . . . .

TALLEST R WAVE is in LEAD V4 = 11 mm

DEEPEST S WAVE is in LEAD V2 = 8 mm

OVERALL QRS AMPLITUDE = 19 mm

25mm/s   10mm/mV   40Hz   005C   12SL 4   CID: 11

My favorite technique for determining if hypertrophy exists is to simply look at the ECG, and note if any of the QRS complexes from one lead are "spearing through" the QRS complexes of another lead, as shown in the example below:

ST. JOSEPH'S HOSPITAL–ER   ROUTINE RETRIEVAL

17 yr
Male   Black

Room:ER
Loc:3   Option:16

Vent. rate   90 BPM
PR interval   136 ms
QRS duration   94 ms
QT/QTc   378/462 ms
P–R–T axes   77 123   58

Normal sinus rhythm
Right atrial enlargement
Right axis deviation
Incomplete right bundle branch block , plus right ventricular hypertrophy
NORMAL SINUS INFERIOR LATERAL CHANGES
Abnormal ECG

QRS COMPLEXES "SPEARING THROUGH" QRS COMPLEXS OF ANOTHER LEAD

QRS COMPLEXES GOING "OFF THE PAGE"

25mm/s   10mm/mV   40Hz   005C   12SL 4   CID: 11   EID:11 EDT:

Although diagnosis of Left Ventricular Hypertrophy (LVH) and Right Ventricular Hypertrophy (RVH) are not achieved solely by interpretation of the 12 Lead ECG, it is good for clinicians to be able to recognize indicators from the ECG that hypertrophy may exist, and then order additional diagnostic testing in order to confirm or rule it out. The table to the right lists indicators used to identify ventricular hypertrophy on the 12 lead ECG.

The Axis of Leads I and V1 are shown in the table to the left. It works like this: In the normal heart, the QRS complex of Lead I is *positive,* and in Lead V1, the QRS in mainly *negative*. When the right ventricle becomes hypertrophic and begins to acquire more than its normal amount of mass, the Lead I – V1 Axis begins to shift: that is, the QRS in Lead I becomes *negative,* and the QRS in V1 becomes *positive.*

Another clue to discovering ventricular hypertrophy is noting if there is atrial hypertrophy in the corresponding ventricle. For example, patients with Left Ventricular Hypertrophy (LVH) often have Left Atrial Hypertrophy, and patients with RVH – you guessed it – often have Right Atrial Hypertrophy.

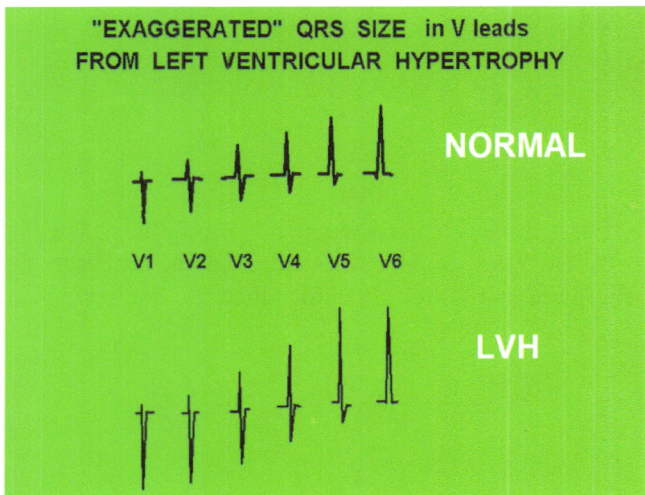

"EXAGGERATED" QRS SIZE in V leads FROM LEFT VENTRICULAR HYPERTROPHY

NORMAL

V1 V2 V3 V4 V5 V6

LVH

Another clue is abnormal R wave progression. In the case of LVH, you may see an "exaggeration" of normal R wave progression. In this case, the deflections of QRS complexes are normal, but there is "extreme amplitude," as demonstrated in the diagram to the left.

In the case of RVH, the right ventricle becomes larger. In cases where there is SYSTOLIC OVERLOAD, the right ventricle acquires more mass. As the right ventricle gains more mass in relationship to the mass of the left ventricle, it begins to "upset" the normal R wave progression. As you can see in the image to the right, when the RV becomes more massive, it can "tip the balance" of R wave progression in the opposite direction. When this occurs, the RV has acquired more mass than the LV.

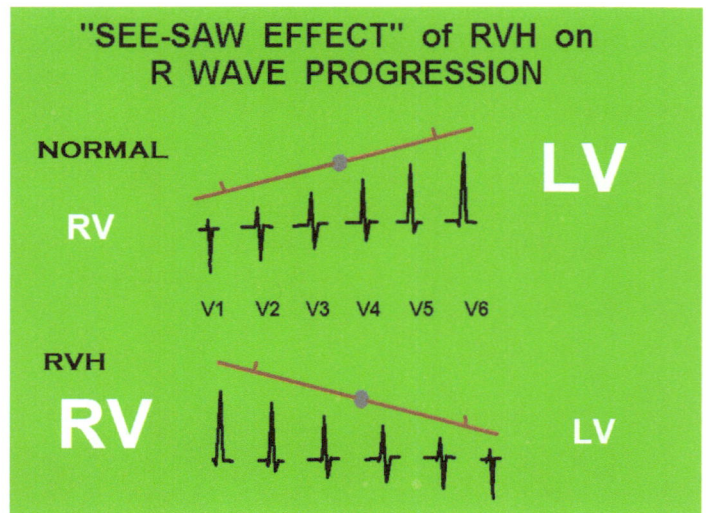

"SEE-SAW EFFECT" of RVH on R WAVE PROGRESSION

CHAMBER ENLARGEMENT

VENTRICULAR STRAIN PATTERNS

☞ T WAVES ARE INVERTED AND ASYMMETRICAL

☞ THERE MAY BE ST SEGMENT DEPRESSION

J POINT

Another indicator seen in cases of systolic overload is the "strain pattern." The T waves become inverted and asymmetrical, as seen to the left. There can also be ST segment depression at the J point.

When there is RVH, a strain pattern may be seen in leads V1 and/or V2. In cases of LVH, the strain pattern will appear in leads V5 and/or V6.

CHAMBER ENLARGEMENT

VENTRICULAR STRAIN PATTERNS

RVH		LVH	
V1	V2	V5	V6

CHAMBER ENLARGEMENT

*MATHEMATICAL FORMULAS FOR DETERMINING LVH and RVH

LVH
- R-WAVE V1 + S-WAVE LEAD III > 25mm
- R-WAVE V5 or V6 > 26mm
- S-WAVE V1 + R-WAVE V5 or V6 > 35mm
- LARGEST R-WAVE + LARGEST S-WAVE in V-LEADS > 45mm

RVH
- R-WAVE V1 + S-WAVE V5 or V6 > 10.5mm
- rSR' in V1 where R' ≥ 10mm

* THIS IS A PARTIAL LIST.

Last but not least are mathematical formulas. We list several of the more popular mathematical formulas to the left. There are many more formulas than the one's we have listed.

WHEN QRS COMPLEXES ARE "TOO SMALL:"

Just as QRS complexes being *too tall* is suggestive of abnormal conditions, so are QRS complexes that are *too small*. The table to the right provides guidelines for determining if the QRS complex is too small.

When QRS complexes are abnormally small, it usually means there is an abnormally high amount of impedance—something is dampening the amount of electrical current reaching the ECG electrodes on the skin surface. It could be excessive body mass, or any of the factors listed in the table below:

QRS AMPLITUDE

CRITERIA FOR MINIMUM AMPLITUDE:

Abnormally LOW QRS VOLTAGE occurs when the OVERALL QRS is:

≤ 0.5 mV (5 mm) IN ANY LIMB LEAD

— *and* —

≤ 1.0 mV (10 mm) IN ANY PRECORDIAL LEAD

OVERALL QRS AMPLITUDE TOO LOW:
(VERTICAL QRS SIZE)

THINK (in absence of obvious OBESITY):

MYOCARDITIS / CONSTRICTIVE PERICARDITIS

EFFUSIONS / TAMPONADE

COPD c̄ HYPERINFLATION

AMYLOIDOSIS (abnormal protein accumulation in organs)

SCLERODERMA (abnormal hardening of skin)

HEMACHROMOTOSIS (excessive iron buildup in blood / organs)

MYXEDEMA (thyroid disorder)

☠ When LOW QRS AMPLITIUDE is noted in patients who exhibit SIGNS OF SHOCK (with or without chest pain) rule out *MYOCARDIITS, CONSTRICTIVE PERICARDITIS, PERICARDIAL EFFUSIONS,* and *PERICARDIAL TAMPONADE.*

☞ COPD is a common cause of low amplitude ECGs. It makes sense if you think about it—air is a poor conductor of electricity—and patients with advanced COPD have *blebs* throughout their lungs, which essentially are large "pockets of air" caused by the breakdown of alveoli.

EVALUATION OF Q WAVES

Small Q waves are frequently seen in many leads, and are considered normal; they're caused by *depolarization of the intraventricular septum.* Q waves that are *too big* are considered *abnormal.* When the entire QRS complex is negative (QS complex), it is considered an abnormal Q wave.

When Q waves exceed the guidelines presented in the table to the right, they are considered *abnormal.* Abnormal Q waves commonly indicate necrosis (old MI) in whatever region of the heart the ECG is viewing. Positive Q waves are also seen in severe cardiomyopathy, myocarditis, hypertrophy, Wolff-Parkinson-White syndrome, left bundle branch block, paced rhythms, and ventricular complexes/rhythms.

Take a closer look at the Q wave guidelines below and on the next page. I suggest committing these guidelines to memory, as your ability to discern between *normal* Q waves and *abnormal* Q waves is an important factor in determining the need for additional testing and making clinical decisions.

Q WAVE RULES - SUMMARY:

- Q WAVES SHOULD BE LESS THAN .40 WIDE (1 mm)

- Q WAVES SHOULD BE LESS THAN 1/3 THE HEIGHT OF THE R WAVE

- Q WAVES CAN BE ANY SIZE IN LEADS III and AVR

- THERE SHOULD BE NO Q WAVES IN LEADS V1, V2, or V3

GENERAL RULES FOR NORMAL Q WAVES - WIDTH

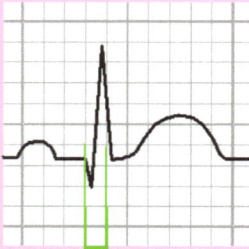

LESS THAN .40 (1 mm) WIDE

GENERAL RULES FOR NORMAL Q WAVES - HEIGHT

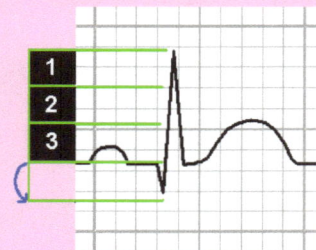

☞ LESS THAN 1/3 THE HEIGHT OF THE R WAVE

NORMAL Q WAVES EXCEPTIONS TO THE RULES

☞ THERE SHOULD BE NO Q WAVES PRESENT IN LEADS: V1 V2 V3

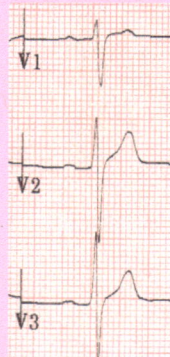

NORMAL Q WAVES EXCEPTIONS TO THE RULES

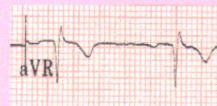

LEAD AVR

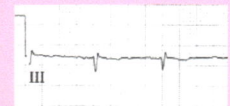

LEAD III

☞ THE Q WAVE CAN BE ANY SIZE

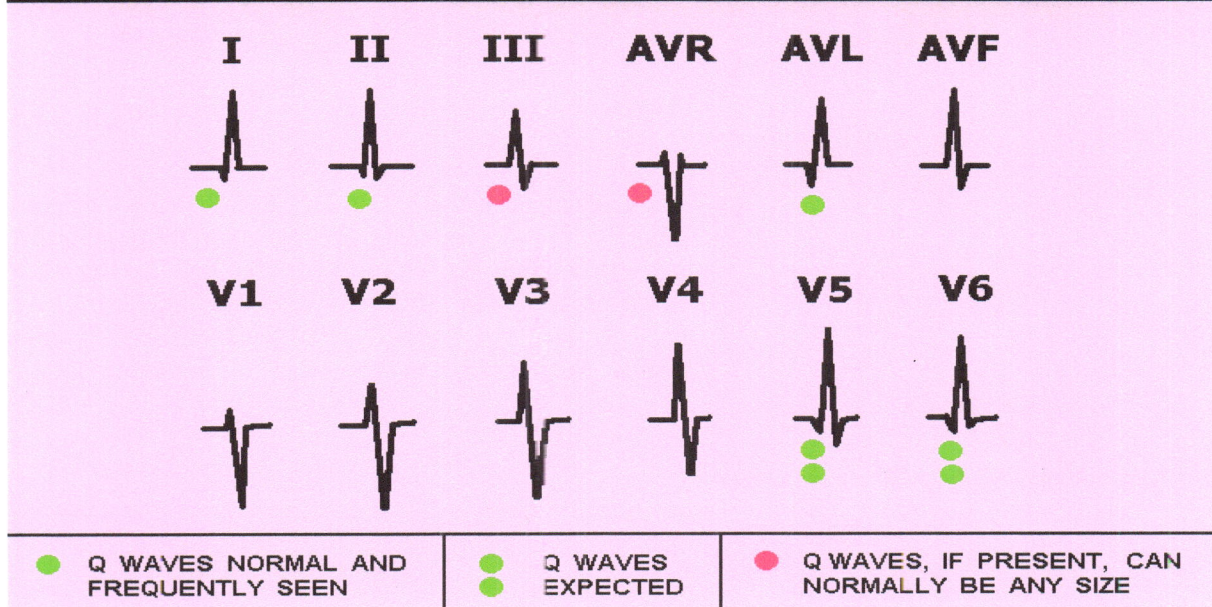

LEADS WHERE Q WAVES ARE NORMAL
- Normal Q WAVES caused by SEPTAL DEPOLARIZATION

| I | II | III | AVR | AVL | AVF |

| V1 | V2 | V3 | V4 | V5 | V6 |

● Q WAVES NORMAL AND FREQUENTLY SEEN

● ● Q WAVES EXPECTED

● Q WAVES, IF PRESENT, CAN NORMALLY BE ANY SIZE

EVALUATION OF THE S-T SEGMENT:

Careful scrutiny of the *J point* (where the QRS and S-T segment intersect), *S-T segment* and *T wave* in every lead of the 12 lead ECG is an essential component of a thorough cardiovascular evaluation. Myocardial ischemia, acute infarction, pericarditis/ myocarditis, hyperkalemia, acute pulmonary embolism, and Brugada syndrome (non-concealed version) – all potentially life-threatening disorders – usually manifest themselves with S-T segment and/or T wave abnormalities on the ECG.

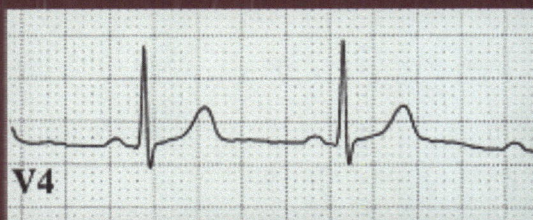

NORMAL J POINT, S-T SEGMENT, and T WAVE CONFIGURATION

V4

● J POINT ISOELECTRIC (within 1mm deviation)
● SLIGHT POSITIVE INCLINATION OF S-T SEGMENT
● UPRIGHT, POSITIVE T WAVE

QRS width is the first issue to consider when evaluating S-T segments and T waves. In cases where QRS width is normal (<120 ms), the criteria used to evaluate S-T segments and T waves is accurate. When QRS complexes are abnormally wide (>120 ms), S-T segments and T waves are distorted, obscuring our assessment capabilities.

The sample ECG strip of lead V4 (above right) is an example of a "textbook normal ECG." Note that the J point is "isoelectric" (or within 1mm of the isoelectric line), the S-T segment has a slight positive inclination, and the T wave is positive, with a "soft, rounded tip."

THE ISOELECTRIC LINE

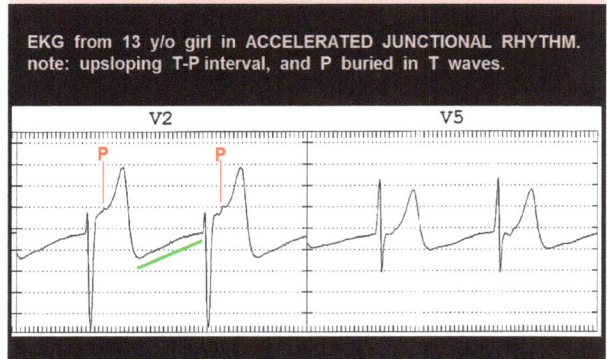

IS MEASURED BETWEEN T and P WAVE, or U and P WAVE

We typically use the ISOELECTRIC LINE to determine if J points and S-T segments are elevated or depressed. The isoelectric line is the "baseline" or "flat line" between heartbeats. It begins at the end of the T wave (or U wave, if U waves are present) and ends when the P wave of the next cardiac cycle begins. We also refer to this as the "T-P Interval."

The problem with the isoelectric line is that it is often not consistently level, as seen in the example to the right.

THE ISOELECTRIC LINE

EKG from 13 y/o girl in ACCELERATED JUNCTIONAL RHYTHM. note: upsloping T-P interval, and P buried in T waves.

THE P-Q JUNCTION

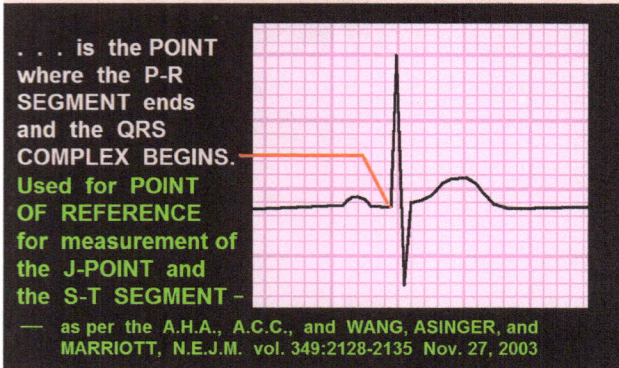

. . . is the POINT where the P-R SEGMENT ends and the QRS COMPLEX BEGINS. Used for POINT OF REFERENCE for measurement of the J-POINT and the S-T SEGMENT –

— as per the A.H.A., A.C.C., and WANG, ASINGER, and MARRIOTT, N.E.J.M. vol. 349:2128-2135 Nov. 27, 2003

According to Wang et al (New England Journal of Medicine, vol 349: p2198-2135, Nov 27, 2003), the P-Q junction is to be used as the point of reference for measurement of J points, S-T segment depression and elevation.

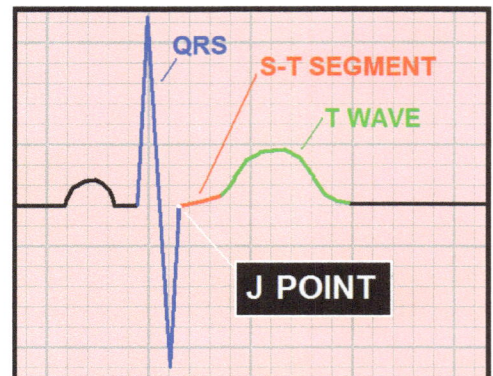

THE J POINT SHOULD BE..

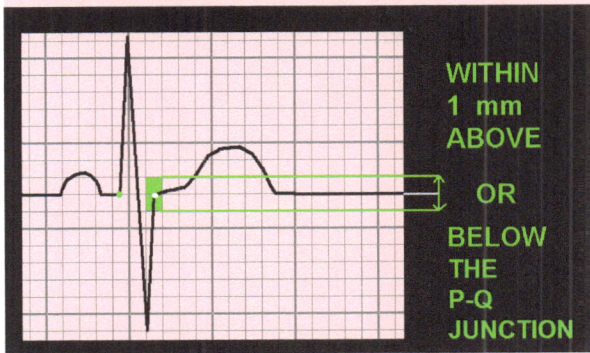

WITHIN 1 mm ABOVE

OR

BELOW THE P-Q JUNCTION

Preferably the J point will be in horizontal alignment with the PQ junction. The commonly accepted normal range is: *the J point should be within one millimeter above or below the level of the P-Q junction.*

The S-T segment should have a slight positive inclination, as seen in the diagram to the right.

THE S-T SEGMENT

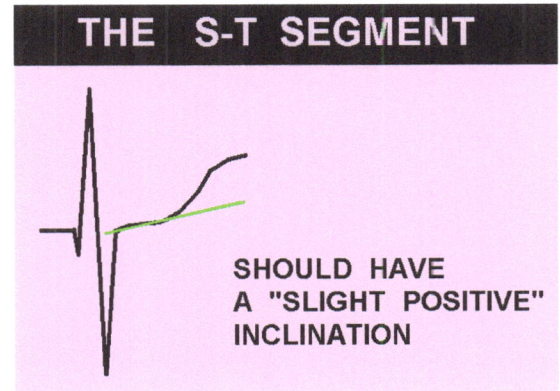

SHOULD HAVE A "SLIGHT POSITIVE" INCLINATION

THE S-T SEGMENT

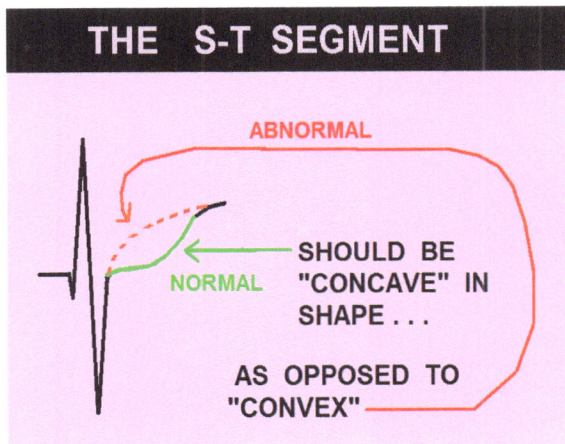

ABNORMAL

SHOULD BE "CONCAVE" IN SHAPE . . .

NORMAL

AS OPPOSED TO "CONVEX"

The S-T segment should be "concave" in shape where it merges with the T wave, as seen in green in the diagram to the left. CONVEX SHAPED S-T SEGMENTS (the dotted red line) CAN BE INDICATIVE OF ACUTE MI, even WITHOUT classic S-T segment elevation.

EVALUATION OF THE T WAVE:

THE T WAVE should have a rounded shape—it should not be pointed. The T wave should be symmetrical—if you draw a vertical line down the center of the T wave, the two halves should look like mirror images of each other.

THE T WAVE

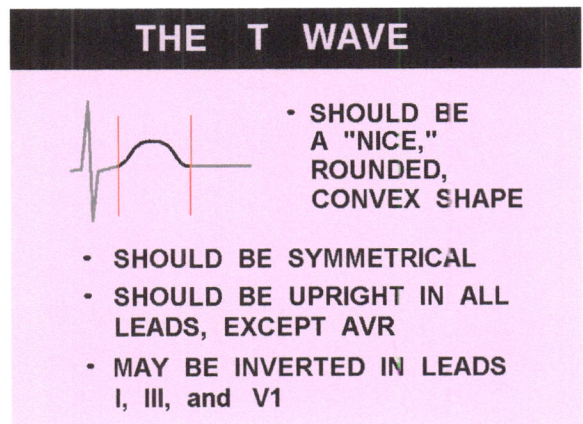

- SHOULD BE A "NICE," ROUNDED, CONVEX SHAPE

- SHOULD BE SYMMETRICAL
- SHOULD BE UPRIGHT IN ALL LEADS, EXCEPT AVR
- MAY BE INVERTED IN LEADS I, III, and V1

59

Leads where the T WAVE may be INVERTED:

Referred by: _____   Unconfirmed

DOS:

I   NORMAL T WAVE INVERTED   T WAVE NORMAL UPRIGHT

aVR   V1   V4

MAY BE INVERTED

T WAVE NORMAL UPRIGHT

II   aVL   V2   V5

T WAVE NORMAL UPRIGHT   MAY BE INVERTED

III   aVF   V3   V6

MAY BE INVERTED

T WAVE AMPLITUDE:

Since many variables can affect T wave amplitude, there is no concrete rule about its vertical size.   I use the guidelines listed to the right as an "alert limit." In the limb leads, the T wave should be equal to or less than 1.0mv (10 mm). The T wve should be equal to or less than 0.5mv (5 mm) in the precordial leads. The T wave should not be taller than the R wave in 2 or more leads.

When I see T waves that exceed these guidelines, I become suspicious that a problem may exist, and begin the process of ruling out potentially lethal conditions, such as hyperkalemia, acute MI, transmural ischemia, and hypertrophy.

THE   T   WAVE

AMPLITUDE GUIDELINES:

- IN THE LIMB LEADS, SHOULD BE LESS THAN 1.0 mv (10 mm)
- IN THE PRECORDIAL LEADS, SHOULD BE LESS THAN 0.5 mv (5 mm)
- SHOULD NOT BE TALLER THAN R WAVE IN 2 OR MORE LEADS.

SPECIFIC S-T SEGMENT and/or T WAVES ABNORMALITIES:

Once abnormal S-T segments and/or T waves have been identified, the next priority is to rule out the potentially life-threatening disorders that can cause such ECG changes.

When abnormal ST segment and/or T wave changes occur during the presence of symptoms suspicious for ACS, STEMI / NSTEMI and Unstable Angina must be aggressively ruled out.

On pages 61 – 65, you will find lists of conditions that are known to cause S-T segment abnormalities. Conditions which are potentially life-threatening are listed in RED, potentially "serious" conditions are listed in YELLOW, and usually benign conditions are listed in BLACK.

S-T SEGMENT ELEVATION - COMMON ETIOLOGIES:

J POINT < 1mm ABOVE P-Q JUNCTION

CONDITION:

- **ACUTE INFARCTION**
- **HYPERKALEMIA**
- **BRUGADA SYNDROME**
- **PULMONARY EMBOLUS**
- **INTRACRANIAL BLEED**
- **MYOCARDITIS / PERICARDITIS**
- **L. VENT. HYPERTROPHY**
- **PRINZMETAL'S ANGINA**
- **L. BUNDLE BRANCH BLOCK**
- **PACED RHYTHM**
- **EARLY REPOLARIZATION & "MALE PATTERN" S-T ELEV.**

ST SEGMENT ELEVATION:

The table above lists eleven conditions known to cause elevation of the ST segment at the J point.

By traditional guidelines, to "qualify" as an ST Segment Elevation MI (STEMI), there must be at least 1mm of ST segment elevation in two or more contiguous leads.   Some published guidelines state there can be up to 2mm of normal ST elevation in the anterior precordial leads.

On the next page, we provide a more detailed look at eight causes of ST elevation: normal "male pattern" ST elevation, Left Bundle Branch Block, Early Repolarization, Left Ventricular Hypertrophy, Acute Pericarditis, Hyperkalemia, Brugada Syndrome, and Acute Anterior Wall MI.

It should be apparent when one studies the ECG patterns displayed on the next page in the "ST Segment Differential Diagnosis" diagram, that in some instances, it could be difficult – if not impossible – to make a specific diagnosis without knowing more about the patient's presenting symptoms, medical history, risk factor profile, and lab values. This is why one major focus of this textbook is to teach clinicians to view the ECG as only "one piece of the diagnostic puzzle," and to be able to "step back and view the totality of the clinical picture" when attempting to make a diagnosis.

This book presents specific, detailed information about diagnosing Left Bundle Branch Block, Left Ventricular Hypertrophy, ST segment elevation MI (STEMI), and Brugada Syndrome. Future textbooks and conference series will provide more information on the other causes of ST elevation.

ST SEGMENT ELEVATION
DIFFERENTIAL DIAGNOSIS

CASE INFORMATION:	I	III	V1	V2	V3	V5	REFERENCE NOTES:
NORMAL "MALE PATTERN" ST ELEVATION - 38 y/o MALE, no CAD							In a study of 529 men ages 16-24, 93% had ST ELEVATION of >1mm in LEADS V1 - V4. 20% of women had the same finding. - J SURAWICZ, el al, J AM COLL CARDIOL 2002;40:1870-76
LEFT BUNDLE BRANCH BLOCK, 46 y/o FEMALE no CAD							A common finding in patients with QRS > 120 ms with LBBB pattern is ST ELEVATION > 1mm. This includes most PACED RHYTHMS (RV Lead)
EARLY REPOLARIZATION 36 y/o MALE no CAD							In many healthy young men (mostly black men) this ST pattern is often noted. - KAMBARA, et al, J AM COLL CARDIOL 1976;38:157-61
LEFT VENTRICULAR HYPERTROPHY 61 y/o FEMALE no CAD							In LVH, the deeper the S WAVE, the GREATER the ST ELEVATION. May present with QS in precordial leads. ST segments CONCAVE - WANG, et al, N ENGL J MED 2003;349:1128-35
PERICARDITIS 41 y/o MALE no CAD							ST ELEVATION diffusely elevated in throughout 12 lead EKG. Often PR segment ↑ aVR and ↓ Lead II. - WANG, et al, N ENGL J MED 2003;349:1128-35
MYOCARDITIS 30 y/o FEMALE no CAD							ST ELEVATION in ACUTE MYOCARDITIS can mimick that of ACUTE MI. - SPODICK et al, CIRCULATION 1995;91:1886-87
HYPERKALEMIA (K+ 8.6) 53 y/o MALE no CAD							HYPERKALEMIA can mimic EKG findings of AMI. Other findings include TALL, PEAKED T WAVES - LEVINE, et al, CIRCULATION 1956;13:29-36
BRUGADA SYNDROME 36 y/o FEMALE no CAD							Genetic disorder responsible for 40-60% of all idiopathic V-FIB. Recognizable V1-V3 pattern. - BRUGADA & BRUGADA et al, J AM COLL CARDIOL 1992;20:1391-96
ACUTE ANTERIOR WALL MI 52 y/o MALE - MID LAD OCCLUSION							ACUTE ST SEGMENT ELEVATION MI (STEMI) characterized by: - ST ELEVATION of >1mm in 2 or more contiguous leads. - ST segments usually CONVEX

S-T SEGMENT DEPRESSION - COMMON ETIOLOGIES:

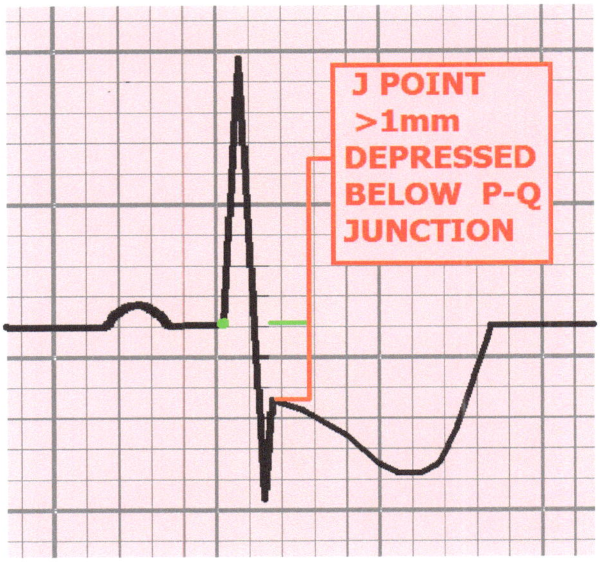

J POINT >1mm DEPRESSED BELOW P-Q JUNCTION

CONDITION:

- **RECIPROCAL CHANGES of ACUTE MI**
- **NON-Q WAVE M.I. (NON-STEMI)**
- **ISCHEMIA**
- **POSITIVE STRESS TEST**
- **VENTRICULAR HYPERTROPHY (STRAIN PATTERN)**
- **WOLFF-PARKINSON-WHITE**
- **OLD MI (NECROSIS vs. ISCHEMIA)**
- **DIGITALIS**
- **R. BUNDLE BRANCH BLOCK**

ST SEGMENT DEPRESSION is caused by numerous conditions, as you can see in the diagram above.

- *Reciprocal ST depression* in acute ST segment elevation MI (STEMI) may or may not be present on an ECG. In cases of STEMI, the presence or absence of reciprocal depression is used to help identify how extensive the MI is (e.g.: *inferior* vs. *inferior-posterior* MI), and to pinpoint the location of the obstruction in the "culprit" artery.
- In cases of *Non-STEMI,* ST elevation is not present on the 12 lead ECG. ST depression is usually – but not always – present. Diagnosis is usually made by the presence of suspicious cardiac-like symptoms, and positive cardiac markers. Typically, there is ST depression in the leads viewing the area of infarct. This type of MI was previously referred to as a "sub-endocardial" or "partial-thickness" MI, due to the infarct not involving the full thickness of myocardial muscle. In cases of isolated posterior wall MI, ST depression will be noted in the anterior leads (V1-V4). In this instance, if posterior leads were placed on the patient's back (leads V7 – V9), we would see ST elevation. But since we typically do not put leads on the patient's back, the standard 12 lead ECG does not directly view the posterior wall.
- ST depression may indicate *ischemia* in the lead being viewed. "ST depression equal to or greater than 0.5 mV (1/2 mm on standard ECG) in the absence of left ventricular hypertrophy is associated with a marked risk for MI, as well as ischemic complications."[5]
- In the "*positive stress test*," we look for ST segments to "drop" in leads which view the ischemic region of the myocardium.
- When *Ventricular Hypertrophy* is caused by the ventricle "straining extra hard" to expel blood, such as through a stenotic valve, a strain pattern (inverted, asymmetrical T wave with J point depression) is often seen.
- In non-concealed forms of *Wolff-Parkinson-White*, which is characterized by the typical short P-R interval, Delta wave and wide QRS complex, we usually see ST depression in several leads. This abnormal ST depression resolves immediately upon successful ablation of the bypass tract.
- In some cases of *old MI,* the signs of ischemia – ST depression, possibly with inverted T waves – never resolves. Why it resolves in some patients and not others is not currently understood.
- Patients on *Digitalis* often have ST depression without ischemia or other identifiable causes.
- *Right Bundle Branch Block* usually always causes ST depression and inverted T waves in the anterior leads. RBBB can mask the markers of anterior wall ischemia, unless there are old "non-ischemic" ECGs available for comparison.

---

[5] Amsterdam, E. et al, Circulation 2010;122:756-776

T WAVE INVERSION - COMMON ETIOLOGIES:

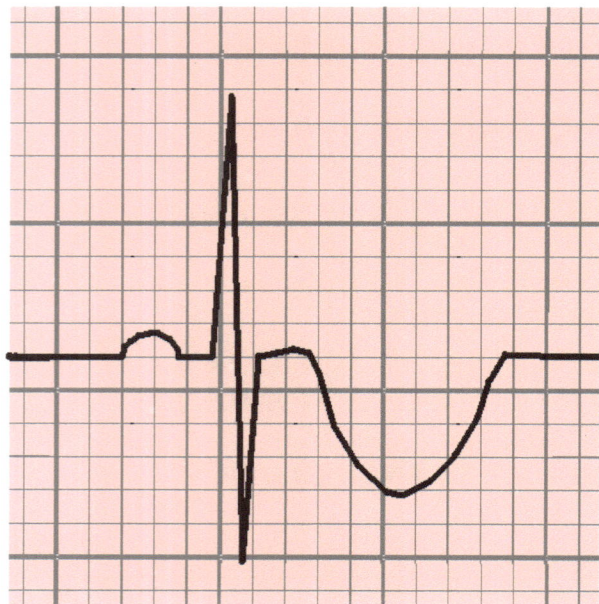

CONDITION:

- **MYOCARDITIS**
- **ELECTROLYTE IMBALANCE**
- **ISCHEMIA**
- **POSITIVE STRESS TEST**
- **CEREBRAL DISORDER**
- **MITRAL VALVE PROLAPSE**
- **VENTRICULAR HYPERTROPHY**
- **WOLFF-PARKINSON-WHITE**
- **HYPERVENTILATION**
- **CARDIOACTIVE DRUGS**
- **OLD MI (NECROSIS vs. ISCHEMIA)**
- **DIGITALIS**
- **R. BUNDLE BRANCH BLOCK**
- **NO OBVIOUS CAUSE**

T WAVE INVERSION is normal in lead AVR. In leads V1, III, and AVL, T wave inversion can occur as a "normal variant." Also, T waves can appear "flat" in these leads. If, however, you note T wave inversion in two or more consecutive leads (two leads that view the same region of the heart), such as limb leads II and III (inferior wall), or leads I and AVL (lateral wall), this should be considered "abnormal." There are several disorders which can cause T wave inversion, some which are have no cardiac etiology.

Large, symmetrical inverted T waves (T amplitude equal to or greater than .20 mV) are consistent with Acute Coronary Syndrome. When patients present with symptoms suspicious for ACS whose ECG features large inverted T waves, ACS must be aggressively ruled out. The distinction between NSTEMI and unstable angina in such patients is based on the presence of elevated cardiac biomarkers.[6]

As is true with S-T segment abnormalities, your first priority when inverted T waves are noted is to rule out potentially life-threatening disorders. Once life-threatening etiologies have been eliminated, you should proceed to rule out other causes, such as those listed in the above diagram. In some cases, exhaustive diagnostic studies may not be able to reveal any cause for the presence of inverted T waves on a patient's ECG. Note that "no obvious cause" is listed on our table.

In cases where the patient has had previous heart damage (necrosis) from an old MI, inverted T waves may be present, even though the patient's "culprit" coronary artery has been opened (stented or bypassed), and there are no new blockages. In these cases, it may be necessary to perform cardiac catheterization to verify that no new blockages exist.

---

[6] Amsterdam, E. et al, Circulation 2010;122:756-776

HYPER-ACUTE T WAVES - COMMON ETIOLOGIES:

CONDITION:

HYPERKALEMIA

ACUTE MI

TRANSMURAL ISCHEMIA

HYPERTROPHY

HYPER-ACUTE T WAVES are defined by their amplitude and shape. Simply stated, when the height of the T wave approaches or exceeds that of the QRS complex, and the tip of the T wave is peaked, so much that it "looks like it would hurt if you sat on it,"[7] or "if you could prick your finger on it,"[8] the T wave is *hyper-acute*.

The presence of hyper-acute T waves is generally an ominous finding. Other than hypertrophy, the common causes of hyper-acute T waves are potentially life threatening disorders, which include *acute MI, hyperkalemia*, and *transmural ischemia*. The presence of hyper-acute T waves warrants an immediate evaluation of the patient to rule out the cause.

☞ One clue that may help identify the cause of a patient's hyper-acute T waves is to note whether they are present GLOBALLY (in nearly all or all leads of the ECG), or limited to one region of the heart (anterior wall, lateral wall, inferior wall). When Hyper-acute T waves are noted *globally*, one should suspect HYPERKALEMIA. When hyper-acute T waves are *noted in one specific region of the heart*, this finding is consistent with blockage of the coronary artery supplying that region (e.g.: anterior wall = LAD blockage, lateral wall = circumflex blockage, inferior wall = RCA blockage).

---

[7] I credit long-time friend and mentor Mike Taigman, author of "Taigman's Advanced Cardiology," for coining this witty and relevant phrase.

[8] a description I heard many times from Dr. Charles Sand during his ACLS lectures at St. Joseph's Hospital in Tampa, Florida

THE Q-T INTERVAL and U WAVES:

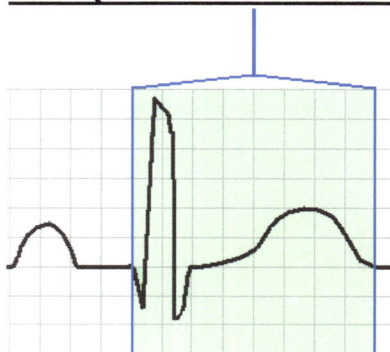

The Q-T Interval is measured from the beginning of the QRS complex to the end of the T wave. It represents the total duration of ventricular depolarization and repolarization. U waves, when present, follow T waves, and are most prevalent in the precordial leads V2 and V3.

VARIES BASED ON PT'S HEART RATE and SEX

ACCURATE QT Interval measurement is a critical component of ECG interpretation. Identification of abnormal prolongation of QT Intervals and/or the presence of abnormally large U waves – combined with appropriate patient management – could save the lives of thousands of patients each year. Long QT Syndrome (LQTS) claims the lives of approximately 3000 people per year,[9] many of whom are young, healthy children and adolescents. The mechanism of sudden death in patients with LQTS is development of Torsades de Pointes, a lethal cardiac dysrhythmia. By formal definition, Long QT Syndromes are characterized by: *prolongation of the corrected QT interval (QTc),* and *clinical findings of syncope or aborted sudden death*. There is often a family history of syncope and/or sudden death.[10]

If diagnosed and properly managed, the incidence of mortality from LQTS could be reduced to nearly zero. Current medical literature indicates that the primary diagnostic finding for LQTS is a prolonged QT interval, which in most cases is readily identifiable on the ECG. In some cases, T wave alterans patterns have been reported. Other documented ECG abnormalities associated with LQTS include abnormally large U waves, and or T/U wave fusion.

After extensive review of patient case studies, current medical journal citations, and textbook descriptions of LQTS, we suggest the following guidelines for QT Interval and U wave evaluation:

Etiology of Long QT Syndromes:
- **Congenital** (14 known subtypes) Genetic mutation results in abnormalities of cellular ion channels
- **Acquired**
  - o Drug Induced
  - o Metabolic/electrolyte induced
  - o Very low energy diets / anorexia
  - o CNS & Autonomic nervous system disorders
- **Miscellaneous**
  - o Coronary Artery Disease
  - o Mitral Valve Prolapse

☞ *Measure QT when patient at resting heart rate.*
Known ECG Indicators of Long QT Syndrome:
- QTc 460ms or longer in females*
- QTc 450ms or longer in males*
- T wave alterans
- U waves >25% of the T wave
- U waves merged with T waves
- U waves >0.1mv (1mm on standard calibrated
- ECG)

ECG Indication of Abnormally SHORT QT Interval:
- QTc less than 390ms

*P. Rautaharju, et al, "Standardization and Interpretation of the ECG, Part IV" JACC2009;53, no. 11:982-991

Suspected LQTS Considerations include:
- Avoidance of Medications that are known to prolong the QT Interval. (refer to "Meds Known to Prolong QT Interval" table on next page).
- Immediate expert consultation, such as with cardiologist / electrophysiologist, in order to rule out LQTS
- Continuous ECG monitoring until LQTS ruled out, or until expert consultant deems it safe to discontinue continuous ECG monitoring

Since the ECG indicators of LQTS are usually easily identified on the 12 Lead ECG, it is imperative that all clinicians who interpret ECGs be familiar with these identifying characteristics. When indicators of LQTS are discovered, we recommend that Suspected LQTS Considerations, listed in the table to the above right, be observed.

---

[9] Fogoros, Richard N, MD, author of "Electrophysiologic Testing."
[10] Jorge McCormack, MD, FACC, "The Role of Genetic Testing in Paediatric Syndromes of Sudden Death," Cardiology in the Young 2009; 19 (supl. 2) 54-65, Cambridge University Press

A more in-depth discussion of LQTS is beyond the scope of this book. Therefore, we will present standard ECG guidelines and alert criteria for the measurement of QT Intervals and U Waves. In the appendix of this book, we provide three case studies where proper application of LQTS knowledge saved the life of a 15 year old boy, a 22 year old girl and her siblings, and that of a 52 year old man.

==QT Interval measurement should be performed in leads where the QT Interval shows the longest; this lead is usually V2 or V3[11]==

Normal QT Interval values are based on the patient's heart rate, and to a lesser extent, the patient's gender.

There are several acceptable ways to calculate the corrected Q-T Interval (QTc). One way is to refer to a chart, like the one seen to the right, which provides the patient's QTc, based on the heart rate and gender of the patient. This method is not always practical, unless you don't mind carrying a chart with you at all times. I'm sure by now, there's an "app" for it, however I haven't checked yet.

THE *QTc INTERVAL

*QTc = Q-T interval, corrected for heart rate

HEART RATE	MALE	FEMALE
150	0.25	0.28
125	0.26	0.29
100	0.31	0.34
93	0.32	0.35
83	0.34	0.37
71	0.37	0.40
60	0.40	0.44
50	0.44	0.48
43	0.47	0.51

FROM: *Annals of Internal Medicine, 1988 109:905.*

Q-T INTERVAL SHOULD BE LESS THAN 1/2 OF THE

R - R INTERVAL *

METHOD WORKS FOR HEART RATES 60 - 100
* IN THIS EXAMPLE WE MEASURED FROM Q-Q, WHICH IS THE SAME DURATION AS R-R.

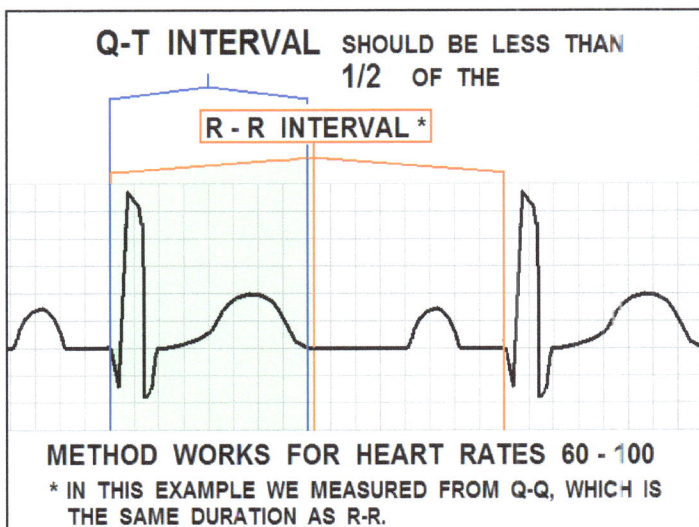

For heart rates between 60-100, use the "Quick Peek" method, shown to the left. This simple method is a favorite of the two electrophysiologists I work with on a regular basis. If it's good enough for them, it's good enough for me!

For heart rates less than 60 or greater than 100, or to calculate the precise corrected QT interval, you can use one of the following mathematical formulas, shown in the table below:

QT CORRECTION FORMULAS:

Bazett's	$QTc = QT/\sqrt{RR}$
Fredericia	$QTc = QT/(RR)1/3$
Framingham	$QTc = QT + 0.154(1 - RR)$
Rautaharju	$QTc = 656/(1 + HR/100)$

U WAVES:

THE U WAVE

REPORTED CAUSES OF U WAVES:

- OFTEN SEEN IN BRADYCARDIAS (RATES BELOW 60)
- HYPOKALEMIA, HYPOCALCEMIA, HYPOMAGNESEMIA
- AFTER-DEPOLARIZATIONS of VENTRICULAR
- HYPOTHERMIA
- DRUGS THAT PROLONG THE QT INTERVAL
- LONG QT SYNDROMES
- REPORTED IN APPROX 15% of ISCHEMIC STROKES

Occasionally, U waves are seen on an ECG. When present, they succeed T waves, which they typically resemble in shape and deflection. They are most prevalent in the precordial leads, most predominantly leads V2 and V3.

The etiology of U waves is most likely from several possible causes. Traditional thought attributes the U wave to "hypokalemia," however with respect to electrolytes, we know that hypocalcaemia, hypomagnesaemia, are also known to cause U waves. Therefore, when U waves are noted, the patient's electrolyte levels should be evaluated.

---

[11] P. Rautaharju, MD, FACC et al, "Standardization and Interpretation of the ECG, Part IV", JACC 2009; Vol 53 No. 11:982-991

Recall that serum magnesium does not accurately reflect intracellular magnesium. If your patient is exhibiting symptoms of low magnesium; for example is presenting with runs of Torsades, sub-normal *intracellular magnesium levels* may be present, despite the reporting of normal *serum magnesium levels* on the electrolyte panel[12].

According to a study performed by Warren Jackman, et. Al., at the University of Oklahoma, U waves are indicative of "early afterdepolarizations," a condition linked to increased incidence of Torsades.

According to Marriott and Cooper[13], when U waves are seen with *deflections opposite that of T waves* (i.e. *positive* T waves with *negative* U waves), it is a sign of possible myocardial ischemia.

My response to seeing U waves on a patient's ECG is to rule out known causes of U waves:
- obtain a thorough patient history, to rule out incidence of syncope and family history of sudden death/ near sudden death.
- evaluate the patient's electrolyte levels, and
- evaluate patient's medications list for meds that prolong the QT Interval.
- rule out hypothermia
- rule out CVA
- monitor the patient's ECG for runs of Torsades.
- Expert consult for LQTS evaluation

The ECG featured to the left provides an example of U waves.

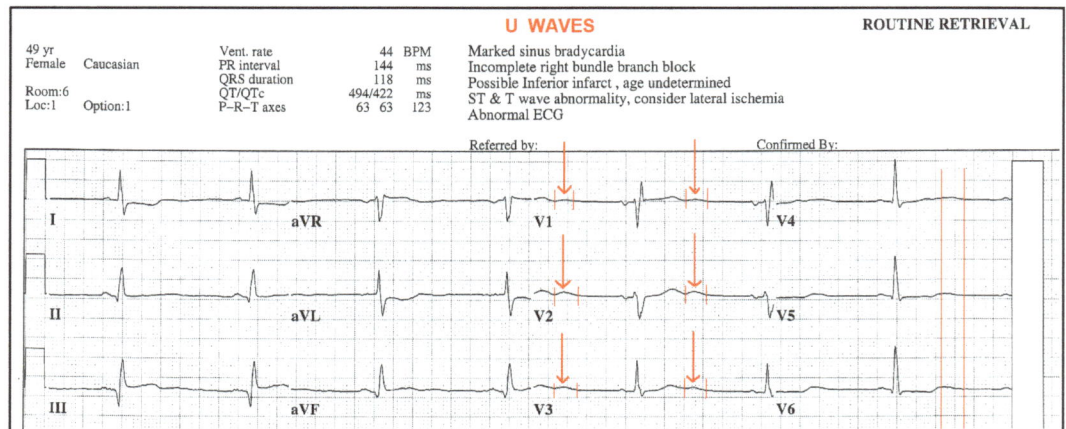

U WAVES		ROUTINE RETRIEVAL

49 yr Female Caucasian Room:6 Loc:1 Option:1

Vent. rate 44 BPM
PR interval 144 ms
QRS duration 118 ms
QT/QTc 494/422 ms
P–R–T axes 63 63 123

Marked sinus bradycardia
Incomplete right bundle branch block
Possible Inferior infarct , age undetermined
ST & T wave abnormality, consider lateral ischemia
Abnormal ECG

Referred by: Confirmed By:

Prolongation of the Q-T interval and/or the presence of abnormal U waves has been linked to an increase incidence of Torsades de Pointes, a potentially fatal dysrhythmia. Patients with a prolonged QT interval should be monitored closely for the development of Torsades. Electrolytes should be checked, with specific emphasis on the patient's Magnesium, Potassium, Calcium and Sodium levels. **Patients with NORMAL serum Potassium levels may have intracellular hypomagnesaemia – therefore we DO NOT withhold administration of Magnesium Sulfate, when Torsades is present.** Abnormal electrolyte levels should be corrected. Patients in Torsades may have no cardiac output and may present in cardiac arrest. **Patients in Torsades who present in cardiac arrest should be managed using the American Heart Association ACLS algorithm for Ventricular Fibrillation. Patients in Torsades whom are hemodynamically unstable should receive an unsynchronized DC countershock, (defibrillation) as per ACLS protocol. Patients in Torsades, who are stable, per AHA ACLS guidelines, should receive Magnesium Sulfate 1 – 2 gm. over 5 to 60 minutes.**

BEWARE of giving MEDS that INCREASE the QT INTERVAL to patients with abnormally prolonged QT intervals and/or abnormal U waves – this practice can lead to TORSADES and CARDIAC ARREST. There are hundreds of medications known to prolong the QT interval, many of which are frequently used, such as Amiodarone, Avalox, Biaxin, Cardene, Corvert, Erythromycin, Geodon, Haloperidol, Levoflaxin, Lithium, Procainamide, Z-pak, Zithromax; many more are listed on page XX in the appendix of this book. Please visit: www.longQT.org and www.azcert.org for additional information, precautions and advice.

---

[12] Rinehart, R et al, Arch Intern Med 1988;148(11):2415-2420
[13] Cooper, J and Marriott, H, "ECG Essentials and Beyond," American College of Cardiovascular Nurses

BUNDLE BRANCH BLOCKS

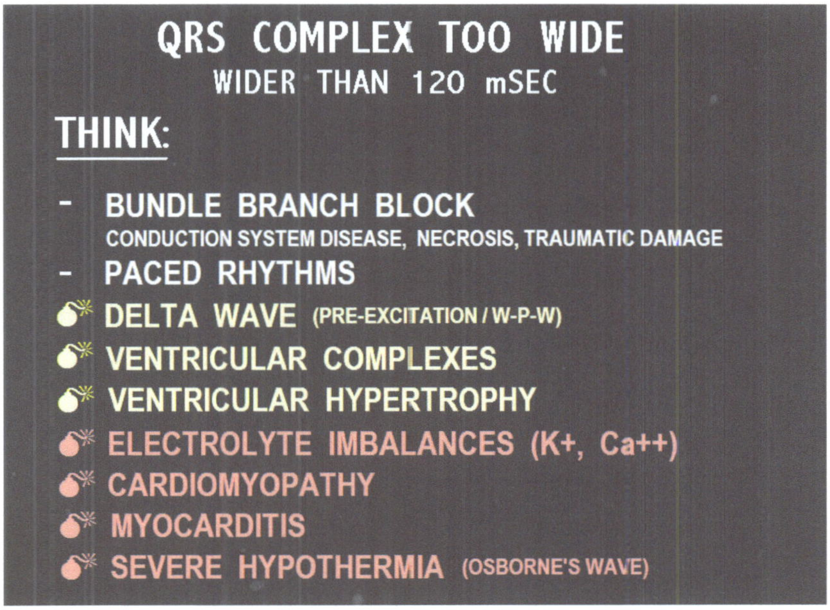

A bundle branch block (BBB) is a delay or blockage of current traveling down either the right or left bundle branch. Because it takes longer for current to go around the blockage, the QRS complex becomes abnormally wide (greater than 120ms).

True bundle branch blocks are caused by diseases that effect cells of the cardiac electrical system, such as Lenhgre's or Lev's disease, necrosis to bundle branch(es) from myocardial infarction, and traumatic damage to bundle branch structures, such as from coronary artery bypass and septal surgeries.

Conditions that cause global myocardial damage, such as hypertrophy, cardiomyopathy, and myocarditis can abnormally widen the QRS because it takes longer for the wave of depolarization to traverse throughout the myocardium. While the mechanism of QRS widening may not be a true blockage within the bundle branches, we tend to classify many wide complex rhythms as bundle branch blocks, or having *bundle branch block patterns.*

Bundle branch blocks can obscure many of the commonly used ECG markers used to identify other serious conditions. For example, patients who have LEFT BUNDLE BRANCH BLOCK always have elevated S-T segments—a finding that makes it difficult to diagnose acute MI with the 12 lead ECG. In cases of RIGHT BUNDLE BRANCH BLOCK, there will frequently be S-T segment depression and inverted T waves, which is a finding often associated with ischemia, NSTEMI and several other conditions.

An abnormally wide QRS can result from several conditions other than bundle branch block. In cases where a patient presents with a newly discovered wide QRS, a thorough evaluation should be performed to rule out potentially lethal causes—especially in cases where the patient is symptomatic. A list of conditions that can cause an abnormally wide QRS is presented in the diagram to the above right.

The main ECG characteristics of BBB include: wide QRS, notching of the QRS complex in certain leads, altered J points, altered S-T segments, and altered T waves.

To identify a BUNDLE BRANCH BLOCK, you must first be sure that the QRS is wide enough to qualify (be greater than 120ms), and must be sure that the rhythm is not originating in the ventricles. If there are P waves on the ECG, and the rhythm is not 3rd degree heart block, the rhythm is most likely originating above the ventricles. You should also rule out *delta waves,* which are associated with Wolff-Parkinson-White syndrome. For an example of delta waves seen with W-P-W, see pages 48, 81 and 84.

I have listed three methods to choose from for identifying Bundle Brach Block patterns. I believe the first two methods are easiest to use, and require only a strip of lead V1. The third method is more complicated, but since it uses V1, V2, V5, and V6, it may provide you with enough information to make a decision in cases where the V1-only methods prove inconclusive.

QRS COMPLEX TOO WIDE
WIDER THAN 120 mSEC

THINK:

- **BUNDLE BRANCH BLOCK**
  CONDUCTION SYSTEM DISEASE, NECROSIS, TRAUMATIC DAMAGE
- **PACED RHYTHMS**
- **DELTA WAVE** (PRE-EXCITATION / W-P-W)
- **VENTRICULAR COMPLEXES**
- **VENTRICULAR HYPERTROPHY**
- **ELECTROLYTE IMBALANCES** (K+, Ca++)
- **CARDIOMYOPATHY**
- **MYOCARDITIS**
- **SEVERE HYPOTHERMIA** (OSBORNE'S WAVE)

Rotate the Rhythm Strip Method:

I refer to this as the *York Hospital Method*, since that is where I first learned of this technique. This method most likely did not originate at York Hospital, so I apologize in advance to the unsung hero who discovered it. If the true identity of the genius who developed this "fine pearl of cardiology" is ever revealed to me, I will appropriately give credit to whom it is due. Until then, I credit my good friend, nursing educator and ECG guru Mike Cooley, MSN, RN, CEN with propagating this simple and accurate technique:

DIAGNOSING BUNDLE BRANCH BLOCKS in LEAD V1

* The "York Hospital" Method:

1. **ROTATE** your rhythm strip (of LEAD V1) CLOCKWISE

2. **DIAGNOSE** -- The side of the ISOELECTRIC LINE that the bulk of the QRS complex rests -- is the side of the heart with the BUNDLE BRANCH BLOCK !

LBBB !

RBBB !

Terminal Phase of QRS in Lead V1 Method:

This is another amazingly simple and accurate technique. With your strip of lead V1, you simply look at the QRS, and determine if the last segment of the QRS is positive (above the isoelectric line), or negative (below the isoelectric line). If the last deflection of the QRS is positive, the patient most likely has a right bundle branch block (RBBB). If the last deflection is negative, the patient most likely has a left bundle branch block (LBBB). Did you ever think it could be this easy? Check it out to the right:

DIAGNOSING BUNDLE BRANCH BLOCK

L.B.B.B.

USING LEAD V1

- QRS WIDER THAN 120 ms
- BEAT IS SUPRAVENTRICULAR IN ORIGIN
- TERMINAL PHASE OF QRS COMPLEX (LAST DEFLECTION)

R.B.B.B.

NEGATIVE = LEFT BUNDLE BRANCH BLOCK

POSITIVE = RIGHT BUNDLE BRANCH BLOCK

Definitive Method:

DIAGNOSING BUNDLE BRANCH BLOCK

USING LEADS V1, V2, and V5, V6:

LOCATING RsR' or RR' COMPLEXES:

| V1 | V2 | V5 | V6 |

RIGHT BUNDLE BRANCH BLOCK

LEFT BUNDLE BRANCH BLOCK

If you're like me, you opt for quick, easy and effective ways to achieve a goal, such as the two techniques we've just presented.

Occasionally, I will come across an ECG that the first two techniques don't fit—such as in cases where the two methods provide conflicting results. In these rare instances, I use the following technique, presented in the image below, as the tie breaker.

To use this technique, you must examine the type of QRS complexes that are in leads V1, V2, V5, and V6. What you're looking for is RSR' or RR' complexes. If you see one or both of these complexes in leads V1 and/or V2, your patient has a RBBB pattern. If you identify RSR' or RR' in V5 and/or V6, your patient has LBBB pattern:

FASCICULAR BLOCKS result from conduction delays in the *anterior* or *posterior fascicles* of the Left Bundle Branch. In most cases of *anterior* or *posterior fascicular* block, patients are often asymptomatic, which usually warrants no immediate corrective action. Patients with fascicular block should undergo periodic ECG evaluation to determine if their conduction disorder is progressively worsening, as can be the case in conduction system diseases, such as Lev-Lenegre Syndrome. In cases of advanced fascicular block, such as Bi-Fascicular or Tri-Fascicular blocks (described below), patients may experience syncope resulting from episodes of high-grade heart block (2nd degree Type II and 3rd degree). Such patients should be considered for pacemaker implantation.

Left Anterior Fascicular Block (LAFB) is when conduction is delayed or blocked within the anterior fascicle of the Left Bundle Branch. ECG identification characteristics include left bundle branch block, slight widening of the QRS complex (typical width 100 – 120ms), a small Q wave in lead I, a deep S wave in lead III, and what I call an "up-down-down" pattern in leads I, II, and III, as shown in the image to the right.

LEFT ANTERIOR FASCICULAR BLOCK

EKG CHARACTERISTICS:

- **LEFT AXIS DEVIATION**
- **QRS WIDTH 100 - 120 ms**
- **"Q1-S3" = Q WAVE, LEAD I and Deep S WAVE, LEAD III**
- **"UP-DOWN-DOWN" PATTERN, LEADS I, II, and III.**

I II III

LEFT POSTERIOR FASCICULAR BLOCK

EKG CHARACTERISTICS:

- **RIGHT AXIS DEVIATION**
- **QRS WIDTH 100 - 120 ms**
- **"S1-Q3" = Deep S WAVE, LEAD I and SMALL Q WAVE, LEAD III**
- **"DOWN-UP-UP" PATTERN, LEADS I, II, and III.**

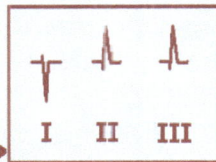

I II III

Left Posterior Fascicular Block (LPFB) is when conduction is – you guessed it – delayed or blocked in the posterior fascicle of the Left Bundle Branch. ECG characteristics include a slight widening of QRS complex (100-120ms), a deep S wave in lead I, a small Q wave in lead III, and what I call an "up-down-down" pattern in leads I, II, and III, as shown in the image to the left.

It is important to determine that the NEGATIVELY deflected QRS complexes (Leads II, III in LAFB; Lead I in LPFB) *are rS complexes and do not have Q waves.* If Q waves are present in the negatively deflected leads, the diagnosis of necrosis, most likely from old MI, should be considered over that of Fascicular Block.

BI-FASCICULAR BLOCKS: In some cases, RIGHT BUNDLE BRANCH BLOCK is seen along with either LAFB or LPFB. When this occurs, it is called "Bi-Fascicular Block." In essence, two of the "three main conduction conduits" between the atria and ventricles are blocked. Patients with this degree of conduction system disease should be monitored carefully for development of high grade heart blocks. Such patients may require pacemaker implantation.

TRI-FASCICULAR BLOCKS: Is defined as "Bi-Fascicular block + 1st or 2nd degree A-V Block." This combination is rarely seen, most likely because patients don't seek medical care until they have developed clinically significant complete heart block. Patients with Tri-Fascicular Block should be considered for permanent pacemaker implantation.

(For example ECGs of the conditions listed on this page, see page 287).

TRIFASICULAR BLOCK

EKG CHARACTERISTICS:

- **RIGHT BUNDLE BRANCH BLOCK**

+

- **LEFT ANTERIOR or POSTERIOR HEMIBLOCK**

+

- **FIRST or SECOND DEGREE HEART BLOCK**

AXIS DEVIATION and ROTATION

☞ **EVALUATE THE AXIS IN BOTH PLANES**

- VERTICAL

" AXIS DEVIATION "

- HORIZONTAL

" AXIS ROTATION "

Another important source of information we use to assist us with diagnosing cardiac abnormalities is the evaluation of the heart's axis in the vertical and horizontal planes.

Axis deviation refers to evaluation of the axis in the vertical (frontal) plane.

Axis rotation refers to evaluation of the axis in the *horizontal plane*. Axis rotation is also referred to as R *wave progression*.

☦ ***REMEMBER . . .***

AXIS DEVIATION is <u>NOT</u> a DIAGNOSIS:

- **It is an observation of the general direction of current flow throughout the myocardium.**

- **Certain conditions, as well as normal variations of how the heart sits in the chest cavity, can cause the AXIS to vary from NORMAL.**

When we evaluate the heart's axis on an ECG, we are making an observation of the general direction of current flow throughout the myocardium. There are several conditions that can cause axis abnormalities: Necrotic tissue from an old MI, enlargement of a heart chamber (hypertrophy), bundle branch blocks and pre-excitation (Wolff-Parkinson-White) are four conditions which commonly effect axis. When we observe axis abnormalities, we need to determine which condition(s) are responsible for the axis change.

To evaluate the *vertical axis*, we utilize the limb leads. Just like so many other things in medicine, there are several ways to do this. I prefer the quickest and easiest method, which uses only LIMB LEADS I and AVF. This method categorizes the vertical axis of all ECGs into one of four categories: *normal, left axis deviation, right axis deviation,* and *far right axis deviation.* (Far right axis deviation is also referred to as "no-man's land" axis deviation).

The downfall of this easy method is that it doesn't provide a precise numerical value for the degree of axis, such as +60 degrees, or -30 degrees. On the bright side, in over 30 years of evaluating ECGs, I cannot recall any situations where I needed to know the exact numerical degree of axis; I only needed to know if the axis was *normal, deviated to the left, the right,* or *far right*.

To use this simple method, look at the table to the right. When the QRS complexes in leads I and AVF are both positive, the axis is normal. If the QRS in lead I is positive, with negative QRS complexes in AVF, we say there is *left axis deviation*. Conversely, if the QRS is negative in lead I and positive in AVF, there is *right axis deviation.* If the QRS complexes in both leads are negative, we say there is *far right axis deviation,* – also known as "*no-man's land*" axis deviation.

☞ **AXIS DEVIATION**

	LEAD I	LEAD AVF
NORMAL	⋀	⋀
LEFT	⋀	⋁
RIGHT	⋁	⋀
FAR RIGHT	⋁	⋁

In the sample ECG below, ***the QRS complexes in limb leads I and AVF are both positive***. As indicated in the table at the bottom of the previous page, the axis is normal. It's that easy!

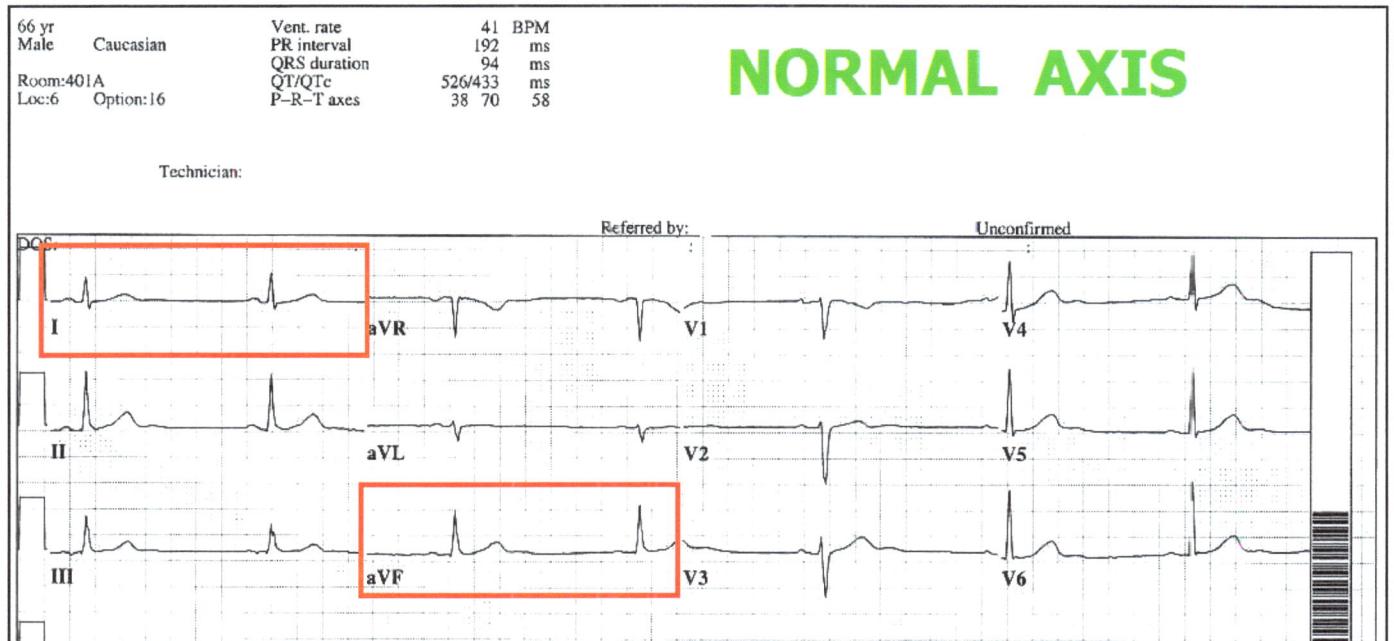

66 yr		Vent. rate	41	BPM
Male	Caucasian	PR interval	192	ms
		QRS duration	94	ms
Room:401A		QT/QTc	526/433	ms
Loc:6	Option:16	P–R–T axes	38 70	58

Technician:

Referred by: Unconfirmed

NORMAL AXIS

I   aVR   V1   V4

II   aVL   V2   V5

III   aVF   V3   V6

On the next few pages, you will see sample ECGs with axis deviation. Once axis deviation is identified, the next step is to rule out each of the disorders that are known to cause that type of axis deviation. Under each sample ECG, you'll find lists of disorders that are known to cause axis deviation.

73

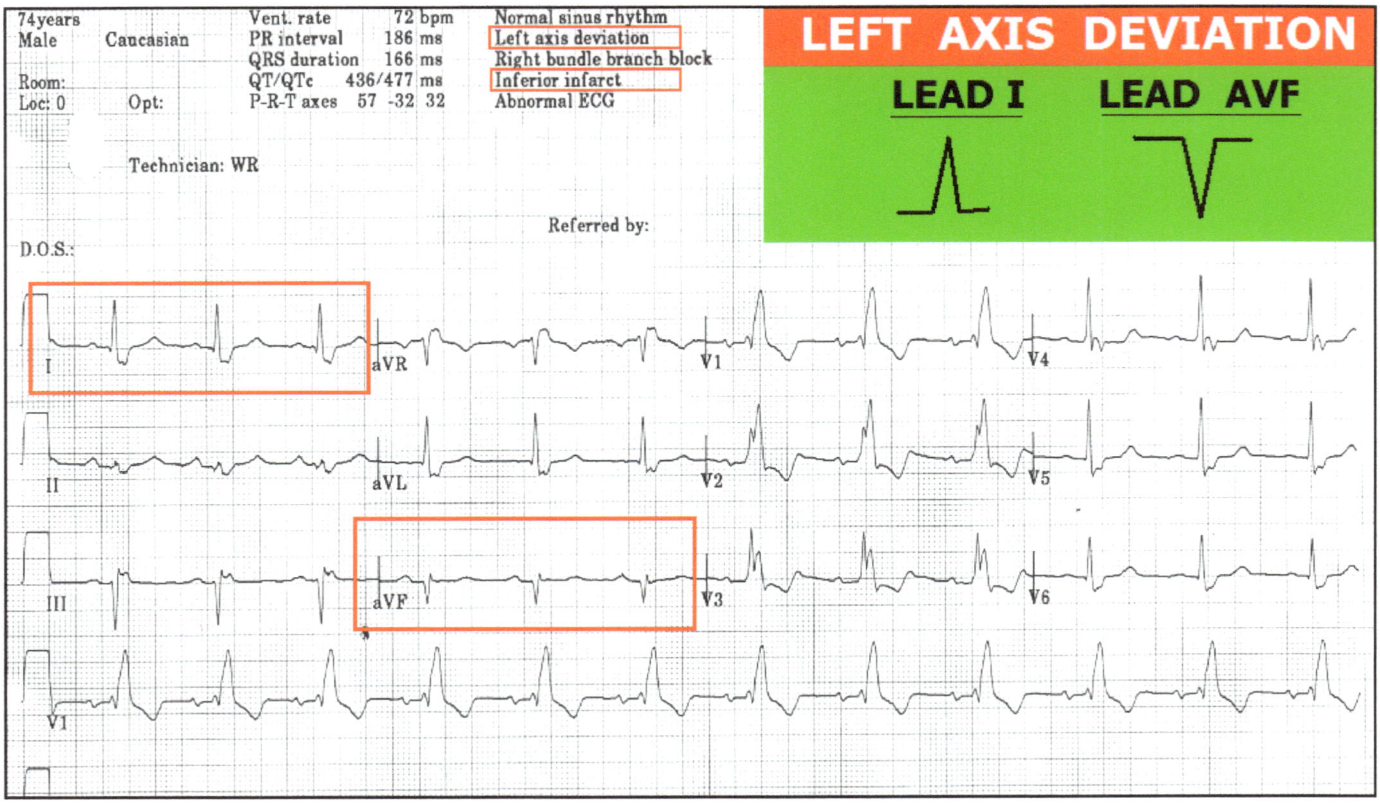

LEFT AXIS DEVIATION

LEAD I   LEAD AVF

I   aVR   V1   V4

II   aVL   V2   V5

III   aVF   V3   V6

V1

COMMON CONDITIONS WHICH *MAY* CAUSE

LEFT AXIS DEVIATION:

☛ **HYPERKALEMIA**

☛ **LEFT BUNDLE BRANCH BLOCK**

☛ **PACEMAKER**

☛ **C.O.P.D.**

☛ **LEFT VENTRICULAR HYPERTROPHY**

☛ **OLD INFERIOR WALL MI**

☛ **LEFT ANTERIOR FASCICULAR BLOCK**

☛ **WOLFF-PARKINSON-WHITE (types A & B)**

In our sample ECG above, which happens to be that of my father, *old inferior wall MI* is the cause of his Left Axis Deviation!

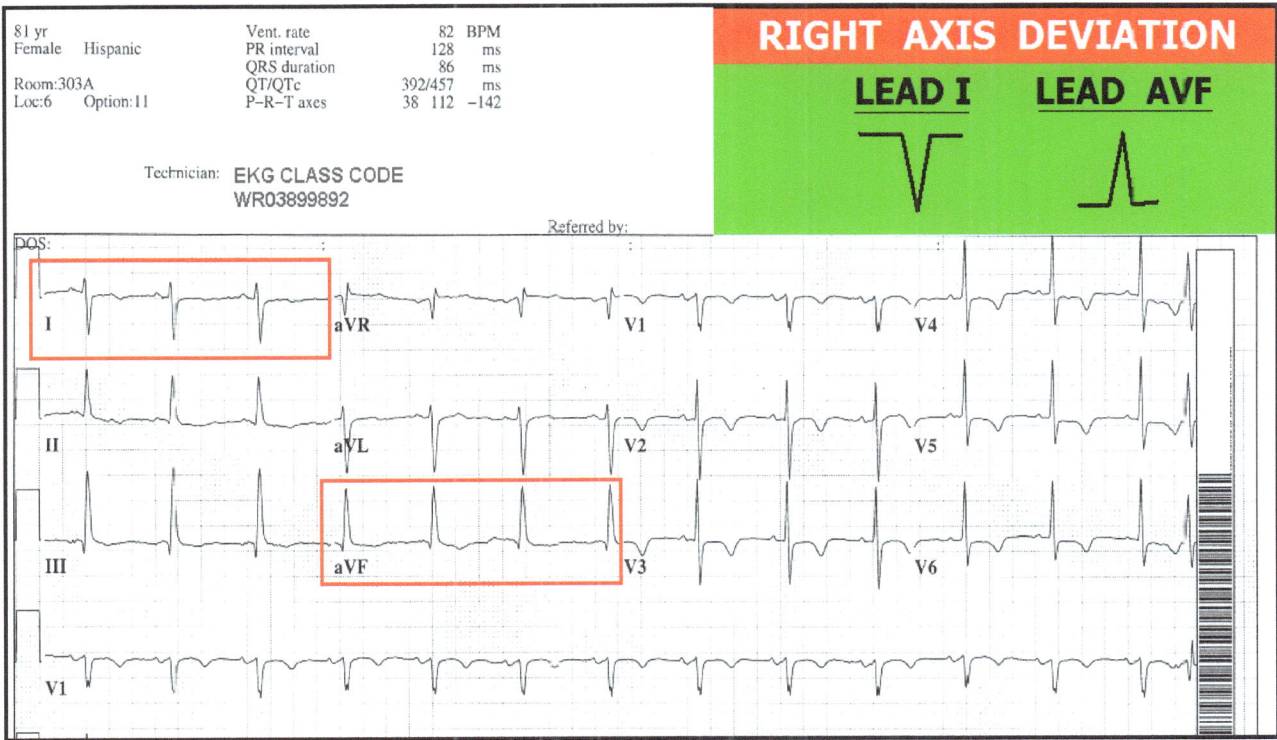

81 yr	Vent. rate	82	BPM
Female Hispanic	PR interval	128	ms
	QRS duration	86	ms
Room:303A	QT/QTc	392/457	ms
Loc:6 Option:11	P–R–T axes	38 112 –142	

Technician: EKG CLASS CODE
WR03899892

Referred by:

RIGHT AXIS DEVIATION

LEAD I   **LEAD AVF**

COMMON CONDITIONS WHICH *MAY* CAUSE
RIGHT AXIS DEVIATION:

- ☛ **PULMONARY EMBOLUS**
- ☛ NORMAL FOR PEDS & TALL, THIN ADULTS
- ☛ RIGHT VENTRICULAR HYPERTROPHY
- ☛ OLD LATERAL WALL MI
- ☛ LEFT POSTERIOR FASICULAR BLOCK
- ☛ DEXTROCARDIA
- ☛ C.O.P.D.
- ☛ ATRIAL / VENTRICULAR SEPTAL DEFECTS

In our sample ECG above, the cause of Right Axis Deviation is *left posterior fascicular block.*

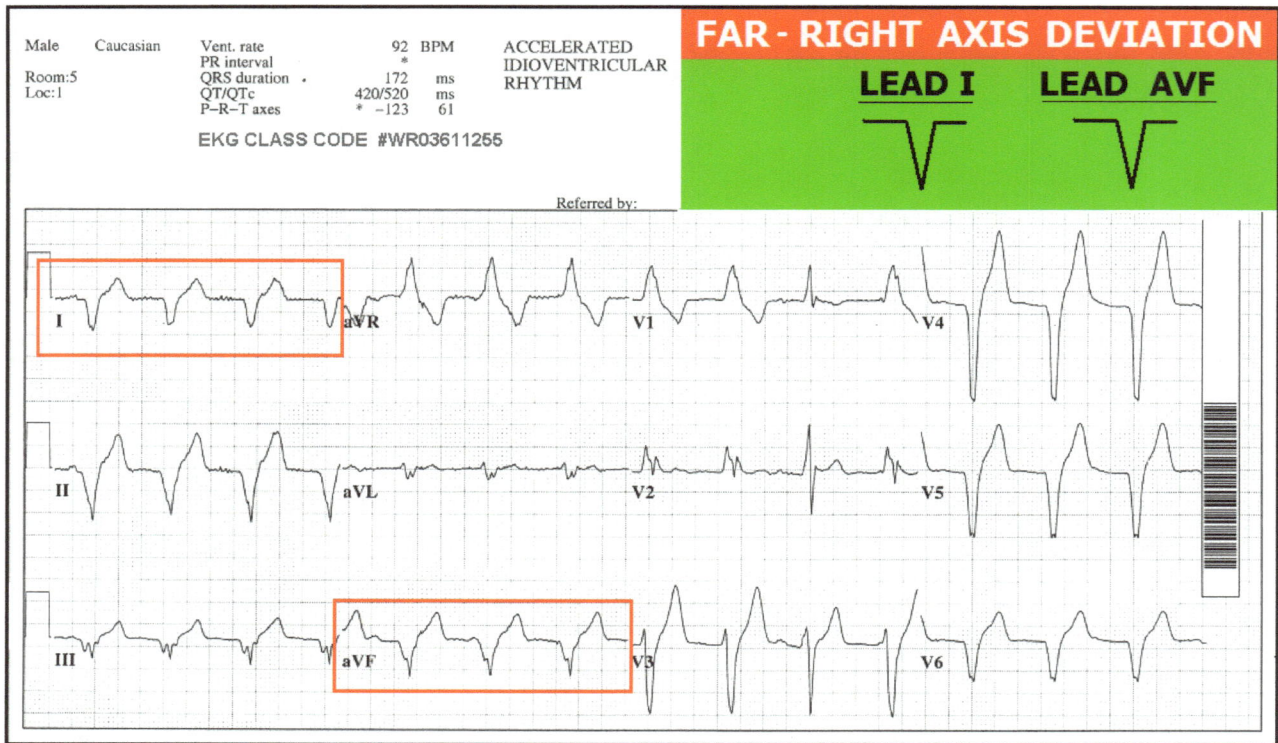

Male	Caucasian	Vent. rate	92	BPM	ACCELERATED
Room:5		PR interval		*	IDIOVENTRICULAR
Loc:1		QRS duration .	172	ms	RHYTHM
		QT/QTc	420/520	ms	
		P–R–T axes	* –123	61	

EKG CLASS CODE #WR03611255

Referred by:

LEAD I   LEAD AVF

I   aVR   V1   V4

II   aVL   V2   V5

III   aVF   V3   V6

COMMON CONDITIONS WHICH *MAY* CAUSE

(NO-MAN'S LAND AXIS)
FAR RIGHT AXIS DEVIATION:

☞ **HYPERKALEMIA**

☞ **VENTRICULAR RHYTHMS**

☞ **LEAD TRANSPOSITION**

☞ **PACEMAKER RHYTHMS**

☞ **C.O.P.D.**

The cause of Far-Right (a.k.a. "No-man's Land") Axis Deviation, is *accelerated idioventricular rhythm.*

AXIS ROTATION is often referred to as *R Wave Progression..* It is a measurement of the *horizontal axis* of the heart. To evaluate the *horizontal axis,* we use the six precordial leads. .

When we say "R wave progression," we are referring to the height of the R wave (the positive deflection), which becomes *progressively larger* as we move from V1 through V6. The image to the right demonstrates R wave progression seen in the normal ECG.

In the normal heart, ventricular depolarization starts as the wave of depolarization travels down the bundle branches. The intraventricular septum is the first region of ventricular muscle to depolarize, and is the cause of small Q waves normally seen on the ECG. As the intraventricular septum depolarizes, current moves *toward* leads V1 and V2, resulting in the small R waves seen on the normal ECG. As current dissipates outward from the septum, the mass of depolarization forces are moving *away* from V1 and V2, resulting in large negative S waves.

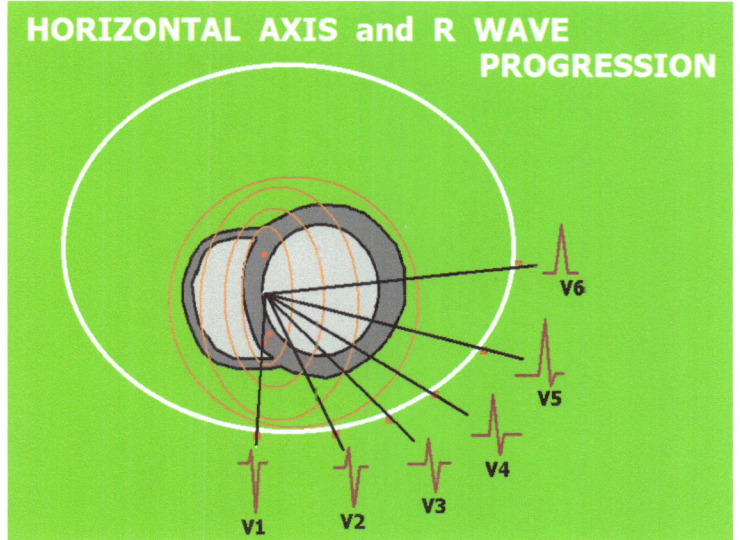

HORIZONTAL AXIS and R WAVE PROGRESSION

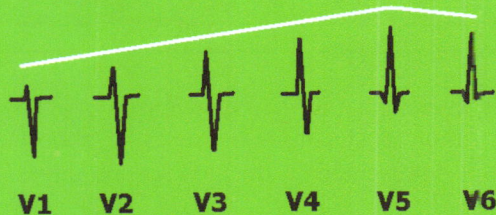

ASSESSING AXIS ROTATION

NORMAL R - WAVE PROGRESSION

V1   V2   V3   V4   V5   V6

From the vantage points of V3 and V4, approximately half of the depolarization wave is moving toward these leads, and half is moving away. This results in QRS complexes that are biphasic.

Since nearly all of the ventricular depolarization wave is moving toward V5 and V6, the QRS complexes in these leads are nearly all positive R waves.

The first step in evaluation of the horizontal axis is to identify which lead *transition* occurs in.

Transition is the lead where the QRS is most biphasic. This should normally occur in V3 or V4. In the example to our left, transition has occurred in V3.

As indicated in our diagram, when transition occurs in V1 or V2, we say, "*transition is shifted toward the right,*" or there is "*early transition.*"

Conversely, when transition occurs in V5 or V6, we say "*transition is shifted toward the left*," or there is "*late transition.*"

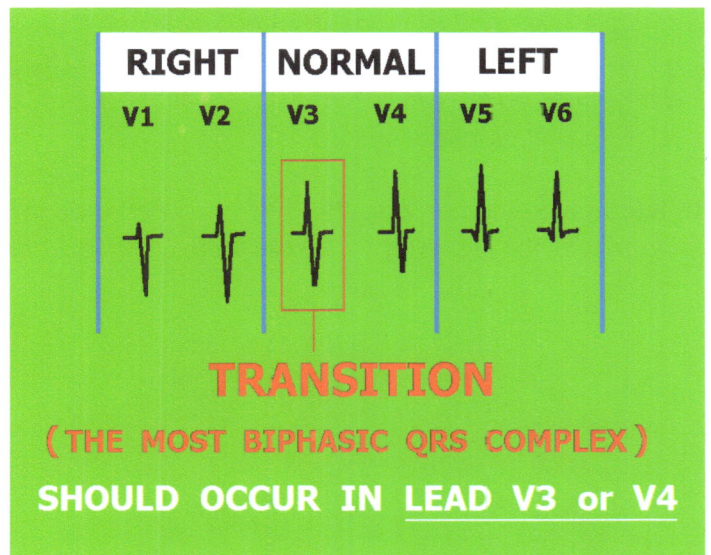

RIGHT		NORMAL		LEFT	
V1	V2	V3	V4	V5	V6

TRANSITION

(THE MOST BIPHASIC QRS COMPLEX)

SHOULD OCCUR IN LEAD V3 or V4

NORMAL TRANSITION

IS BETWEEN LEADS V3 and V4

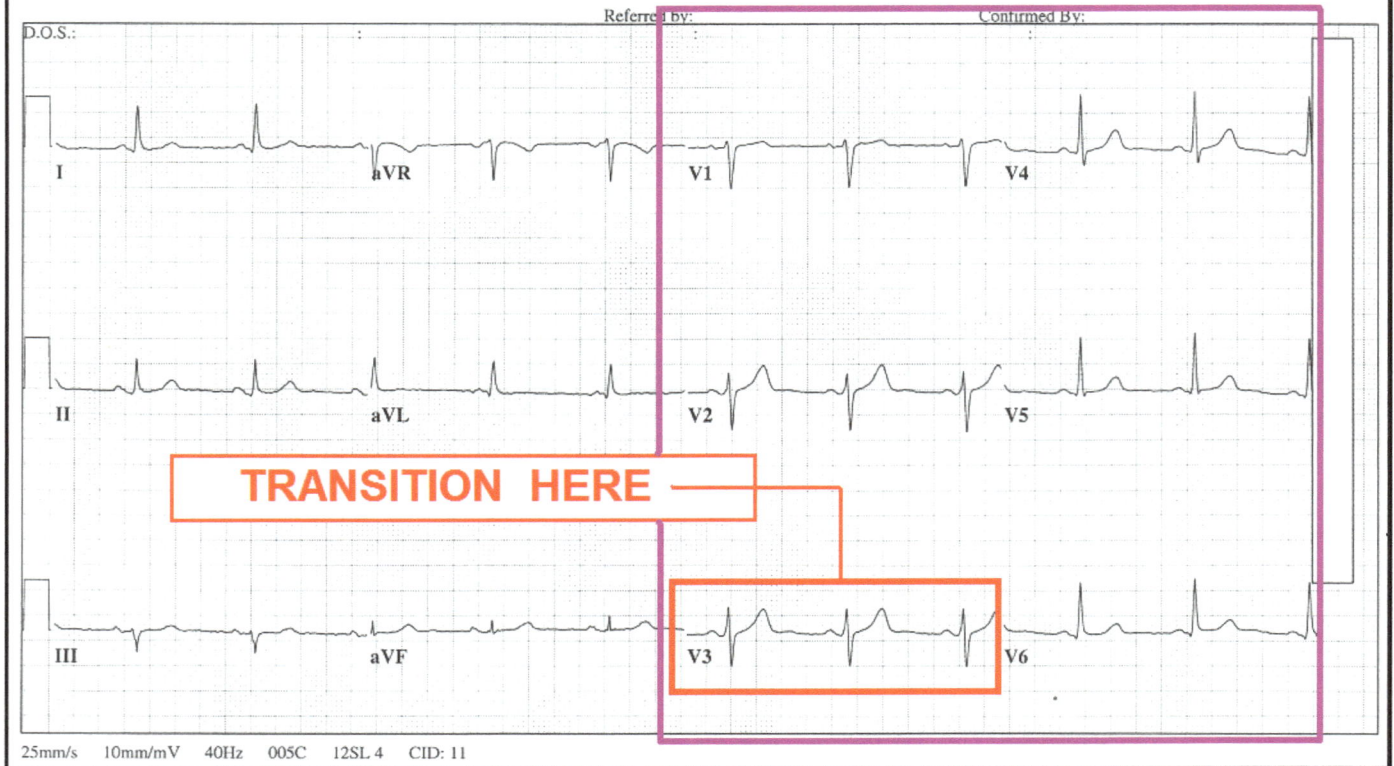

TRANSITION HERE

25mm/s   10mm/mV   40Hz   005C   12SL 4   CID: 11

Whenever abnormal R wave progression is identified, we must investigate further to determine if any abnormal conditions are present. This task is simplified if you know the four most common causes of abnormal R wave progression, which are presented below, with discussion and examples presented on the next several pages.

The four conditions which most commonly cause abnormal R wave progression are:

1. Bundle Branch Blocks
2. Myocardial Necrosis (Old MI): Anterior and Posterior
3. Ventricular Hypertrophy
4. Wolff-Parkinson-White

In addition to memorizing the four most common causes of abnormal R wave progression, it is helpful to memorize the saying: *"Transition shifts toward hypertrophy and away from necrosis."*

By knowing the four conditions which commonly cause abnormal R wave progression, you can simply start with the first condition listed, which is bundle branch block, and rule it out. Is the QRS wide enough to indicate bundle branch block? If the answer is "no, the QRS is too narrow," move on to the next condition. It is simply a process of ruling out each condition.

On the next several pages, we arrive at the cause of each patient's abnormal R wave progression by using the "helpful clues" we have provided, as seen below. Using these "clues" will help you to arrive at the most likely cause of your patient's abnormal R wave progression.

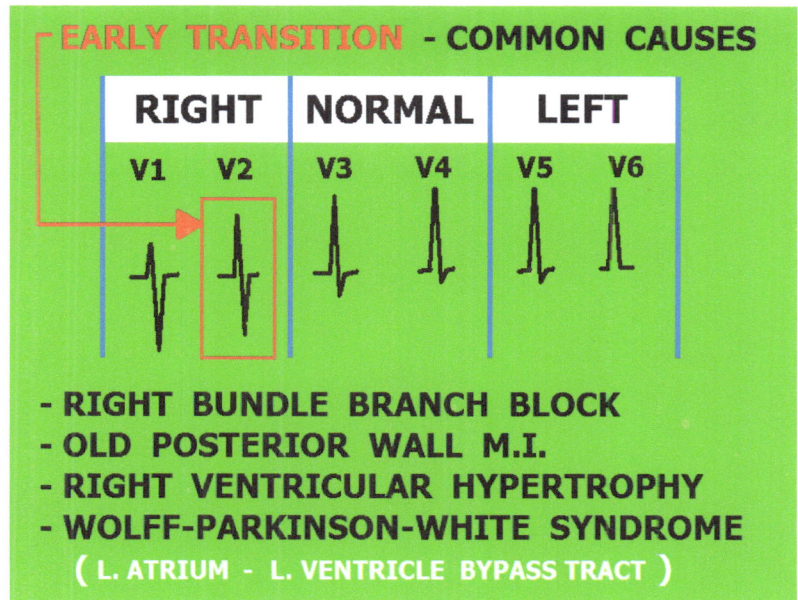

EARLY TRANSITION - COMMON CAUSES

RIGHT		NORMAL		LEFT	
V1	V2	V3	V4	V5	V6

- RIGHT BUNDLE BRANCH BLOCK
- OLD POSTERIOR WALL M.I.
- RIGHT VENTRICULAR HYPERTROPHY
- WOLFF-PARKINSON-WHITE SYNDROME
(L. ATRIUM - L. VENTRICLE BYPASS TRACT)

COMMON CAUSES OF EARLY TRANSITION
....SOME HELPFUL CLUES:

1. Right Bundle Branch Block (RBBB)

- QRS wider than 120ms
- Supraventricular rhythm (normal P : QRS relationship)
- RSR' or RR' ("notching") in V1, V2, and/or V3

2. Old Posterior Wall MI

- Usually accompanied by OLD INFERIOR WALL MI
- Does NOT abnormally widen the QRS complex

3. Right Ventricular Hypertrophy (RVH)

- Corresponding Right Atrial Hypertrophy (RAH)
- Right Axis Deviation (RAD)
- QRS in LEAD I more NEGATIVE than POSITIVE (R<S)

4. Wolff-Parkinson-White (WPW)

- Short P-R Interval
- Presence of Delta Waves
- Wide QRS complexes

The next two pages contain ECGs with early transition, where we have utilized the "helpful clues" from the above table to identify the underlying abnormal condition.

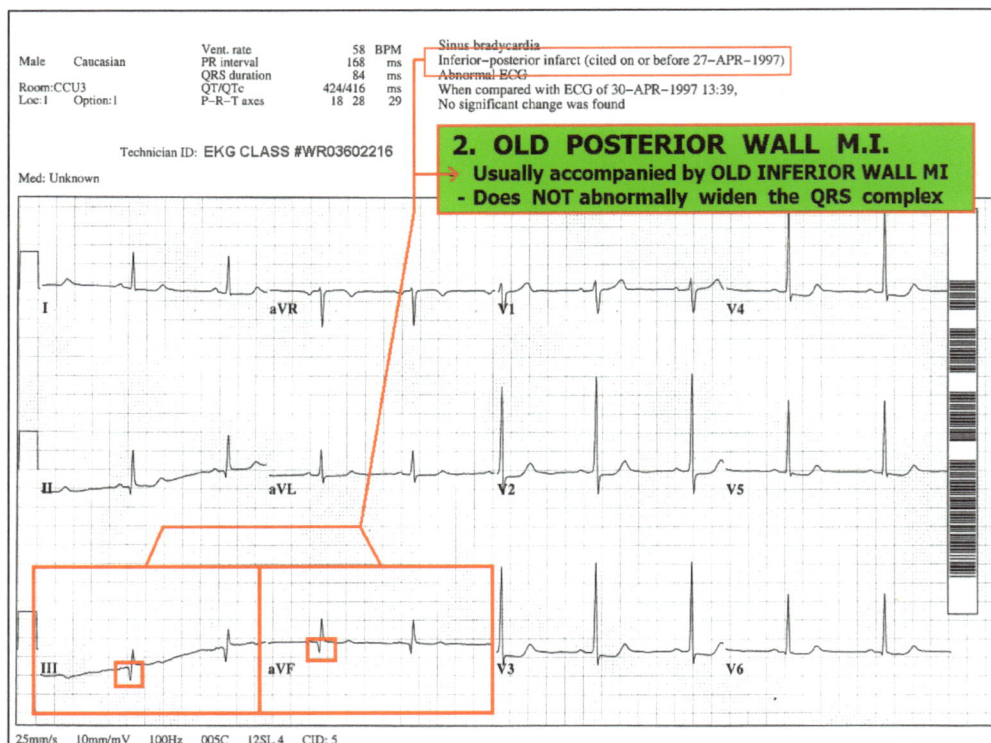

ECG annotations (left ECG):

74 years		Vent. rate	72 bpm	Normal sinus rhythm
Male	Caucasian	PR interval	186 ms	Left axis deviation
		QRS duration	166 ms	Right bundle branch block
Room:		QT/QTc	436/477 ms	Inferior infarct, age undetermined
Loc: 0	Opt:	P-R-T axes	57 -32 32	Abnormal ECG

Technician: WR

D.O.S.:

Referred by: Unconfirmed

P Waves precede each QRS w/ reg. P-R int.

1. RIGHT BUNDLE BRANCH BLOCK
- QRS wider than 120ms
- Supraventricular origin QRS complexes
- RSR' or RR' ("notching") in V1, V2, and/or V3

40 Hz   25.0 mm/s   10.0 mm/mV   4 by 2.5s + 3 rhythm lds   MACVU 003C   12SL™ v250

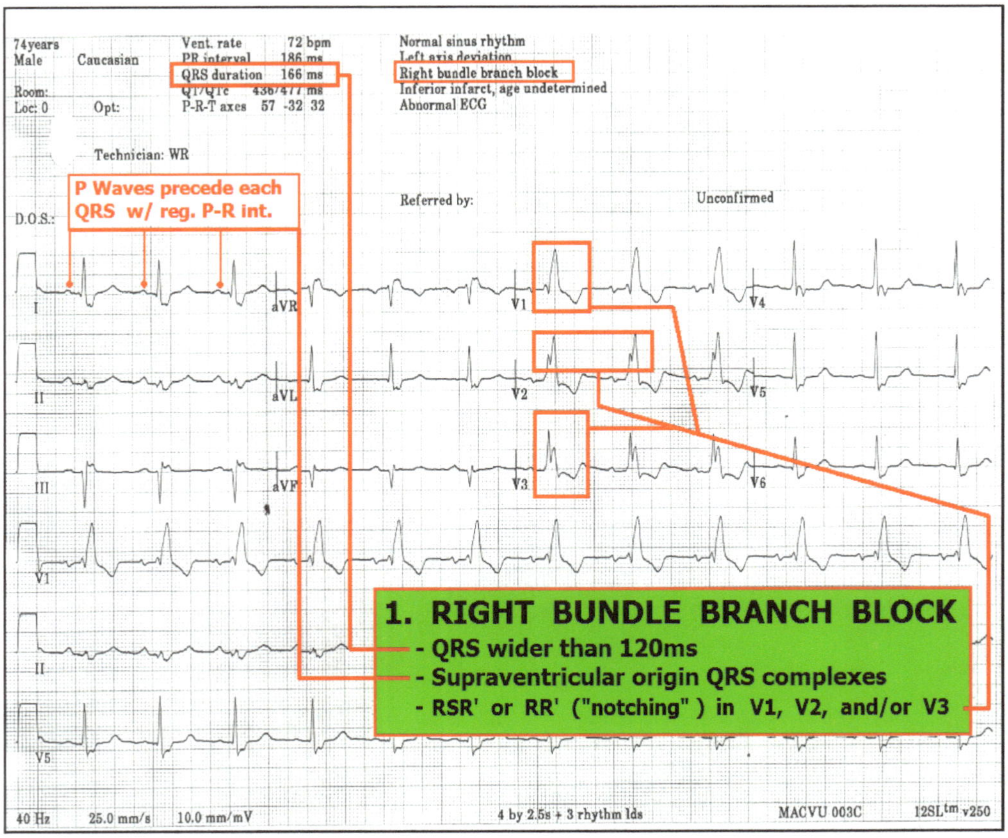

In the ECG to the left, we see that transition is VERY early...that it, the QRS complexes have already transitioned to "positive" *before* V1.

We also immediately note the QRS complexes are abnormally wide, greater than 120ms.

There are P waves preceding each QRS, with normal and consistent P-R intervals, letting us see there is a relationship between the atria and ventricles.

In V2 and V3, we see notching. When you add up the clues, they point to Right Bundle Branch Block, which is the cause of this patient's early transition.

In the ECG to the right, transition occurs between V1 and V2. Narrow QRS complexes are noted, ruling out RBBB as the cause. There are no signs of HYPERTROPHY or W-P-W.

We *do* note there are *significant Q waves* in leads III and aVF, which view the inferior wall of the left ventricle, indicating old inferior wall MI as a likely diagnosis.

Since the same arteries which supply the inferior wall also supply the posterior wall, it is very common to see posterior wall infarction together with inferior wall infarction, which is this patient's diagnosis.

ECG annotations (right ECG):

Male	Caucasian	Vent. rate	58 BPM	Sinus bradycardia
		PR interval	168 ms	Inferior-posterior infarct (cited on or before 27-APR-1997)
Room:CCU3		QRS duration	84 ms	Abnormal ECG
Loc:1	Option:1	QT/QTc	424/416 ms	When compared with ECG of 30-APR-1997 13:39,
		P-R-T axes	18 28 29	No significant change was found

Technician ID: EKG CLASS #WR03602216

Med: Unknown

2. OLD POSTERIOR WALL M.I.
- Usually accompanied by OLD INFERIOR WALL MI
- Does NOT abnormally widen the QRS complex

25mm/s   10mm/mV   100Hz   005C   12SL 4   CID: 5

In the ECG to the right, we note the positive R waves in V1 are larger than the negative S waves, which is an abnormal finding.

We also note the Lead I and V1 Axis is abnormal, a finding associated with RVH. (the QRS should be upright in I and negative in V1).

We also see abnormally tall P waves in Lead II and V1 (taller than 2mm), indicating Right Atrial Hypertrophy (RAH), and there is Right Axis Deviation.

These findings are all consistent with RVH, which is the patient's diagnosis.

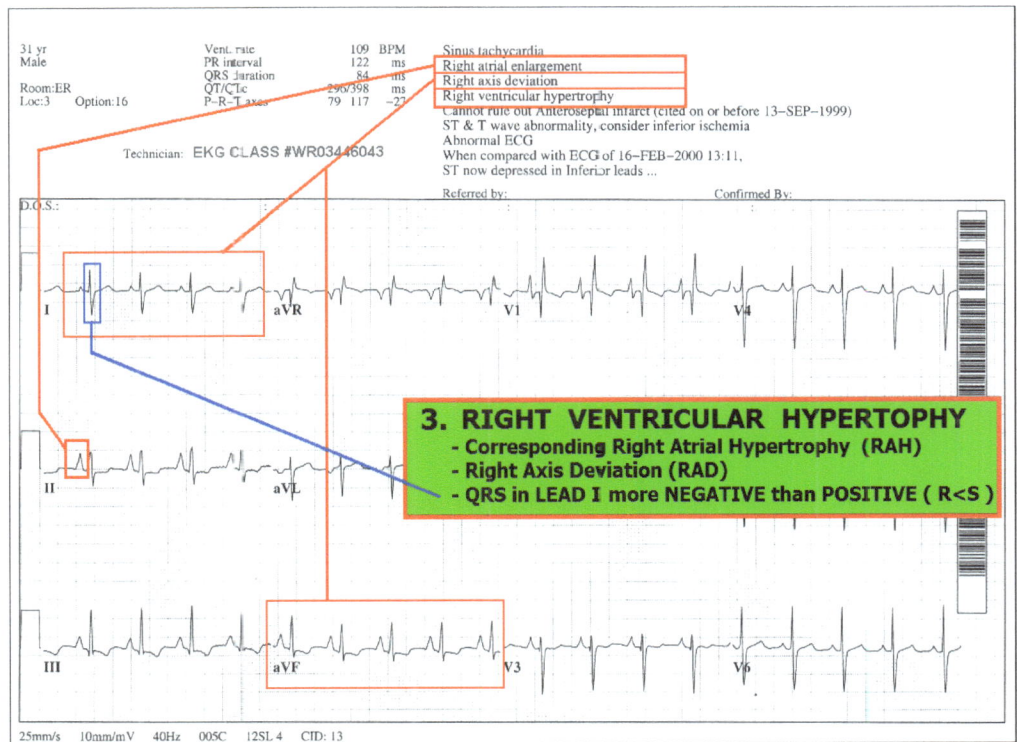

3. RIGHT VENTRICULAR HYPERTOPHY
- **Corresponding Right Atrial Hypertrophy (RAH)**
- **Right Axis Deviation (RAD)**
- **QRS in LEAD I more NEGATIVE than POSITIVE (R<S)**

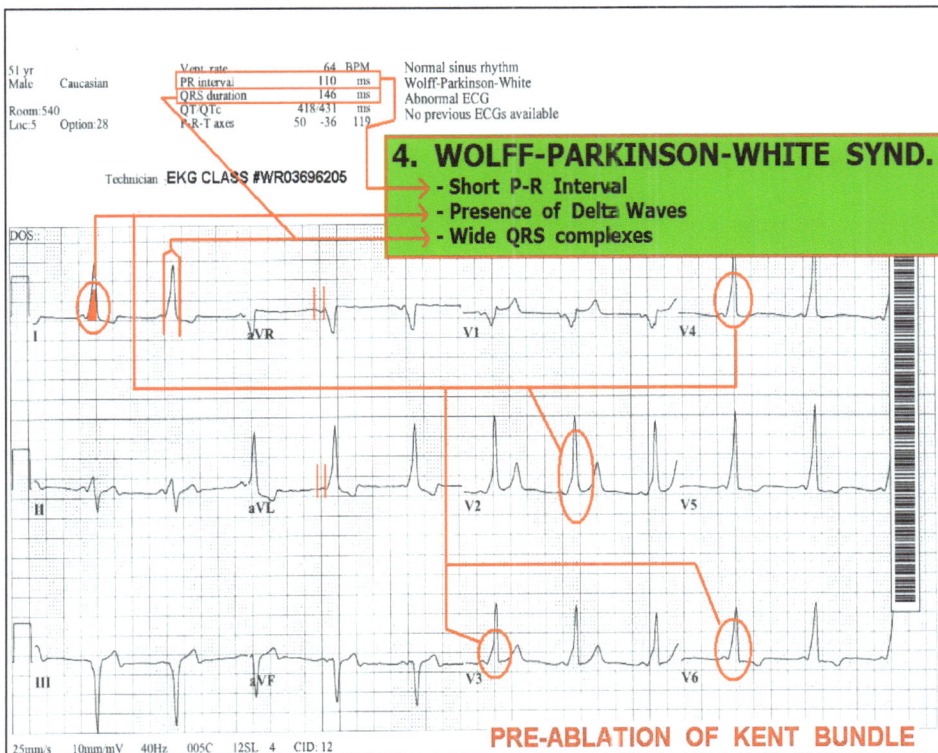

4. WOLFF-PARKINSON-WHITE SYND.
- **Short P-R Interval**
- **Presence of Delta Waves**
- **Wide QRS complexes**

PRE-ABLATION OF KENT BUNDLE

In the ECG to the left, transition occurs between leads V1 and V2. In fact, V2 is completely positive (only an R wave).

All the traditional indicators of Wolff-Parkinson-White (WPW) syndrome are present: *an abnormally short P-R interval* (less than 120ms), *delta waves,* and *abnormally wide QRS complexes* (>120ms). Delta waves are seen in the earliest segment of the QRS complex, when the bypass tract causes early depolarization of ventricular muscle at its point of insertion. Delta waves are characterized by "a visible change in the angulation of the first segment of the QRS complex." As you can see by the example in Lead I, the delta wave, shaded red, truly has a triangular "delta" shape.

Note the term, "Kent Bundle," used in the above ECG. In earlier ECG curricula, the term "Kent Bundle" was used to describe *bypass tracts.*

By now you may have noticed that the same conditions which cause *early transition* are the *inverse* of those which cause *late transition*. For example, *right bundle branch block* causes *early transition*; *left bundle branch block* causes *late transition*. *Old posterior wall M.I.* causes *early transition*; *old anterior wall M.I.* causes *late transition*, etc.

The next two pages contain ECGs with late transition, where the "clues" listed from the table below are used to identify the cause of late transition.

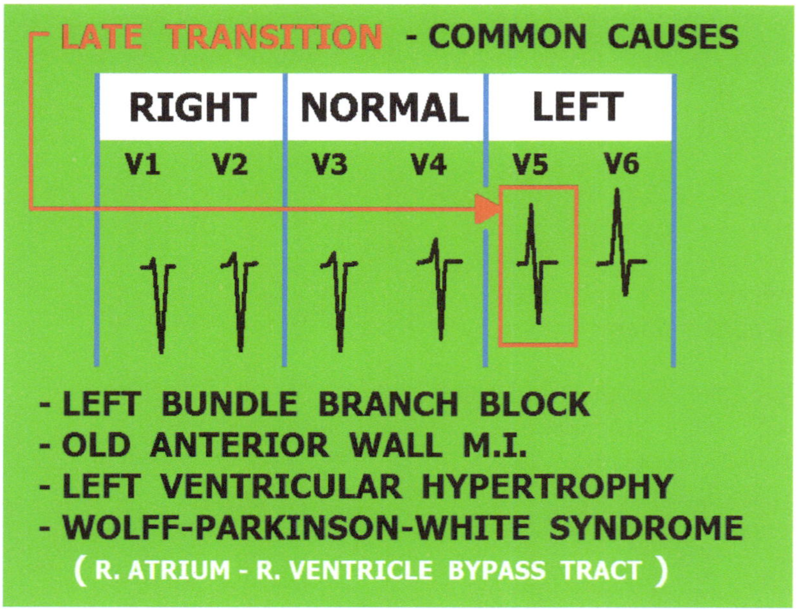

LATE TRANSITION - COMMON CAUSES

RIGHT	NORMAL	LEFT
V1 V2	V3 V4	V5 V6

- LEFT BUNDLE BRANCH BLOCK
- OLD ANTERIOR WALL M.I.
- LEFT VENTRICULAR HYPERTROPHY
- WOLFF-PARKINSON-WHITE SYNDROME
  (R. ATRIUM - R. VENTRICLE BYPASS TRACT)

COMMON CAUSES OF LATE TRANSITION
....SOME HELPFUL CLUES:

1. Left Bundle Branch Bock (LBBB)
- Supraventricular Rhythm
- QRS wider than 120 ms (.12 sec)
- RsR' or RR' ("notching") in V5 and/or V6

2. Old Anterior MI
- Q Waves in V1, V2, and /or V3
- Other causes of LATE TRANSITION ruled out

3. Left Ventricular Hypertrophy (LVH)
- Corresponding Left Atrial Hypertrophy (LAH)
- T wave Strain Pattern V5 / V6
- Intrinsicoid Deflection in V5 / V6 > 45 ms
- V1 S wave + V5 or V6 R wave > 35 mm
- R or S wave in any LIMB LEAD > 20mm

4. Wolff-Parkinson-White (Type B)
- Presence of DELTA waves
- Short P-R Interval (< 120 ms)
- Wide QRS (> 120 ms)

In the ECG to the right, we see that transition is late, occurring in V5.

We note the QRS complexes are abnormally wide, greater than 120ms.

There are P waves preceding each QRS, with normal and consistent P-R intervals, letting us see there is a relationship between the atria and ventricles.

In V5 and V6, we see notching. Admittedly, the notching is subtle, but it's there. This ECG shows "classic" Left Bundle Branch Block in a patient with no CAD or hypertrophy. Also note there is ST segment elevation in leads V1 to V3.

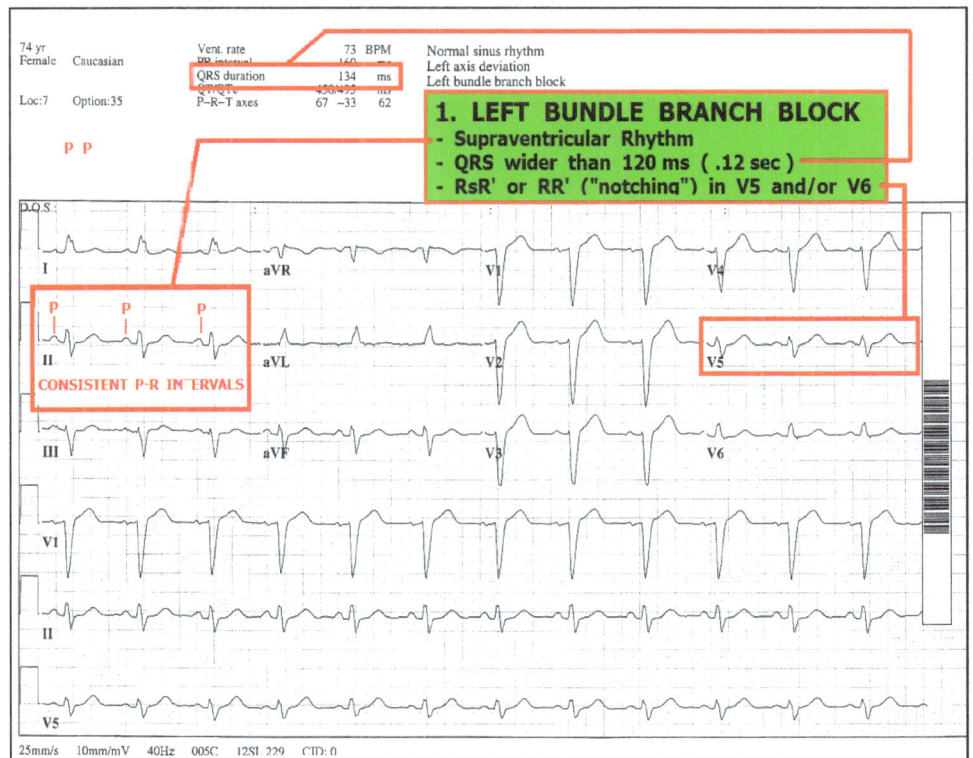

74 yr
Female   Caucasian

Loc:7   Option:35

Vent. rate	73	BPM
PR interval	160	
QRS duration	134	ms
QT/QTc	450/495	ms
P–R–T axes	67	–33	62

Normal sinus rhythm
Left axis deviation
Left bundle branch block

1. LEFT BUNDLE BRANCH BLOCK
- Supraventricular Rhythm
- QRS wider than 120 ms (.12 sec)
- RsR' or RR' ("notching") in V5 and/or V6

CONSISTENT P-R INTERVALS

25mm/s   10mm/mV   40Hz   005C   12SI 229   CID: 0

---

91 yr
Female   Caucasian

Room:3
Loc:1   Option:1

Vent. rate	87	BPM
PR interval	156	ms
QRS duration	80	ms
QT/QTc	332/399	ms
P–R–T axes	45	4	96

Normal sinus rhythm
Possible Anterior infarct
Abnormal ECG

Technician ID: EKG CLASS # WR03110848

2. OLD ANTERIOR WALL M.I.
- Q waves in V1, V2, V3 and/or V4
- other causes of LATE TRANSITION ruled out

25mm/s   10mm/mV   100Hz   005C   12SI 4   CID: 5

In the ECG to the left, transition occurs between V4 and V5. Narrow QRS complexes are noted, ruling out LBBB as the cause. There are no signs of HYPERTROPHY or W-P-W.

We *do* note QS complexes in V1 and V2, which view the anterior-septal wall of the left ventricle, indicating old septal wall MI as a likely diagnosis.

Even though there are no Q waves in V3 and V4, since transition occurs late, with Q waves seen in V1 – V2, and there are no other obvious causes of late transition (LBBB, hypertrophy and WPW are ruled out), old anterior wall MI should be suspected.

The first thing that you notice when you view the ECG to the right is that QRS complexes from one lead "spear through" QRS complexes from other leads. When this happens, it almost means ventricular hypertrophy is present.

Another clue is the presence of left atrial hypertrophy: the P waves in Lead II are abnormally large, and are negative in V1.

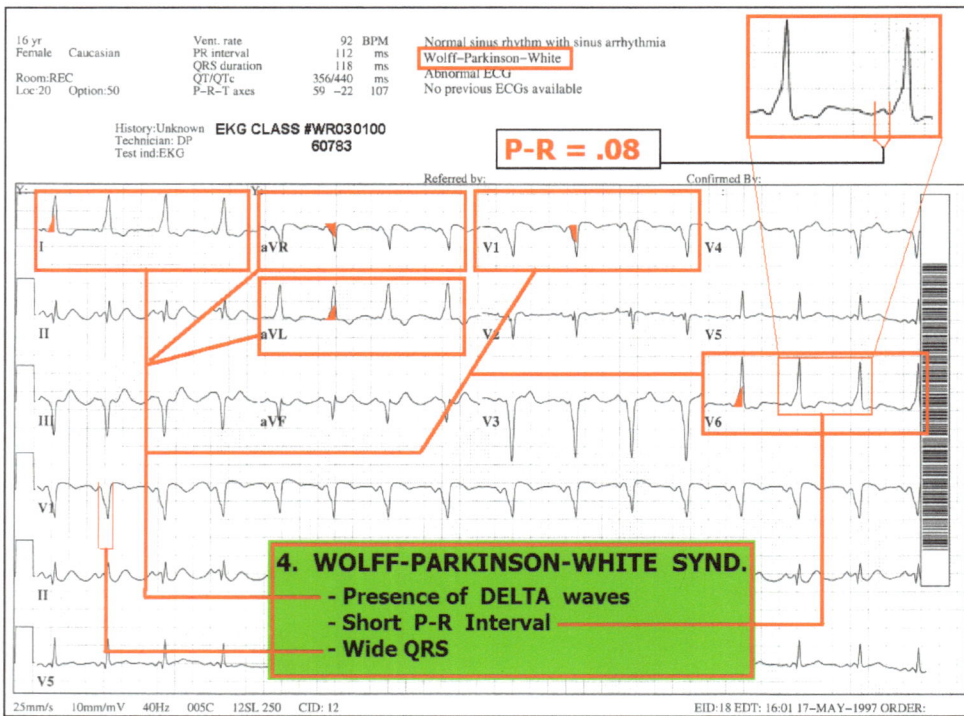

53 yr
Male

Room:ER
Loc.:3   Option:23

EKG CLASS #WR03896717

Vent. rate   115   BPM
PR interval   160   ms
QRS duration   92   ms
QT/QTc   316/437   ms
P–R–T axes   76 –39   59

**UNEDITED COPY – REPORT IS COMPUTER GENERATED ONLY. WITHOUT PHYSICIAN INTERPRETATION
Sinus tachycardia
Possible Left atrial enlargement
Left axis deviation
Left ventricular hypertrophy
Abnormal ECG
No previous ECGs available

S wave V1 = 14 mm
R wave V5 = 22 mm
TOTAL = 36 mm
= LVH

R-wave = 22 mm

3. LEFT VENTRICULAR HYPERTROPHY
- Corresponding Left Atrial Hypertrophy (LAH)
- T wave Strain Pattern V5 / V6
- Intrinsicoid Deflection in V5 / V6 > 45 ms
- V1 S wave + V5 or V6 R wave > 35 mm
- R or S wave in any LIMB LEAD > 2.0 mV (20 mm)

25mm/s   10mm/mV   40Hz   005C   I2SL 233   CID: 7   EID:28 EDT: 11:27   -NOV-   ORDER:

16 yr
Female   Caucasian

Room:REC
Loc:20   Option:50

History:Unknown   EKG CLASS #WR030100
Technician: DP   60783
Test ind:EKG

Vent. rate   92   BPM
PR interval   112   ms
QRS duration   118   ms
QT/QTc   356/440   ms
P–R–T axes   59 –22   107

Normal sinus rhythm with sinus arrhythmia
Wolff-Parkinson-White
Abnormal ECG
No previous ECGs available

P-R = .08

4. WOLFF-PARKINSON-WHITE SYND.
- Presence of DELTA waves
- Short P-R Interval
- Wide QRS

25mm/s   10mm/mV   40Hz   005C   12SL 250   CID: 12   EID:18 EDT: 16:01 17-MAY-1997 ORDER:

In the ECG to the left, transition occurs between leads V4 and V5.

All the traditional indicators of Wolff-Parkinson-White (WPW) syndrome are present: *an abnormally short P-R interval* (less than 120ms), *delta waves,* and *abnormally wide QRS complexes* (>120ms). Note that delta waves can be seen in leads with negative QRS deflections as well as those with positive deflections.

Note the patient's age of 16. Many WPW patients with non-concealed WPW are discovered when the patient has a "routine" ECG performed, such as during a comprehensive physical exam.

Many WPW patients experience episodes of tachycardia, some with very high rates. This young lady had episodes of SVT with rates of 280. After ablation of the bypass tract, her 12 lead ECG became normal.

ECG EVALUATION - A STRUCTURED APPROACH

A structured approach to ECG evaluation simply means that you follow an organized checklist of things to evaluate when you read an ECG.

Employing such methodology helps you to stay focused, and reduces the likelihood that you'll miss something significant. In the practice of ECG interpretation, the most subtle abnormality can be the only clue that your patient suffers from a life-threatening condition, and if overlooked, can have catastrophic results. The traditional format for reviewing ECGs, presented in numerous textbooks, is shown in the diagram to the right:

☞ ECG EVALUATION
THE TRADITIONAL FORMAT

- **RATE**
  - ☐ BRADY, NORMAL, or TACHY
  - ☐ HOW WILL RATE EFFECT PT'S HEMODYNAMIC STATUS?
- **RHYTHM**
  - ☐ REGULAR, IRREGULAR, or IRREGULARLY IRREGULAR
  - ☐ IDENTIFY FOCUS: SINUS, JUNCTIONAL, or VENTRICULAR
  - ☐ IDENTIFY RHYTHM: (SR, A-FIB, FLUTTER, HEART BLOCK, etc.)
- **AXIS**
  - ☐ DEVIATION: NORMAL, LEFT, RIGHT, FAR RIGHT
  - ☐ ROTATION: SHIFT TO L or R
- **HYPERTROPHY**
  - ☐ ATRIAL: R and/or L
  - ☐ VENTRICULAR
  - ☐ CONSIDER CAUSE OF HYPERTROPHY (VAVLE DISORDERS, PULONARY DISEASE, HYPERTENSION, CONGENITAL DEFECTS)
- **ISCHEMIA / INFARCTION / NECROSIS**
  - ☐ INDENTIFY AREA OF HEART INVOLVED
  - ☐ CONSIDER COMMON ARTERIES THAT SERVE EFFECTED AREA
  - ☐ ANTICIPATE FAILURES OF ASSO. STRUCTURES / ACTION PLAN !

As a new paramedic in the early 1980s, I carried a small laminated card imprinted with this "traditional" ECG checklist. Following it helped me to stay focused, especially when reading the complicated ECGs of patients with multiple cardiac abnormalities.

☞ ECG EVALUATION
EMERGENT "CATH LAB" APPROACH

- **RATE**
  - ☐ BRADY, NORMAL, or TACHY ? (PACE / CARDIOVERT)
  - ☐ HOW WILL RATE EFFECT PT'S HEMODYNAMIC STATUS ?

- **QRS WIDTH**
  - ☐ PACEMAKER RHYTHM (USELESS FOR STEMI / ISCHEMIA EVAL.)
  - ☐ LBBB (NEW LBBB vs. PREVIOUSLY DIAGNOSED ? - LOW EF ?)
  - ☐ VENTRICULAR RHYTHM ? (V-TACH: MONO or POLYMORPHIC)
  - ☐ DELTA WAVES ?!? (W-P-W: NO AV NODAL BLOCKERS !!!!)
  - ☐ ACUTE HYPERKALEMIA ? (TALL, PEAKED T WAVES)
  - ☐ PROLONGED Q-T INTERVAL ?
  - ☐ BRUGADA SYNDROME ? (RBBB, V1-V3 "TRIANGULAR" S-T ELEV.)

- **ISCHEMIA / INFARCTION / NECROSIS**
  (EVALUATION of J POINT, S-T SEGMENTS, T WAVES)
  - ☐ IDENTIFY AREA OF HEART INVOLVED
  - ☐ IDENTITY SUSPECTED "CULPRIT" ARTERY
  - ☐ CONSIDER SIZE OF MI (CARDIOGENIC SHOCK ?)
  - ☐ ANTICIPATE FAILURE OF ASSOCIATED STRUCTURES
  - ☐ SIGNIFICANT Q WAVES ? - OLD MI vs. CURRENT EVOLVING MI

- **AXIS**
  - ☐ ROTATION: LATE R WAVE PROGRESSION - OLD ANTERIOR MI ?
    EARLY R WAVE PROGR. - OLD POSTERIOR MI ?

- **then CONTINUE WITH TRADITIONAL FORMAT . . .**

After a decade of working in a fast-paced, high-volume interventional cardiac catheterization and electrophysiology lab, I realized my "structured approach" to evaluating ECGs had evolved from the "traditional" format, to what I call the "emergent cath lab approach," which is featured in the diagram to the left. Using this approach," the clinician quickly zooms in on *conditions that are imminently life-threatening*."

The basic philosophy to this approach is once you have ruled out conditions that are imminently life-threatening, you have time to perform a careful, more thorough evaluation, and focus on non-emergent conditions.

THE COMPUTER-DERIVED DIAGNOSIS

DO NOT accept the ECG computer-derived diagnosis at face value. If you read the computer generated interpretation, you must perform a *line-by-line validation* of each diagnosis listed – and then look for ones it missed.

While ECG interpretation software continues to improve, accepting these diagnoses as accurate without validating it for yourself could be a mortal mistake for your patient, as demonstrated in the examples featured on the next two pages. Each of the example ECGs have enough clues present for a competent ECG interpreter to correctly diagnose each disorder.

(If you've ever been "burned" by the ECG computer, you'll quickly learn to think of it like the nasty little fellow in the diagram to the right)!

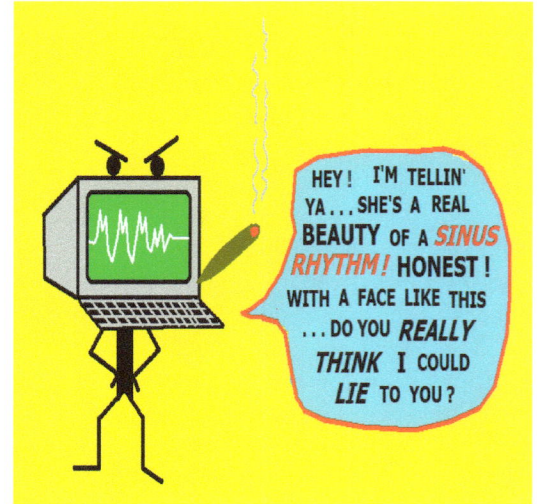

COMPUTER MISDIAGNOSIS of ECGs:

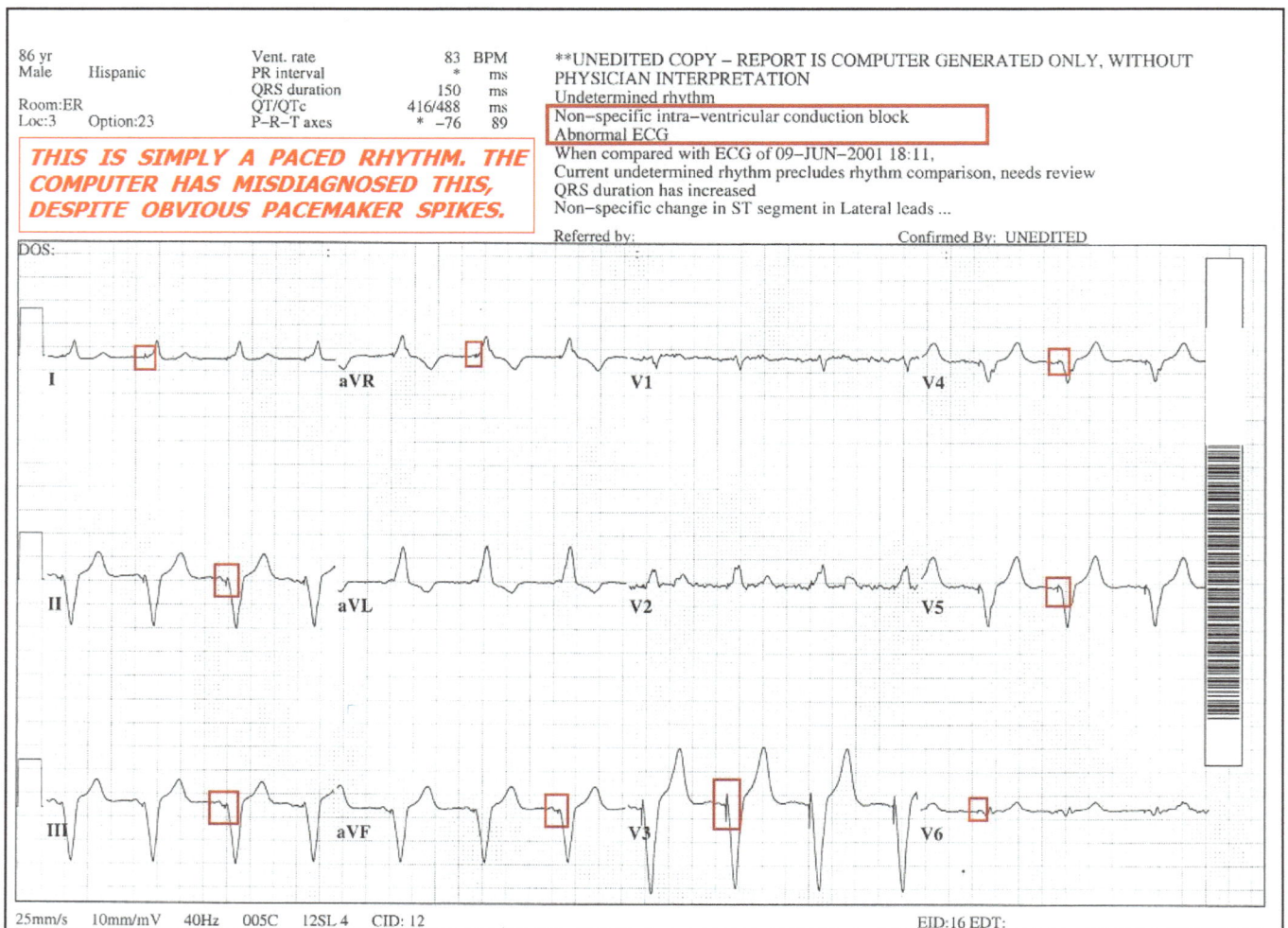

86 yr		Vent. rate	83	BPM
Male	Hispanic	PR interval	*	ms
		QRS duration	150	ms
Room:ER		QT/QTc	416/488	ms
Loc:3	Option:23	P–R–T axes	* –76	89

**UNEDITED COPY – REPORT IS COMPUTER GENERATED ONLY, WITHOUT PHYSICIAN INTERPRETATION
Undetermined rhythm
Non–specific intra–ventricular conduction block
Abnormal ECG
When compared with ECG of 09–JUN–2001 18:11,
Current undetermined rhythm precludes rhythm comparison, needs review
QRS duration has increased
Non–specific change in ST segment in Lateral leads ...

Referred by: Confirmed By: UNEDITED

THIS IS SIMPLY A PACED RHYTHM. THE COMPUTER HAS MISDIAGNOSED THIS, DESPITE OBVIOUS PACEMAKER SPIKES.

25mm/s   10mm/mV   40Hz   005C   12SL 4   CID: 12   EID:16 EDT:

COMPUTER MISDIAGNOSES OF ECGs:

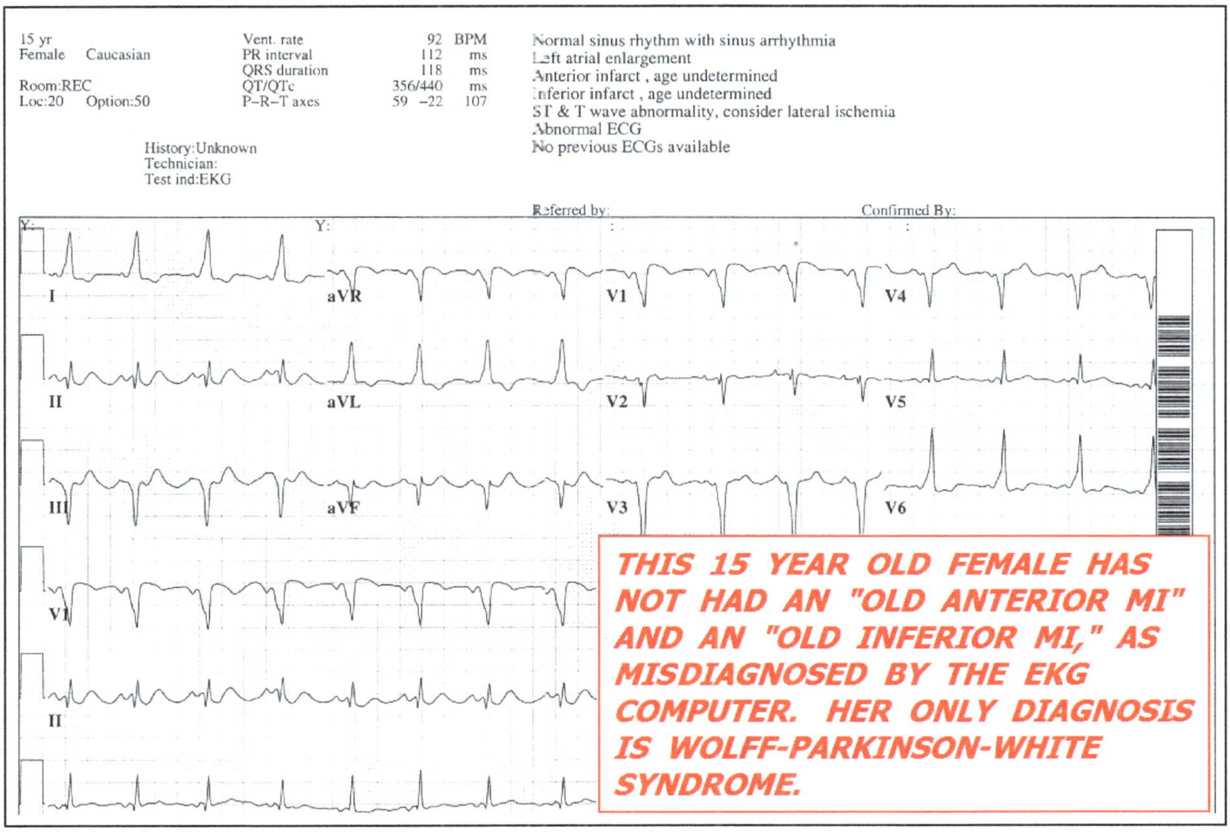

15 yr
Female Caucasian
Room:REC
Loc:20 Option:50
Vent. rate 92 BPM
PR interval 112 ms
QRS duration 118 ms
QT/QTc 356/440 ms
P-R-T axes 59 -22 107
Normal sinus rhythm with sinus arrhythmia
Left atrial enlargement
Anterior infarct , age undetermined
Inferior infarct , age undetermined
ST & T wave abnormality, consider lateral ischemia
Abnormal ECG
No previous ECGs available
History:Unknown
Technician:
Test ind:EKG
Referred by:
Confirmed By:
I
aVR
V1
V4
II
aVL
V2
V5
III
aVF
V3
V6
V1
II
THIS 15 YEAR OLD FEMALE HAS NOT HAD AN "OLD ANTERIOR MI" AND AN "OLD INFERIOR MI," AS MISDIAGNOSED BY THE EKG COMPUTER. HER ONLY DIAGNOSIS IS WOLFF-PARKINSON-WHITE SYNDROME.

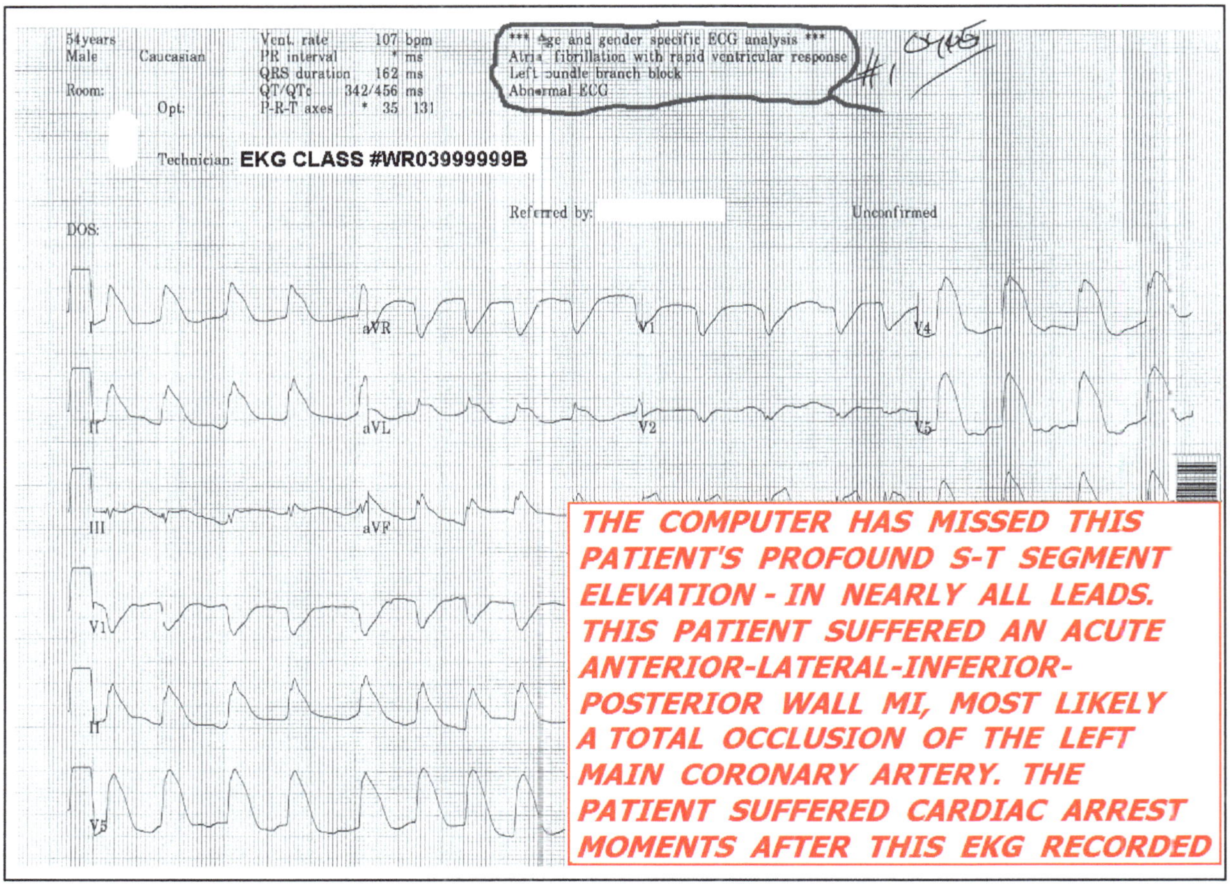

54years
Male Caucasian
Room:
Opt:
Vent. rate 107 bpm
PR interval * ms
QRS duration 162 ms
QT/QTc 342/456 ms
P-R-T axes * 35 131
*** Age and gender specific ECG analysis ***
Atrial fibrillation with rapid ventricular response
Left bundle branch block
Abnormal ECG
#1
Technician: EKG CLASS #WR03999999B
Referred by:
Unconfirmed
DOS:
I
aVR
V1
V4
II
aVL
V2
V5
III
aVF
V1
II
V5
THE COMPUTER HAS MISSED THIS PATIENT'S PROFOUND S-T SEGMENT ELEVATION - IN NEARLY ALL LEADS. THIS PATIENT SUFFERED AN ACUTE ANTERIOR-LATERAL-INFERIOR-POSTERIOR WALL MI, MOST LIKELY A TOTAL OCCLUSION OF THE LEFT MAIN CORONARY ARTERY. THE PATIENT SUFFERED CARDIAC ARREST MOMENTS AFTER THIS EKG RECORDED

☞ REVIEW QUESTIONS:

REINFORCE YOUR KNOWLEDGE OF ESSENTIAL CONCEPTS:

(Review questions originate from highlighted text and graphic images)

Basic Concepts of 12 Lead ECG Interpretation

40 yr	Vent. rate	64	BPM
Male	PR interval	130	ms
	QRS duration	96	ms
Room:ER	QT/QTc	396/408	ms
	P–R–T axes	40 11	61

For question 15 through 20, refer to the ECG to the right.

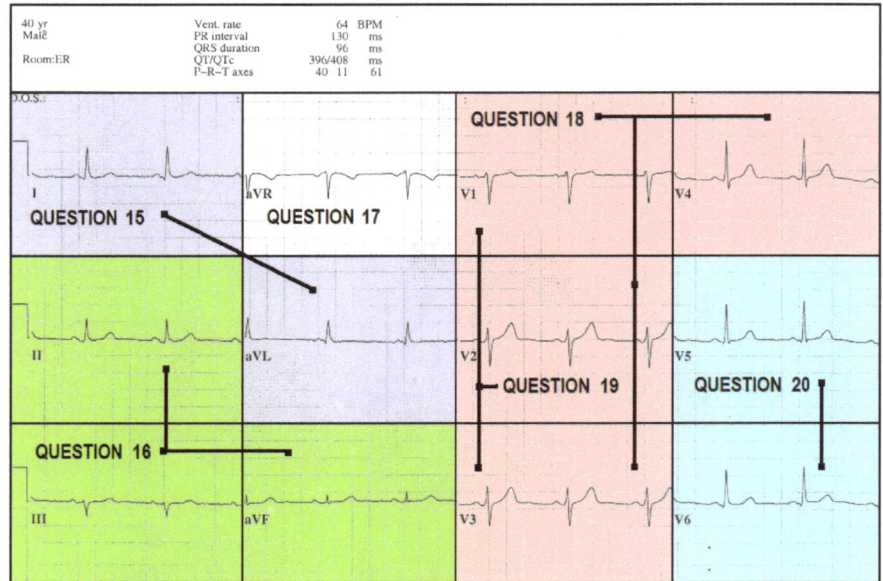

QUESTION 18
QUESTION 15
QUESTION 17
QUESTION 16
QUESTION 19
QUESTION 20

I   aVR   V1   V4
II   aVL   V2   V5
III   aVF   V3   V6

15. (p. 40) The region of the heart viewed by ECG leads I and aVL (shaded purple) can be supplied by arteries that branch off of the *left anterior descending* or *circumflex arteries,,* or a *ramus artery* that branches off of the Left Main Coronary Artery.
    a. True
    b. False

16. (p. 40) Leads II, III, and aVF (shaded green) view the _____ of the left ventricle, which receives its blood supply from the _____.
    a. anterior wall: left anterior descending artery
    b. posterior wall: right coronary artery or circumflex artery
    c. lateral wall: circumflex artery
    d. inferior wall: right coronary artery or circumflex artery

17. (p. 42) Lead aVR views the *basilar septum*, and receives its blood supply from the large *first septal perforator* which arises off of the *proximal left anterior descending artery (LAD)*. When ST segment elevation is seen in Lead aVR in acute MI, it is associated with blockage of the proximal LAD, and in some cases, the LMCA, and results in _____.
    a. extensive anterior-septal wall MI
    b. inferior-posterior wall MI
    c. lateral wall MI
    d. right ventricular wall MI

18. (p. 41) Leads V1 – V4 (shaded pink) view the _____ wall of the left ventricle, which receives its blood supply from the _____.
    a. anterior wall: left anterior descending artery
    b. posterior wall: right coronary artery or circumflex artery
    c. lateral wall: circumflex artery
    d. inferior wall: right coronary artery or circumflex artery

19. (p. 41) Leads V1 – V3 also view the _____ wall of the left ventricle via ***reciprocal changes***.
  a. anterior
  b. posterior
  c. lateral
  d. inferior

20. (p. 42) Leads V5 and V6 (shaded light blue) view the _____ wall of the left ventricle.
  a. anterior
  b. posterior
  c. lateral
  d. inferior

21. (p. 42) Leads II, III, and aVF view the region of the heart supplied by the _____ artery in 75-80% of the population, and the _____ artery in 10-15% of the population.
  a. right coronary, circumflex
  b. left anterior descending, diagonal
  c. first septal perforator, inferior
  d. circumflex, ramus

22. (p. 43) The standard 12 Lead ECG has two significant "blind spots," which are the:
  a. right ventricle and left ventricle
  b. anterior wall and posterior wall
  c. posterior wall and right ventricle
  d. lateral wall and posterior wall

23. (p. 46) Indications for obtaining an 18 lead ECG are any time there is ST elevation in the inferior leads (II, III, and aVF), and/or ST depression in the anterior leads (V1-V4).
  a. True
  b. False

24. (p. 49) The P-R interval should not be shorter than _____ ms or longer than _____ ms.
  a. 100, 400
  b. 120, 200
  c. 150, 300
  d. 120, 280

25. (p. 51) When QRS complexes are wider than _____ms, J Points, ST segments and T waves can become altered, making them unreliable for evaluating the presence of ischemia and infarction.
  a. 80
  b. 100
  c 110
  d. 120

26. (p. 56) Small Q waves are normally seen in some leads. As a general rule, Q waves should not be wider than 40ms (1mm on standard ECG). Regarding Q wave amplitude (vertical height), it should not be larger than 1/3 the size of the R wave.
  a. True
  b. False

27. (p. 56) Q waves can be any size in leads _____ and _____, and be considered normal.
  a. II and V6
  b. III and aVR
  c. I and V1
  d. I and aVF

28. (p. 56) No Q waves, of any size, should ever be seen in leads ____, _____, and _____.
    a. V1, V2, and V3
    b. aVR, aVL, aVF
    c. II, III, and aVF
    d. V4, V5, and V6

29. (p. 57) If the QRS complexes are of normal width, we must evaluate the J Point, _____, and T wave in every lead to evaluate for the presence of myocardial ischemia and infarction.
    a. P wave
    b. U wave
    c. P-R interval
    d. ST segment

For questions 30 and 31, refer to the images to the right.

IMAGE A

ST SEGMENT

IMAGE B

ST SEGMENT

30. (p. 59) The ST Segment in IMAGE A is an example of:
    a. a concave ST segment, which is normal
    b. a convex ST segment, which can be seen in the early phase of Acute MI, before the J point elevates
    c. a depressed ST segment, which could indicate ischemia
    d. a down-sloping ST segment, which could indicate ischemia

31. (p. 59) The ST Segment in IMAGE B is an example of:
    a. a concave ST segment, which is normal
    b. a convex ST segment, which can be seen in the early phase of Acute MI, before the J point elevates
    c. a depressed ST segment, which could indicate ischemia
    d. a down-sloping ST segment, which could indicate ischemia

32. (p. 65) Common causes of hyperacute T waves include: hyperkalemia, _____, transmural ischemia and hypertrophy.
    a. pericarditis
    b. alcohol intoxication
    c. diabetic ketoacidosis
    d. acute myocardial infarction

33. (p. 66) The "Quick Peek Method" for checking the Q-T Interval states that for heart rates between 60 – 100, the Q-T Interval should be less than_____.
    a. 1/3 the size of the QRS complex
    b. half of the R-R Interval
    c. ¼ the size of the patient's P-R Interval
    d. half the patient's heart rate divided by the width of the QRS complex, in millimeters

34. (p. 67) Prolonged Q-T Intervals can cause _____, which is a potentially lethal dysrhythmia for which A.H.A. ACLS advocates the use of Magnesium Sulfate to treat.
   a. asystole
   b. atrial fibrillation
   c. Torsades de Pointes
   d. sinus tachycardia

35. (p. 69, 71) _____ causes ST segments to be elevated continuously, making it difficult to diagnose STEMI.
   a. Left Bundle Branch Block
   b. Right Bundle Branch Block
   c. 2nd Degree Type II Heart Block
   d. H&R Block

36. (p. 69, 71) _____ causes ST depression and T wave inversion in the anterior precordial leads, making it difficult to diagnose myocardial ischemia.
   a. Left Bundle Branch Block
   b. Right Bundle Branch Block
   c. 2nd Degree Type II Heart Block
   d. H&R Block

For test questions
37 – 39
refer to
PRACTICE ECG 1

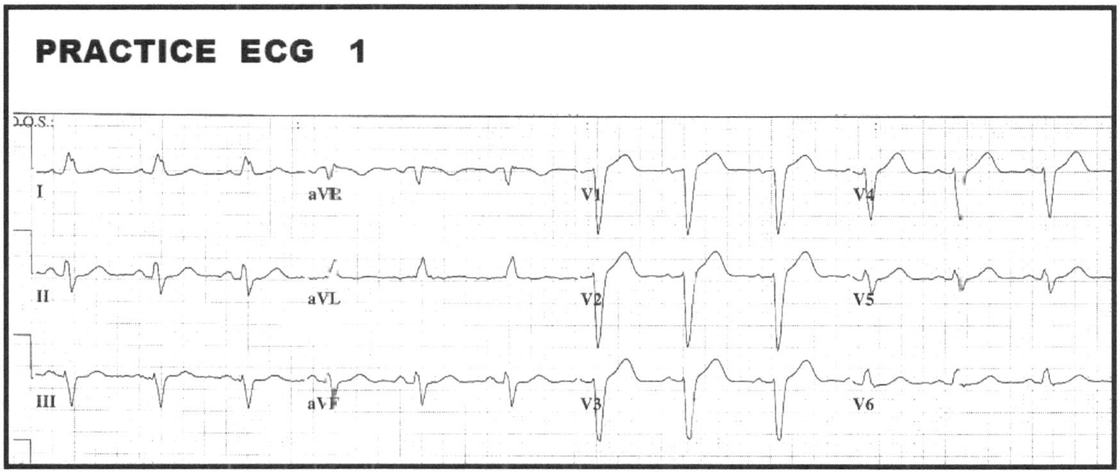

PRACTICE ECG 1

37. (p. 70-71) The cause of this patient's wide QRS complexes is:
   a. Right Bundle Branch Block
   b. Left Bundle Branch Block
   c. Ventricular Escape Rhythm
   d. Wolff-Parkinson-White Syndrome

38. (p. 72) Regarding the vertical axis, this patient's ECG shows _____.
   a. a normal axis
   b. Left Axis Deviation
   c. Right Axis Deviation
   d. Far Right, or "No Man's Land" Axis Deviation

39. (p. 77) Regarding assessment of the horizontal axis, (or "R wave progression), transition occurs in Lead_____ and which means the horizontal axis is _____.
   a. V1 or V2: shifted to the right, or is "early."
   b. V3 or V4: normal
   c. V5 or V6: shifted to the left, or is "late."
   d. I'm truly LOST and I DON'T KNOW.

For test questions 40 – 42, refer to PRACTICE ECG 2

PRACTICE ECG 2

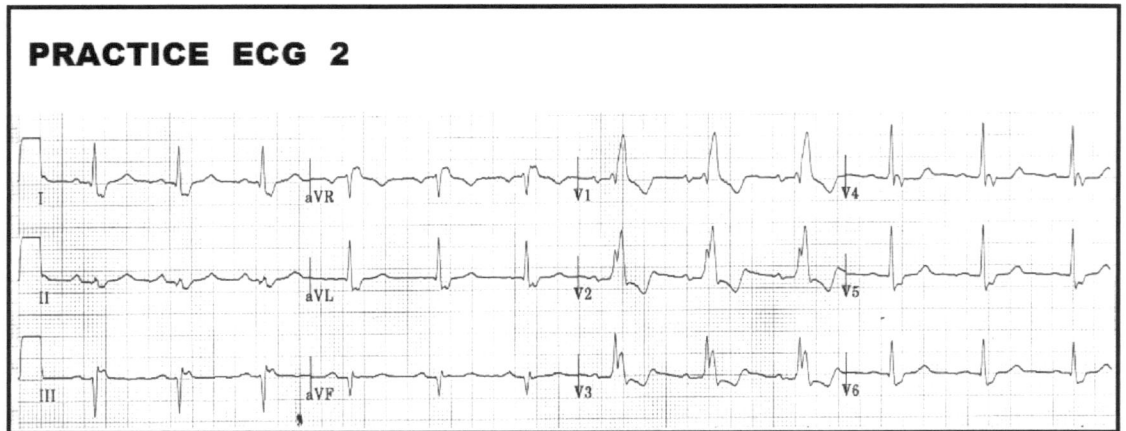

40. (p. 70-71) The cause of this patient's wide QRS complexes is:
   a. Right Bundle Branch Block
   b. Left Bundle Branch Block
   c. Ventricular Escape Rhythm
   d. Wolff-Parkinson-White Syndrome

41. (p. 72) Regarding the vertical axis, this patient's ECG shows _____.
   a. a normal axis
   b. Left Axis Deviation
   c. Right Axis Deviation
   d. Far Right, or "No Man's Land" Axis Deviation

42. (p. 77) Regarding assessment of the horizontal axis, (or "R wave progression), transition occurs in Lead_____, which means the horizontal axis is _____.
   a. before Lead V1: shifted to the right, or is "early."
   b. V3 or V4: normal
   c. after Lead V6: shifted to the left, or is "late."
   d. I've had enough of this. I want to take the rest of the day off!

43. (p. 78) The four most common causes of Abnormal R Wave Progression are:
   a. Bundle Branch Blocks
   b. _____
   c. Ventricular Hypertrophy
   d. Wolff-Parkinson-White Syndrome

      1. Old Anterior or Posterior Wall MI
      2. Atrial Hypertrophy
      3. AV Nodal Blocks
      4. Long Q-T Syndrome

92

PATIENT ASSESSMENT - PHASE I:

RULE OUT LIFE-THREATENING CONDITIONS:

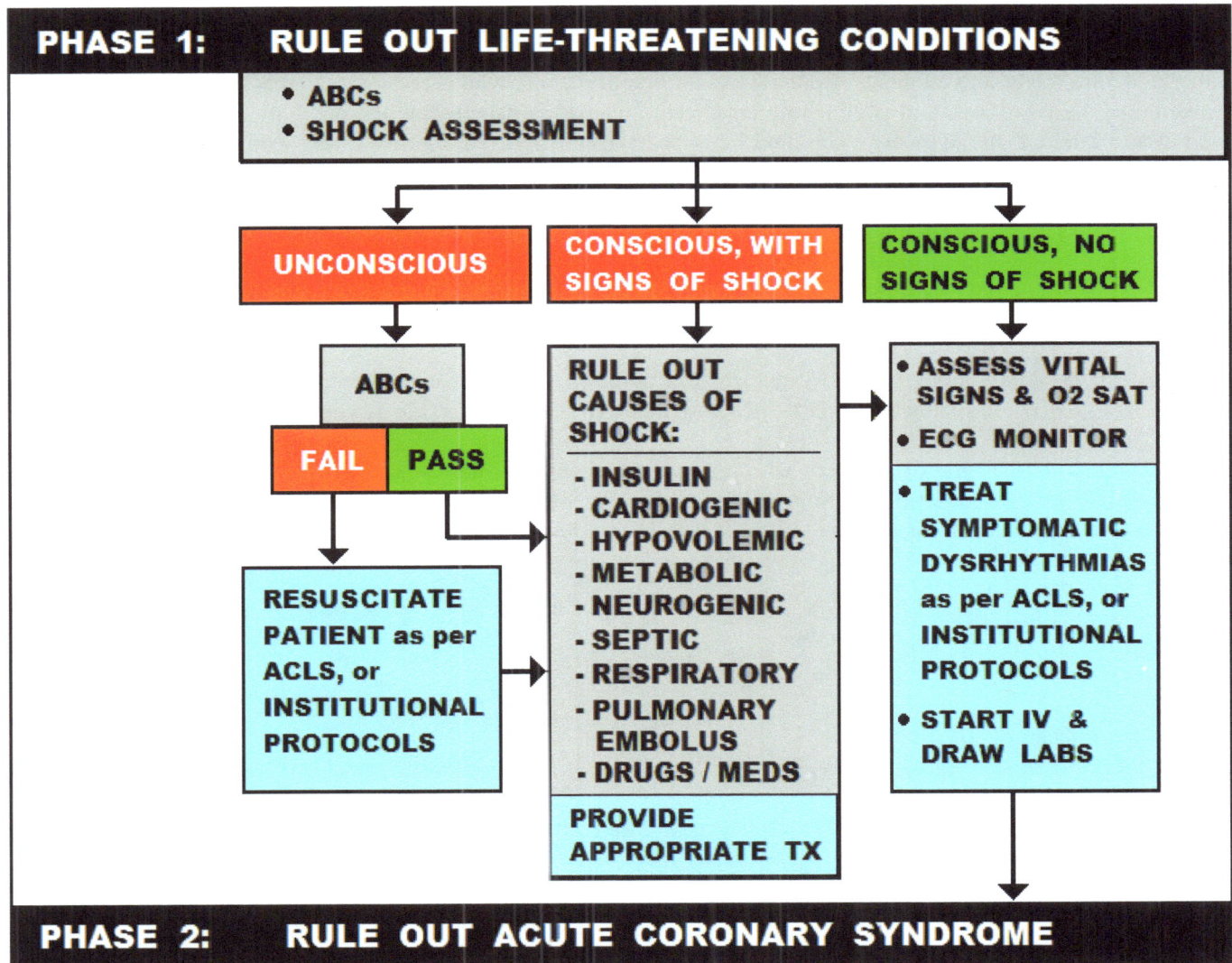

PHASE 1:   RULE OUT LIFE-THREATENING CONDITIONS

- ABCs
- SHOCK ASSESSMENT

UNCONSCIOUS

CONSCIOUS, WITH SIGNS OF SHOCK

CONSCIOUS, NO SIGNS OF SHOCK

ABCs

FAIL   **PASS**

RESUSCITATE PATIENT as per ACLS, or INSTITUTIONAL PROTOCOLS

RULE OUT CAUSES OF SHOCK:

- INSULIN
- CARDIOGENIC
- HYPOVOLEMIC
- METABOLIC
- NEUROGENIC
- SEPTIC
- RESPIRATORY
- PULMONARY EMBOLUS
- DRUGS / MEDS

PROVIDE APPROPRIATE TX

- ASSESS VITAL SIGNS & O2 SAT
- ECG MONITOR

- TREAT SYMPTOMATIC DYSRHYTHMIAS as per ACLS, or INSTITUTIONAL PROTOCOLS
- START IV & DRAW LABS

PHASE 2:   RULE OUT ACUTE CORONARY SYNDROME

Phase one begins the moment you make visual contact with the patient. The phase one assessment should take less than a minute to complete, unless the need to provide life-saving treatment interrupts the process.

The phase one assessment consists of:

ABCs
Shock Assessment
Vital signs and SAO2
ECG monitor – determine heart rhythm

THE ABCs and SHOCK ASSESSMENT are usually conducted concurrently, because in most cases, you complete both evaluations simultaneously before you reach the patient's side. Here are two examples:

You walk into the patient's room. As you proceed through the doorway, you see your patient sitting up in his bed, which is located across the room. He looks at you and nods, acknowledging your presence. As you approach, you note he appears calm and alert. His skin color is normal; he does not appear diaphoretic, and his breathing is unlabored. From these observations, you determine the ABCs and shock assessment are complete: the patient's airway is open, he is breathing adequately, he has a pulse, and he is not currently exhibiting signs of inadequate tissue perfusion (shock).

In the second scenario, you make visual contact with your patient, who is conscious and is sitting upright. You also notice he is restless, and is clutching his chest. His skin is pale, ashen and diaphoretic. His breathing is rapid and labored; his eyes are wide, and he appears frightened. Experience tells you that the ABCs are currently present, and that your patient is probably in shock. You know you must work rapidly to determine the cause of shock and intervene before his condition deteriorates further. When you arrive at his bedside, you touch his skin; it is cold and clammy.

In both examples, you have completed the ABCs and Shock Assessment in just a few seconds – *the amount of time it took you to walk across the room and reach the patient's side.*

In the case of an unconscious patient, visualize skin color as you approach. When you reach the patient's side, manually assess the ABCs. Pay attention to the temperature of the patient's skin as you proceed.

When you reach the bedside of a patient who meets the criteria for shock -- *pale, ashen skin, anxious or lethargic behavior*, and *rapid or labored breathing* -- touch the patient's forehead with the back of your hand to assess temperature, and then check for a radial pulse. If the *skin is abnormally cool*, and the *radial pulse quality is poor or absent*, the patient is in a state of shock, or hypo-perfusion. At this point, action must be quickly taken to *identify the cause* and *initiate therapeutic intervention.*

The visual indicators of shock, listed in the table to the right, are triggered by the release of epinephrine and norepinephrine, which result in *accelerated heart* and *respiratory rates*, peripheral vaso-constriction (*cool, pale, diaphoretic skin*), and in the early stages of shock, *restlessness and anxiety.** As cerebral perfusion decreases, the patient's level of consciousness decreases to lethargy, and eventually, unconsciousness.

SHOCK ASSESSMENT

LOC:	ANXIOUS RESTLESS LETHARGIC UNCONSCIOUS		AWAKE ALERT & ORIENTED
SKIN:	PALE / ASHEN CYANOTIC COOL DIAPHORETIC		NORMAL HUE WARM DRY
BREATHING:	TACHYPNEA		NORMAL
PULSE:	WEAK / THREADY TOO FAST or SLOW		STRONG
STATUS:	💣 SHOCK 💣		NORMAL

* One notable exception to this rule is *spinal shock*, which results in autonomic system dysreflexia; patients in spinal shock do not typically display pale, clammy, diaphoretic skin or elevated heart rates.

Think of shock as "the corridor to death," because everyone who dies goes through shock to get there. Granted, for those who suffer mortal injuries, the period of shock may be very brief and irreversible. When a patient is found to be in shock, it is our job to find the cause and reverse it: *we must reach into the corridor to death and pull the patient back.*

Conversely, when a patient is alert, relaxed, with warm, dry skin, and is breathing normally, the patient is rarely in shock. Of course, lack of shock-like signs and symptoms does not mean that no lethal conditions exist; it just means that at the moment, the patient is stable.

ASSESS VITAL SIGNS, and SAO2:

(Delegate this task to another team member while you proceed to ECG monitoring)

Obtain the patient's *blood pressure, palpable pulse* and *respiratory rates,* and *oxygen saturation.*

☞ If your patient is *unconscious, presents with signs of shock,* and/or has *verbalized complaints that could be of cardiac origin,* ECG monitoring should be implemented immediately to determine if any dysrhythmias are present.

IMPLEMENT CONTINUOUS ECG, ETCO2 and SAO2 MONITORING:

The primary goal of ECG monitoring is to determine the presence of:

> **Potentially lethal heart rhythms,** such as *ventricular tachycardia, Torsades de pointes, high grade heart blocks,* etc.
> **Ventricular heart rates *too fast* or *too slow*** to maintain hemodynamic stability. A general guideline is whenever ventricular rates are *LESS THAN 50* or *GREATER THAN 150,* and signs of shock are present, consider *ventricular heart rate* as a probable cause.

Follow American Heart Association's *Advanced Cardiac Life Support* (ACLS) guidelines, or your institutions protocols to treat potentially lethal heart rhythms, and/or correct ventricular heart rates which are too fast or too slow to maintain hemodynamic stability.

☞ Remember that end-title CO2 (ETCO2) values reflect immediate changes to your patient's ventilatory status. If you patient stops breathing, the ETCO2 value will immediately drop, while your patient's oxygen saturation value may remain "normal" for up to a minute or more.

START IV and DRAW LAB SAMPLES:

(Delegate this task to another team member – while you continue on to Phase Two assessment; *Ruling out Acute Coronary Syndrome*)

The IV should be started above the hand veins. For example, it is recommended for the administration of IV Adenosine, an antecubital IV site, (or a central intravenous line), should be used. For suspected AMI patients, use a 3-way adapter, and consider a 2^(nd) IV line, time permitting.

For suspected cardiac patients, obtain the following STAT lab assays:
   Cardiac markers (Troponin I, T, or Troponin I ultra) and/or (CK, CK-MB)
   Basic metabolic (electrolyte) panel (BMP)
   Magnesium (Mg++) level (unless included in electrolyte panel)
   Complete blood count (CBC)
   B-type Natriuretic Peptide (BNP)
Optional studies:
   Lipid panel (total cholesterol, LDL, HDL, VLDL, triglycerides)
   C-Reactive Protein (CRP)

☞ **Serum Magnesium Levels**: A "normal" magnesium level in your patient's lab profile does not necessarily indicate normal intracellular magnesium levels. Serum magnesium levels reflect only a small part of the total body content of Magnesium. The intracellular content can be low, despite normal serum levels in a person with clinical magnesium deficiency.[14] If your patient is experiencing ECG characteristics indicative of low intracellular magnesium, such as lengthening of the QT interval with runs of Torsades de Pointes, despite the presence of "normal" serum magnesium levels, the administration of one to two grams of magnesium sulfate should be considered. *In plain English, if your patient is having runs of Torsades de Pointes, do not withhold magnesium just because the serum magnesium level is normal.* When a low serum magnesium level is observed, it is a good indicator that your patient's intracellular magnesium level is also low.

---

* We advocate point-of-care (POC) testing, such as the Troponin I ultra (cTnI-u). *These testing units produce accurate results within 20 minutes.* (Bayer Diagnostics/Siemens Medical)

---

[14] Rinehart, R. et al, Arch Intern Med. 1988;148(11):2415-2420.

PATIENT ASSESSMENT - PHASE TWO:

RULE OUT ACUTE CORONARY SYNDROME (ACS):

During the phase one assessment, we evaluated the patient for the presence of imminent life-threatening conditions, and provided any necessary therapeutic interventions. The priority of the phase two assessment is ruling out the presence of Acute Coronary Syndrome, or ACS. Next to problems with the ABCs and shock, ACS is the next most commonly lethal condition which could affect the well-being of your patient. The American Heart Association's Advanced Cardiac Life Support (ACLS) curriculum categorizes ACS into the first three categories listed below. A fourth and fifth category, *stable angina* and *asymptomatic myocardial ischemia*, also presented here, are usually *chronic conditions*, and therefore do not fall into the *acute* coronary syndrome classification.

STEMI: (S-T segment elevation myocardial infarction). *STEMI is an acute myocardial infarction identified on the 12 lead ECG with two or more contiguous leads displaying S-T segment elevation of greater than 1mm. Patients usually exhibit cardiac symptoms* (typical or atypical), and *cardiac markers* elevate as injury and necrosis to myocardial cells occurs.

NSTEMI: (Non S-T segment elevation myocardial infarction). **NSTEMI is an acute myocardial infarction which does not *present with S-T segment elevation*.** There is often **S-T segment depression**, either from subendocardial (non Q wave producing) myocardial infarction, or from transmural **posterior wall infarction**, which does not typically show S-T elevation on the standard 12 lead ECG. The ECG may only exhibit subtle abnormalities, or it may be **normal**. **Patients usually exhibit cardiac symptoms** (typical or atypical). In nearly all cases, abnormal elevation of **cardiac markers** is the factor which defines the diagnosis of NSTEMI.

Unstable Angina: An ischemic condition which exists when the patient exhibits symptoms of ACS, which may occur at rest. In cases where the patient has a prior history of stable angina, there is a change or worsening of the usual pattern of angina. Symptoms abate with rest, nitrates, O2 and/or the administration of GP IIb/IIIa inhibitors. If S-T elevation is present on the 12 lead ECG, it is usually transient and disappears when the patient's symptoms subside (Prinzmetal's angina). Typically, the ECG exhibits one or more of the "ischemic patterns" described on page 134, or the ECG may be normal. Cardiac markers are negative or borderline. Unstable angina is usually caused by a partially-occlusive, platelet-rich thrombus.

Stable Angina: An ischemic condition in which ACS symptoms are triggered by physical (or in some cases emotional) stress. The symptoms follow a predictable pattern. Patients can usually articulate the activities which typically elicit symptoms, and what is usually necessary to alleviate them. There may be associated ECG changes, or the ECG may be normal. Cardiac markers are negative. Stable angina is usually caused by partially occlusive, stable plaque

Asymptomatic Myocardial Ischemia: The patient does not report any symptoms. Many cases of asymptomatic myocardial ischemia are discovered when an abnormal ECG is recorded during a routine physical exam, other screening process, or a patient with a *significant risk factor profile* is identified by an astute health care professional who begins an aggressive cardiac work-up. Cardiac markers are normal. CRP may be elevated. This condition is usually caused by non-occlusive, stable plaque.

☞   Please note, as we progress through the "Ruling Out ACS" section of our book, we mention utilization of other diagnostic modalities, such as CT Coronary Angiography, Echocardiography, and others, where appropriate. Because the focus of this textbook is *interpretation of the ECG*, we do not provide any explanations of how to interpret or utilize the data obtained from other diagnostic modalities.

The PHASE TWO Assessment consists of:

Rapid, targeted patient assessment:
        Presence of Typical or Atypical ACS symptoms?
        Auscultate Heart and Lung sounds
12 lead ECG evaluation
Evaluation of cardiac markers
Consider/Rule Out other lethal causes of chest pain: aortic dissection and pulmonary embolus
STAT Chest X-Ray
ACS risk stratification
Consider need for additional testing (exercise stress test, echo, coronary CT angio, cardiac cath, etc.)

☞ It is noteworthy to mention that each component of the *phase two assessment* listed above is of equal importance; for any one component can yield the key piece(s) of information that leads to a rapid, accurate – and possibly lifesaving – diagnosis. Therefore, the clinician should be methodical in obtaining this information, and should not be tempted to take shortcuts in the patient evaluation process. As we will demonstrate in our case studies, omitting part of this assessment can result in misdiagnosis – and catastrophic outcomes – for your patients.

The presence of two or more positive assessment findings listed in the "Quadrad of ACS" correlates with a high incidence of Acute Coronary Syndrome. Patients under the age of 40 presenting with ACS symptoms who have 4 or more risk factors for CAD are 22.5 times more likely to have ACS.[15] This should serve as the impetus for aggressively pursing additional diagnostic testing to definitively rule out ACS. For example: *your patient presents with vague symptoms which are **atypical for ACS**, but when you factor into this "clinical equation" the **presence of multiple significant risk factors**, an **ECG which shows "non-specific abnormalities**," and **lab results which show normal cardiac markers but elevated levels of C-Reactive Protein,** you decide to order a cardiac echo and a CT coronary angiogram.*

"THE QUADRAD of ACS"

☑ **PRESENTING SYMPTOMS**
☑ **ECG ABNORMALITIES**
☑ **CARDIAC MARKERS**
☑ **RISK FACTOR PROFILE**

A **POSITIVE** finding in **TWO** or MORE of the above categories indicates it is **EXTREMELY LIKELY** that ACS is present . . . . steps must be AGGRESSIVELY TAKEN to definitively RULE OUT the PRESENCE of ACS !

☞ As validated by multiple ACS risk stratification tools – such as TIMI, GRACE, and PURSUIT – the more *positive findings* that a patient has in the areas of ***presenting symptoms, ECG abnormalities, cardiac markers*** and ***risk factors,*** the higher the likelihood that ACS is present. A new ACS patient evaluation tool, known as the Simple ACS (SACS) Score, is currently in the process of scientific validation. The SACS Score is based solely on the "Quadrad of ACS," and is shown on page 157. You can learn more about the SACS Score by accessing the National Institutes of Health (NIH) website: www.clinicaltrials.gov. In the search window, enter the NIH study ID, which is: NCT00947804.

---

[15] Han, JH et al., "Role of Cardiac Risk Factors in diagnosis of ACS," Ann Emerg Med 2007 Feb;49:145-52

SUMMARY OF ACUTE CORONARY SYNDROMES & CORONARY ARTERY DISEASE

CLASSIFICATION	CONDITION	SYMPTOMS	ECG	LABS
ACUTE CORONARY SYNDROME	**STEMI** S-T SEGMENT ELEVATION MI	• ACUTE CORONARY SYNDROME (ACS) SYMPTOMS ARE PRESENT • ONSET OF SYMPTOMS DURING REST or EXERTION	• S-T SEGMENT ELEVATION IN 2 or more CONTIGUOUS LEADS • RECIPROCAL S-T DEPRESSION MAY or MAY NOT BE PRESENT	POSITIVE CARDIAC MARKERS

	NSTEMI NON- S-T SEGMENT ELEVATION MI	• SYMPTOMS NOT EFFECTED BY POSITION, MOVEMENT or RESPIRATION
		• SYMPTOMS NOT RELIEVED BY REST or NITRATES
			• ECG FINDINGS MAY BE CONSTANT, or INTERMITTENT (with symptoms):
			  ■ ISCHEMIC PATTERNS: S-T SEGMENT DEPRESSION and/or INVERTED T WAVES, or OTHER ISCHEMIC PATTERNS (SEE DIAGRAM, PAGE 115)
			  ■ HYPERACUTE T WAVES
				POSITIVE CARDIAC MARKERS

	UNSTABLE ANGINA	• NEW ONSET OF CARDIAC CHEST PAIN /ACS SYMPTOMS, or • ONSET OF CARDIAC CHEST PAIN / ACS SYMPTOMS WHILE AT REST, or • CHANGE IN PATTERN OF PREVIOUSLY STABLE ANGINA	• IF S-T ELEVATION IS PRESENT, IT SHOULD SUBSIDE WITH REST (PRINZMETAL'S ANGINA) • ECG MAY BE NORMAL	CARDIAC MARKERS NEGATIVE or BORDERLINE
NON-ACUTE CORONARY ARTERY DISEASE	STABLE ANGINA	PATIENT HAS EXERTIONAL CHEST PAIN, WHICH SUBSIDES WITH REST and/or REST AND NITRATES. SYMPTOMS ARE PREDICTABLE and FOLLOW A "USUAL PATTERN"	• PATTERNS OF ISCHEMIA MAY BE PRESENT, or • ECG MAY BE NORMAL	CARDIAC MARKERS NORMAL CRP and/or CHOLEST. MAY BE ELEVATED
	ASYMPTOMATIC CORONARY ARTERY DISEASE	NONE. THE PATIENT MAY HAVE NOTHING MORE THAN "POSITIVE" RISK FACTORS		

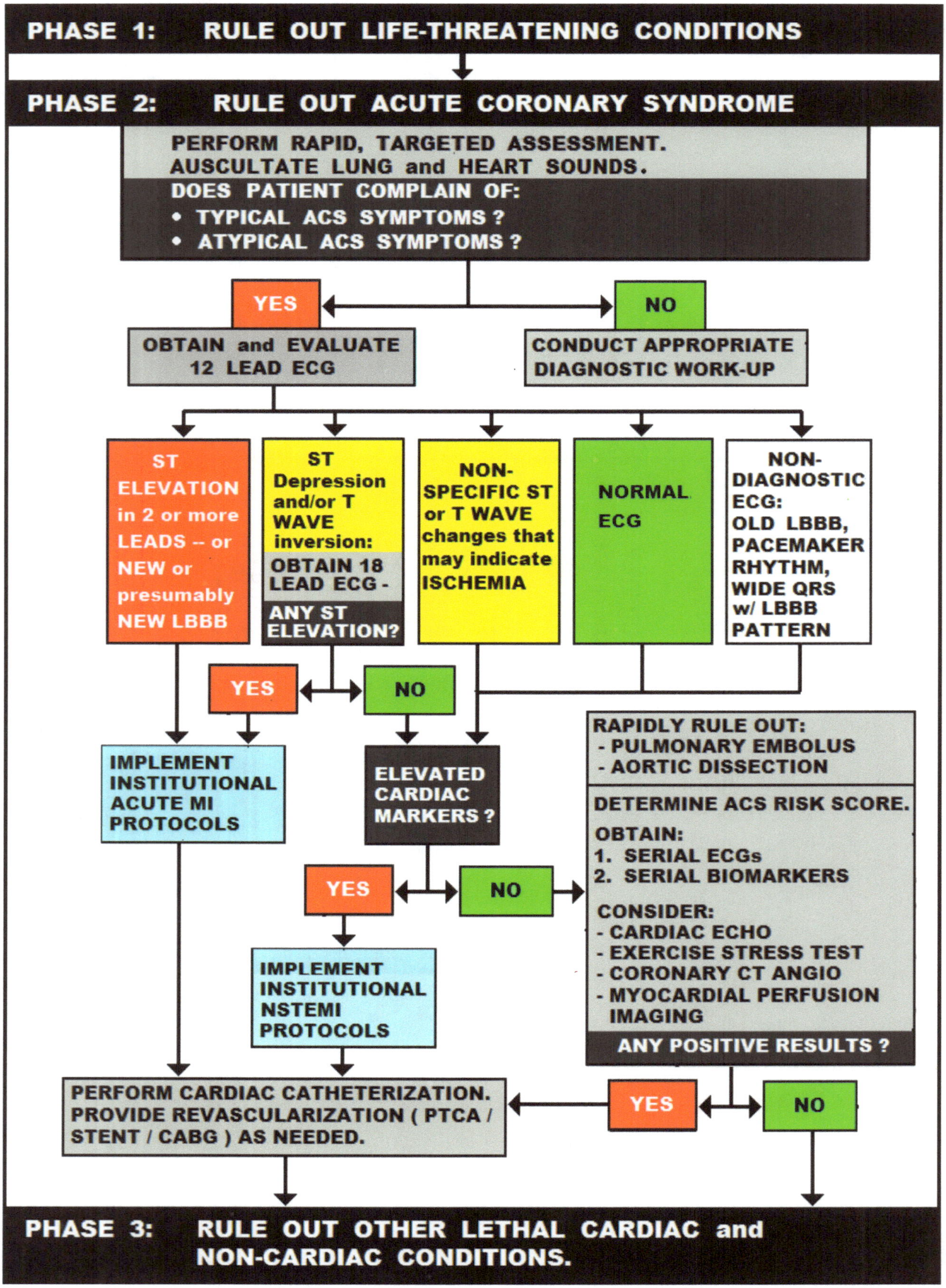

PHASE 1: RULE OUT LIFE-THREATENING CONDITIONS

PHASE 2: RULE OUT ACUTE CORONARY SYNDROME

PERFORM RAPID, TARGETED ASSESSMENT. AUSCULTATE LUNG and HEART SOUNDS.

DOES PATIENT COMPLAIN OF:
- **TYPICAL ACS SYMPTOMS ?**
- **ATYPICAL ACS SYMPTOMS ?**

YES → **OBTAIN and EVALUATE 12 LEAD ECG**

NO → **CONDUCT APPROPRIATE DIAGNOSTIC WORK-UP**

| ST ELEVATION in 2 or more LEADS -- or NEW or presumably NEW LBBB | ST Depression and/or T WAVE inversion: OBTAIN 18 LEAD ECG - ANY ST ELEVATION? | NON-SPECIFIC ST or T WAVE changes that may indicate ISCHEMIA | NORMAL ECG | NON-DIAGNOSTIC ECG: OLD LBBB, PACEMAKER RHYTHM, WIDE QRS w/ LBBB PATTERN |

YES **NO**

IMPLEMENT INSTITUTIONAL ACUTE MI PROTOCOLS

ELEVATED CARDIAC MARKERS ?

RAPIDLY RULE OUT:
- **PULMONARY EMBOLUS**
- **AORTIC DISSECTION**

DETERMINE ACS RISK SCORE.

OBTAIN:
1. **SERIAL ECGs**
2. **SERIAL BIOMARKERS**

CONSIDER:
- **CARDIAC ECHO**
- **EXERCISE STRESS TEST**
- **CORONARY CT ANGIO**
- **MYOCARDIAL PERFUSION IMAGING**

ANY POSITIVE RESULTS ?

YES **NO**

IMPLEMENT INSTITUTIONAL NSTEMI PROTOCOLS

PERFORM CARDIAC CATHETERIZATION. PROVIDE REVASCULARIZATION (PTCA / STENT / CABG) AS NEEDED.

YES **NO**

PHASE 3: RULE OUT OTHER LETHAL CARDIAC and NON-CARDIAC CONDITIONS.

CONDUCT RAPID, TARGETED PATIENT ASSESSMENT:

Ascertain the patient's chief complaint and primary symptoms. Listen for KEYWORDS, such as **chest pain, chest pressure, "heaviness in the chest,"** and **shortness of breath**. In a study conducted by Louis Graff et al, 77.8% of patients presenting with Acute Myocardial Infarction (AMI) presented with *chest pain* and/or *shortness of breath*.[16]

DEFINING TYPICAL SYMPTOMS of ACS:

☞ **TYPICAL SYMPTOMS of ACUTE CORONARY SYNDROME:**

✓ **CHEST PAIN** - DESCRIBED AS . . .
- "HEAVINESS, PRESSURE, DULL PAIN, TIGHTNESS"
- CENTERED IN CHEST, SUBSTERNAL
- MAY RADIATE TO SHOULDERS, JAW, NECK, LEFT or RIGHT ARM
- NOT AFFECTED by:
  - MOVEMENT
  - POSITION
  - DEEP INSPIRATION

✓ **SHORTNESS OF BREATH**
- MAY or MAY NOT BE PRESENT

✓ **NAUSEA / VOMITING**
- MAY or MAY NOT BE PRESENT

The moment the patient states any complaints which arouse your suspicion that ACS may be present, **OBTAIN A STAT 12 LEAD ECG.**

Be aware that the patient's symptoms may be *intermittent,* and may have abated by the time of patient evaluation. *Intermittent symptoms of ACS are often indicative of Unstable Angina or imminent AMI.* Therefore, you should proceed aggressively with the patient evaluation process until ACS and *significant coronary artery disease* have been definitively ruled out.

Although most ACS patients describe their chest pain as a "dull, pressure-like sensation," a recent multi-center chest pain study identified that 22% of patients presenting with symptoms described their chest pain as "sharp" or "stabbing" in nature, and 7% who experienced chest pain reproducible on palpation were eventually diagnosed with ACS.[17]

---

[16] Graff, L, et al, "Triage of patients for rapid (5 minute) ECG: a rule based on presenting chief complaints," *Ann. Emerg. Med.,* December 2000;36:554-560

[17] Amsterdam, E, et al, "AHA Scientific Statement- Testing of Low Risk Patients Presenting to the Emergency Department With Chest Pain:" Circulation 2010;122:756-776

ATYPICAL SYMPTOMS of ACS and THE "SILENT" MI:

A more challenging patient to assess and diagnose in a timely manner are the Acute MI patients who present without any typical chest pain symptoms (e.g. chest pain, pressure, discomfort, heaviness, etc.). These folks often seek medical attention for other reasons; they feel bad, they know something is wrong, and they may not realize the problem is with their heart. They complain of *atypical symptoms*. Fortunately, we've been able to identify a common profile for patients whom are at higher risk to experience AMI without chest pain, and a list of the most common symptoms they complain of.

To facilitate memorization of the patient profiles for those at high risk for "silent MI, [18]" and the symptoms they commonly complain of, we developed the sentence, "*our SHREWD MINDS FACED the biggest challenge.*" The acronym **SHREWD** represents the profiles of AMI patients most likely to present without chest symptoms, and **MINDS FACED** are acronyms representing the atypical symptoms most often complained of.

Acute MI patients who present without chest pain* are SHREWD:	* The information listed in the table to the immediate left resulted from a study conducted by John G. Canto, MD, MSPH, et. al., of the University of Alabama. The study consisted of 434,877 patients diagnosed with AMI between 1994 and 1998 in 1,674 US hospitals. Study results were published in the Journal of the American Medical Association (JAMA) on June 28, 2000, Vol. 283, No. 24, pages 3223-3229
Stroke (previous history of) **H**eart failure (previous history of) **R**ace (non-white) **E**lderly (age 75+) **W**omen **D**iabetes mellitus	

Common atypical complaints associated with AMI without chest pain include:

Malaise (weakness)	**F**atigue
Indigestion	**A**bdominal pain
Nausea	**C**old sweats
Dizziness	**E**levated heart rate
Syncope	**D**sypnea

Regarding AMI patients who present without chest pain, there are several other relevant points to emphasize[19]:
"Without chest pain" also meant there was NO abnormal symptoms of neck/jaw/shoulder or arm discomfort.
Approximately 1/3 of all AMI patients in the study (142,445 out of 434,877) presented without chest pain.
Patients without chest pain were 2X more likely to experience sudden cardiac arrest (8.5 vs. 4.3%).
Patients without chest pain had more than twice the rate of in-hospital mortality (23.3 vs. 9.3%).
Patients without chest pain had a higher incidence of CHF requiring medical intervention (29.3 vs. 15.0%).
Patients without chest pain were more likely to present with pulmonary edema and a higher Killip classification.

It should be universally understood that there is a higher incidence of misdiagnosis / late diagnosis of AMI in the "silent MI" and atypical symptom subgroups, and a significantly increased delay in these patients receiving appropriate treatment.

---

[18] "Prevalence, Clinical Characteristics, and Mortality Among Patients With AMI Presenting Without Chest Pain," JG Canto, MD, MSPH, et al, JAMA 2000; 283 no. 24: p. 3223-29
[19] ibid

Effect of Having Multiple Risk Factors for AMI Without Chest Pain

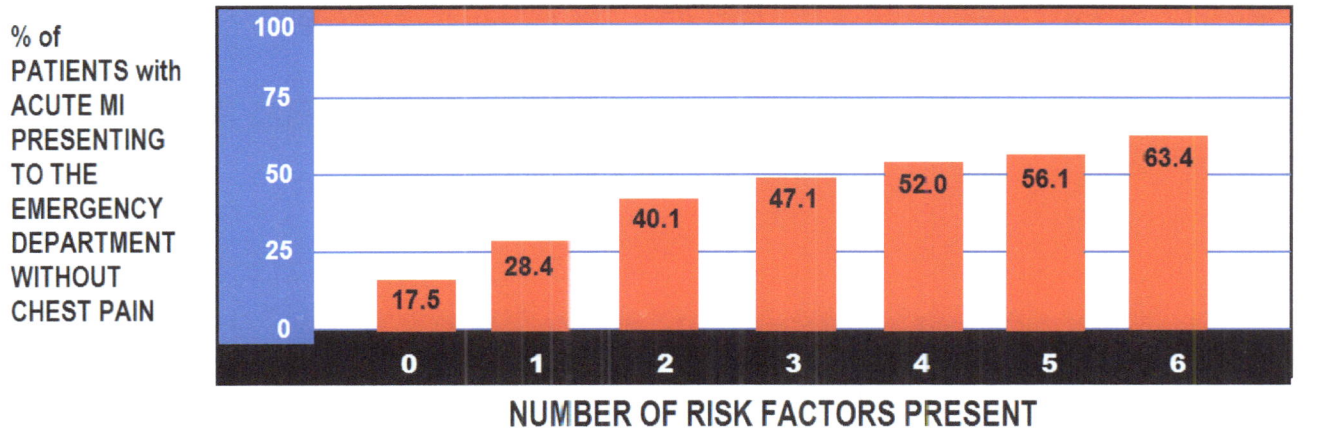

% of PATIENTS with ACUTE MI PRESENTING TO THE EMERGENCY DEPARTMENT WITHOUT CHEST PAIN

Number of Risk Factors	%
0	17.5
1	28.4
2	40.1
3	47.1
4	52.0
5	56.1
6	63.4

NUMBER OF RISK FACTORS PRESENT

RISK FACTORS INCLUDE: **S**troke (previous), **H**eart failure (previous), **R**ace (non-white), **E**lderly (age 75+), **W**omen, **D**iabtetes

DATA SOURCE: J. CANTO, MD, MSPH, et al, JAMA 2000 ; 283 : 3223 - 3229

Data supplied by the above chart advises us that when multiple risk factors for AMI without chest pain are present, the likelihood that patients will present without chest pain increases significantly. For patients with four or more risk factors for "silent MI," the likelihood that they will present to the ED having AMI without chest pain is greater than 50%.

With respect to female patients, a study consisting of 515 post-myocardial infarction female patients was conducted by Jean C. McSweeney, et.al,[20] and published in Circulation in 2003. This study found that *ONLY 29.7% OF FEMALE PATIENTS HAD CHEST PAIN PRIOR TO THEIR AMI, and* **43% OF THESE PATIENTS DID NOT HAVE ANY CHEST PAIN AT ANY TIME DURING THEIR MYOCARDIAL INFARCTION!**

The tables below illustrate the symptoms experienced by female MI patients *before* their MI (below, left) and *during* their MI (below, right).

WOMEN'S MAJOR SYMPTOMS *PRIOR* TO THEIR HEART ATTACK:	
UNUSUAL FATIGUE	71 %
SLEEP DISTURBANCE	48 %
SOB	42 %
INDIGESTION	39 %
ANXIETY	36 %

APPROXIMATELY 78 % OF WOMEN REPORTED EXPERIENCING AT LEAST ONE OF THESE SYMPTOMS FOR MORE THAN ONE MONTH EITHER DAILY OR SEVERAL TIMES PER WEEK PRIOR TO THEIR MI.

WOMEN'S MAJOR SYMPTOMS DURING THEIR HEART ATTACK:	
SHORTNESS OF BREATH	58 %
WEAKNESS	55 %
UNUSUAL FATIGUE	43 %
COLD SWEAT	39 %
DIZZINESS	39 %

☞ *43 % HAD NO CHEST PAIN AT ANY TIME DURING THEIR MI !*

Circulation, 2003:108;2619-2623

Case study 2, beginning on page 172 provides an example of atypical ACS symptoms of female patients.

---

[20] Jean C. McSweeney, et.al, University of Arkansas, published in *Circulation, 2003;108:2619-2623*

DIFFERENTIATION of STABLE ANGINA vs. UNSTABLE ANGINA:

In *stable angina*, patients usually have been previously diagnosed with coronary artery disease, and have *predictable* symptoms: that is, every time they engage in certain activities, they experience chest pain, which subsides with rest.

In *unstable angina*, the patient typically describes *symptoms which are new*, or *a change in the usual pattern of symptoms*, or that *symptoms have come on during rest*.

The table below summarizes the difference in symptoms of *stable* vs. *unstable angina*:

stable angina vs. unstable angina

stable angina		unstable angina
1. SYMPTOMS START DURING PHYSICAL EXERTION.	**VS.**	1. SYMPTOMS MAY START AT ANY TIME, EVEN DURING REST
2. SYMPTOMS ARE "PREDICTABLE"		2. SYMPTOMS ARE *NEW*, *DIFFERENT*, or *WORSE* THAN PREVIOUS EPISODES

In cases of unstable angina, the ECG may exhibit abnormalities, or it may be *perfectly normal.*

In cases where the ECG is normal, it is often the *high index of suspicion* – based on other factors, such as a significant *risk factor profile*, and/or *persistent symptoms* that prompt the clinician to pursue *additional diagnostic testing*, which reveals the presence of critical arterial blockages – and ultimately saves the life of a patient.

See Case Study 17, on page 268, for an example of a physician making the diagnosis of unstable angina – despite the presence of a normal ECG – and discovering advanced triple-vessel disease.

AUSCULTATE HEART and LUNG SOUNDS:

Conduct a rapid assessment of the patient's **heart** and **lung sounds**. The presence of *fluid in the lungs* (fine and/or coarse crackles), is a deciding factor in selection of appropriate treatment modalities in cases of patients suffering from acute MI with accompanying hypotension. (a table of "basic heart sounds" is located on page 18).

The presence of pulmonary edema combined with a new systolic murmur can signify the presence of *Acute Papillary Muscle Rupture* or *Ventricular Septal Rupture*, conditions which can rapidly be fatal if not quickly discovered and appropriately treated.

OBTAIN and EVALUATE a 12 LEAD ECG for ACS:

At the first indication that ACS may be present, a 12 lead ECG should immediately be obtained and evaluated.

☞   The moment you decide that a 12 LEAD ECG is necessary, **OBTAIN A COPY OF THE PATIENT'S PREVIOUS ECG(s), if available, for comparison.**   If many old ECGs exist, get the most recent two, and the oldest one.

☞   **"Obtain and interpret a 12 lead ECG *within the first ten minutes of patient contact* in all suspected ACS cases."**   This is a clinical standard of practice defined in the American Heart Association's Advanced Cardiac Life Support curriculum.

With the newly recorded ECG in hand, determine if it is of DIAGNOSTIC QUALITY. If the QRS complexes are TOO WIDE (>120ms), the ECG MARKERS of ACS can be altered.   Follow the guidelines listed in the table below:

If the QRS complexes are within normal limits (width <120 ms.), proceed to STEP 2 – EVALUATE the ECG for ACS, on page 112.

STEP 1 - EVALUATE WIDTH OF QRS:

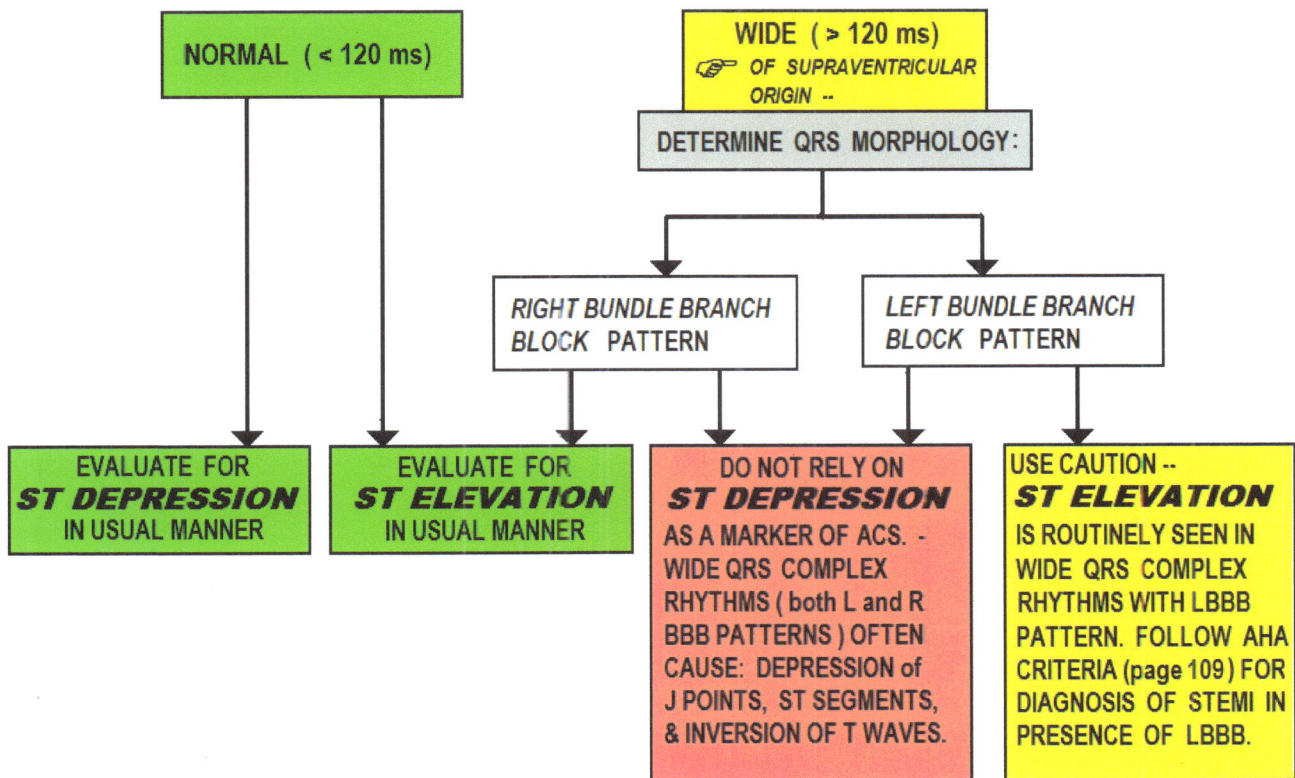

NORMAL (< 120 ms)

WIDE (> 120 ms)
☞ OF SUPRAVENTRICULAR ORIGIN --

DETERMINE QRS MORPHOLOGY:

RIGHT BUNDLE BRANCH BLOCK PATTERN

LEFT BUNDLE BRANCH BLOCK PATTERN

EVALUATE FOR
ST DEPRESSION
IN USUAL MANNER

EVALUATE FOR
ST ELEVATION
IN USUAL MANNER

DO NOT RELY ON
ST DEPRESSION
AS A MARKER OF ACS. - WIDE QRS COMPLEX RHYTHMS (both L and R BBB PATTERNS) OFTEN CAUSE: DEPRESSION of J POINTS, ST SEGMENTS, & INVERSION OF T WAVES.

USE CAUTION --
ST ELEVATION
IS ROUTINELY SEEN IN WIDE QRS COMPLEX RHYTHMS WITH LBBB PATTERN. FOLLOW AHA CRITERIA (page 109) FOR DIAGNOSIS OF STEMI IN PRESENCE OF LBBB.

The table below demonstrates how conditions such as *Ventricular Hypertrophy, Wolff-Parkinson-White syndrome, Pacemaker generated rhythms* and *ventricular rhythms* – in addition to Bundle Branch Blocks – can alter the ECG markers of ACS.

CONDITIONS WHICH ALTER THE ECG MARKERS
of ACUTE CORONARY SYNDROME

RIGHT BUNDLE BRANCH BLOCK	LEFT BUNDLE BRANCH BLOCK
W-P-W BYPASS TRACT, LEFT LATERAL WALL 49 y/o MALE	SAME PATIENT AS ON LEFT - IMMEDIATELY AFTER RF ABLATION OF BYPASS TRACT
W-P-W BYPASS TRACT, RIGHT ANTERIOR/ LATERAL WALL 14 y/o MALE	SAME PATIENT AS ON LEFT - IMMEDIATELY AFTER RF ABLATION OF BYPASS TRACT
PACEMAKER - RIGHT VENTRICULAR APEX	PACEMAKER TURNED OFF HERE
RIGHT VENTRICULAR HYPERTROPHY (Strain Pattern)	LEFT VENTRICULAR HYPERTROPHY (Strain Pattern)
VENTRICULAR TACHYCARDIA FOCUS: LEFT FASICULAR, 17 y/o FEMALE	VENTRICULAR TACHYCARDIA- FOCUS: RIGHT VENTRICULAR APEX

Remember that many conduction disorders are **intermittent,** such as *bundle branch blocks, Wolff-Parkinson-White*, and *pacemaker rhythms*. By carefully observing the ECGs of these patients, you may observe periods where **normally conducted QRS complexes resume**, providing you with the opportunity to record *diagnostic quality ECGs*.

WIDE QRS COMPLEX RHYTHMS with RBBB PATTERN:

> **Common causes of wide QRS complexes with RIGHT BUNDLE BRANCH BLOCK aberration include:**
>
> **Right Bundle Branch Block**
> **Right Ventricular Hypertrophy**
> **Wolff-Parkinson-White (WPW) Syndrome (with left-sided bypass tract)**
> **Left Ventricular Pacing**
> **Ventricular Rhythms (usually of left ventricular origin)**

ST SEGMENT DEPRESSION and *T WAVE INVERSION* are typically caused by RBBB pattern QRS widening, an effect which mimics ECG findings of ischemia and NSTEMI. *This effect renders the ECG unreliable for diagnosing ischemia and NSTEMI.*

ST SEGMENT ELEVATION is not typically caused by RBBB; therefore, when it is present on an ECG with RBBB, STEMI should be suspected until proven otherwise.

The following three ECGs are from patients with STEMI, confirmed by elevation of cardiac markers and discovery of total coronary arterial occlusion with thrombus during emergency cardiac catherization:

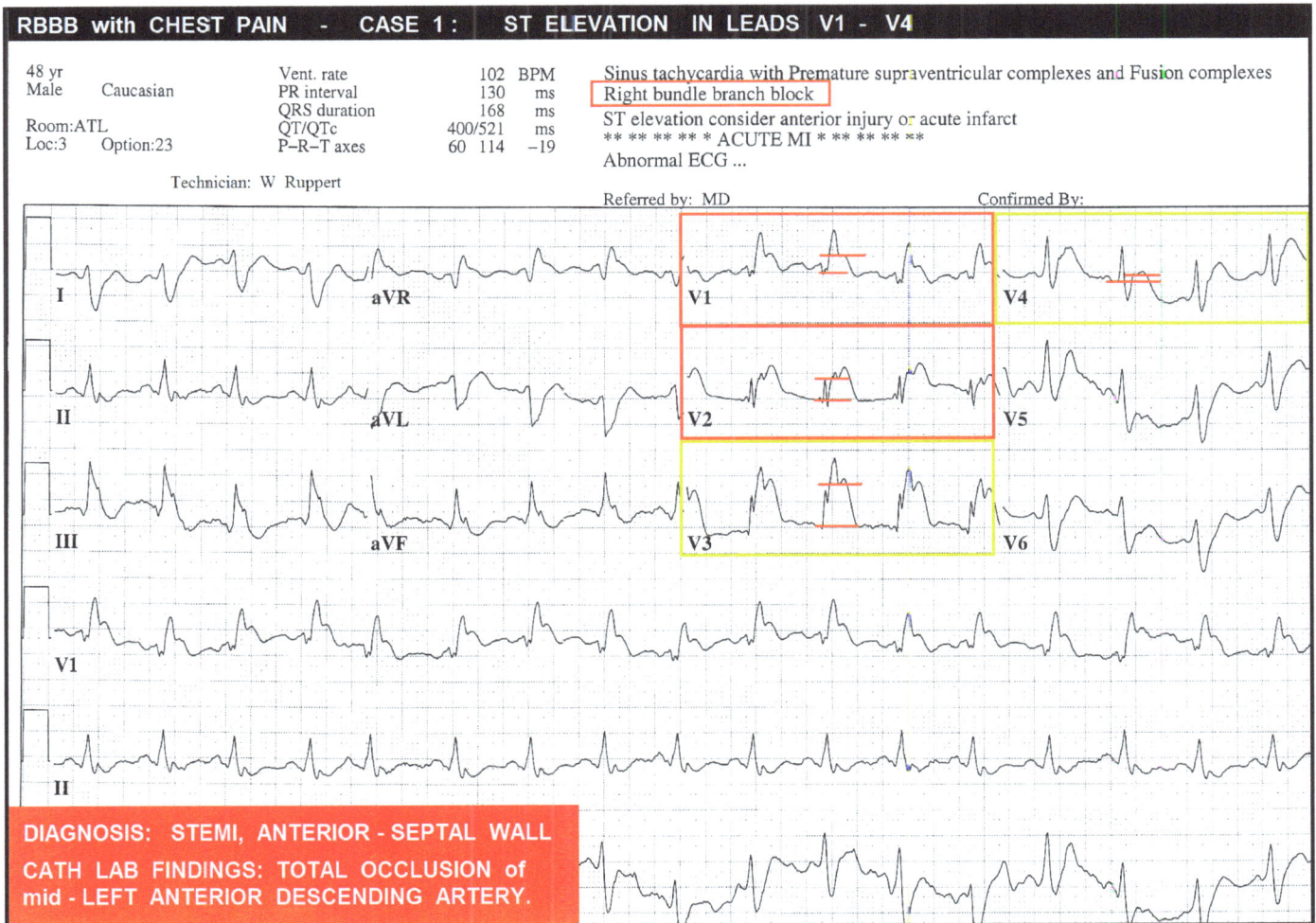

The patient whose ECG is shown above underwent successful thrombectomy and PCI with drug-eluting stent to the mid section of the Left Anterior Descending artery.

RBBB with CHEST PAIN - CASE 2: ST ELEVATION LEADS II, III, aVF - WITH RECIPROCAL ST DEPRESSION in LEADS V1 - V6

25 yr		Vent. rate	67	BPM	Sinus rhythm with 1st degree A–V block
Male	Caucasian	PR interval	258	ms	Right bundle branch block
		QRS duration	136	ms	ST elevation consider inferior injury or acute infarct
		QT/QTc	398/420	ms	** ** ** ** * ACUTE MI * ** ** ** **
Loc:3	Option:23	P–R–T axes	44 94 82		Abnormal ECG

Referred by: MD   Confirmed By: UNEDITED DR.

DIAGNOSIS: STEMI - INFERIOR-POSTERIOR WALL

CATH LAB FINDINGS: TOTAL OCCLUSION of DOMINANT RIGHT CORONARY ARTERY

The patient whose ECG is shown above underwent successful PCI with drug-eluting stent to the mid-right coronary artery, with restoration of TIMI grade III flow to the posterior descending and posterior lateral arterial distributions.

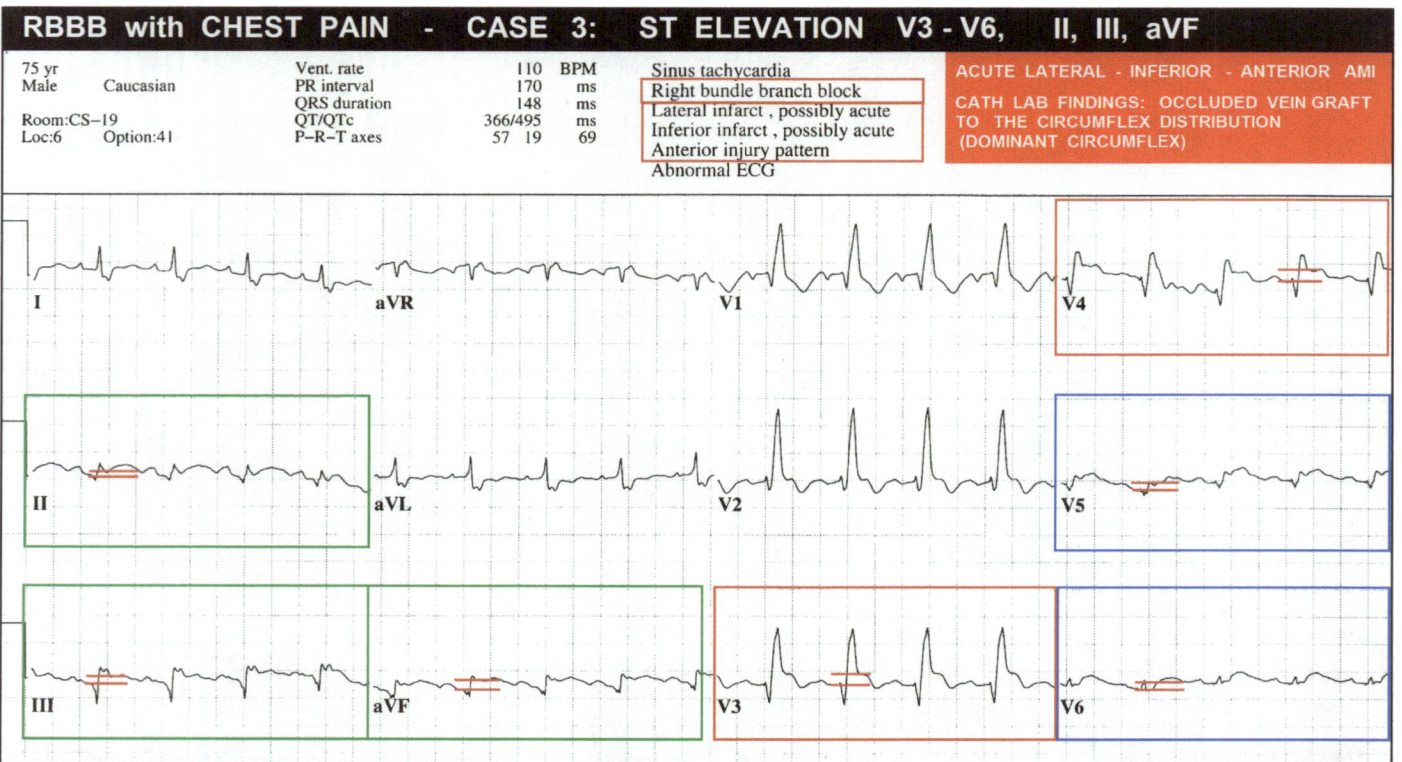

RBBB with CHEST PAIN - CASE 3: ST ELEVATION V3 - V6, II, III, aVF

75 yr		Vent. rate	110	BPM	Sinus tachycardia
Male	Caucasian	PR interval	170	ms	Right bundle branch block
		QRS duration	148	ms	Lateral infarct , possibly acute
Room:CS–19		QT/QTc	366/495	ms	Inferior infarct , possibly acute
Loc:6	Option:41	P–R–T axes	57 19 69		Anterior injury pattern
					Abnormal ECG

ACUTE LATERAL - INFERIOR - ANTERIOR AMI

CATH LAB FINDINGS: OCCLUDED VEIN GRAFT TO THE CIRCUMFLEX DISTRIBUTION (DOMINANT CIRCUMFLEX)

SUMMARY: As demonstrated in the three example ECGs, Right Bundle Branch Block does not obscure ST elevation in any region of the myocardium viewed by the standard 12 Lead ECG. ST elevation in cases of inferior, anterior, and lateral MI are easily detectable by evaluating J points and ST segments in the usual manner.

WIDE QRS COMPLEX RHYTHMS with LBBB PATTERN:

Common causes of wide QRS complexes with LEFT BUNDLE BRANCH BLOCK aberrancy include:
Left Bundle Branch Block **Left Ventricular Hypertrophy** **Wolff-Parkinson-White (WPW) syndrome (with right-sided bypass tract)** **Right Ventricular Pacing** **Ventricular Rhythms (usually of right ventricular origin)**

ST SEGMENT ELEVATION is almost always seen *continuously* on ECGs with LBBB aberrancy, an effect which complicates our ability to diagnose STEMI, NSTEMI, or ischemia.

When patients present **with ACS symptoms whose 12 lead ECG shows LBBB**, use the American Heart Association recommended guidelines, shown in the table to the right, for diagnosing STEMI:

A.H.A. ACLS GUIDELINES

1. If patient has a CONFIRMED HISTORY of LBBB, rely on:
   - CARDIAC MARKERS
   - SYMPTOMS
   - RISK FACTOR PROFILE
   - HIGH INDEX OF SUSPICION

   for diagnosis of STEMI

2. If patient has:

   a) previously NORMAL ECGs (no LBBB)
   -- or --
   b) no old ECGs available for comparison

   consider diagnosis as STEMI until proven otherwise.

☞ HELPFUL INDICATORS FOR ECG DIAGNOSIS OF STEMI in the presence of LBBB:

- ST ELEVATION > 5 mm
- COMPARE J POINT, ST SEGMENTS and T WAVES of previous ECG with LBBB to NEW ECG.
- CONVEX ST SEGMENT = poss. MI CONCAVE ST SEGMENT = normal
- CONCORDANT ST changes (1 mm or > ST DEPRESSION V1 - V3 or ST ELEVATION LEADS II, III, AVF)
- ST ELEVATION in LEADS II, III, and/or AVF

N. ENGL. J. MED v 348; p933 - 940 - Zimetbaum, et. al.

According to Zimetbaum, et al,[21] the indicators listed in the table to the left are reliable in the ECG diagnosis of STEMI when left bundle branch block is present:

---

[21] Zimetbaum, et.al,; New England Journal of Medicine: vol 348; p933 - 940

The ECG below is from a 58 year old female who presented to the ED with "continuous substernal chest pressure" and shortness of breath for approximately 30 minutes:

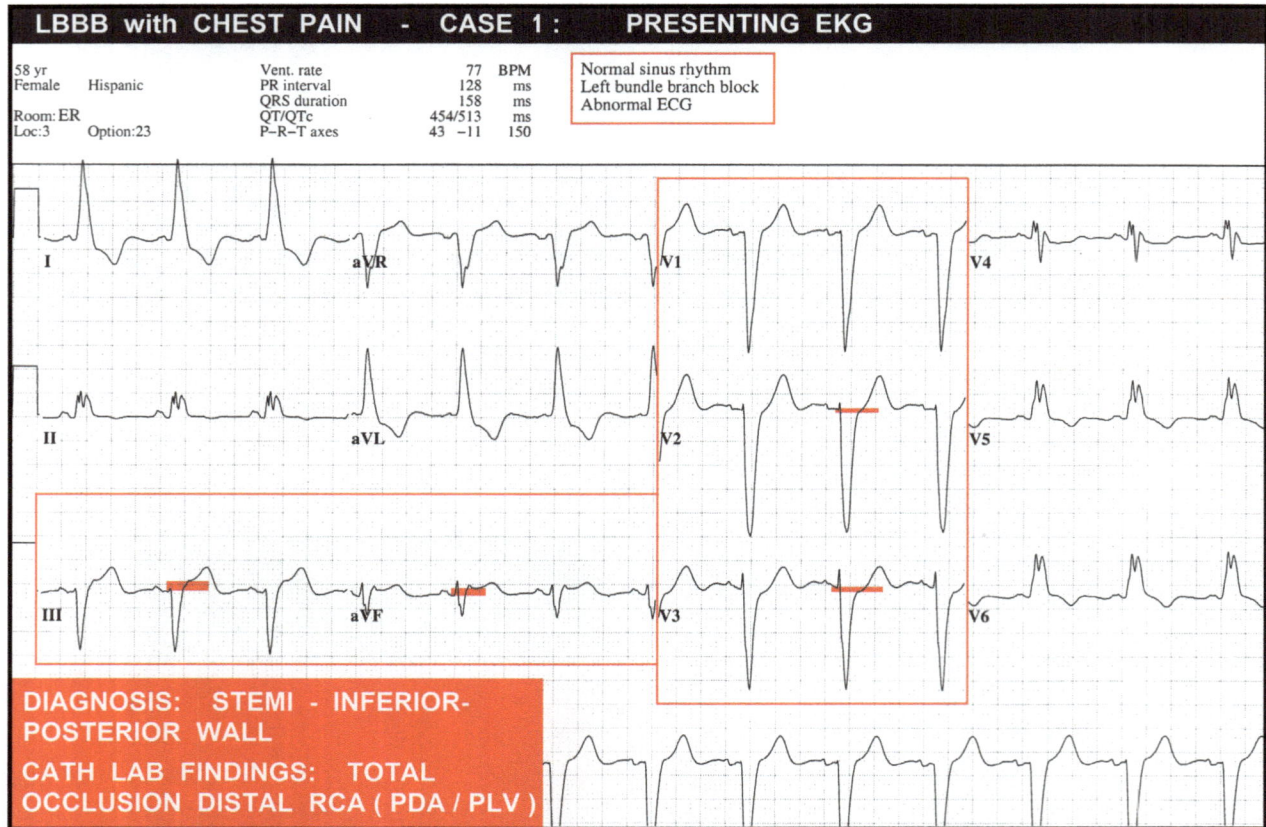

LBBB with CHEST PAIN - CASE 1:   PRESENTING EKG

58 yr
Female   Hispanic

Room: ER
Loc:3   Option:23

Vent. rate	77	BPM
PR interval	128	ms
QRS duration	158	ms
QT/QTc	454/513	ms
P-R-T axes	43 -11	150

Normal sinus rhythm
Left bundle branch block
Abnormal ECG

DIAGNOSIS: STEMI - INFERIOR-POSTERIOR WALL

CATH LAB FINDINGS: TOTAL OCCLUSION DISTAL RCA (PDA / PLV)

Note **ST elevation in leads III and aVF**, and **"minimal" ST depression in leads V2 and V3** – which are obvious changes from the ECG below, recorded during a hospital admission 7 months earlier. *Also note that in the ECG above, the computer does not capture any of these ECG changes.*

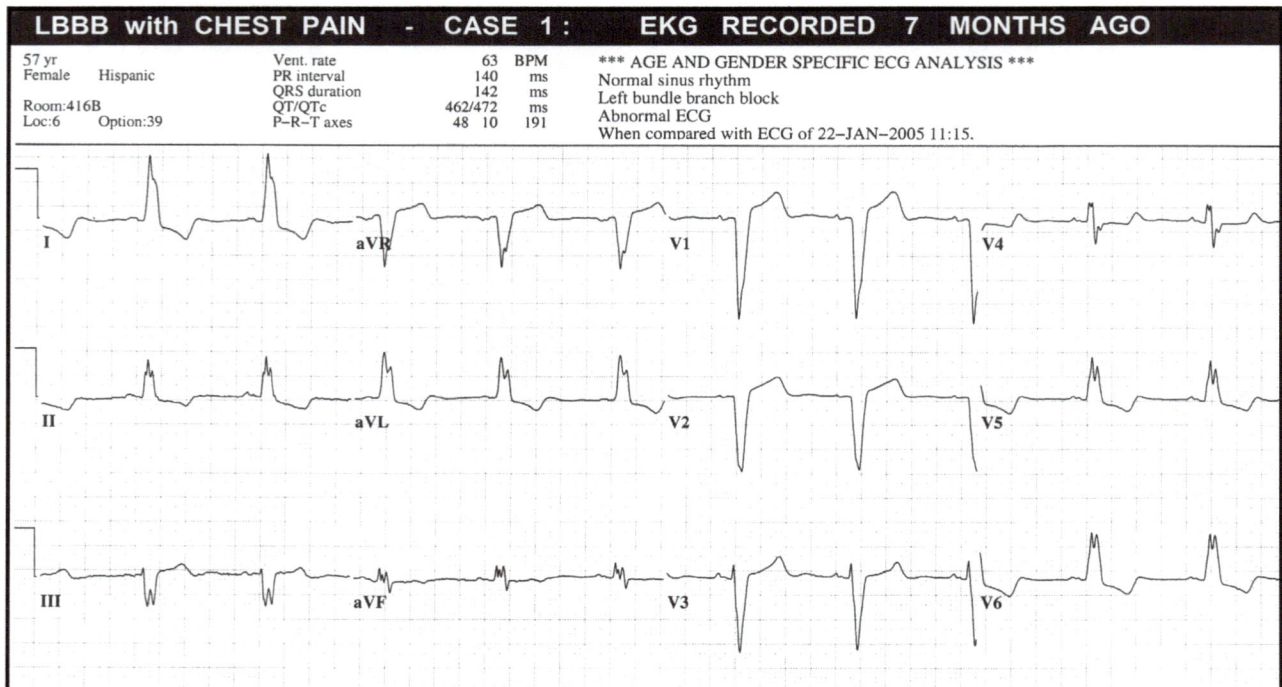

LBBB with CHEST PAIN - CASE 1:   EKG RECORDED 7 MONTHS AGO

57 yr
Female   Hispanic

Room:416B
Loc:6   Option:39

Vent. rate	63	BPM
PR interval	140	ms
QRS duration	142	ms
QT/QTc	462/472	ms
P-R-T axes	48 10	191

*** AGE AND GENDER SPECIFIC ECG ANALYSIS ***
Normal sinus rhythm
Left bundle branch block
Abnormal ECG
When compared with ECG of 22-JAN-2005 11:15.

110

Since ST elevation in the precordial leads is *normal* and *expected* when LBBB is present, it becomes noteworthy when the J point is *isoelectric* or *depressed* in the presence of LBBB. The image to the right compares this patient's J points in lead V3. There is an impressive 3.5mm difference between the old and new ECGs. This represents a negative deflection of 3.5mm in the new ECG. When the patient's **ST elevation** in inferior leads III and aVF is taken into consideration, *the negative deflection of 3.5mm in lead V3 is most likely indicative of posterior injury.*

Based on the patient's symptoms and ECG changes, she was taken immediately to the cardiac catheterization suite, where a total thrombus occlusion of the distal circumflex artery was discovered in a co-dominant system. After successful thrombectomy and PCI, TIMI III flow was restored to the patient's posterior lateral distribution, **validating the initial ECG finding of inferior-posterior MI.**

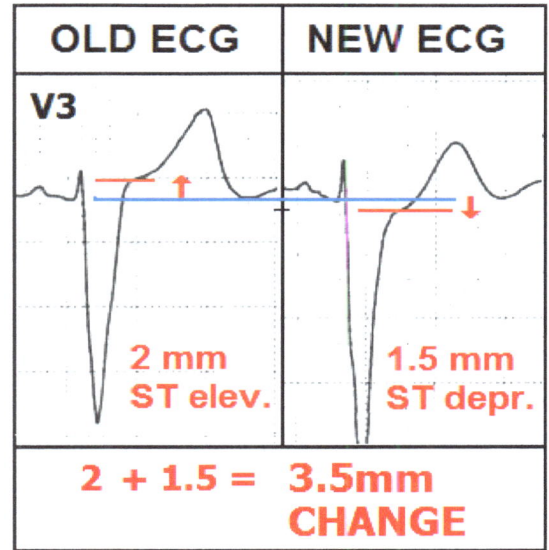

OLD ECG	NEW ECG
V3	
2 mm ST elev.	1.5 mm ST depr.
2 + 1.5 = 3.5mm CHANGE	

In another case study, a 46 year old male presented with *"severe sub-sternal chest pressure for the last several hours."* The pain was not affected by *position, movement,* or *deep inspiration,* and was a "10" on a scale of 1-10. The patient stated that up until this event, he did not recall ever having a 12 lead ECG recorded. His ECG below shows a **presumably new LBBB** – that when combined with his current chest pain, made his diagnosis "rule out acute anterior-septal wall MI." He was taken STAT to the cath lab, where a total proximal occlusion of the Left Anterior Descending artery was discovered. He underwent successful PCI.

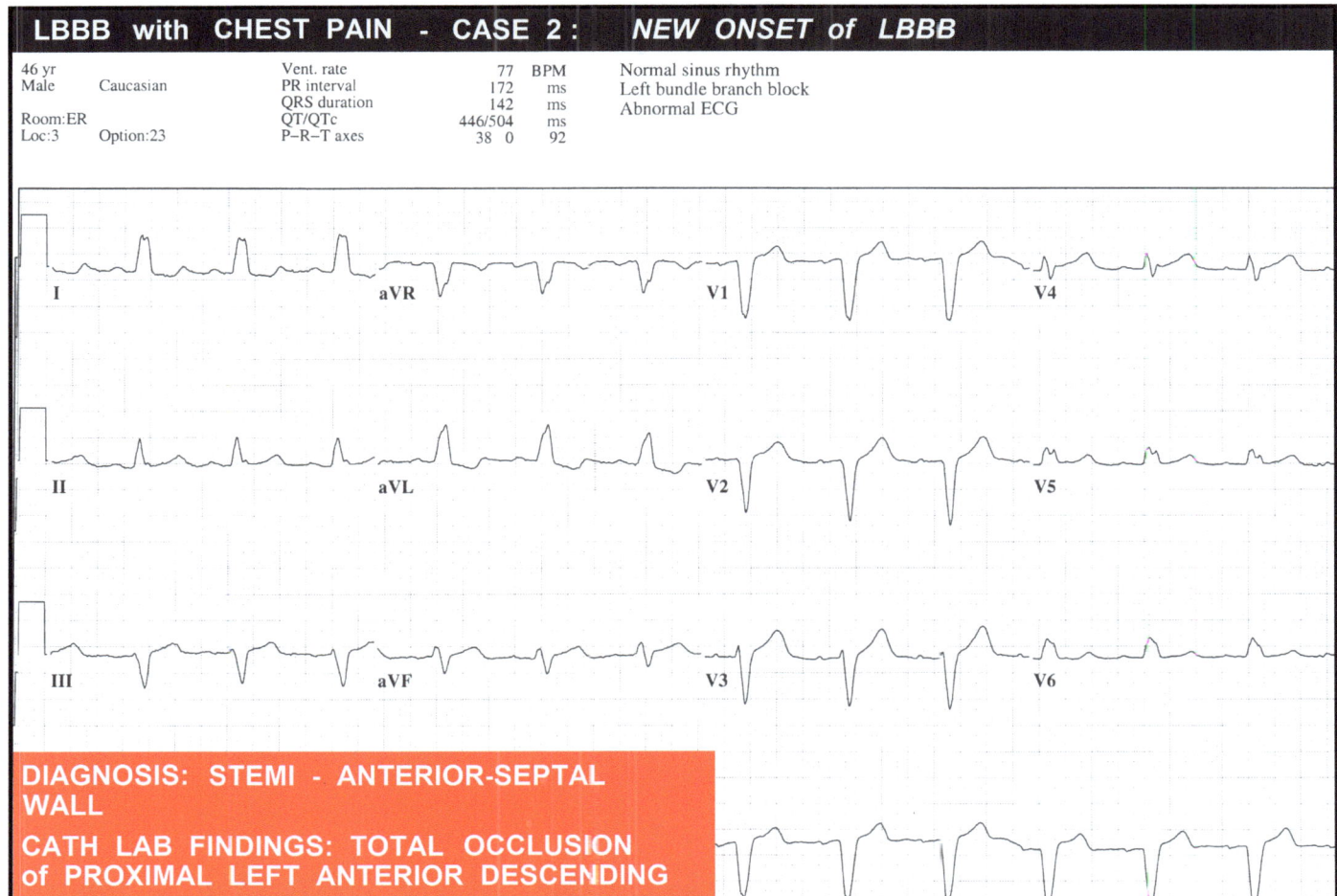

LBBB with CHEST PAIN - CASE 2: *NEW ONSET of LBBB*

46 yr				
Male	Caucasian	Vent. rate	77 BPM	Normal sinus rhythm
		PR interval	172 ms	Left bundle branch block
		QRS duration	142 ms	Abnormal ECG
Room:ER		QT/QTc	446/504 ms	
Loc:3	Option:23	P–R–T axes	38 0 92	

I aVR V1 V4

II aVL V2 V5

III aVF V3 V6

DIAGNOSIS: STEMI - ANTERIOR-SEPTAL WALL

CATH LAB FINDINGS: TOTAL OCCLUSION of PROXIMAL LEFT ANTERIOR DESCENDING

STEP 2 - EVALUATE the ECG for ACS

THE ECG MARKERS USED FOR DETERMINING THE PRESENCE OF ACUTE CORONARY SYNDROME INCLUDE:

- J POINTS
- ST SEGMENTS
- T WAVES

CAREFULLY SCRUTINIZE THESE MARKERS IN EVERY LEAD OF THE 12 LEAD ECG, TO DETERMINE IF THEY ARE *NORMAL* or *ABNORMAL*.

Use the criteria presented in the diagram to the right as a template for defining normal parameters for *J points, ST segments* and *T waves*.

THE J POINT is point where the *QRS complex ends* and the *ST segment begins*. It is usually easy to discern, except in cases where the ST segment is "slurred." The J point should be within 1mm of the isoelectric line. To determine the isoelectric line, traditional ECG interpretation standards rely on the T-P interval (flatline between complexes) to determine what is "isoelectric."

NORMAL ST - T WAVES

- WHEN QRS WIDTH IS NORMAL (< 120 ms)

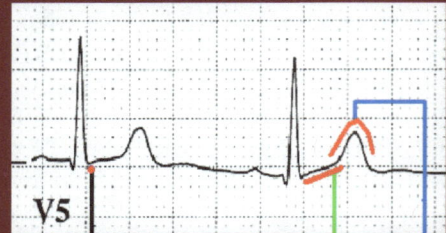

ASSESS: V5

- J POINT: ISOELECTRIC (or < 1 mm dev.)
- ST SEG: SLIGHT, POSITIVE INCLINATION
- T WAVE: UPRIGHT, POSITIVE

☞ in EVERY LEAD EXCEPT aVR !!

THE P-Q JUNCTION

. . . is the POINT where the P-R SEGMENT ends and the QRS COMPLEX BEGINS. Used for POINT OF REFERENCE for measurement of the J-POINT and the S-T SEGMENT –

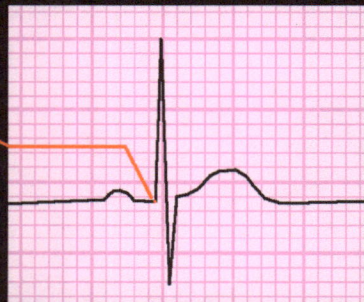

The P-Q JUNCTION. Perhaps a more accurate determination of the isoelectric plane – especially in cases where the TP interval fluctuates, or contains excessive artifact – is to use the *PQ junction*. According to Wang, Asinger and Marriott et al,[22] the P-Q junction is to be used as the point of reference for measurement of J points, S-T segment depression and elevation.

---

[22] Wang, Asinger, and Marriott et al, New England Journal of Medicine, vol 349: p2198-2135, Nov 27, 2003

THE ST SEGMENT should not be flat; it should have a slight positive inclination, as seen here ------------------------------►

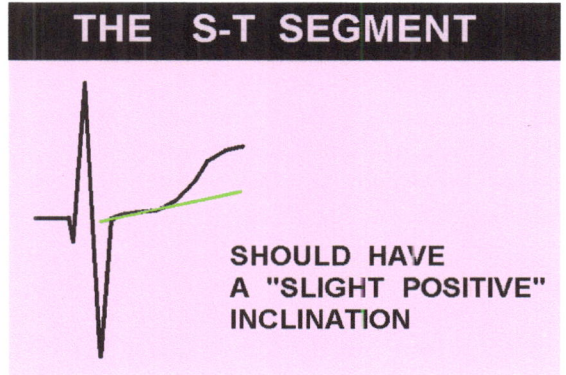

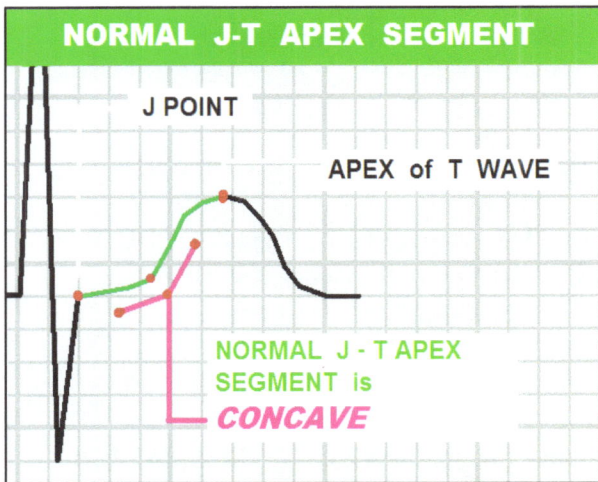

THE S-T SEGMENT

SHOULD HAVE
A "SLIGHT POSITIVE"
INCLINATION

NORMAL J-T APEX SEGMENT

J POINT

APEX of T WAVE

NORMAL J - T APEX
SEGMENT is
CONCAVE

◄-----**THE J-T APEX SEGMENT** is comprised of the *S-T segment* and the *first half of the T wave*. Its starting point is the J point, and it terminates at the apex (peak) of the T wave. *The normal J-T Apex segment is CONCAVE.*

☞ The relevance of evaluating the J-T APEX SEGMENT is to identify the earliest onset of STEMI. Frequently, there are discernable changes to the J-T Apex segment prior to the occurrence of S-T segment elevation at the J point.

THE T WAVE should have a smooth, rounded shape. It should be symmetrical—if you draw a vertical line down the center of the T wave, the two halves should look like mirror images of each other. It should be upright (positive) in all leads, except aVR. As a normal variant, the T wave may be inverted in leads aVL, III and V1, as demonstrated in the example below:

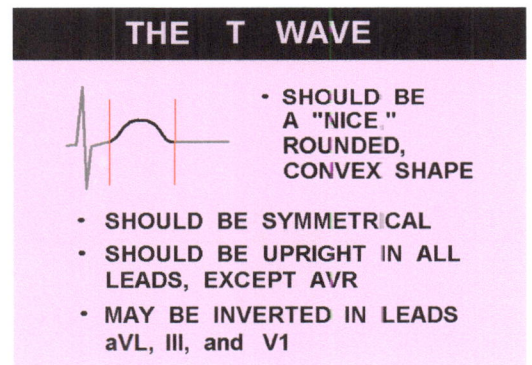

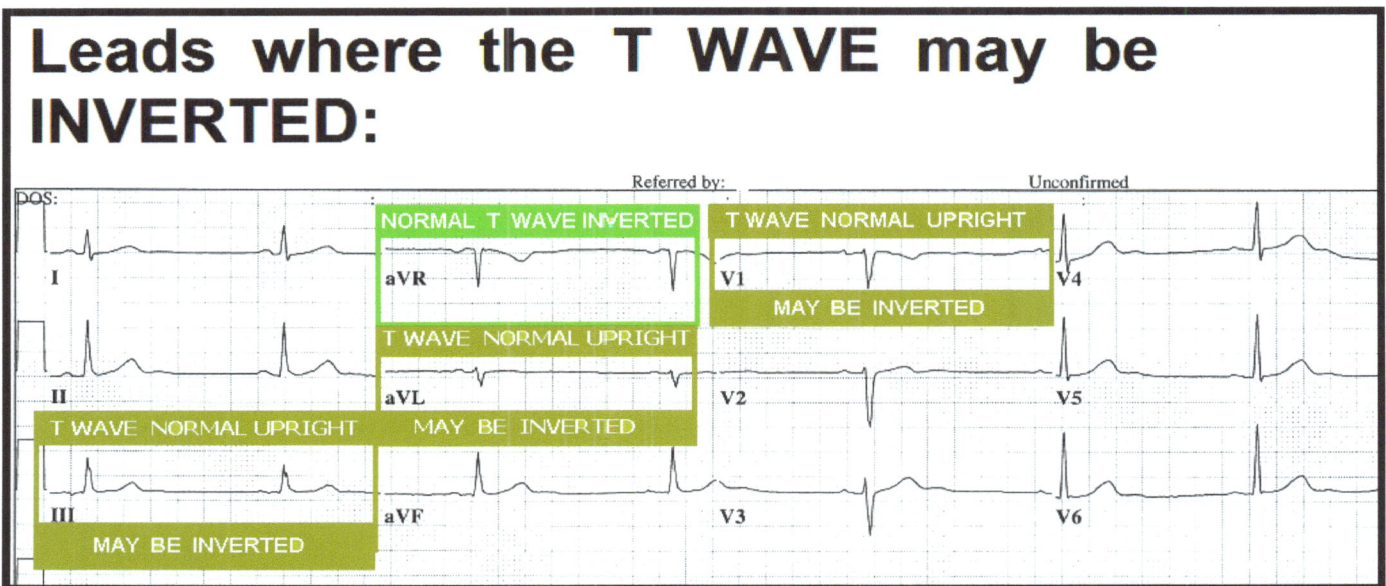

THE T WAVE

- SHOULD BE
  A "NICE"
  ROUNDED,
  CONVEX SHAPE
- SHOULD BE SYMMETRICAL
- SHOULD BE UPRIGHT IN ALL
  LEADS, EXCEPT AVR
- MAY BE INVERTED IN LEADS
  aVL, III, and V1

Leads where the T WAVE may be INVERTED:

Referred by: _____   Unconfirmed _____

DOS:

I

NORMAL T WAVE INVERTED

aVR

T WAVE NORMAL UPRIGHT

V1

T WAVE NORMAL UPRIGHT

V4

MAY BE INVERTED

II

T WAVE NORMAL UPRIGHT

aVL

MAY BE INVERTED

V2

V5

T WAVE NORMAL UPRIGHT

III

MAY BE INVERTED

aVF

V3

V6

T WAVE AMPLITUDE can be affected by many variables. There is no concrete rule about vertical size of the T wave. Use the guidelines listed to the right as an "alert limit." When T waves exceed these guidelines, be suspicious that one of the potentially lethal conditions which cause *hyperacute T waves* may exist, and begin the process of ruling them out.

(See HYPERACUTE T WAVES, page 120).

THE T WAVE

AMPLITUDE GUIDELINES:

- IN THE LIMB LEADS, SHOULD BE LESS THAN 1.0 mv (10 mm)
- IN THE PRECORDIAL LEADS, SHOULD BE LESS THAN 0.5 mv (5 mm)
- SHOULD NOT BE TALLER THAN R WAVE IN 2 OR MORE LEADS.

To evaluate an ECG for Acute Coronary Syndrome, carefully scrutinize the *J POINTS*, *ST SEGMENTS*, and *T WAVES* in every lead of the 12 lead ECG, applying the rules presented in this section. Be aware that *any deviation* from what is herein described as *normal* should be considered *abnormal*, and could signify the presence of *ACUTE CORONARY SYNDROME, non-acute ischemia*, or one of the conditions listed in "Differential Diagnosis of Abnormal ST Segments and T Waves," beginning on page 125.

☞ SIMPLY STATED, if it is *NOT NORMAL* it is *ABNORMAL!*

EVALUATE for S-T SEGMENT ELEVATION 40ms BEYOND the J POINT:

To help clinicians identify acute MI in cases where there are *J-T Apex segment abnormalities* and/or *hyper-acute T waves* without significant ST elevation at the J point, the American Heart Association presented *"J point plus 40ms"* in its ACLS curriculum revisions for the year 2000. This change calls for clinicians to assess for ST elevation *40ms after the J point*, as illustrated in the diagram to the right --------------------------->

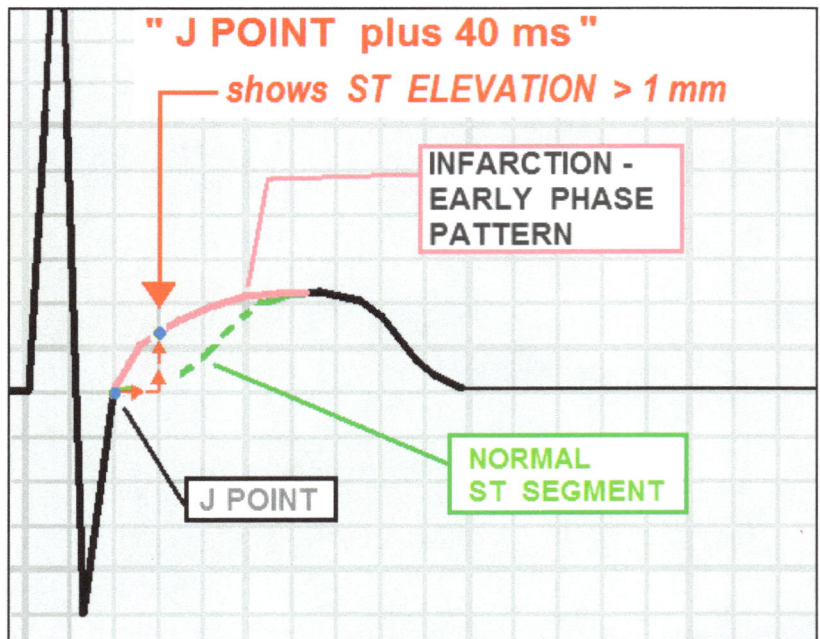

" J POINT plus 40 ms "
— shows ST ELEVATION > 1 mm

INFARCTION - EARLY PHASE PATTERN

J POINT

NORMAL ST SEGMENT

The table below features common J Point, ST Segment and T Wave abnormalities associated with ACUTE CORONARY SYNDROME, in patients with diagnostic quality ECGs (QRS complexes with durations less than 120ms):

13 ECG PATTERNS of ACS & ISCHEMIA
-- J POINT, ST SEGMENT, and T WAVE ABNORMALITIES --

!	S-T SEGMENT ELEVATION at J POINT	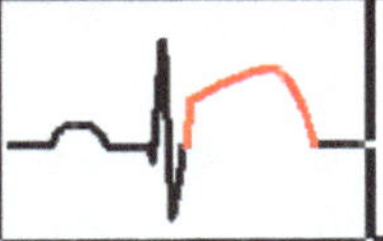	- ACUTE MI - ACUTE PERICARDITIS / MYOCARDITIS - EARLY REPOLARIZATION
!	FLAT or CONVEX J-T APEX SEGMENT	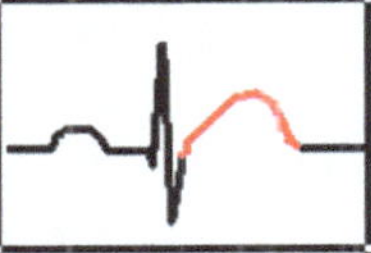 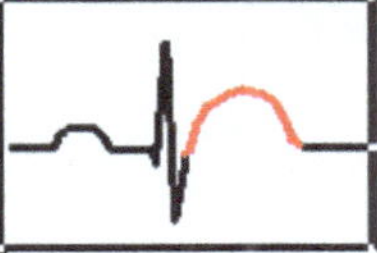	- ACUTE MI - ISCHEMIA
!	HYPER-ACUTE T WAVE	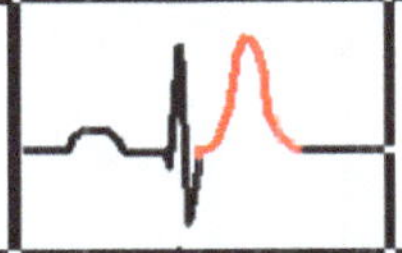	- HYPERKALEMIA - TRANSMURAL ISCHEMIA - ACUTE MI - HYPERTROPHY
!	DEPRESSED J pt. DOWNSLOPING ST and INVERTED T	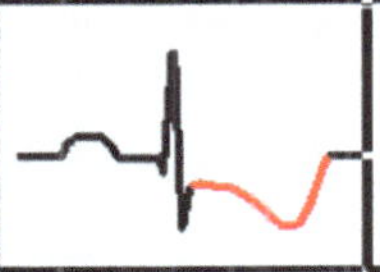	- ACUTE (NON-Q WAVE) MI - ACUTE MI - (RECIPROCAL CHANGES) - ISCHEMIA
	INVERTED T WAVE	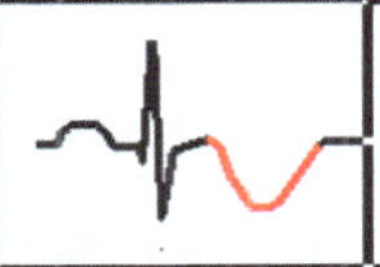	- MYOCARDITIS - ELECTROLYTE IMBAL. - ISCHEMIA
	SHARP S-T T ANGLE	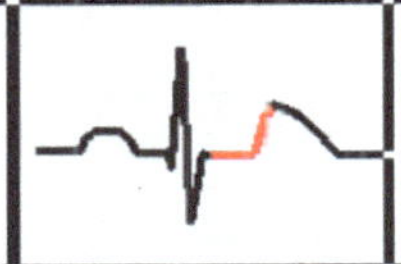	- ACUTE MI (NOT COMMON) - ISCHEMIA
	BI-PHASIC T WAVE (WELLEN'S)	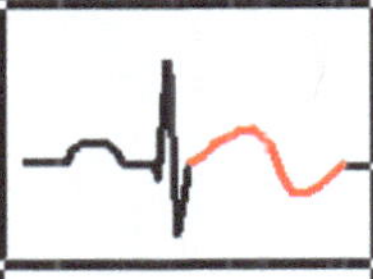	- SUB-TOTAL LAD LESION - VASOSPASM - HYPERTROPHY
	DEPRESSED J POINT with UPSLOPING ST	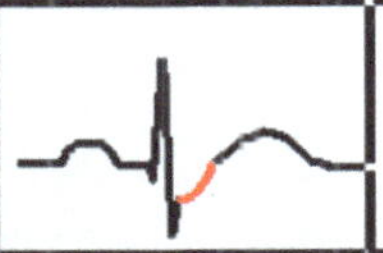	- ISCHEMIA
	DOWNSLOPING S-T SEGMENT	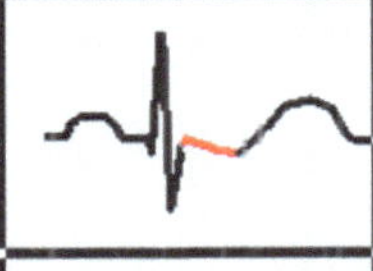	- ISCHEMIA
?	FLAT S-T SEGMENT > 120 ms	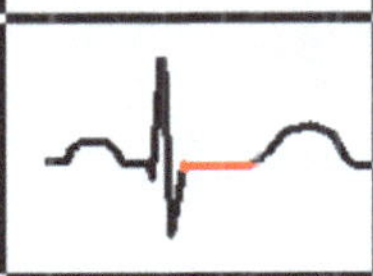	- ISCHEMIA
?	LOW VOLTAGE T WAVE WITH NORMAL QRS	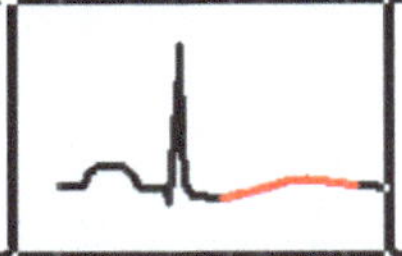	- ISCHEMIA
?	U WAVE POLARITY OPPOSITE THAT OF T WAVE	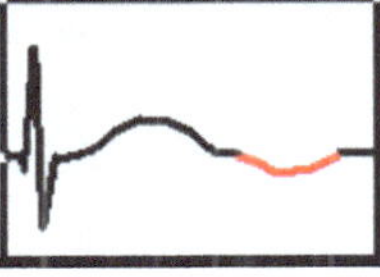	- ISCHEMIA

115

ECG DIAGNOSIS OF ACUTE MI:

Traditional ECG training teaches us to look for obvious "ST segment elevation in two or more contiguous leads" in order to diagnose ACUTE MI on the 12 Lead ECG. This is appropriate; however there are other less obvious ECG markers of AMI – often overlooked by the ECG's computer – which clinicians must be aware of and look for.

Changes to the ***ST segment*** and ***first half of the T wave*** (a.k.a. "The J – T Apex segment") are routinely observed in the Cardiac Cath Lab during PTCA and stent deployment. Balloon inflations, typically ranging between 15 and 60 seconds, often cause the J-T Apex segment to flatten or assume a convex shape, as seen in our example below. These subtle changes often precede "classic" ST segment elevation at the J point. The case study on page 118 provides a good example.

During NORMAL STATES of PERFUSION, the J POINT is ISOELECTRIC and the ST SEGMENT has a CONCAVE appearance. When measured 40 ms beyond the J POINT (noted by the RED DOT), the ST SEGMENT elevation is less than 1mm.

Both figures were recorded from a 54 year old male while resting (figure A), and during PTCA of the Left Anterior Descending artery (figure B).

fig A

During a 20 second BALLOON OCCLUSION of the patient's LAD during routine PTCA, the ST segment assumes a CONVEX shape. When measured 40 ms beyond the J POINT, the ST segment is elevated > 1 mm. This phenonemon is seen routinely in the cath lab prior to the occurance of ST ELEVATION at the J POINT during PTCA and STENTING.

fig B

NOTE: J POINT does NOT ELEVATE !

ECG MARKERS of ACUTE M.I.

EARLY or PRE-INFARCTION	ACUTE INFARCTION	EVOLVING INFARCTION
• HYPERACUTE T WAVES	• S-T SEGMENT ELEVATION	• ABNORMAL Q WAVES
• FLAT or CONVEX J-T APEX SEGMENTS	• S-T SEGMENT DEPRESSION	• ABNORMAL R-WAVE PROGRESSION in PRECORDIAL LEADS

On the next several pages, we present and discuss the "ECG Markers of Acute MI" in detail, and reinforce essential concepts with Case Studies from the Cardiac Cath Lab.

116

PRE-INFARCTION PATTERNS - ABNORMAL J-T APEX SEGMENTS:

In the earliest phases of acute MI, the J-T Apex segment may change – *often without significantly elevating or depressing the J point* – a subtle change which is sometimes missed by ECG interpretation software and clinicians alike.

The image to the right overlays three variations of J-T Apex Segments; *concave, flat,* and *convex.* The *concave* pattern, shown in green, is normal. The *flat J-T apex segment*, in orange, is abnormal, as is the *convex J-T apex segment,* which is shown in red. *Flat* and *Convex J-T apex segments* may indicate acute myocardial infarction.

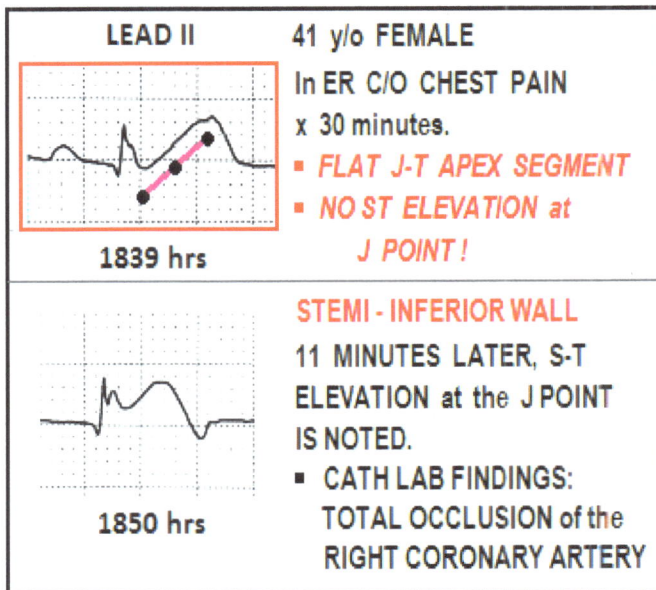

J - T APEX SEGMENT VARIATIONS

ABNORMAL - *CONVEX*

ABNORMAL - *FLAT*

NORMAL - *CONCAVE*

PATTERNS of EARLY INFARCTION
-- FLAT and CONVEX J-T APEX SEGMENTS

LEAD II

41 y/o FEMALE
In ER C/O CHEST PAIN
x 30 minutes.
- FLAT J-T APEX SEGMENT
- NO ST ELEVATION at
  J POINT !

1839 hrs

STEMI - INFERIOR WALL
11 MINUTES LATER, S-T
ELEVATION at the J POINT
IS NOTED.
- CATH LAB FINDINGS:
  TOTAL OCCLUSION of the
  RIGHT CORONARY ARTERY

1850 hrs

The image to the left is from a patient who presented to the ED complaining of chest pain. Her first ECG did not show ST elevation; however an astute physician noticed the odd appearance of the J-T apex segment. In this case, the J-T Apex Segment is FLAT, making it difficult to discern where the ST segment ends and the T wave begins. Eleven minutes later, a second ECG was obtained, demonstrating clearly defined S-T segment elevation at the J point. She was taken emergently to the Cardiac Cath Lab, where a total occlusion of her right coronary artery was discovered.

In another case, a 53 year old male presented to the ED with typical ACS type chest pain. His ECG (in image to the right) featured CONVEX J-T APEX SEGMENTS in leads I and aVL. We were fortunate to have an old ECG available for comparison; he had been hospitalized a year prior, and an ECG was recorded during that visit. The ED physician compared the two, and quickly concluded the patient should visit the Cath Lab, STAT. An ECG recorded just before he was wheeled to the Cath Lab showed elevation of his S-T segment at the J point. We found a large thrombus in his circumflex artery. Fortunately for him, he had a small, non-dominant circumflex, which minimized his area of infarct. Thrombectomy and stenting of the circumflex artery resolved his symptoms.

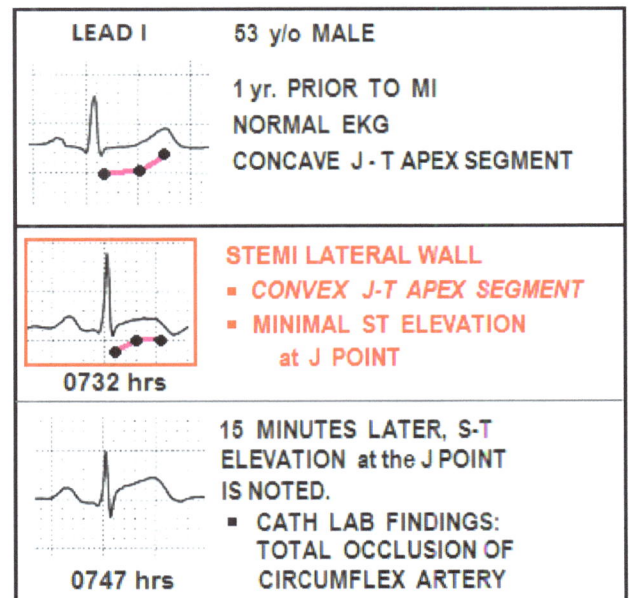

LEAD I

53 y/o MALE

1 yr. PRIOR TO MI
NORMAL EKG
CONCAVE J - T APEX SEGMENT

STEMI LATERAL WALL
- CONVEX J-T APEX SEGMENT
- MINIMAL ST ELEVATION
  at J POINT

0732 hrs

15 MINUTES LATER, S-T
ELEVATION at the J POINT
IS NOTED.
- CATH LAB FINDINGS:
  TOTAL OCCLUSION OF
  CIRCUMFLEX ARTERY

0747 hrs

CHIEF COMPLAINT and SIGNIFICANT HISTORY:

56 y/o **MALE** presents to **ED** with complaint of "**INTERMITTENT SUBSTERNAL & SUB-EPIGASTRIC PRESSURE**" x 3 HOURS. **PMHx** of **ESOPHAGEAL REFLUX.** NO other significant past medical history.

RISK FACTOR PROFILE:

- ✺ **FAMILY HISTORY** - father died of MI at age 62
- ☑ **PREVIOUS CIGARETTE SMOKER** - quit 15 years ago.
- ☑ **CHOLESTEROL - DOES NOT KNOW;** "never had it checked."
- ☑ **OBESITY**

PHYSICAL EXAM: Patient supine on exam table, mildly anxious, currently complaining of "mild indigestion," skin is warm, pale, dry; REST OF EXAM is UNREMARKABLE.

VITAL SIGNS: BP 142/94, P 80, R 20, SAO2 98%

LABS: JUST OBTAINED, RESULTS NOT AVAILABLE YET.

The ECG below was recorded within minutes of the patient's arrival. When measured at the J point, ST elevation is minimal.

NOTICE the computer's interpretation of this ECG is "NORMAL ECG" -- it did not notice the CONVEX J-T APEX SEGMENTS!

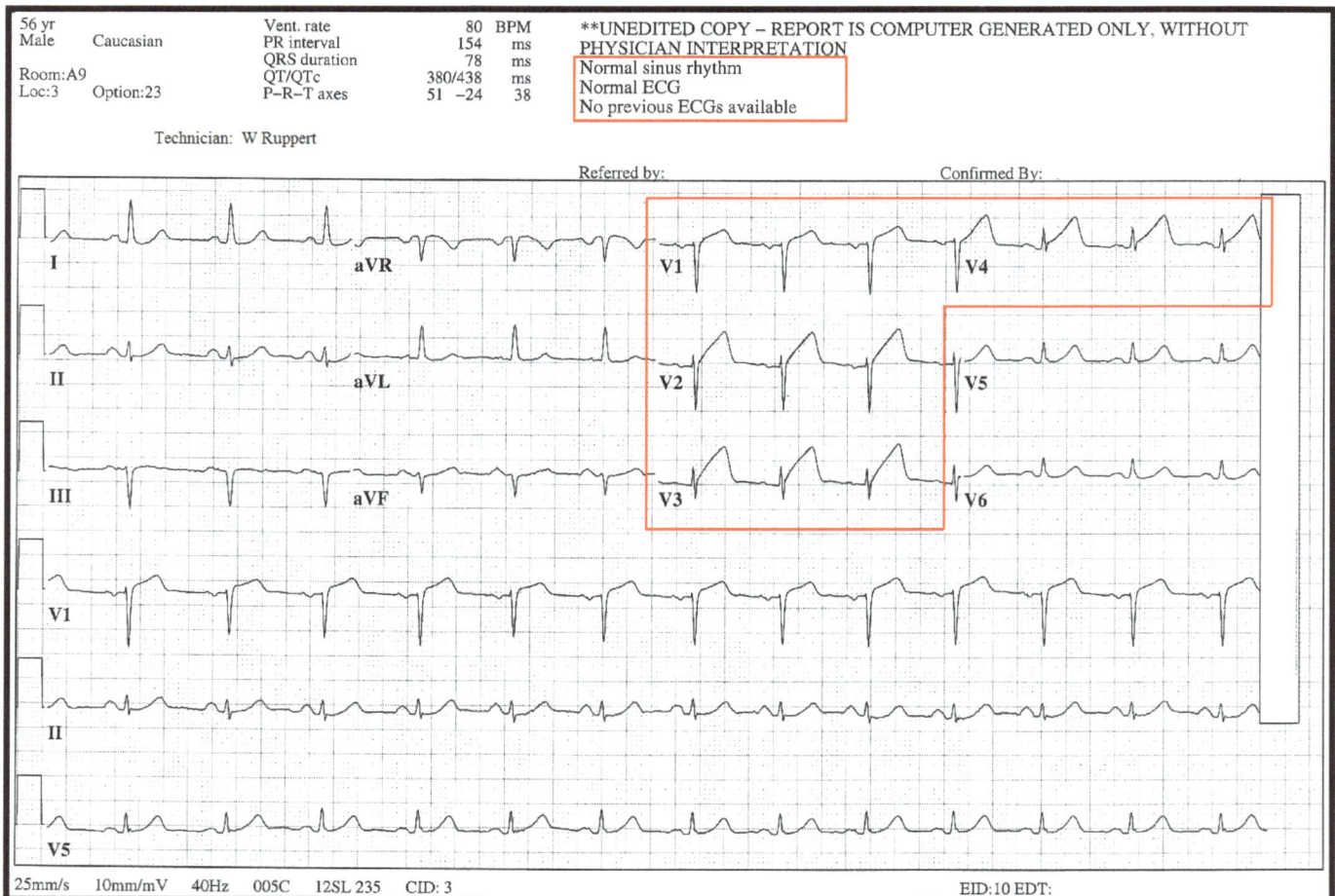

56 yr		Vent. rate	80	BPM
Male	Caucasian	PR interval	154	ms
		QRS duration	78	ms
Room:A9		QT/QTc	380/438	ms
Loc:3	Option:23	P–R–T axes	51 –24 38	

Technician: W Ruppert

**UNEDITED COPY – REPORT IS COMPUTER GENERATED ONLY, WITHOUT PHYSICIAN INTERPRETATION
Normal sinus rhythm
Normal ECG
No previous ECGs available

Referred by: Confirmed By:

25mm/s   10mm/mV   40Hz   005C   12SL 235   CID: 3   EID:10 EDT:

When *J POINT PLUS 40ms* guidelines are applied, *ST segment elevation is 2.0mm,* as seen in the amplified view of lead V2:

The patient was taken STAT to the cardiac cath lab, where the angiogram shown below was obtained. Based on the findings of critical stenosis discovered in the patient's left anterior descending, circumflex, ramus, and right coronary arteries (RCA image not shown), he was transferred immediately to the Cardiac Surgery suite where successful quadruple CABG was performed.

measurement of ST elevation:

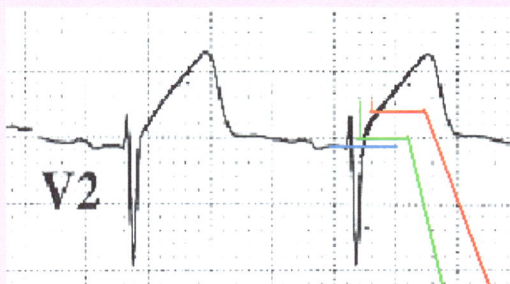

V2

at J POINT = 1.0 mm
at J POINT + 40 ms = 2.0 mm

ACUTE MI = S-T elev. > 1.0 mm

CASE STUDY: 56 y/o male with INTERMITTENT "CHEST HEAVINESS" . . . .

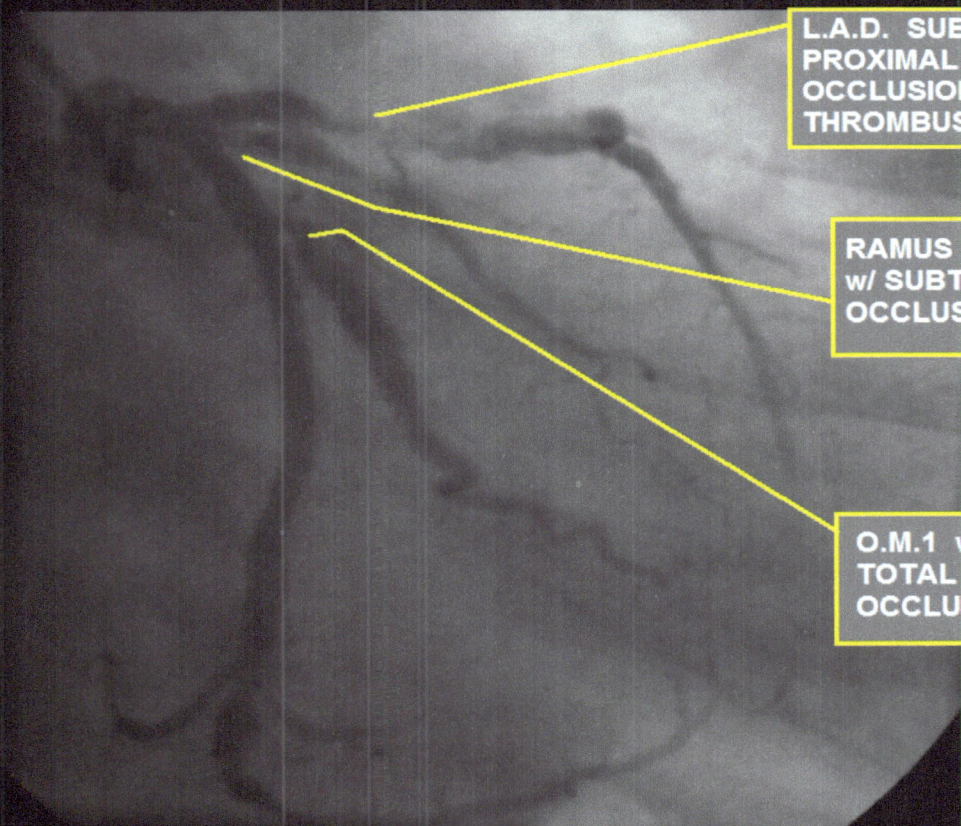

L.A.D. SUBTOTAL PROXIMAL OCCLUSION WITH THROMBUS

RAMUS ARTERY w/ SUBTOTAL OCCLUSION

O.M.1 w/ SUB-TOTAL OCCLUSION

TREATMENT PLAN : EMERGENCY CORONARY ARTERY BYPASS SURGERY (4 VESSEL)

PRE-INFARCTION PATTERNS - HYPER-ACUTE T WAVES:

Hyper-acute T waves are sometimes observed on the ECGs of patients during the onset of Acute MI. As shown in the diagram to the right, other causes of hyper-acute T waves include *transmural ischemia, hyperkalemia,* and *ventricular hypertrophy.* Note that the first three conditions – *hyperkalemia, acute MI* ("early phase pattern"), and *transmural ischemia* are potentially life-threatening conditions – *making the presence of hyperacute T waves a disconcerting finding!*

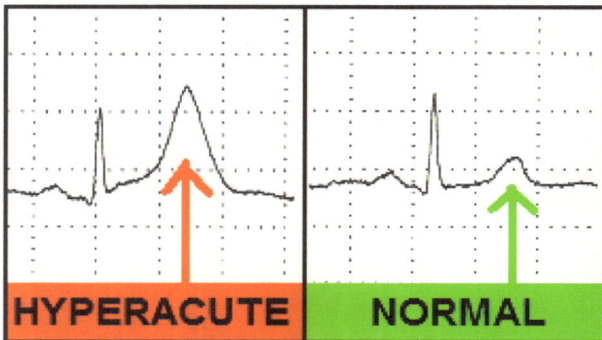

HYPER-ACUTE T WAVES - COMMON ETIOLOGIES:

CONDITION:

- **HYPERKALEMIA**
- **ACUTE MI**
- **TRANS-MURAL ISCHEMIA**
- **HYPERTROPHY**

HYPERACUTE | NORMAL

The diagram above illustrates a *hyper-acute T wave* (lead V5) in a patient with a sub-totally occluded proximal Left Anterior Descending artery (above right image). The normal T wave was recorded 15 minutes after successful PCI to this lesion.

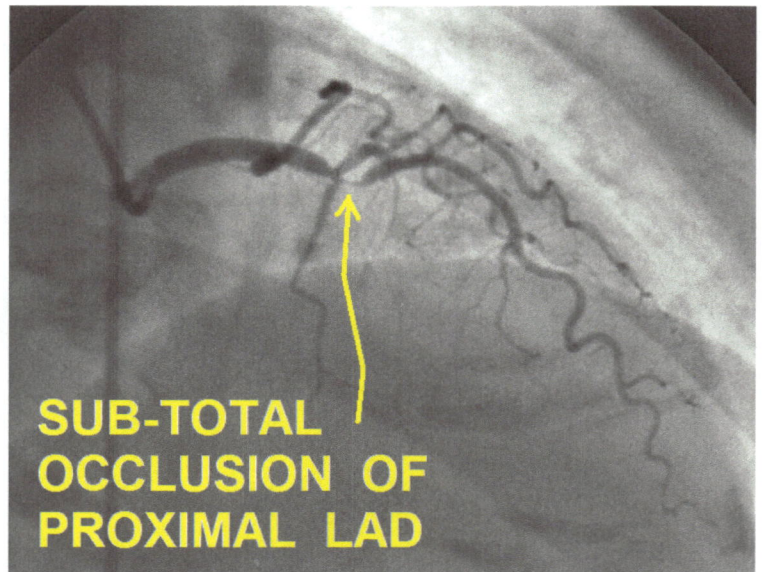

SUB-TOTAL OCCLUSION OF PROXIMAL LAD

☞   *Hyper-acute T waves* may not be recognized as *abnormal* by your ECG Machine's **ECG interpretation software** – which is what occurred during our CASE STUDY, shown on the next page. *This incident demonstrates why clinicians should not accept the ECG machine's computerized interpretation at face value.*

CASE STUDY: HYPERACUTE T WAVES

CHIEF COMPLAINT and SIGNIFICANT HISTORY:

30 y/o male presents to ER via EMS, c/o sudden onset of dull chest pain x 40 min. Pain level varies, not effected by position, movement or deep inspiration. No associated symptoms.

RISK FACTOR PROFILE: NONE. CHOLESTEROL UNKNOWN.

PHYSICAL EXAM: Patient is supine on exam table, CAO x 4, anxious, restless, skin pale, cool, dry. Patient c/o chest pressure, "7" on 1 - 10 scale, uneffected by position, movement, deep inspiration. Lungs clear. HS: NL S1, S2, no rubs, murmurs, gallops

VITAL SIGNS: BP 136/88   P 90   R 20   SAO2 98%

DIAGNOSTIC TESTING: 1st TROPONIN I - ultra: <0.07

The patient's first ECG was taken within 10 minutes of the patient's arrival in the emergency department. ***Note that the computer's interpretation declares this a "normal ECG."*** The J points in the anterior leads are elevated between 2 – 3 mm in leads V1 through V3, well within the "normal" range for "male pattern ST elevation[23]." The initial ED physician's diagnosis was "Early Repolarization." Approximately 17 minutes after arriving in the ED, the patient demonstrated V-Fib, and was defibrillated x 1 at 360 joules, with return of sinus rhythm with pulse. A STAT 2-D echo was performed, which revealed anterior wall hypokinesis. At this point, based on the above findings, a "CODE STEMI" was activated by the ED physician, and the patient was taken immediately to the cardiac catheterization lab.

30 yr				
Male	Black	Vent. rate	88	BPM
		PR interval	164	ms
		QRS duration	90	ms
Room: ER		QT/QTc	370/447	ms
Loc:	Option:	P–R–T axes	61 62 53	

Normal sinus rhythm
Normal ECG
No previous ECGs available   ← NOTE COMPUTER INTERPRETATION

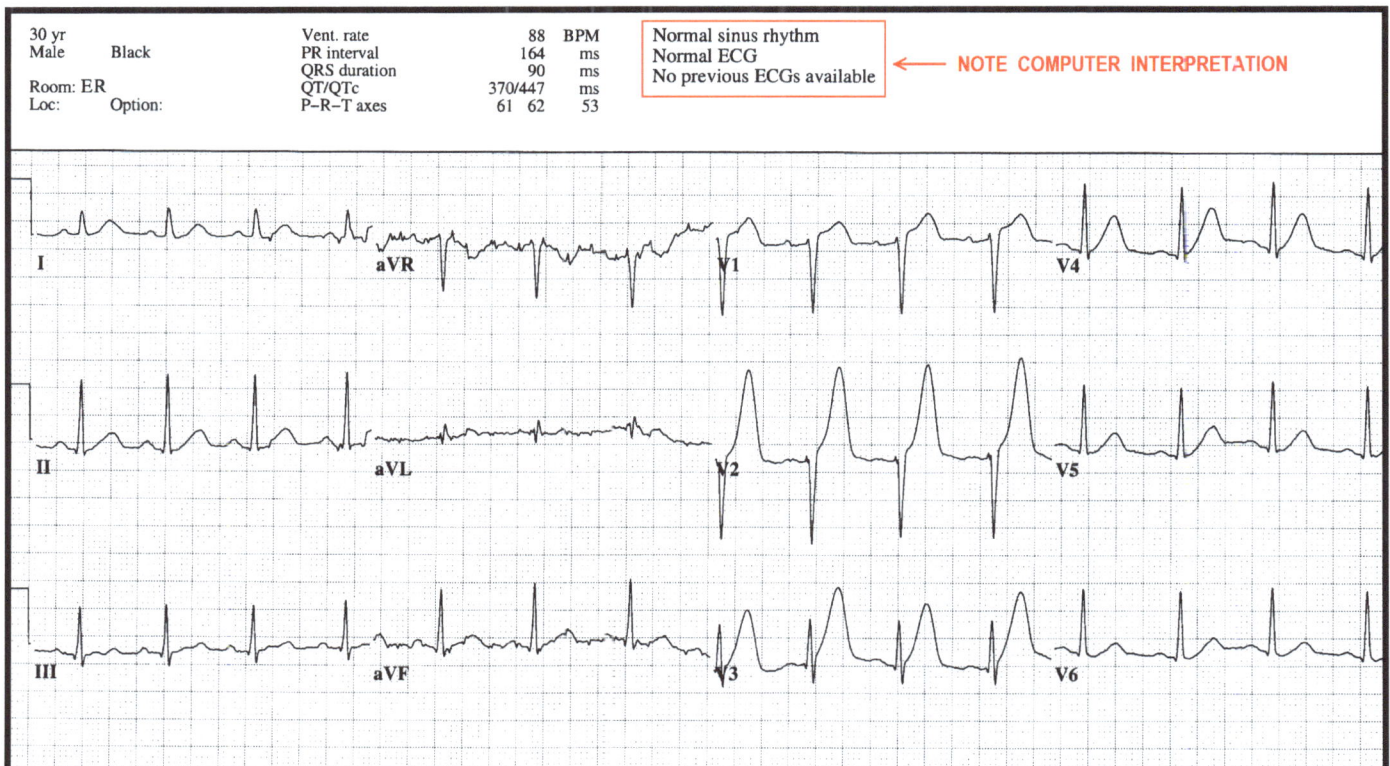

[23] J Surawicz, et al, J Am Coll Cardiol 2002;40:1870-76

30 yr		Vent. rate	88	BPM	Normal sinus rhythm
Male	Black	PR interval	164	ms	Normal ECG
		QRS duration	90	ms	No previous ECGs available
Room: ER		QT/QTc	370/447	ms	**HIGHLIGHTED AREAS =**
Loc:	Option:	P–R–T axes	61 62	53	**HYPERACUTE T WAVES**

CORONARY ARTERIAL DISTRIBUTIONS:
V1 - V4 = LEFT ANTERIOR DESCENDING (LAD)
I, AVL = DIAGONAL (DIAG) off the LAD or
OBTUSE MARGINAL (OM) off CIRCUMFLEX (CX)
V5, V6 = CIRCUMFLEX
II, III, AVF = RIGHT CORONARY ARTERY or CX

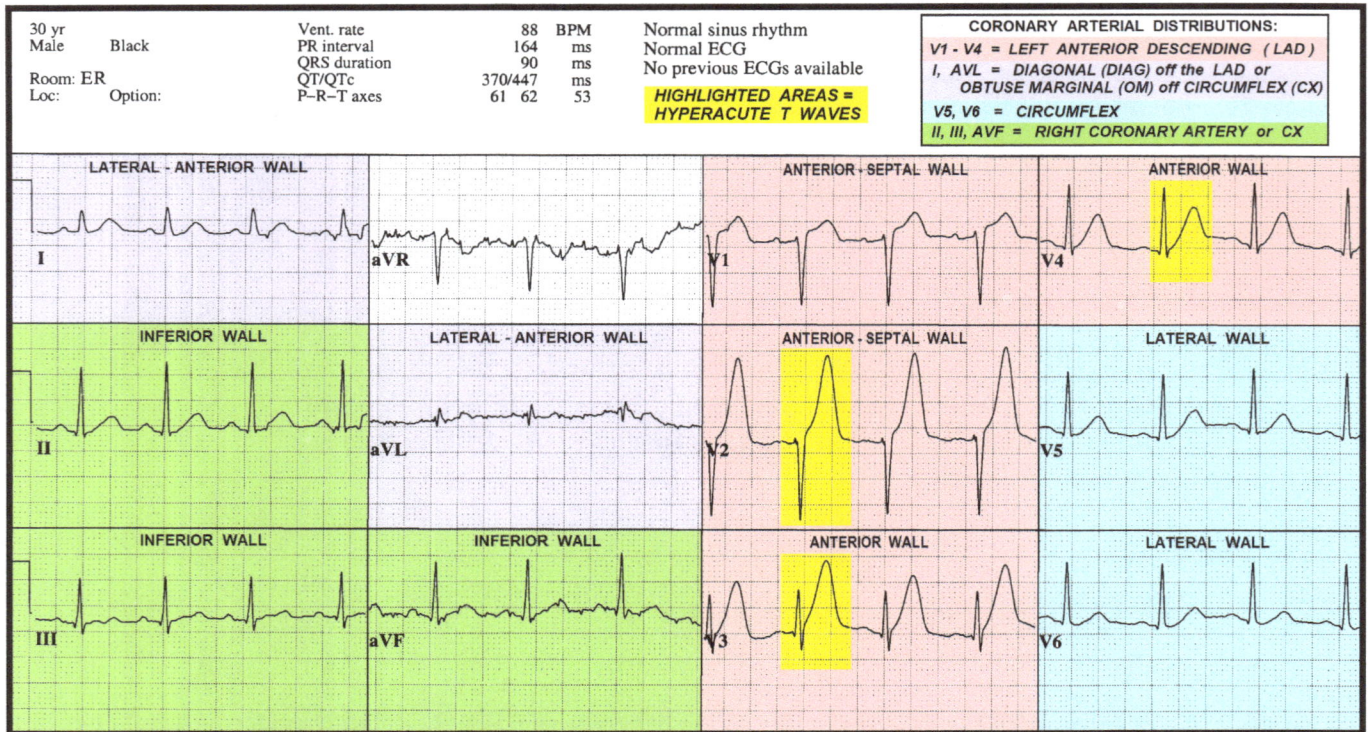

> ☞ Of the four conditions which cause HYPERACUTE T WAVES (*hyperkalemia, acute MI, transmural ischemia, and ventricular hypertrophy*), **significant arterial blockage** is the cause of *acute MI* and *transmural ischemia*. One helpful clue that points to a possible diagnosis of *anterior wall ischemia* in this case study is the observation that *hyperacute T waves are only seen in one arterial distribution* – that is, they are only seen in leads that view the ANTERIOR WALL, which receives its blood supply from the left anterior descending artery. Another helpful clue in this case study is that *the patient is complaining of symptoms consistent with AMI.*

In the cardiac catherization lab, a total proximal occlusion of the *left anterior descending artery* was discovered (below, left image). The patient underwent successful PTCA and stenting to the LAD (below, right image). It is also interesting to note that this patients ONLY ECG indicator of Acute MI was the presence of hyperacute T waves; at no time did he develop "typical" ST segment elevation.

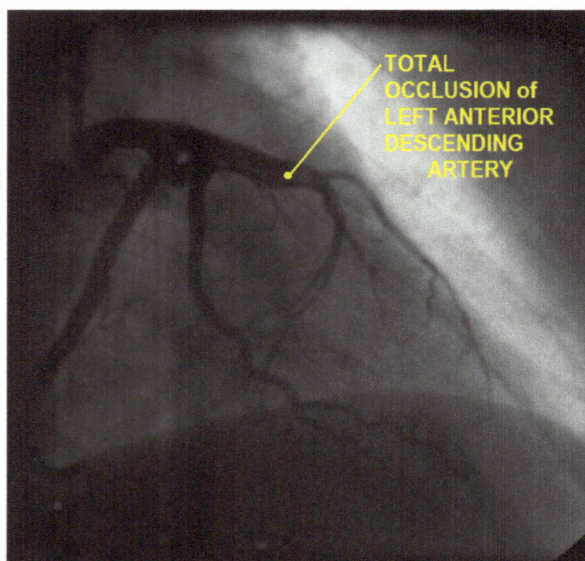

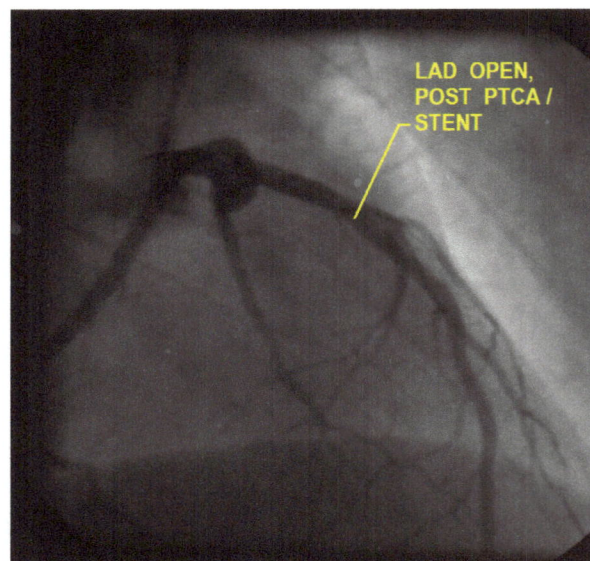

Case study contributed by: John Toole, MD, FACC

ACUTE MYOCARDIAL INFARCTION - STEMI:

As stated in the previous section, *"Pre-Infarction Patterns,"* ST SEGMENT ELEVATION may be preceded by HYPERACUTE T WAVES, FLAT or CONVEX J-T APEX SEGMENTS – or ST SEGMENT ELEVATION may occur as the first ECG abnormality of AMI. In the example below, *primary ST Segment elevation* is the first indicator of arterial obstruction, and *occurs within seconds of inflation of the PTCA balloon*:

S-T SEGMENTS ELEVATE WITHIN SECONDS OF CORONARY ARTERY OCCLUSION:

I

II

IN THIS CASE, a normal response to balloon occlusion of the RIGHT CORONARY ARTERY during PTCA in the CARDIAC CATH LAB

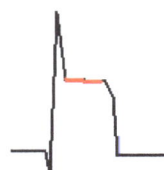

Reciprocal S-T Segment Depression *may* or *may not* be present during AMI. The presence of S-T Depression on an ECG which exhibits significant S-T elevation is a fairly reliable indicator that AMI is the diagnosis – and often *indicates a proximal arterial blockage* (see CASE STUDY 3, page 178). **However the *lack of Reciprocal S-T Depression* DOES NOT rule out AMI.**

S-T Segments may be downsloping, flat, or upsloping:

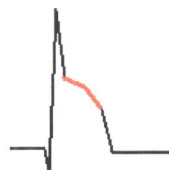

DOWNSLOPING   FLAT   UPSLOPING
S-T SEGMENT   S-T SEGMENT   S-T SEGMENT

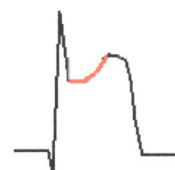

The table below features samples of ST elevation taken from the ECGs of patients experiencing AMI. Angiographic findings in the Cardiac Cath Lab for each patient revealed total obstruction of a coronary artery. Notice the difference in the appearance of ST segments: some are UPSLOPING, some are relatively FLAT, and some feature DOWNSLOPING ST segments:

ST SEGMENT ELEVATION in ACUTE MI:

The following samples are from patients with ACUTE MI, as confirmed by discovery of total arterial occlusion in the Cardiac Cath Lab:

			"TOOMBSTONE" PATTERN	"FIREMAN'S HAT" PATTERN
V5 - ANTERIOR LATERAL MI	V4 - ANTERIOR LATERAL MI	aVL - ANTERIOR LATERAL MI	V2 - ANTERIOR LATERAL MI	V3 - ANTERIOR LATERAL MI
"TOOMBSTONE" PATTERN				"FIREMAN'S HAT" PATTERN
V4 - ANTERIOR LATERAL MI	V5 - ANTERIOR LATERAL MI	V5 - ANTERIOR LATERAL MI	II - INFERIOR POSTERIOR MI	aVF - INFERIOR POSTERIOR MI
III - INFERIOR MI	III - INFERIOR POSTERIOR MI	III - INFERIOR MI	III - INFERIOR MI	II - INFERIOR POSTERIOR MI

As a GENERAL GUIDELINE, the following ECG characteristics appear to correlate with an extensive area of myocardial injury during STEMI:

High J point of ST elevation ("tombstones" or "fireman's hat" ST elevation- see above)
Multiple zones of infarct (ANTERIOR-LATERAL, INFERIOR-POSTERIOR-LATERAL, etc).
Presence of RECIPROCAL ST DEPRESSION: usually indicates a proximal occlusion of the blocked artery (as opposed to a mid- or distal occlusion).
ST elevation in aVR (often means PROXIMAL LAD and/or LEFT MAIN CORONARY ARTERY occlusion
ST elevation in Leads I and aVL: with ANTERIOR MI = PROXIMAL LAD occlusion; with LATERAL MI = PROXIMAL CIRCUMFLEX occlusion; and INFERIOR MI = PROXIMAL OCCLUSION of a DOMINANT CIRCUMFLEX artery.

DIFFERENTIAL DIAGNOSIS of ST ELEVATION:

Note in the table below, there are numerous conditions that can cause ST segment elevation which can mimic that of ACS. As you study the ECG patterns below, notice that discerning ST elevation caused by AMI versus that of other etiologies may be extremely difficult – or impossible to do – in some cases.

☞ For the full 12 Lead ECGs of ST SEGMENT ELEVATION caused by conditions other than STEMI, see "12 Lead ECGs of STEMI Mimics," beginning on page 273.

ST SEGMENT ELEVATION
DIFFERENTIAL DIAGNOSIS

CASE INFORMATION:	I	III	V1	V2	V3	V5	REFERENCE NOTES:
NORMAL "MALE PATTERN" ST ELEVATION - 38 y/o MALE, no CAD							In a study of 529 men ages 16-24, 93% had ST ELEVATION of >1mm in LEADS V1 - V4. 20% of women had the same finding. - J SURAWICZ, el al, J AM COLL CARDIOL 2002;40:1870-76
LEFT BUNDLE BRANCH BLOCK, 46 y/o FEMALE no CAD							A common finding in patients with QRS > 120 ms with LBBB pattern is ST ELEVATION > 1mm. This includes most PACED RHYTHMS (RV Lead)
EARLY REPOLARIZATION 36 y/o MALE no CAD							In many healthy young men (mostly black men) this ST pattern is often noted. - KAMBARA, et al, J AM COLL CARDIOL 1976;38:157-61
LEFT VENTRICULAR HYPERTROPHY 61 y/o FEMALE no CAD							In LVH, the deeper the S WAVE, the GREATER the ST ELEVATION. May present with QS in precordial leads. ST segments CONCAVE - WANG, et al, N ENGL J MED 2003;349:1128-35
PERICARDITIS 41 y/o MALE no CAD							ST ELEVATION diffusely elevated in throughout 12 lead EKG. Often PR segment ↑ aVR and ↓ Lead II. - WANG, et al. N ENGL J MED 2003;349:1128-35
MYOCARDITIS 30 y/o FEMALE no CAD							ST ELEVATION in ACUTE MYOCARDITIS can mimick that of ACUTE MI. - SPODICK et al, CIRCULATION 1995;91:1886-87
HYPERKALEMIA (K+ 8.6) 53 y/o MALE no CAD							HYPERKALEMIA can mimic EKG findings of AMI. Other findings include TALL, PEAKED T WAVES - LEVINE, et al, CIRCULATION 1956;13:29-36
BRUGADA SYNDROME 36 y/o FEMALE no CAD							Genetic disorder responsible for 40-60% of all idiopathic V-FIB. Recognizable V1-V3 pattern. - BRUGADA & BRUGADA et al, J AM COLL CARDIOL 1992;20:1391-96
ACUTE ANTERIOR WALL MI 52 y/o MALE - MID LAD OCCLUSION							ACUTE ST SEGMENT ELEVATION MI (STEMI) characterized by: - ST ELEVATION of >1mm in 2 or more contiguous leads. - ST segments usually CONVEX

When patients with known chronic conditions that elevate ST segments, such as LVH or LBBB present with symptoms of AMI, it is imperative that clinicians expediently and thoroughly rule out AMI. The chronic ST elevation of these patients may "mask" ST elevation caused by AMI. Here is where having OLD ECGs to compare today's ECG to, and thoroughly evaluating each component of the **Quadrad of ACS – symptoms, risk factor profile, ECG,** and **cardiac markers –** will aid you in rapidly ruling out STEMI. Use of a validated ACS Risk Stratification tool, such as the Modified TIMI ACS Risk Score, will aid you in attaining a higher degree of diagnostic accuracy.

4. EVOLVING MI – THE DEVELOPMENT of SIGNIFICANT Q WAVES and R –WAVE PROGRESSION ABNORMALITIES:

During the early phase of STEMI, the J-T Apex segments may become flat or convex, and T waves may become hyper acute. Or, the ECG may progress directly to elevated J points and ST segment elevation. During the active phase of AMI, cardiac cells are still alive; however since no oxygen or glucose is being supplied to cells in the infarct zone, cell metabolism converts from *aerobic* to *anaerobic*. The cell is able to remain alive for a short period of time by metabolizing its remaining glycogen reserves. During AMI, ATP production nearly halts, cell contractions ceases, and metabolic waste products accumulate. If circulation is not restored over a period of hours, as glycogen reserves are depleted, cell death occurs. Since dead cells are unable to propagate electrical impulses, Q waves become visible in ECG leads that view the regions of cardiac cell necrosis. The table below describes different states of cardiac cell perfusion:

CARDIAC CELL PERFUSION STATES

NORMAL STATE OF PERFUSION

ARTERIAL BLOCKAGES	→ NONE SIGNIFICANT
CELLULAR OXYGENATION	→ NORMAL
CELLULAR METABOLISM	→ AEROBIC
CELLULAR FUNCTION	→ NORMAL CONTRACTION

EKG: J POINT ISOELECTRIC, ST SEG "SLIGHT, POSTIVE INCLINATION, T WAVE POSITIVE, UPRIGHT.

ISCHEMIA

ARTERIAL BLOCKAGES	→ PARTIAL OBSTRUCTION
CELLULAR OXYGENATION	→ INSUFFICIENT
CELLULAR METABOLISM	→ AEROBIC
CELLULAR FUNCTION	→ REDUCED CONTRACTION
PATIENT SYMPTOMS	→ *POSSIBLE*, WITH EXERTION

EKG: J POINT DEPRESSED, ST SEGMENT VARIES, T WAVE VARIES

INFARCTION

ARTERIAL BLOCKAGES	→ TOTAL OBSTRUCTION
CELLULAR OXYGENATION	→ NONE
CELLULAR METABOLISM	→ ANAEROBIC *CELL BEGINS TO BURN GLYCOGEN RESERVES*
CELLULAR FUNCTION	→ STOPS CONTRACTING
PATIENT SYMPTOMS	→ *TYPICAL or ATYPICAL ACS Sx*

EKG – INDICATIVE: J POINT ELEVATES, ST SEGMENT CONVEX, T WAVE POSITIVE, MAY ENLARGE
EKG – RECIPROCAL: J POINT DEPRESSES, ST SEGMENT DOWNSLOPING, T WAVE INVERTED

NECROSIS

ARTERIAL BLOCKAGES	→ TOTAL OBSTRUCTION
CELLULAR OXYGENATION	→ NONE
CELLULAR METABOLISM	→ *CELL DIES WHEN GLYCOGEN RESERVES DEPLETED.*
CELLULAR FUNCTION	→ NONE. CELL DEAD.
PATIENT SYMPTOMS	→ *POSS. HYPOTENSION, DEATH*

EKG – INDICATIVE: J POINTS, ST SEGMENTS NORMALIZE; ABNORMAL Q WAVES FORM
EKG – RECIPROCAL: J POINTS, ST SEGMENTS NORMALIZE; ABNORMAL TALL R WAVES FORM

Usually within the first hour of AMI, abnormal Q waves on the ECG are not evident. As the process of cell death ensues, usually over a period of several hours, Q waves begin to form. If perfusion is not restored, QRS complexes may progress to totally negative waveforms; "QS" complexes.

When this process occurs in ANTERIOR WALL MI, the formation and deepening of Q waves in the anterior leads will alter the normal progression of R waves, leading to "delayed R wave progression."

Whether evaluating the ECG of a patient currently experiencing AMI, or reading the ECG of an asymptomatic patient, we must evaluate for evidence of myocardial cell necrosis; specifically for the presence of abnormal Q waves, and/or abnormal R wave progression in the precordial leads.

EVALUATION OF Q WAVES

Small Q waves are frequently seen in many leads, and are considered normal; they're caused by *depolarization of the intraventricular septum*. Q waves that are *too big* are considered *abnormal*. When the entire QRS complex is negative (QS complex), it is considered an abnormal Q wave.

When Q waves exceed the guidelines presented in the table to the right, they are considered *abnormal*. Abnormal Q waves commonly indicate necrosis (old MI) in whatever region of the heart the ECG is viewing. Positive Q waves are also seen in severe cardiomyopathy, myocarditis, hypertrophy, Wolff-Parkinson-White syndrome, left bundle branch block, paced rhythms, and ventricular complexes/rhythms.

Q WAVE RULES - SUMMARY:

- Q WAVES SHOULD BE LESS THAN .40 WIDE (1 mm)

- Q WAVES SHOULD BE LESS THAN 1/3 THE HEIGHT OF THE R WAVE

- Q WAVES CAN BE ANY SIZE IN LEADS III and AVR

- THERE SHOULD BE NO Q WAVES IN LEADS V1, V2, or V3

The ECG below was taken one year prior to the patient's acute INFERIOR WALL STEMI. Note that there are NO abnormal Q waves present.

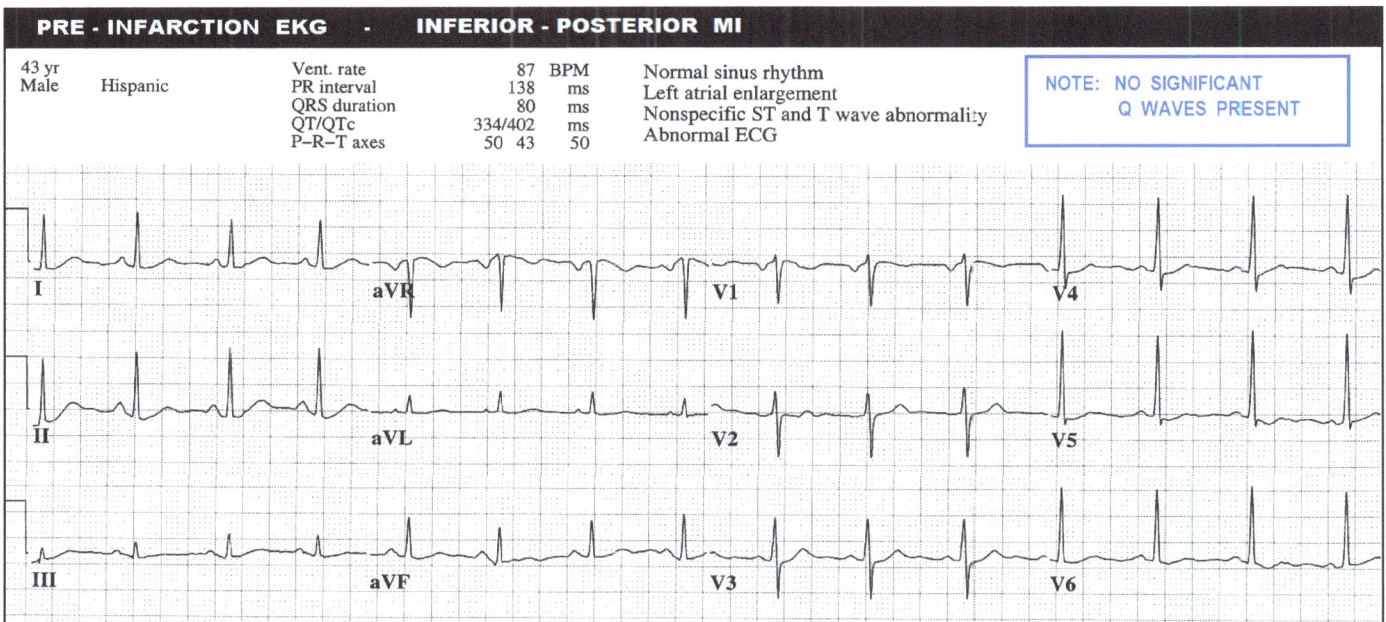

PRE - INFARCTION EKG - INFERIOR - POSTERIOR MI

43 yr Male	Hispanic	Vent. rate	87	BPM	Normal sinus rhythm
		PR interval	138	ms	Left atrial enlargement
		QRS duration	80	ms	Nonspecific ST and T wave abnormality
		QT/QTc	334/402	ms	Abnormal ECG
		P–R–T axes	50 43	50	

NOTE: NO SIGNIFICANT Q WAVES PRESENT

The ECG on the next page was recorded in the ER 5 minutes after the patient arrived, with a chief complaint of "chest pressure of varying intensity for several hours." The appearance of abnormal Q waves helps to corroborate the patient's claim that the symptoms have persisted for several hours.

44 yr		Vent. rate	83	BPM	Normal sinus rhythm
Male	Hispanic	PR interval	130	ms	
		QRS duration	86	ms	Inferior infarct , possibly acute
		QT/QTc	362/425	ms	Lateral injury pattern
		P–R–T axes	53 70	98	** ** ** ** * ACUTE MI * ** ** ** **

SIGNIFICANT ST ELEVATION, INFERIOR LEADS

D.O.S.:

ABNORMAL Q WAVES - INFERIOR LEADS

The ECG below was recorded approximately 6 hours after the ECG above. Note ST segments have resolved, and Q waves are now dominant in all inferior leads.

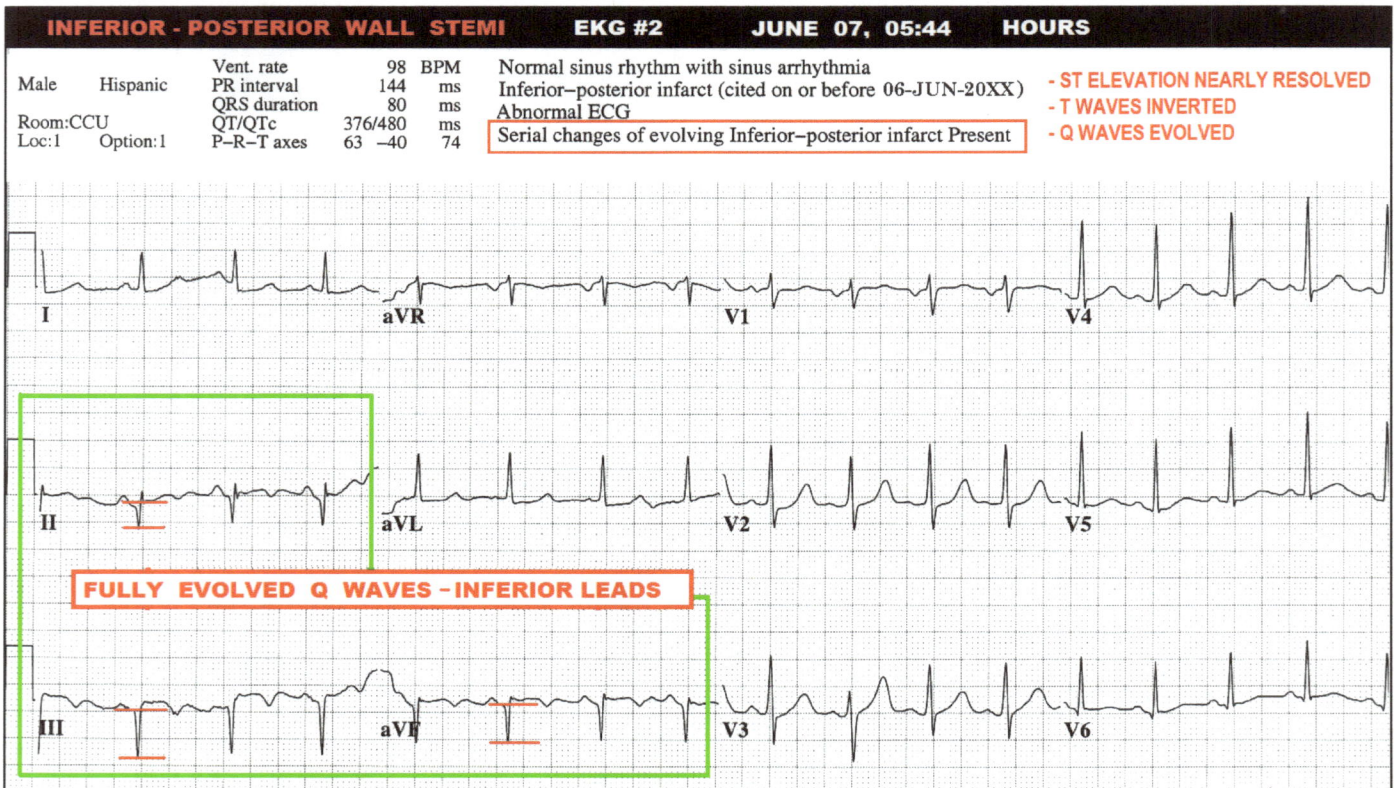

Male	Hispanic	Vent. rate	98	BPM	Normal sinus rhythm with sinus arrhythmia
		PR interval	144	ms	Inferior–posterior infarct (cited on or before 06-JUN-20XX)
		QRS duration	80	ms	Abnormal ECG
Room:CCU		QT/QTc	376/480	ms	
Loc:1	Option:1	P–R–T axes	63 –40	74	Serial changes of evolving Inferior–posterior infarct Present

- ST ELEVATION NEARLY RESOLVED
- T WAVES INVERTED
- Q WAVES EVOLVED

FULLY EVOLVED Q WAVES – INFERIOR LEADS

EVALUATION OF R WAVE PROGRESSION

In the Basic 12 Lead ECG Concepts chapter of this book we presented Axis Rotation, a.k.a. Evaluation of R Wave Progression. As a reminder, QRS complexes in lead V1 are mainly negative, with only small positive R waves. As we progress through the precordial leads from V1 through V6, R waves become taller, and the negative deflecting S waves become smaller. In simpler terms, the QRS complexes become more positive.

Also recall that when we evaluate the precordial leads for R Wave Progression, we note which lead features the most *biphasic QRS complex*. The lead which is most biphasic is called "*transition*." In the normal ECG, transition occurs in V3 or V4. If transition occurs in V1 or V2, we say there is "early transition," and if transition occurs in leads V5 or V6, we say there is "late transition."

(If you need to review the causes of abnormal R wave progression, see pages 77 - 84).

Also recall that one of the four common causes of abnormal transition is myocardial necrosis, or "old MI."

Early transition can indicate *posterior wall necrosis*. Conversely, *late transition*, also called "*poor R wave progression*" can indicate *anterior wall necrosis*.

Just as Q waves develop during evolving myocardial infarction, R wave progression changes as myocardial tissue becomes necrotic.

LATE TRANSITION DUE TO ANTERIOR WALL NECROSIS:

The following 6 ECGs demonstrate how Q waves form and R wave progression becomes delayed during the evolution of anterior wall ST segment elevation MI (STEMI):

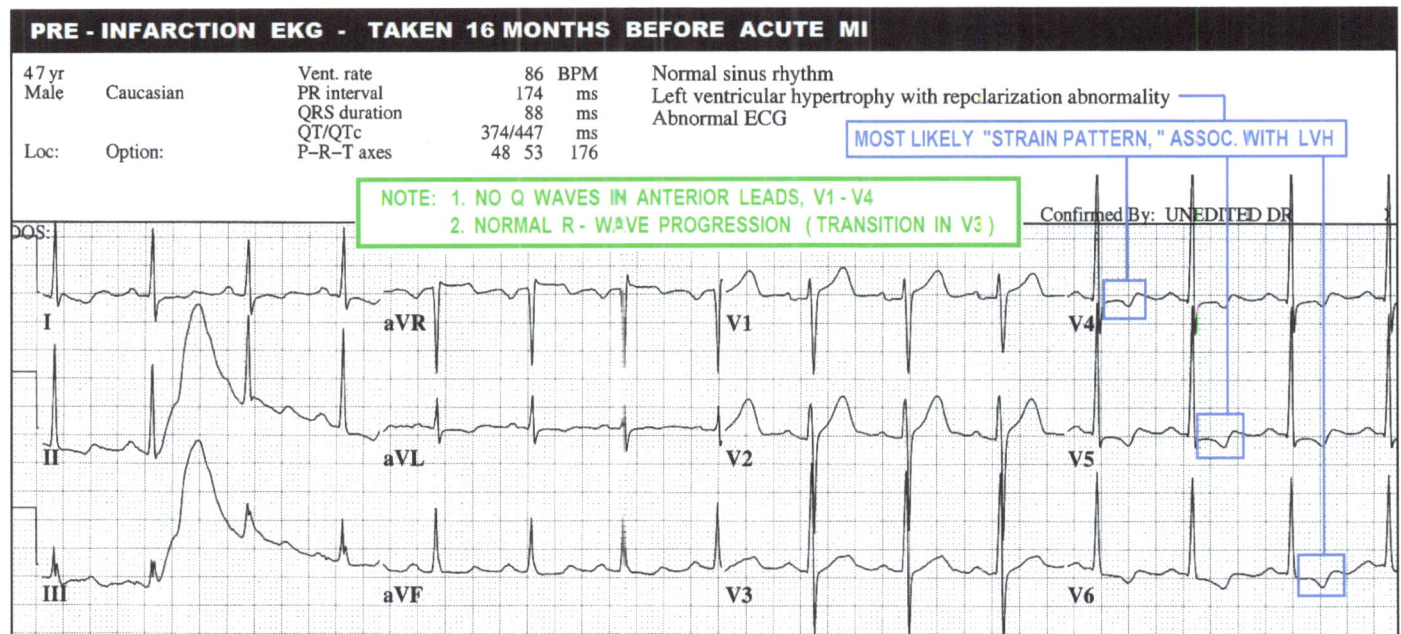

PRE - INFARCTION EKG - TAKEN 16 MONTHS BEFORE ACUTE MI

47 yr		Vent. rate	86 BPM	Normal sinus rhythm
Male	Caucasian	PR interval	174 ms	Left ventricular hypertrophy with repolarization abnormality
		QRS duration	88 ms	Abnormal ECG
		QT/QTc	374/447 ms	
Loc:	Option:	P–R–T axes	48 53 176	

MOST LIKELY "STRAIN PATTERN," ASSOC. WITH LVH

NOTE: 1. NO Q WAVES IN ANTERIOR LEADS, V1 - V4
2. NORMAL R - WAVE PROGRESSION (TRANSITION IN V3)

Confirmed By: UNEDITED DR

In the above ECG, taken approximately 16 months before the patient's acute anterior wall MI, R wave progression is normal. Transition is in V3. No Q waves are present in the precordial leads.

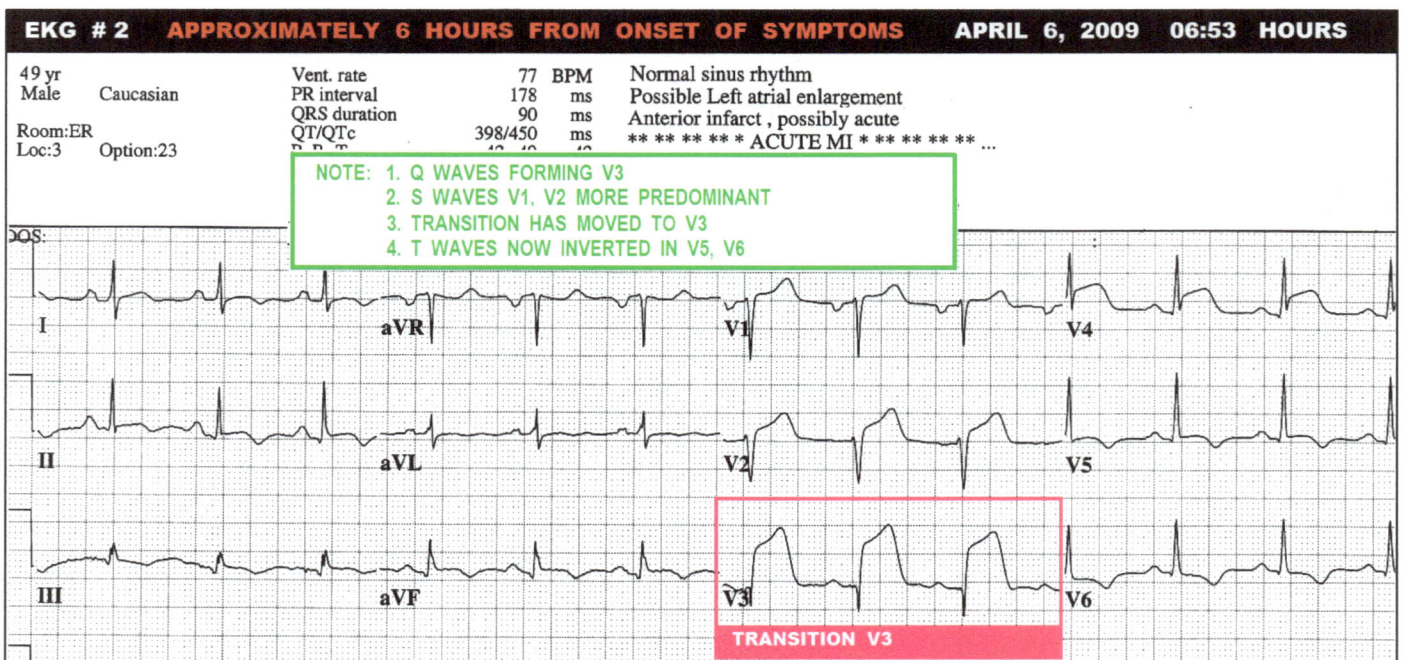

EKG #1 UPON ARRIVAL IN E.D. - CHEST PAIN x 40 MINUTES   APRIL 6, 2009   01:14 HOURS

49 yr		Vent. rate	91	BPM	Normal sinus rhythm
Male	Caucasian	PR interval	172	ms	Left atrial enlargement
		QRS duration	86	ms	Cannot rule out Inferior infarct , new
		QT/QTc	350/430	ms	Anterior injury pattern
Loc:3	Option:23	P-R-T axes	41 17 -15		** ** ** ** ** ACUTE MI ** ** ** ** **

EKG TAKEN UPON ARRIVAL IN EMERGENCY DEPARTMENT.
- CHEST PAIN x 40 MINUTES
- ST ELEVATION V1 - V4

NOTE: 1. NO Q WAVES IN V1 - V4
       2. TRANSITION IS BETWEEN V2 and V3

TRANSITION BETWEEN V2 - V3

The patient presented to the emergency department with substernal chest pressure and shortness of breath approximately thirty minutes after his symptoms started. The above ECG was recorded within ten minutes of the patient's arrival in the triage area. Profound ST segment elevation is noted in V2 – V4, with subtle ST changes in leads I, aVL, and V5. QS vs. rS complexes seen in lead V2.

EKG #2   APPROXIMATELY 6 HOURS FROM ONSET OF SYMPTOMS   APRIL 6, 2009   06:53 HOURS

49 yr		Vent. rate	77	BPM	Normal sinus rhythm
Male	Caucasian	PR interval	178	ms	Possible Left atrial enlargement
		QRS duration	90	ms	Anterior infarct , possibly acute
Room:ER		QT/QTc	398/450	ms	** ** ** ** ** ACUTE MI ** ** ** ** ** ...
Loc:3	Option:23				

NOTE: 1. Q WAVES FORMING V3
       2. S WAVES V1, V2 MORE PREDOMINANT
       3. TRANSITION HAS MOVED TO V3
       4. T WAVES NOW INVERTED IN V5, V6

TRANSITION V3

ECG #2, shown above, was recorded approximately 6 hours after ECG 1. Note the change in V3 – Q waves are now evident. Transition has shifted from "between V2 and V3 to V3 only.

49 yr		Vent. rate	94	BPM	Normal sinus rhythm
Male	Caucasian	PR interval	168	ms	Cannot rule out Inferior infarct
		QRS duration	86	ms	Anterior infarct , possibly acute
Room:CSU14		QT/Q~			
Loc:1	Option:1	P–R–			

NOTE: 1. Q WAVES (QS COMPLEXES) NOW IN V1 - V4
2. TRANSITION HAS MOVED TO BETWEEN V4 - V5
3. ST SEGMENT ELEVATION RESOLVING

I   aVR   V1   V4
TRANSITION BETWEEN V4 - V5
II   aVL   V2   V5
III   aVF   V3   V6

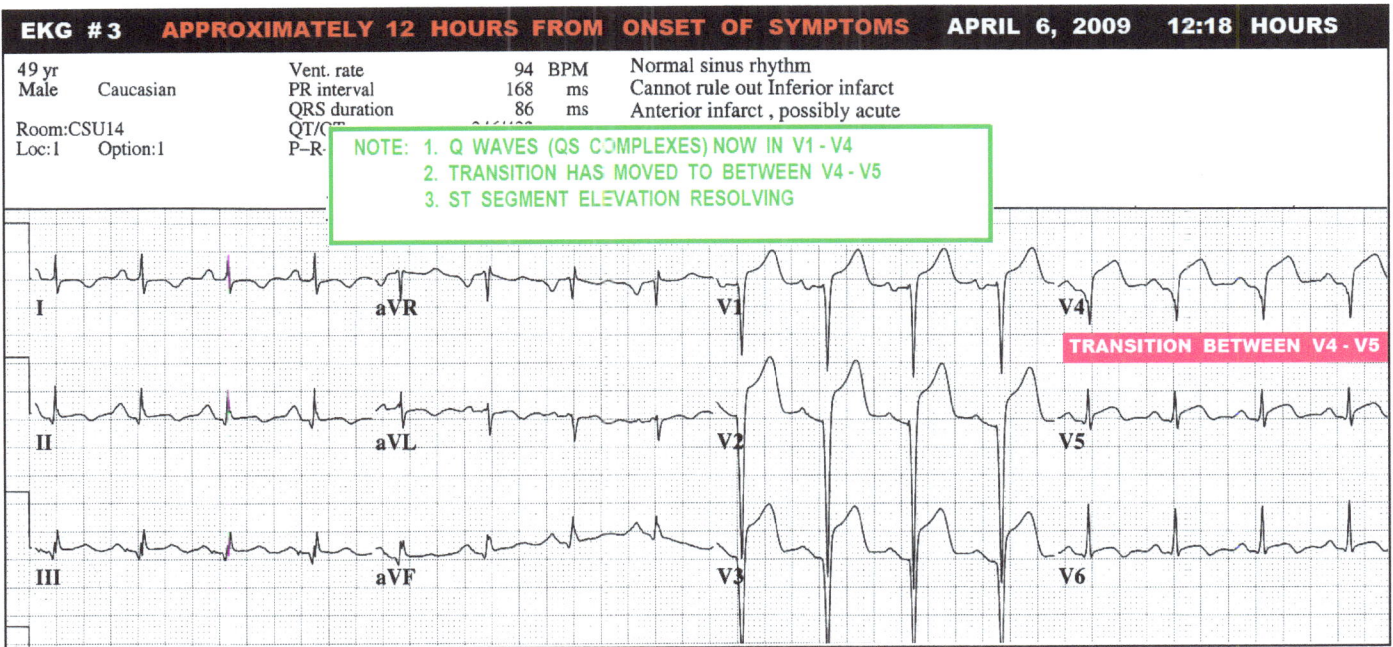

ECG 3, taken approximately six hours after ECG 2, shows significant changes: Clearly defined QS complexes are now seen in leads V1 through V4. There are NO R waves visible now in any of the anterior leads: V1 through V4. Transition has shifted from V3 to half-way between V4 and V5.

49 yr		Vent. rate	86	BPM	Normal sinus rhythm
Male	Caucasian	PR interval	174	ms	Anterior infarct , possibly acute
		QRS duration	78	ms	Lateral injury pattern
Room:CS1		QT/QTc	360/430	ms	** ** ** ** * ACUTE MI * ** ** ** **
Loc:5	Option:28	P–R–T axes			

NOTE: 1. Q WAVES IN LEADS V2 - V5
2. ST ELEVATION NOW IN V5
3. TRANSITION HAS SHIFTED TO V6
4. ST ELEVATION IN ANTERIOR LEADS RESOLVING

I   aVR   V1   V4
II   aVL   V2   V5
III   aVF   V3   V6
TRANSITION V6

ECG 4, taken 7 hours after ECG 3, shows marked changes consistent with evolving anterior wall MI: QS complexes now noted in V1 through V5. Transition has shifted to V6; very "delayed."

On the next page, the ECG was taken one year after our patient's acute anterior wall MI.   This ECG represents the "classic old anterior wall MI" ECG: QS complexes in Leads V1 – V4, very delayed R wave progression (no R waves seen until Lead V6).

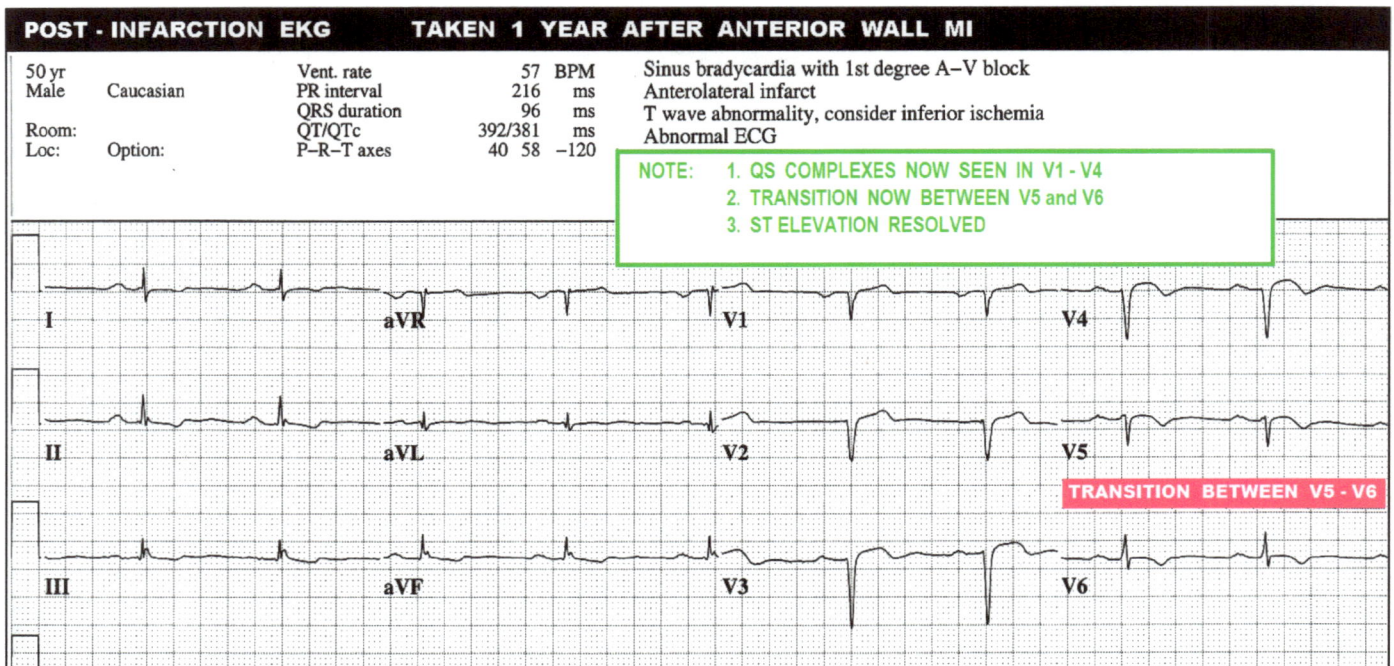

POST - INFARCTION EKG   TAKEN 1 YEAR AFTER ANTERIOR WALL MI

50 yr		Vent. rate	57	BPM
Male	Caucasian	PR interval	216	ms
		QRS duration	96	ms
Room:		QT/QTc	392/381	ms
Loc:	Option:	P–R–T axes	40 58 –120	

Sinus bradycardia with 1st degree A–V block
Anterolateral infarct
T wave abnormality, consider inferior ischemia
Abnormal ECG

NOTE: 1. QS COMPLEXES NOW SEEN IN V1 - V4
2. TRANSITION NOW BETWEEN V5 and V6
3. ST ELEVATION RESOLVED

TRANSITION BETWEEN V5 - V6

EARLY TRANSITION DUE TO POSTERIOR WALL NECROSIS:

The next two ECGs demonstrate how posterior wall necrosis results in early transition. The first ECG, seen below, is the patient's pre-infarction ECG. Note that transition is in V3, which is normal.

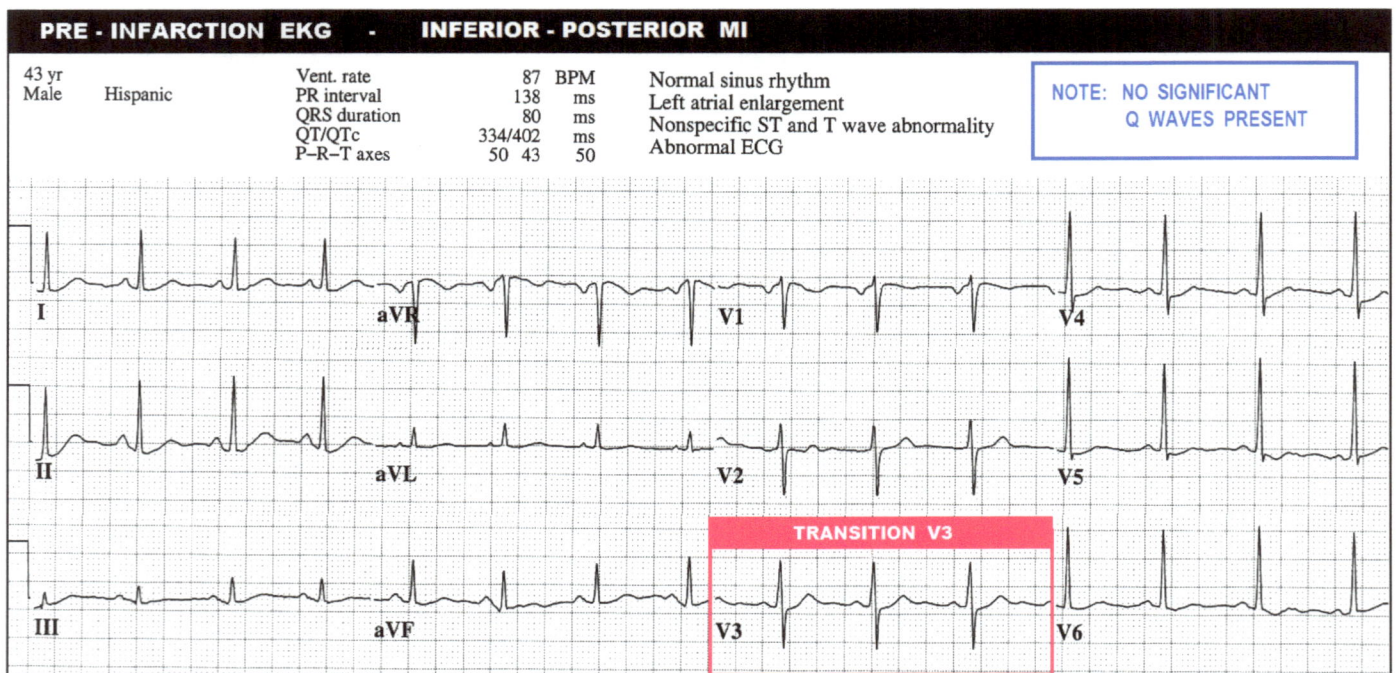

PRE - INFARCTION EKG   -   INFERIOR - POSTERIOR MI

43 yr		Vent. rate	87	BPM
Male	Hispanic	PR interval	138	ms
		QRS duration	80	ms
		QT/QTc	334/402	ms
		P–R–T axes	50 43 50	

Normal sinus rhythm
Left atrial enlargement
Nonspecific ST and T wave abnormality
Abnormal ECG

NOTE: NO SIGNIFICANT
Q WAVES PRESENT

TRANSITION V3

132

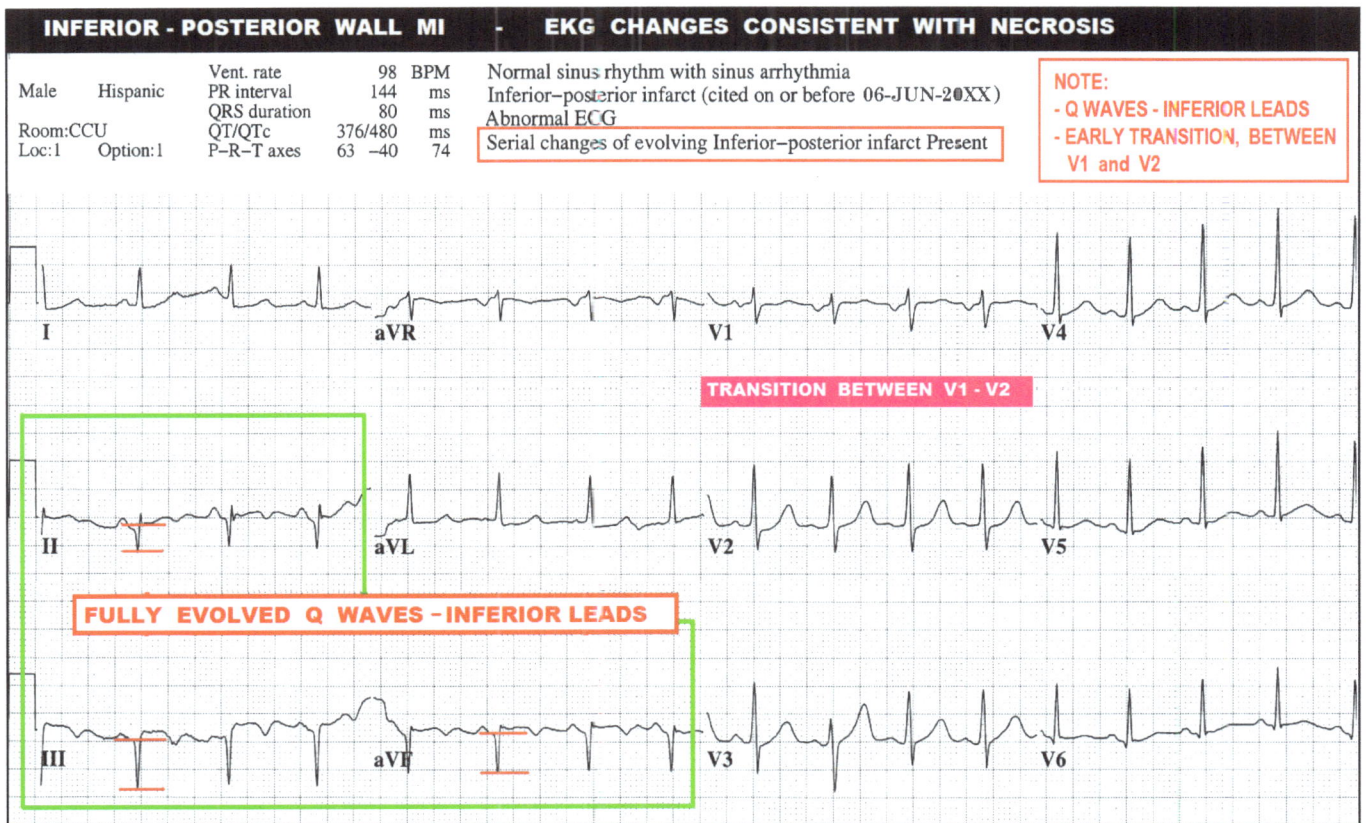

INFERIOR - POSTERIOR WALL MI - EKG CHANGES CONSISTENT WITH NECROSIS

		Vent. rate	98	BPM	Normal sinus rhythm with sinus arrhythmia
Male	Hispanic	PR interval	144	ms	Inferior–posterior infarct (cited on or before 06-JUN-20XX)
		QRS duration	80	ms	Abnormal ECG
Room:CCU		QT/QTc	376/480	ms	Serial changes of evolving Inferior–posterior infarct Present
Loc:1	Option:1	P–R–T axes	63 –40	74	

NOTE:
- Q WAVES - INFERIOR LEADS
- EARLY TRANSITION, BETWEEN V1 and V2

TRANSITION BETWEEN V1 - V2

FULLY EVOLVED Q WAVES – INFERIOR LEADS

After the patient's inferior-posterior MI is almost fully evolved, note the change in transition: it has moved from V3 to somewhere between V1 and V2. This change, from normal to early transition, is our only clue on the 12 lead ECG that this patient incurred necrosis to the posterior wall of his left ventricle.

In most cases of *Posterior Wall MI*, Inferior Wall MI is also present. This is due to the fact that the "culprit artery" – the one with the blockage – feeds both regions of the heart.

(See pages 79 - 80 to review early transition caused by old posterior wall MI).

ECG PATTERNS ASSOCIATED WITH NSTEMI and ISCHEMIA:

The patterns of NSTEMI and ischemia are presented together, because the ECG findings are often identical; it is the presence of POSITIVE CARDIAC MARKERS that formally distinguish NSTEMI patients from those with myocardial ischemia.

ISCHEMIA

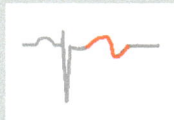

BI-PHASIC T WAVE

- SUB-TOTAL OCCLUSION of LEFT ANTERIOR DESCENDING ARTERY (when noted in V1-V4)
- LEFT VENTRICULAR HYPERTROPHY
- COCAINE INDUCED VASOSPASM

BI-PHASIC T WAVES

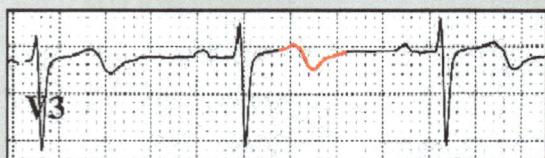

58 y/o MALE WITH SUB-TOTAL OCCLUSIONS OF THE LEFT ANTERIOR DESCENDING ARTERY

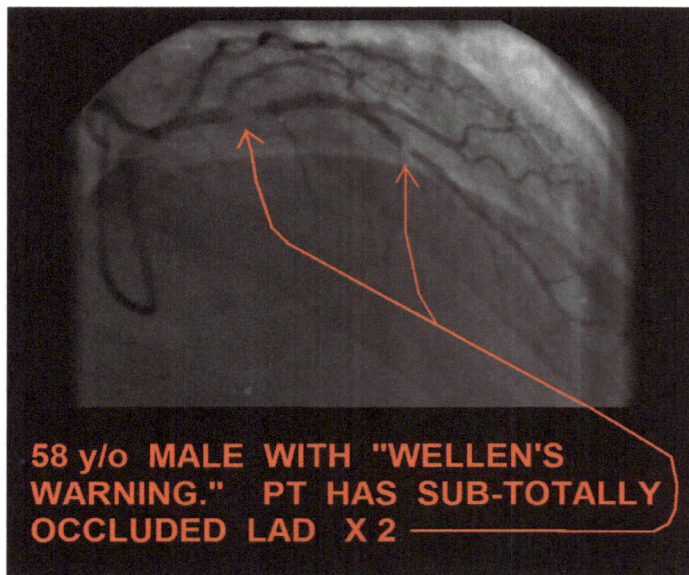

Biphasic T waves are associated with the three conditions listed in the diagram to the left.[24]

When observed in the anterior chest leads (V1 – V4), the *biphasic T wave*, which has been described as one component of "Wellen's Syndrome[25]," has been associated with high incidence of sub-total occlusions of the proximal left anterior descending artery. This finding has been observed by the author on numerous occasions, including the case of the 58 year old male, whose ECG tracing and cath lab angiogram are seen in the two images below:

58 y/o MALE WITH "WELLEN'S WARNING." PT HAS SUB-TOTALLY OCCLUDED LAD X 2

The patterns displayed in the diagram to the right are fairly reliable indicators of ischemia. *S-T depression with an inverted T wave* is considered a "classic" sign of ischemia, and is frequently seen in "positive" stress tests.

Symmetrical, inverted T waves equal or greater than .20 mV (4mm on standard ECG) are consistent with ACS[26]

☞ Remember that other conditions can result in S-T segment depression and inverted T waves. See the diagram located on page 63 for lists of these other conditions.

ISCHEMIA   HELPFUL PATTERNS . . .

J POINT DEPRESSION (> 1 mm)

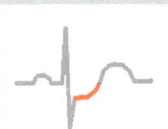

INVERTED T WAVES

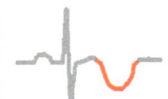

J POINT DEPRESSION + INVERTED T WAVES

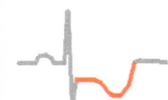

---

[24] Cooper, J and Marriott, HJL: 12 Lead Intermediate ECG Readings; Am Coll of Cardiov Nursing, 2005
[25] Marriott, Henry JL: Emergency Electrocardiography: p 35. Trinity Press, 1997
[26] Amsterdam, Erza et. al "AHA Scientific Statement," Circulation 2010; 122:756-776

OBTAINING SERIAL ECGs:

ACS can not be safely or accurately ruled out with one normal ECG and one normal set of cardiac markers.

Patients with UA/NSTEMI, and in some cases those with a *sub-total occlusion of a coronary artery who are in the early stages of acute MI* will present with *intermittent symptoms*, and their *initial ECGs and labs may be normal – especially if the patient is symptom-free at the time of examination.*

According to Anderson et al, "*an ECG recorded during an episode of symptoms is particularly valuable. Transient ST-segment changes equal to or greater than 0.5mm which are recorded during a symptomatic episode at rest, which resolve when symptoms abate is strongly suggestive of acute ischemia, and is associated with a very high probability of severe underlying CAD.*"[27]

The following *serial ECG protocol* is the one I use for patients with persistent ACS symptoms. This intense monitoring regimen has yielded the discovery of multiple patients with *dynamic ECG changes*, resulting in quicker diagnoses – and shorter door-to-treatment intervals!

"By obtaining SERIAL ECGs, you effectively turn a two-dimensional study into a 3-D object: you add the dimension of TIME to the study of your patient's cardiac electrical activity."

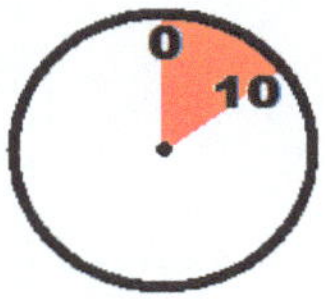

OBTAIN and INTERPRET FIRST ECG within 10 MINUTES of patient arrival.

☞ **If first ECG is NEGATIVE or INCONLUSIVE in patients whom ARE CURRENTLY experiencing ACS SYMPTOMS --**

OBTAIN SERIAL ECGs:

- **1 ECG every 15 minutes for FIRST HOUR**
- **1 ECG every 30 minutes for NEXT 2 HOURS**
- **1 ECG every 60 minutes for NEXT 4 HOURS**
- **1 ECG every 4 - 6 hours for remainder of first 24 hours.**

☞ **OBTAIN an ECG EVERY TIME THE PATIENT REPORTS CHANGE(S) in SYMPTOMS.**

---- COMPARE the J POINTS, ST SEGMENTS, and T WAVES of each newly recorded ECG with the previous ECGs.

☞ **IMPLEMENT CONTINUOUS ECG MONITORING of any LEAD(S) where the 12 LEAD ECG demonstrates ST - T WAVE ABNORMALITIES which could be CONSISTENT WITH ACUTE CORONARY SYNDROME !**

While the diagram to the right presents a very aggressive approach with respect to the time intervals and number of ECGs obtained, it is consistent with guidelines published in the American Heart Association's Scientific Statement released in August, 2010. Another perhaps more effective method to discover ACS-induced ECG abnormalities is to employ continuous ST segment monitoring for suspected ACS patients.[28]

---

[27] J Anderson et al., "ACC/AHA Guidelines for Mgmt of UA/NSTEMI," Circulation 2007; e170

[28] E Amsterdam et al, "AHA Scientific Statement- Testing of Low Risk Patients Presenting to the Emergency Department With Chest Pain:" Circulation 2010;122:756-776

To demonstrate the necessity of obtaining and comparing serial ECGs, we obtained the next four ECGs from a 33 year old male, who presented to the ED with a chief complaint of "coughing and chest pain." The patient was about to be discharged when a veteran ED physician discerned that the chest pain – which many would have written off as "pleuritic" – was indeed suspicious for ACS, and *had an onset prior to that of the coughing episodes.*

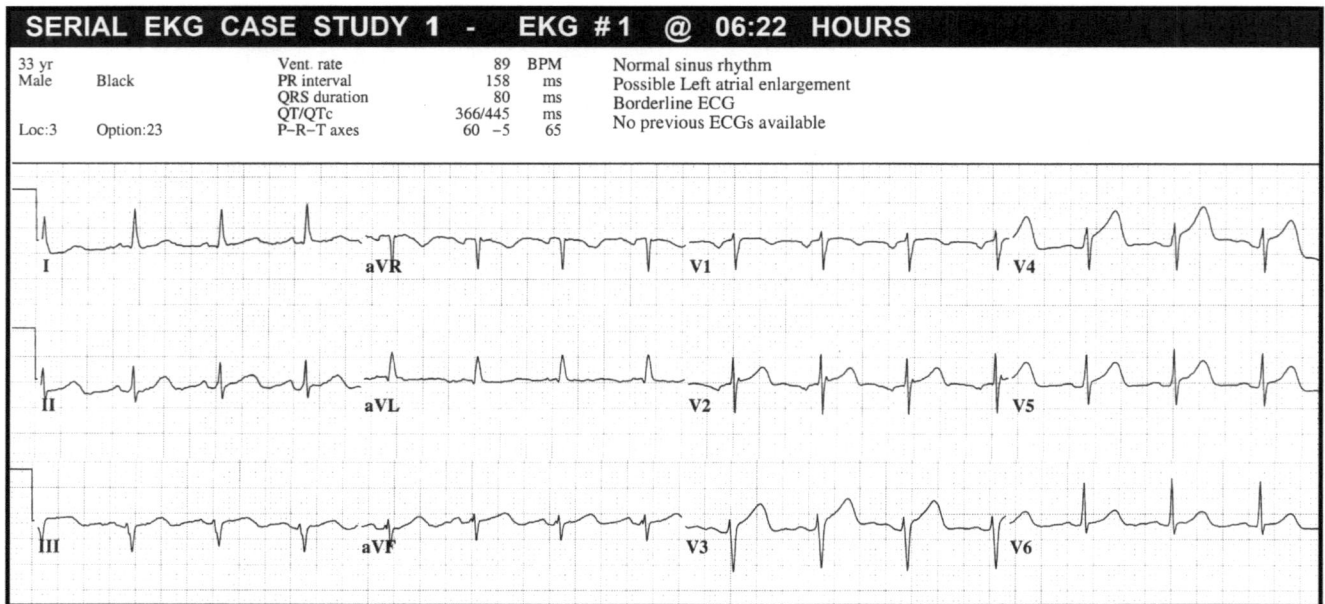

SERIAL EKG CASE STUDY 1 - EKG #1 @ 06:22 HOURS

33 yr Male	Black			
		Vent. rate	89	BPM
		PR interval	158	ms
		QRS duration	80	ms
		QT/QTc	366/445	ms
Loc:3	Option:23	P–R–T axes	60 –5	65

Normal sinus rhythm
Possible Left atrial enlargement
Borderline ECG
No previous ECGs available

When the above ECG was recorded, the patient was pain-free. The ST elevation seen in the precordial leads was believed to be "normal male pattern ST elevation," a finding of concave ST segments and J point elevation of 1-3mm in the precordial leads.[29] In terms of prevalence, this finding was observed to be present in 91% of 6014 healthy men in the Air Force.[30]

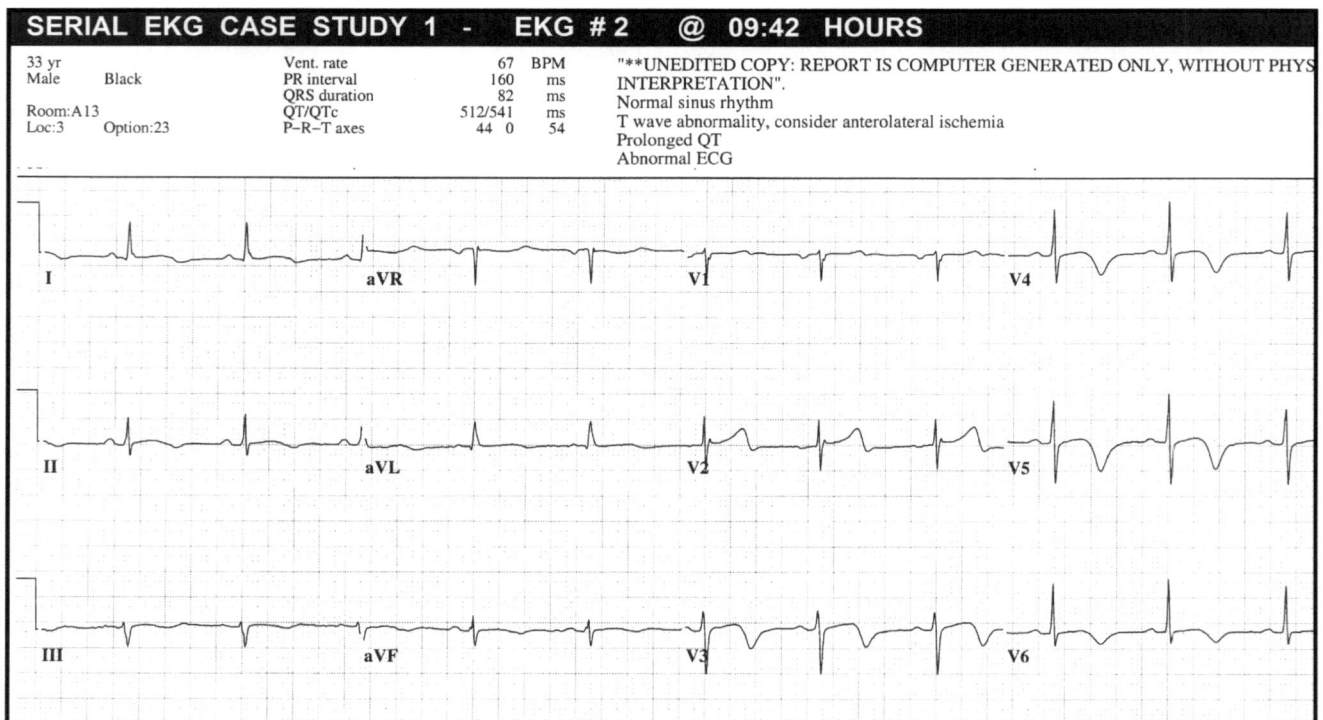

SERIAL EKG CASE STUDY 1 - EKG #2 @ 09:42 HOURS

33 yr Male	Black			
		Vent. rate	67	BPM
		PR interval	160	ms
		QRS duration	82	ms
Room:A13		QT/QTc	512/541	ms
Loc:3	Option:23	P–R–T axes	44 0	54

"**UNEDITED COPY: REPORT IS COMPUTER GENERATED ONLY, WITHOUT PHYS INTERPRETATION".
Normal sinus rhythm
T wave abnormality, consider anterolateral ischemia
Prolonged QT
Abnormal ECG

[29] Wang, Asinger, and Marriott et al., N Engl J Med 2003; 349:2128-2129
[30] Hiss et al., Am J Cardiol 1960;6:200-231

The patient remained pain-free at the time the second ECG (bottom of previous page) was recorded. Of concern are *dynamic J point, ST segment, and T wave changes* in nearly all leads, when compared to ECG 1. Based on this finding, coupled with the patient's complaint of intermittent chest pain, the patient was admitted to the hospital, with the diagnosis of ***chest pain, rule out ACS.***

SERIAL EKG CASE STUDY 1 - EKG # 3 @ 12:12 HOURS					

33 yr		Vent. rate	64	BPM	Normal sinus rhythm
Male	Black	PR interval	160	ms	Marked T wave abnormality, consider anterolateral ischemia
		QRS duration	84	ms	Prolonged QT
		QT/QTc	514/530	ms	Abnormal ECG
Loc:7	Option:35	P–R–T axes	45 3	91	When compared with ECG of 05–NOV–2008 05:12.

The patient complained of chest pain during the recording of the 3rd ECG (above), and the 4th ECG (below). Note the evolving, dynamic J point, ST segment, and T wave changes in all leads, with the most changes seen in the anterior leads, V1 – V4, and lengthening of the QT interval.

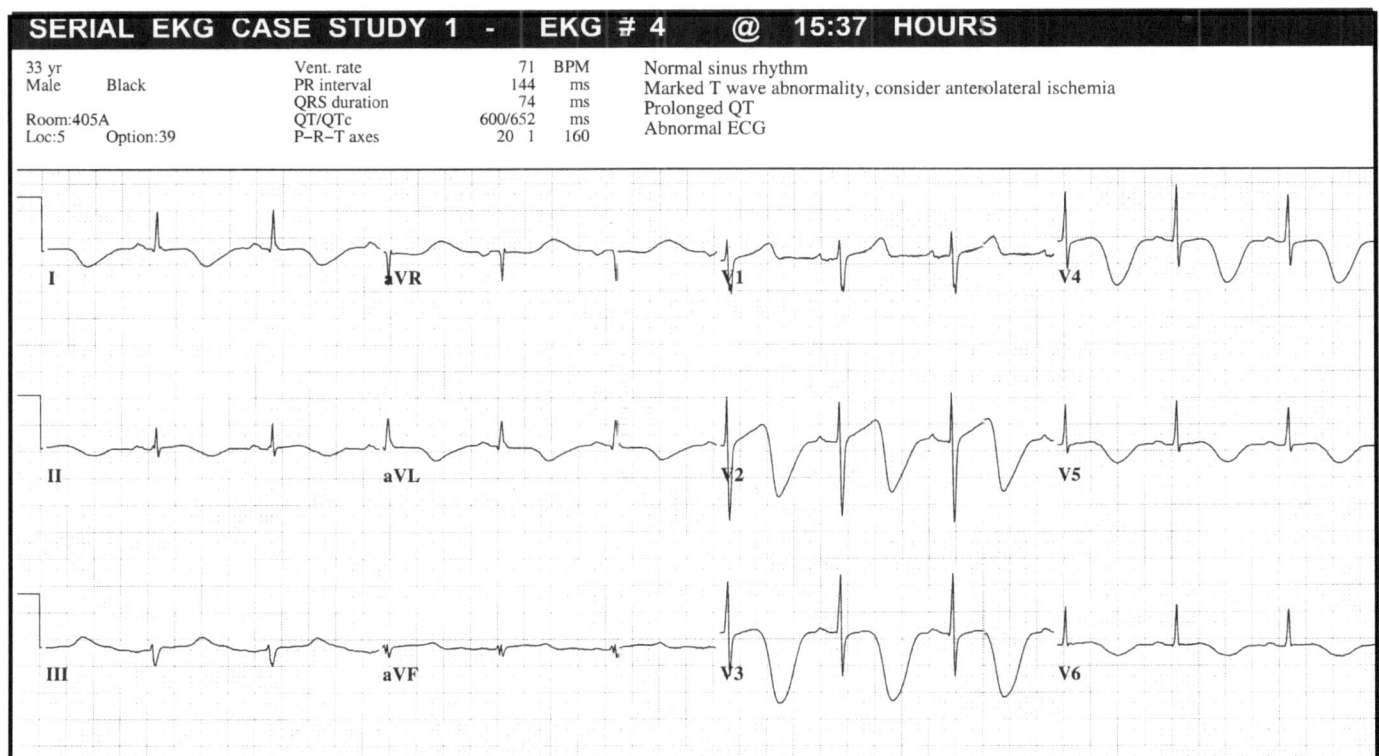

SERIAL EKG CASE STUDY 1 - EKG # 4 @ 15:37 HOURS					

33 yr		Vent. rate	71	BPM	Normal sinus rhythm
Male	Black	PR interval	144	ms	Marked T wave abnormality, consider anterolateral ischemia
		QRS duration	74	ms	Prolonged QT
Room:405A		QT/QTc	600/652	ms	Abnormal ECG
Loc:5	Option:39	P–R–T axes	20 1	160	

137

Based on the evolving, dynamic ECG changes, the patient was taken to the cardiac catheterization lab, where the following angiography was obtained:

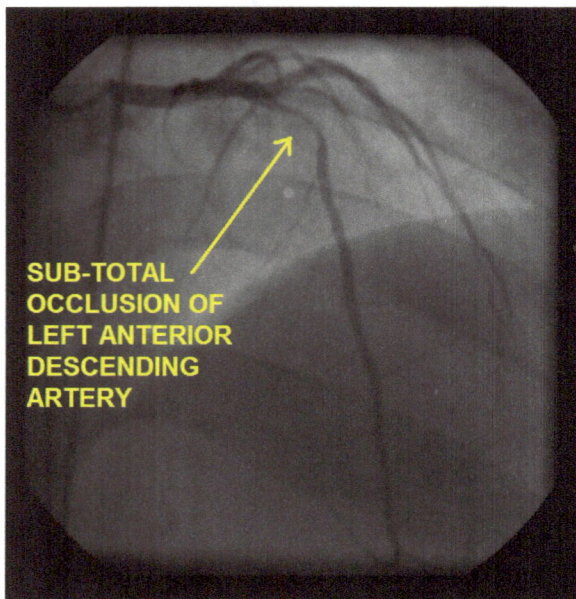

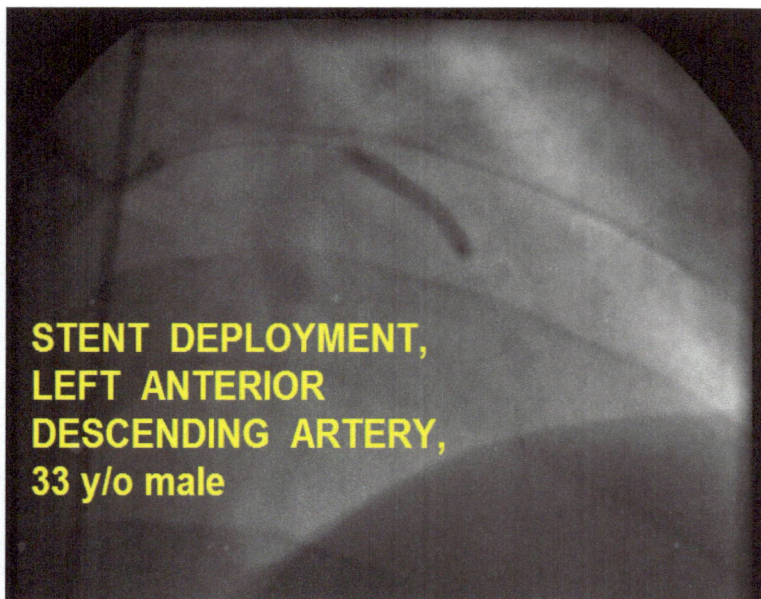

As seen in the above left image, the patient had a 95-99% occlusion of the proximal left anterior descending artery. This finding is consistent with the marked J point, ST segment and T wave changes noted in leads V1-V4 noted in ECG 3 and ECG 4.

After successful PCI, the patient was discharged 2 days later. *This case study highlights the importance of carefully and systematically obtaining a thorough history and physical, and the value of obtaining serial ECGs --* especially in cases such as this, where the patient's *visual presentation of youth and deceptive appearance of health,* combined with a complaint of "coughing" could serve as a deterrent, and lead a less-vigilant clinician into "taking shortcuts" in the patient evaluation process – *and in this case, could have lead to a catastrophic outcome for this 33 year old male.*

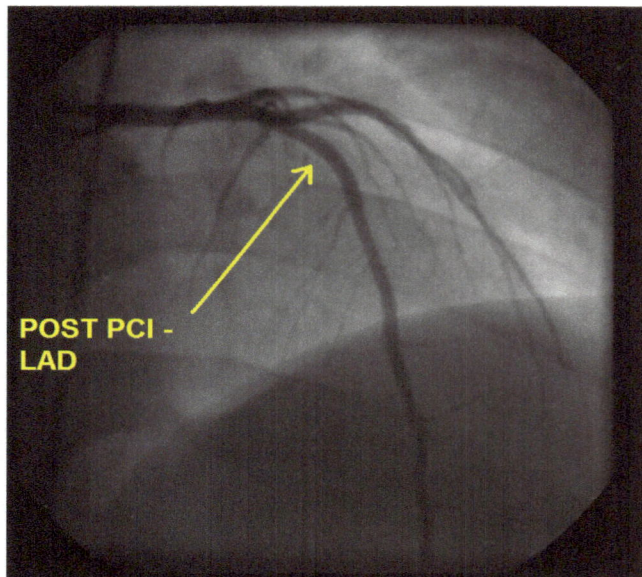

This patient's case study is a good example of Wellen's Syndrome[31], which includes:

ST and T wave changes in the anterior precordial leads (V1 – V4).
Biphasic T waves
Inverted T waves
No abnormal Q waves
Normal R wave progression
Normal or minimally elevated cardiac markers

ECG abnormalities may be present during episodes of chest pain, and may be present during asymptomatic periods.
ECG changes associated with high incidence of critical stenosis in the proximal Left Anterior Descending artery.

Case Study contributed by Charles Sand, MD, FACEP, FACP

---

[31] Rhinehardt, J, et al, Am J Emerg Med 2002 Nov;20(7):638-43.

CARDIAC MARKERS and other ESSENTIAL LABS:

Interpretation of key lab values is often the determining factor in correctly diagnosing an acute, life-threatening cardiac disorder. *Cardiac markers* are a key diagnostic factor in cases such as ***chest pain with LBBB*** and ***Non-STEMI***, and when differentiating between serious disorders, such as ***acute Pericarditis*** vs. ***STEMI***.

In cases of ***hyperkalemia*** vs. ***STEMI,*** treatment interventions are markedly different for each condition. The time wasted when STEMI interventions are initiated for a patient whose S-T elevation is caused by ***acute hyperkalemia*** can be deadly. A simple electrolyte panel helps to clarify which treatment protocols are indicated.

The following lab assays are frequently essential to accurately diagnosing cardiovascular disorders. We include descriptions and normal ranges for each of the following:

Assessing Myocardial Injury:
>Troponin-I, ultra-Troponin-I, Troponin-T
>CPK, CK-MB, CK Index
>Myoglobin

Assessing Heart Failure
>B-type natriuretic peptide (BNP)

Serum electrolytes:
>Potassium (K+)
>Magnesium (Mg++)
>(recall that a "normal" serum Mg++ level does not rule out low intracellular magnesium: please refer to page 96 for more information).

Risk Factor Assessment:
>C-reactive protein (CRP)
>Cholesterol panels (Total cholesterol, HDL, LDL, VLDL)
>Triglycerides

The normal ranges listed in this book are for *adult patients without known renal or hepatic disease*, and are quoted from multiple sources. Because NORMAL VALUES vary from institution to institution based on *laboratory equipment manufacturers' specifications*, *REFER TO YOUR INSTITUTION'S PRINTED LAB VALUES to determine if a patient's assay is normal or abnormal.*

CARDIAC MARKERS
RISE - PEAK - NORMALIZE TIME APPROXIMATIONS

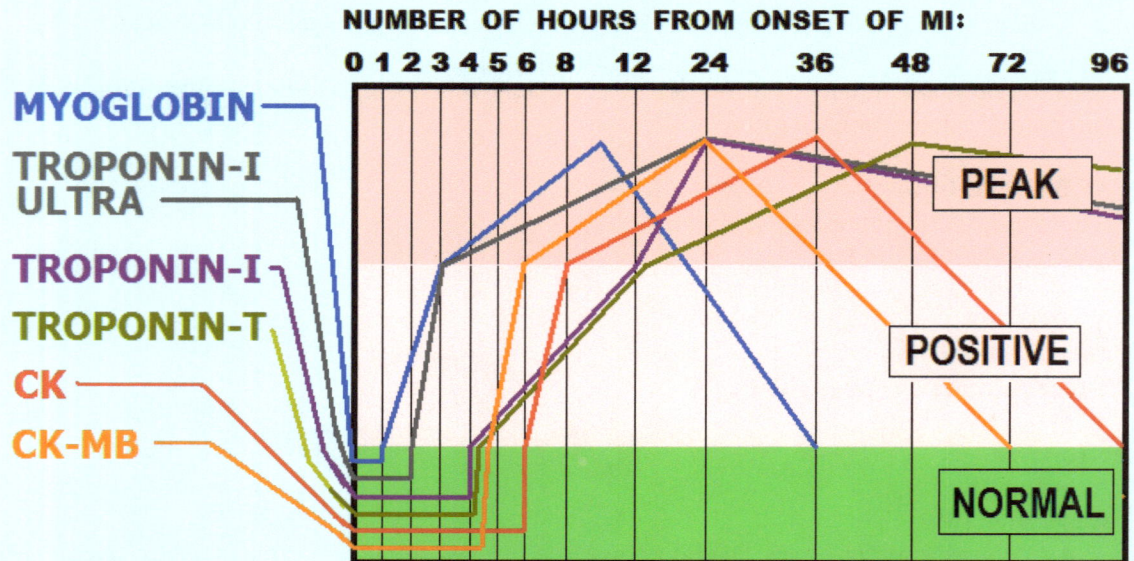

NUMBER OF HOURS FROM ONSET OF MI:

0 1 2 3 4 5 6 8 12 24 36 48 72 96

MYOGLOBIN
TROPONIN-I ULTRA
TROPONIN-I
TROPONIN-T
CK
CK-MB

PEAK
POSITIVE
NORMAL

CARDIAC MARKERS
RISE - PEAK - NORMALIZE TIME APPROXIMATIONS

NUMBER OF HOURS FROM ONSET OF MI:

	RISES (POSITIVE) -	PEAKS -	RETURNS TO NORMAL
MYOGLOBIN	1 - 3	8 - 10	24 - 36
TROPONIN-I ULTRA	2 - 3	10 - 24	5 - 10 days
TROPONIN-I	4 - 12	10 - 24	5 - 10 days
TROPONIN-T	4 - 12	12 - 48	5 - 15 days
CK	6 - 8	24 - 36	3 - 4 days
CK-MB	4 - 6	10 - 24	3 days

ASSESSMENT of MYOCARIAL INJURY:

MYOGLOBIN:

- *MARKER OF ACUTE CARDIAC AND SKELETAL MUSCLE INJURY - **NOT CARDIAC SPECIFIC** . . .*

MYOGLOBIN is a heme protein found in cardiac and skeletal muscle tissue. In cases of AMI, levels rise within 1 - 3 hours, making it the first marker to elevate during AMI. MYOGLOBIN is rapidly cleared from the body, so a "normal" level does not rule out AMI. Myoglobin levels PEAK in 8 - 12 hours, and normalize in 24 - 36 hours.* TO BE CONSIDERED "POSITIVE" FOR AMI, a second assay must be drawn ONE HOUR from the first positive test result - and must at least DOUBLE in value from the first sample.

MYOGLOBIN VALUES (ng/ml):

0 - 130	NORMAL
> 130	ABNORMAL*
--->	TO BE CONSIDERED POSITIVE FOR ACUTE MI, 2nd ASSAY, 1 HOUR AFTER FIRST, MUST DOUBLE IN VALUE

* Range used by St. Joseph's Hospital lab, Tampa, FL, 07/2008

CARDIAC TROPONIN I - ultra (cTnI - u):

- *MARKER OF MYOCARDIAL CELL DAMAGE*

TROPONIN - I	CARDIAC SPECIFIC
TROPONIN - T	CROSS-REACTIVE (SKELETAL and CARDIAC)
TROPONIN - C	STRIATED MUSCLE

TROPONIN I - ultra has been documented to have 99% specificity in the diagnosis of AMI. Point-of-care test units (Bayer Diagnositics / Seimens Medical) produce results in 20 minutes. Tests results show positive in as little as 3 hours from the onset of MI.

TROPONIN I - ultra VALUES (ng/ml) *:

< 0.07	NORMAL
0.07 - 0.10	MILD ELEVATION
0.11 - 0.78	MYOCARDIAL INJURY
> 0.78	MYOCARDIAL INFARCTION

* Values published by WORLD HEALTH ORGANIZATION

ASSESSMENT of MYOCARIAL INJURY:

CARDIAC TROPONIN - I (cTnI):

- MARKER OF MYOCARDIAL CELL DAMAGE

--->
TROPONIN - I	**CARDIAC SPECIFIC**
TROPONIN - T	**CROSS-REACTIVE** (SKELETAL and CARDIAC)
TROPONIN - C	**STRIATED MUSCLE**

TROPONIN I is released when there is MYOCARDIAL CELL NECROSIS.   Levels rise within 4 - 12 hours, peak in 10 - 24 hours, and return to baseline in 5 - 10 days.* Common causes of elevated TROPONIN-I include: STEMI, NSTEMI, PTCA, MYOCARDITIS, CARDIOVERSION, CPR, RENAL FAILURE, & PULMONARY EMBOLUS

TROPONIN-I VALUES (ng/ml):

< 0.4	**NORMAL (NO MYOCARDIAL DAMAGE)**
0.4 - 1.5	**SUGGESTIVE of MILD MYOCARDIAL INJURY**
> 1.5	**CONSISTENT WITH ACUTE MI**

* Current Control Trials, Cardiovascular Medicine, 2001; 2(2): p. 75-84

CARDIAC TROPONIN - T (cTnt):

- MARKER OF MYOCARDIAL CELL DAMAGE

TROPONIN - I	**CARDIAC SPECIFIC**
TROPONIN - T	**CROSS-REACTIVE** (SKELETAL and CARDIAC)
TROPONIN - C	**STRIATED MUSCLE**
--->

TROPONIN T is released when there is MYOCARDIAL CELL DAMAGE, or SKELETAL MUSCLE DAMAGE. Newer methods of processing Troponin T assays have increased specificity for its use as a CARDIAC MARKER to nearly identical to that of TROPONIN I.*   cTnt rises to positive levels in 4 - 12 hrs., peaks in 12 - 48 hrs., and returns to baseline in 5 - 15 days post MI.**   RENAL FAILURE and PULONARY EMBOLUS may also elevate cTnt levels.

TROPONIN T values   (ng/ml):

< 0.4	**NORMAL (NO MYOCARDIAL DAMAGE)**
0.4 - 1.5	**SUGGESTIVE of MILD MYOCARDIAL INJURY**
> 1.5	**CONSISTENT WITH ACUTE MI**

 * M. Luscher, et.al., "Circulation," 1997: 96; p2578-2585
** "Taber's Encyclopedic Medical Dictionary," 20th Ed., 2005, p 2434

ASSESSMENT of MYOCARIAL INJURY:

CK, CK-MB, and CK INDEX:

- MARKER OF MYOCARDIAL CELL DAMAGE

| CREATINE KINASE (CK) —— NON CARDIAC SPECIFIC |
| CK-MB ISOENZYME ———— CARDIAC SPECIFIC |

CK levels rise whenever there is significant TISSUE DAMAGE --
anywhere in the body. When testing for AMI / ACS, obtain both the CK
and CK-MB assays. When the CK is elevated from MYOCARDIAL
DAMAGE, the CK-MB level will also be elevated. TOTAL CK LEVELS
RISE IN 8 HOURS, and CK-MB RISES IN 4 - 6 HOURS FROM
THE ONSET OF ACUTE MI.*

CK LEVELS:		CK-MB LEVELS:		CK INDEX:**
30 - 220	NORMAL	0 - .05	NORMAL	(CK-MB/CK x 100)
> 220	TISSUE DAMAGE, (NOT CARDIAC SPECIFIC)	> .05	MYOCARDIAL INJURY / INFARCTION	> 2.5 is SUGGESTIVE of MI

  * Heger, Niemann & Criley, "Cardiology, 5th Ed.," p: 134, 2004, Lippincott
 ** Heger, Niemann & Criley, "Cardiology, 5th Ed.," p: 134, 2004, Lippincott

ASSESMENT OF HEART FAILURE:

B-TYPE NATRIURETIC PEPTIDE (BNP)

- MARKER OF HEART FAULURE

BNP is one of four known natriuretic peptides (ANP, BNP, CNP
and DNP).   BNP is released from the heart ventricles, most
predominantly the LEFT VENTRICLE during CARDIAC VOLUME
or PRESSURE OVERLOAD.*

BNP VALUES   (pg/ml) :

< 100	——————	NORMAL
100 - 499	——————	MILD - MODERATE FAILURE.
500 - 700	——————	MODERATE - SEVERE FAILURE
> 700	——————	DECOMPENSATING FAILURE
> 1000	——————	often seen w/ PULMONARY EDEMA

  * R.E. Hobbs, MD, "Cleveland Clinic Journal of Medicine," vol. 70, p.333-336

POTASSIUM (K$^+$) :

- ELECTROLYTE ESSENTIAL to CARDIAC AUTOMATICITY

Abnormal variations in a patient's SERUM POSTASSIUM (K+) level (hypokalemia and hyperkalemia) can rapidly lead to ABNORMAL CARDIAC RHYTHMS and ultimately CARDIAC ARREST and DEATH. Common conditions which alter a patient's K+ levels include: use of diuretics (e.g. Furosemide), renal failure, severe vomiting and diarrhea, and tricyclic antidepressant overdose. In addition to patients afflicted with the above listed conditions, all suspected ACS patients should have routine monitoring of their SERUM ELECTROLYTE LEVELS.

POTASSIUM LEVELS (mEq / L) :

< 3.0	CRITICAL HYPOKALEMIA
3.0 - 3.4	HYPOKALEMIA
3.5 - 5.5	NORMAL
5.6 - 6.6	HYPERKALEMIA
> 6.6	CRITICAL HYPERKALEMIA

MAGNESIUM (Mg++) :

- ELECTROLYTE ESSENTIAL to CARDIAC AUTOMATICITY

Like Potassium, Magnesium is an essential electrolyte to cardiac automaticity. When abnormal levels of Mg++ are present, instability of the myocardial electrical system commonly results. Hypomagnesemia may lead to LETHAL VENTRICULAR DYSRHYTHMIAS, such as Torsades de Pointes and Ventricular Fibrillation. Be alert for abnormal Magnesium levels whenever the patient has abnormal POTASSIUM levels, and / or exhibits abnormal amounts of VENTRICULAR ECTOPY and / or VENTRICULAR RHYTHMS, and when Q-T intervals are abnormal).

MAGNESIUM LEVELS (mEq / L) :

< 1.6	LOW
1.6 - 2.4	NORMAL
> 2.4	ELEVATED

Remember that a normal *serum magnesium* level does not rule out an abnormally low *intracellular magnesium* level. Please see page 96 for more information.

* C-REACTIVE PROTEIN (CRP):

- MARKER OF MYOCARDIAL INFLAMMATION

CRP is not a cardiac enzyme. It is a marker of acute inflammation. It may be used as a BASELINE RISK ASSESSMENT TOOL. It also has value in guaging the severity of an acute MI.

ACUTE MI - CRP LEVEL (days after onset of MI):

DAY 1 - LEVEL >15 = MORE PRONE TO CHF
DAY 3 - LEVEL >85 = HIGH MORTALITY RATE

CRP VALUES:

< 0.83	= LOW
0.83 - 2.07	= LOW / MODERATE
2.08 - 3.85	= MODERATE
3.85 - 6.05	= HIGH / MODERATE
> 6.05	= HIGH

* Erza A. Amsterdam, MD., Preventive Cardiology, 2003: Spring; 6(2): 70

* C-REACTIVE PROTEIN (CRP):

- MARKER OF MYOCARDIAL INFLAMMATION

CRP is not a cardiac enzyme. It is a marker of acute inflammation. It may be used as a BASELINE RISK ASSESSMENT TOOL. It also has value in guaging the severity of an acute MI.

CRP AS RISK FACTOR ASSESSMENT TOOL:

- Draw two samples, 14 days apart.
- Average the two values together and compare to chart below (reported in mg / dl):

< 1.0	=	LOW RISK
1.0 - 3.0	=	AVERAGE RISK
> 3.0	=	HIGH RISK

* Erza A. Amsterdam, MD., Preventive Cardiology, 2003: Spring; 6(2): 70

RISK FACTOR ASSESSMENT:

LIPID PROFILE VALUES *

	TOTAL CHOLESTEROL	LDL	HDL	TRIGLYCERIDES
OPTIMAL	< 200	< 100	> 60	< 150
NEAR OPTIMAL	200-239	100-129	40-59	150-199
BORDERLINE		139-159		200-499
HIGH	> 240	> 160	< 40	> 500

VLDL: < 36   HOMOCYSTEINE: < 10

* NATIONAL INSTITUTES of HEALTH; publication number : 01-3305

☞ REVIEW QUESTIONS:
REINFORCE YOUR KNOWLEDGE OF ESSENTIAL CONCEPTS:

44.   (p. 98) The "Quadrad of ACS" includes:
  a. patient's age, symptoms, risk factor profile, ECG findings
  b. symptoms, risk factor profile, ECG findings, cardiac markers
  c. symptoms, risk factor profile, ECG findings, cardiac echo
  d. symptoms, cholesterol profile, ECG findings, cardiac markers

45. (p. 105) Whenever a decision is made to obtain an ECG on your patient, you should immediately remember to _____.
  a. obtain the patient's billing account number so he/she gets billed for it
  b. advise the patient he/she has "the right to refuse an ECG."
  c. obtain copies of any old ECGs to compare the new one to
  d. hide the ECG from the patient unless he/she signs a HIPAA waiver allowing you to show it to him/her.

46.   (p. 107) When ST segment elevation is seen on an ECG with Right Bundle Branch Block (RBBB), you should:
  a. suspect and rule out STEMI: RBBB does not cause ST elevation, nor does it mask it.
  b. do nothing: RBBB causes chronic ST segment elevation
  c. ask the patient for his autograph; ST elevation has never been seen with RBBB
  d. prepare for immediate synchronized cardioversion; the patient is obviously in Ventricular Tachycardia

47.   (p. 109) Left Bundle Branch Block does NOT cause chronic ST segment elevation on the ECG
  a. True
  b. False

48.   (p. 109) Per American Heart Association (AHA), a patient who presents with chest pain and a presumably new Left Bundle Branch Block should be treated as an acute Anterior-Septal Wall MI until proven otherwise.
  a. True
  b. False

49.   (p. 114) When you evaluate each lead of a 12 Lead ECG for ST segment elevation, the AHA recommends that you measure for ST elevation:
  a. at the J point
  b. 40ms (1mm) after the J point
  c. 200ms (5mm) after the J point
  d. at the peak of the T wave

PRACTICE ECG 3

For questions 50 - 52 refer to PRACTICE ECG 3

50.   (p. 120) The abnormality seen in the yellow highlighted boxes is:
   a. Hyperacute T waves
   b. ST segment depression
   c. Not an abnormality; the ECG is normal
   d. Biphasic T waves

51.   (p. 122) The region of the heart with the suspected abnormality is the _____ which receives its blood supply from the _____.
   a. anterior wall, right coronary artery
   b. lateral wall, circumflex artery
   c. posterior wall, right coronary artery or circumflex artery
   d. anterior wall, left anterior descending artery

52.   (p. 120) The finding of hyperacute T waves may indicate which of the following:
   a. the early phase of acute myocardial infarction
   b. hyperkalemia
   c. trans-mural ischemia
   d. all of the above

53.   (p. 123) "Official" guidelines for diagnosing ST Segment Elevation MI (STEMI) is **significant *ST segment elevation in two or more contiguous leads***. Significant ST elevation is defined as:
   a. 1mm or more in the limb leads, and 2mm or more in the precordial leads
   b. 2mm or more in the limb leads, and 3mm or more in the precordial leads
   c. 3mm or more in the limb leads, and 4mm or more in the precordial leads
   d. 5mm or more in the limb leads, and 10mm or more in the precordial leads

PRACTICE ECG 4

For questions
54-56
refer to
PRACTICE
ECG 4

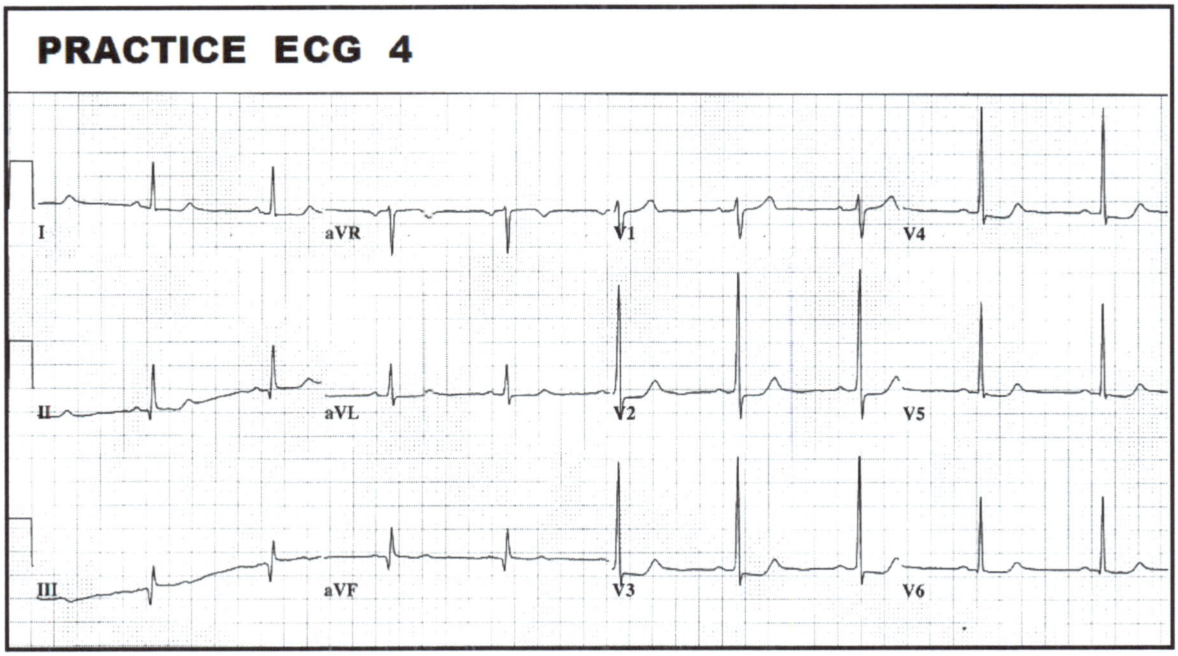

54.   (p. 127) Abnormal Q waves are seen in which leads?
   a. lateral leads, V5 and V6
   b. lateral-anterior leads I and aVL
   c. Inferior leads III and aVF
   d. Anterior leads V1 – V4

55.   (p. 77) Transition is seen _____, which is _____.
   a. between V1 and V2, early
   b. between V3 and V4, normal
   c. between V5 and V6, late
   d. before V1, very early

56.   (p. 80) The cause of early transition in this ECG is most likely from:
   a. Right Bundle Branch Block
   b. Old Posterior Wall MI
   c. Right Ventricular Hypertrophy
   d. Wolff-Parkinson-White Syndrome

PRACTICE ECG 5

For questions 57-60 refer to PRACTICE ECG 5

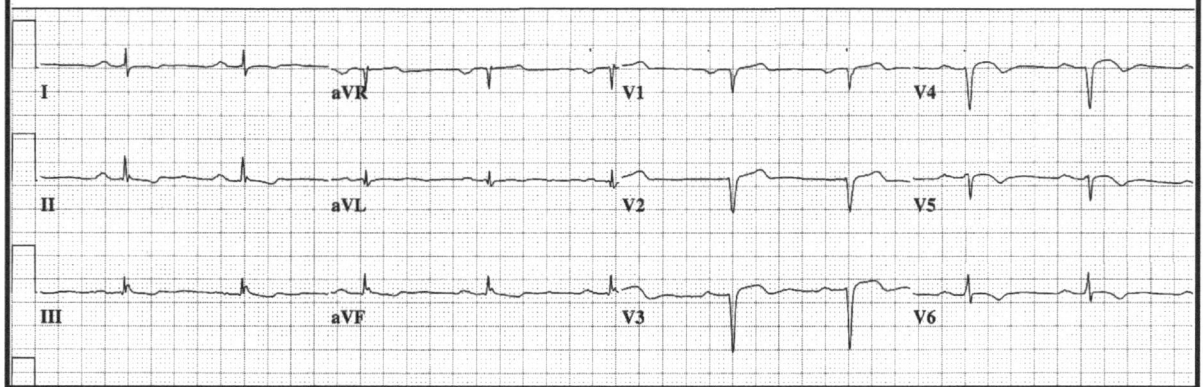

I   aVR   V1   V4

II   aVL   V2   V5

III   aVF   V3   V6

57. (p. 133) Abnormal Q waves are seen in which leads?
   a. lateral leads, V5 and V6
   b. lateral-anterior leads I and aVL
   c. Inferior leads III and aVF
   d. Anterior leads V1 – V4

58. (p. 77) Transition is seen _____, which is _____.
   a. between V1 and V2, early
   b. between V3 and V4, normal
   c. between V5 and V6, late
   d. before V1, very early

59. (p. 83) What most likely is the cause of abnormal R wave progression in this ECG?
   a. Left Bundle Branch Block
   b. Old Anterior Wall MI
   c. Left Ventricular Hypertrophy
   d. Wolff-Parkinson-White Syndrome

60. (p. 42, 134) Based on leads which show inverted T waves, which region(s) of the heart could be ischemic?
   a. Inferior-Lateral
   b. Anterior-Septal
   c. Posterior
   d. Anterior-Lateral

150

SERIAL CARDIAC MARKERS:

In cases of ACS without obvious ST elevation on the ECG, the finding of *rising* and/or *elevated cardiac markers* should expedite the decision to provide more aggressive anti-ischemic therapy. With the advent of assays which are becoming faster, more sensitive and more precise, it is possible to identify and exclude AMI within 6 hours of the onset of symptoms, as opposed to the traditional method of obtaining serial measurements every 6 or 8 hours.[32]

The diagram below features an example protocol for collecting serial cardiac markers on patients whom initially present with ACS symptoms. This protocol incorporates a *multi-marker approach*. When Myoglobin (very early marker, but not cardiac specific) is combined with and Troponin or CK-MB (later markers, but with improved specificity), MI can be *excluded* within 6 hours of the onset of symptoms, with reported sensitivity of 95% and a high negative predictive value.[33] This is achieved by drawing initial baseline measurements, and repeat sampling in 90 minutes.

To *reasonably* exclude MI, we are looking for *no significant rise* in Myoglobin and a normal cTn or CK-MB at the 90 minute mark.

If the second Myoglobin value is 2x or more the baseline value at the 90 minute mark, MI should be strongly suspected. This is especially true if there is a slight increase in cTn or CK-MB. If cTn or CK-MB falls into the *positive* range, *acute myocardial infarction* should be considered as the working diagnosis. (This would be the case if there was any significant delay between onset of symptoms and the initial patient exam – a fairly common scenario).

The third set of samples is obtained 60 minutes after the second, or approximately 2.5 hours from baseline sampling. If cTn-Ultra testing is utilized (POC testing apparatus, marketed by Bayer Diagnostics/Siemens Medical), test results typically show *positive* in 2-3 hours after the onset of MI. This means that a reliable positive diagnosis of AMI can be made 2.5 hours after initial patient contact – even if the patient arrived at the ED minutes after becoming symptomatic.

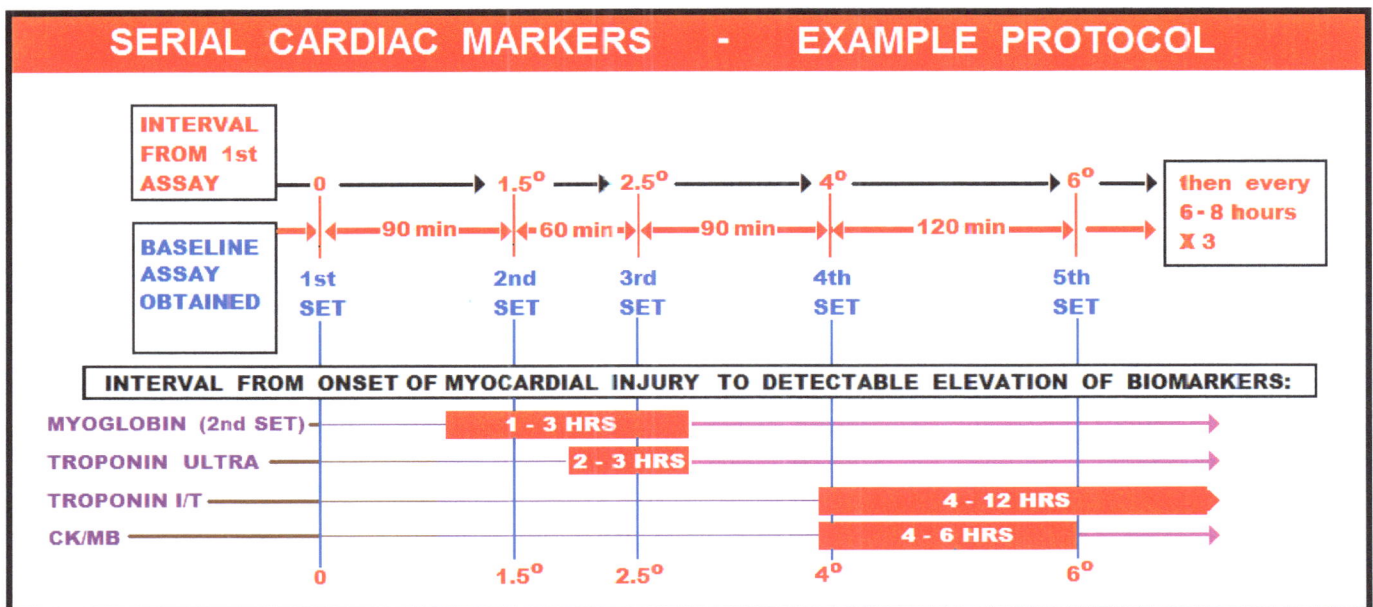

---

[32] J Anderson et al., "ACC/AHA Guidelines for Mgmt of UA/NSTEMI," Circulation 2007; e175
[33] J Anderson et al., "ACC/AHA Guidelines for Mgmt of UA/NSTEMI," Circulation 2007; e175

RISK STRATIFICATION for CORONARY ARTERY DISEASE / ACS:

The purpose of risk factor stratification in the population of patients presenting to the ED with ACS-like symptoms is to identify the subgroup of patients with a higher probability of having ischemic cardiovascular disease.

There are several valid ACS risk stratification tools available; the Modified Thrombolysis In Myocardial Infarction (TIMI) ACS score, Global Registry of Acute Myocardial Events (GRACE) and Platelet glycoprotein IIb/IIIa in Unstable angina: Receptor Suppression Using Integrilin (PURSUIT) scores. All three scoring methods have been validated in scientific studies for predicting outcomes in high-risk patients.

TIMI, (presented on the next page) is the most widely used of the latter three scores. It is the least complicated, and relies on information readily obtained during rapid patient evaluation. In the population of patients presenting to the ED whom appear to be in the low-risk category, additional risk stratification is often necessary.[34] This is due to frequent incidence of patients with low scores (0-2) who are found to have significant obstructive coronary artery disease. In the case studies we selected for inclusion in this book, several patients with severe CAD and ACS had low TIMI Scores upon arrival in the ED. For this reason, we decided to exclude TIMI scores from our case studies; instead, we simply indicate which factors in the "Quadrad of ACS" were present: *ACS-like symptoms, ECG abnormalities, 3 or more CAD risk factors*, and *positive cardiac biomarkers*. In addition, we have developed a model ACS risk stratification tool, the "Simple Acute Coronary Syndrome (SACS) Score, which is currently in the process of scientific validation (see page 157).

RISK FACTORS
for the development of
CORONARY ARTERY DISEASE:

- 💣 HEREDITY
- 💣 ↑ LDL and ↓ HDL CHOLESTEROL PROFILES
- 💣 SMOKING
- 💣 DIABETES MELLITUS
- ● OBESITY
- ● PHYSICAL INACTIVITY
- ● HYPERTENSION
- ● AGE - OVER 65
- ● MALE
- ● HIGH STRESS

per the AMERICAN HEART ASSOCIATION

Regardless of whether your patient evaluation protocol includes utilization of an ACS risk stratification scoring tool, evaluation of your patient's *risk factor profile* must be factored into your clinical decision-making process. The factors listed in the diagram to the left are known precursors to the development of coronary artery disease. Ongoing data produced by the American Heart Association serves to refine our knowledge of risk factors and their relationship to CAD. The first four risk factors in this list – heredity, high LDL and/or low LDL cholesterol, smoking, and diabetes mellitus – are what I have learned to call *"the big four"* risk factors, and appear to play a strong role in the development of CAD.

The presence of multiple risk factors during patient evaluation should alert you to the possibility that significant cardiovascular disease may be present; this should factor into your decision-making process with respect to the *pursuit of additional diagnostic testing* when patients present with symptoms which are suspicious for coronary artery disease.

☞ When patients under 40 with 4 or 5 risk factors present to the ED with ACS symptoms, *they are 22.5 times more likely to have ACS.*[35]

[34] Erza Amsterdam, MD et al, Circulation 2010;122:756-776
[35] Han, JH et al., "Role of Cardiac Risk Factors in diagnosis of ACS," Ann Emerg Med 2007 Feb;49:145-52

The Modified TIMI Risk Score:

The TIMI Risk Score is featured in the AHA Advanced Cardiac Life Support (ACLS) curriculum,[36] and is used at the St. Joseph's Hospital Heart Institute, where I am currently affiliated, in Tampa, Florida.

The TIMI Risk Stratification Score is a modified version of the original 14 point *TIMI Risk Score for STEMI,* which was developed and validated in multiple medication trials, for use in predicting *mortality associated with STEMI.*[37] Of the fourteen criteria in the original TIMI score, the ACS Risk Stratification version uses seven:

Thrombolysis In Myocardial Infarction (TIMI) ACS Risk Stratification Tool:

One point is assigned for each positive value in the seven criteria listed below:

- ☐ Age 65 or older
- ☐ Chest pain / pressure within the last 24 hours
- ☐ 3 or more major risk factors:
  - o Family history of CAD
  - o Diabetes Mellitus
  - o Hypercholesterolemia
  - o Smoking
  - o Hypertension
- ☐ Previously diagnosed coronary artery disease
- ☐ Aspirin taken in last 24 hours
- ☐ ST segment deviation (elevation or depression) equal to or greater than 0.5 mm
- ☐ Elevated Troponin level (any above your institution's normal ranges).

TOTAL SCORE (0 - 7)

	Risk of Death, MI, or Urgent Need for Revascularization Within Next 14 Days:	Risk Status:
0 - 2	5 - 8 %	LOW
3 - 4	13 - 20 %	INTERMEDIATE
5 - 7	26 - 41 %	HIGH

INFORMATION IN ABOVE TABLE FROM: "HANDBOOK OF EMERGENCY CARDIOVASCULAR CARE," AMERICAN HEART ASSOCIATION, 2006; p 38

☞

For more information on the Modified TIMI ACS Risk Stratification Score, and a WEALTH of valuable information with respect to all aspects of ACS patient evaluation and treatment, please visit: www.TIMI.org. This website bears testament to the *extensive, impressive* and *invaluable contributions* of **Eugene Braunwald, MD** to advancements in cardiovascular medicine.

On the following page is a flow chart illustrating how the TIMI Risk Score is incorporated into the clinical decision making process at St. Joseph's Hospital Heart Institute in Tampa, Florida:

---

[36] AHA ACLS curriculum, "Handbook of Emerg Cardiovascular Care," 2006; p38
[37] RL Soiza et al., QJ Med 2006;99:81-87

St. Joseph's Hospital Emergency Center Chest Pain Management
PASSION Pilot

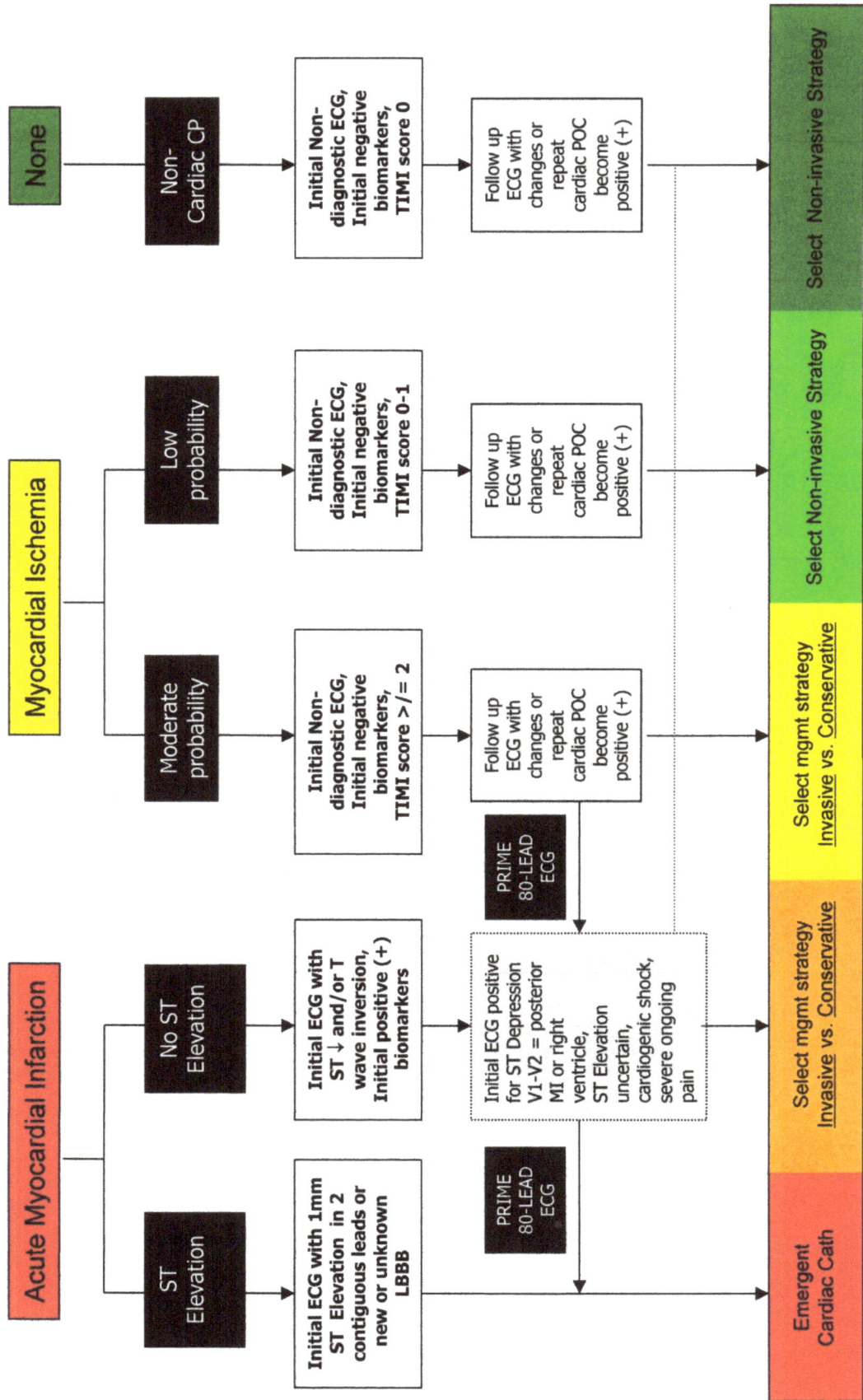

Acute Myocardial Infarction

- ST Elevation
  - Initial ECG with 1mm ST Elevation in 2 contiguous leads or new or unknown LBBB
    - PRIME 80-LEAD ECG
- No ST Elevation
  - Initial ECG with ST ↓ and/or T wave inversion, Initial positive (+) biomarkers
    - Initial ECG positive for ST Depression V1-V2 = posterior MI or right ventricle, ST Elevation uncertain, cardiogenic shock, severe ongoing pain

Myocardial Ischemia

- Moderate probability
  - Initial Non-diagnostic ECG, Initial negative biomarkers, TIMI score >/= 2
    - Follow up ECG with changes or repeat cardiac POC become positive (+)
      - PRIME 80-LEAD ECG
- Low probability
  - Initial Non-diagnostic ECG, Initial negative biomarkers, TIMI score 0-1
    - Follow up ECG with changes or repeat cardiac POC become positive (+)

None

- Non-Cardiac CP
  - Initial Non-diagnostic ECG, Initial negative biomarkers, TIMI score 0
    - Follow up ECG with changes or repeat cardiac POC become positive (+)

- Emergent Cardiac Cath
- Select mgmt strategy Invasive vs. Conservative
- Select mgmt strategy Invasive vs. Conservative
- Select Non-invasive Strategy
- Select Non-invasive Strategy

PROVIDED BY: Pamela K. Jones, Cardiovascular Clinical Outcomes Coordinator, St. Joseph's Hospital, Tampa, FL

CASE STUDY: IMPORTANCE of RISK FACTORS

CHIEF COMPLAINT and SIGNIFICANT HISTORY:

62 y/o MALE presents to cardiologist's office with intermittent ACS symptoms (chest heaviness, dyspnea).   - Pt. DOES NOT correlate symptoms with exertion.

RISK FACTOR PROFILE:

- **FAMILY HISTORY** - both parents + CAD before age 65
- **PREVIOUS CIGARETTE SMOKER** - 20+ yrs., quit 15 years ago
- **HIGH CHOLESTEROL** - Dx 5 yrs ago, taking STATIN med since.
- **DIABETES** - Controlled with diet and oral meds.

PHYSICAL EXAM: Patient supine on exam table, skin warm, dry, color NL

Patient is asymptomatic, all systems WNL

VITAL SIGNS: BP 153/88, P 80, R 16, SAO2 99%

DIAGNOSTIC TESTING: EKG NORMAL, EXERCISE STRESS TEST PASSED.

62 yr		Vent. rate	78	BPM
Male	Caucasian	PR interval	202	ms
		QRS duration	82	ms
Room: CCRA		QT/QTc	384/437	ms
Loc:	Option:	P–R–T axes	51 10	11

Normal sinus rhythm
Normal ECG

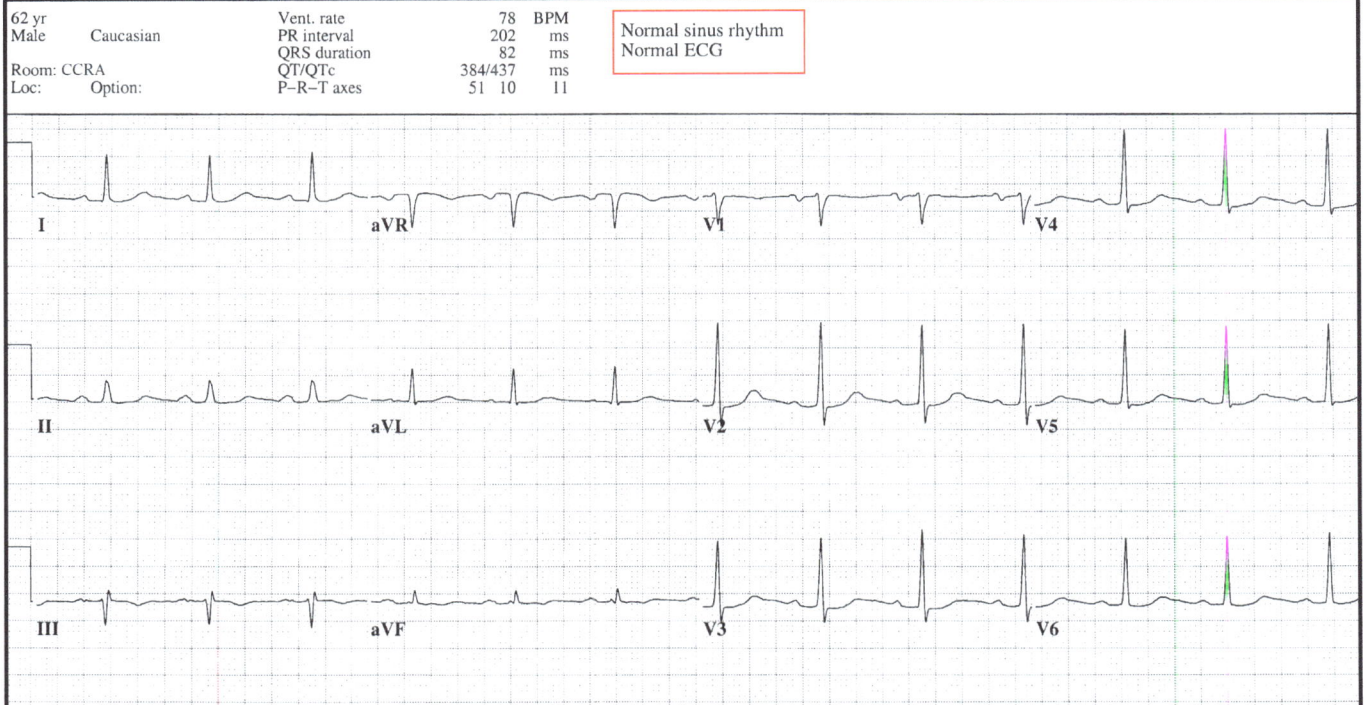

I   aVR   V1   V4

II   aVL   V2   V5

III   aVF   V3   V6

Despite the patient's successful "passing" of the Exercise Stress Test, the cardiologist was not convinced that his patient was free of obstructive coronary artery disease (CAD). The doctor advised his patient that cardiac catheterization would be necessary to definitely rule out obstructive CAD.

The patient's HMO refused to authorize cardiac catheterization based on the patient's normal ECG and Exercise Stress Test results. The cardiologist refused to accept the HMO's denial, and informed the patient he would waive his fee in order to gain the patient's consent. The patient agreed to proceed with the cardiac catheterization. The results are shown below:

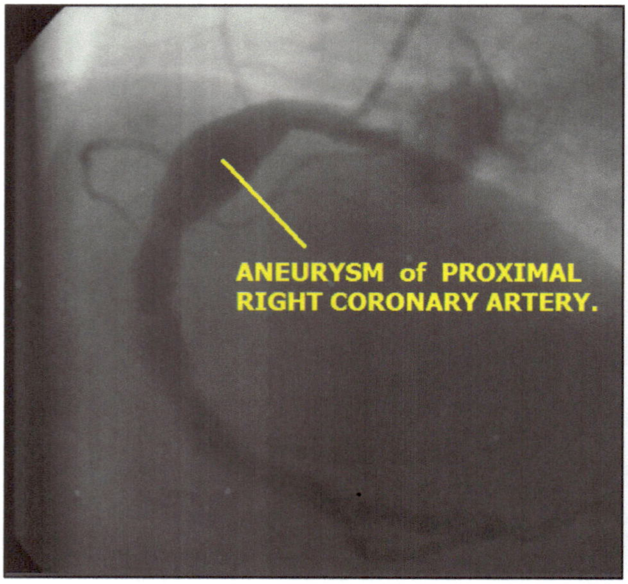

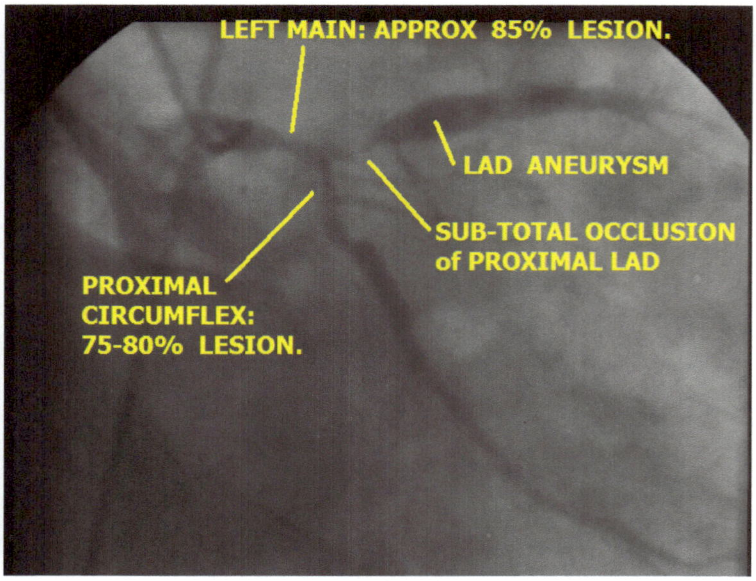

Once presented with the above coronary angiography, the HMO agreed to cover the patient's cardiac catheterization and coronary artery bypass surgery. The following day, the patient underwent successful quadruple coronary artery bypass surgery.

Case Study contributed by Querubin "Ben" Mendoza, MD

The Simple Acute Coronary Syndrome (SACS) Score:

Simple Acute Coronary Syndrome Score:

SYMPTOMS		POINTS ASSIGNED	TOTAL POINTS
CHECK ONE:	◆ **TYPICAL ACS - eg:** - CHEST PAIN (pressure / heaviness / dull) (may radiate to neck/ shoulders/ jaw/ arm) - DYSPNEA (may or may not be present)	**2**	
	◆ **ATYPICAL ACS - eg:** EPIGASTRIC PAIN / UNUSUAL FATIGUE / WEAKNESS / DIZZINESS / DIB COLD SWEATS / NAUSEA / PALPITATIONS	**1**	
	◆ **NONE RELEVANT**	**0**	
ECG			
CHECK ONE:	◆ **ST ELEVATION** (≥ 1mm @ J POINT plus 40 ms) ◆ **HYPERACUTE T WAVES** - and/or - ◆ **CONVEX ST SEGMENTS** -- ANY of ABOVE in 2 or more contiguous leads ◆ **NEW or PRESUMABLY NEW LBBB**	**2**	
	NEW or PRESUMABLY NEW: ◆ **ST DEPRESSION** (>0.5 mm @ J POINT) and/or ◆ **INVERTED or BIPHASIC T WAVES** and/or ◆ **PREVIOUSLY UNDIAGNOSED Q WAVES** **&/or ABNORMAL R WAVE PROGRESSION** (CONSISTENT WITH MYOCARDIAL INJURY /NECROSIS) ◆ **DYNAMIC ST SEGMENT** and/or **T WAVE** **CHANGES** IN SERIAL ECGs (any of the above IN 2 or MORE CONTIGUOUS LEADS)	**1**	
	◆ **NORMAL or NON-DIAGNOSTIC ECG**	**0**	
RISK FACTORS for CORONARY ARTERY DISEASE			
CHECK ALL THAT APPLY:	◆ **PREVIOUSLY DIAGNOSED CORONARY ARTERY DISEASE** (CAD) **and / or**	**1**	
	◆ **FAMILY HISTORY** ◆ **DIABETES** ◆ ↑ **LDL and/or** ↓ **HDL**	**3 or MORE RISK FACTORS:**	
	◆ **SMOKING** ◆ **AGE: 65 or MORE** ◆ **HYPERTENSION**	**NO Hx OF CAD & LESS THAN 3 RISK FACTORS:**	**0**	
CARDIAC MARKERS			
CHECK ONE:	◆ **TROPONIN** and/or **CK/MB** - ANY ELEVATION ABOVE YOUR INSTITUTION'S NORMAL RANGE:	**1**	
	◆ **NORMAL**	**0**	
TOTAL SCORE ⟶			

While screening approximately 300 case studies for inclusion in this book, we discovered several incidents where the TIMI Risk Score did not correlate with the patient's diagnosis. This observation prompted us to develop the SACS score, shown to the left.

The SACS score is an easy-to-use, practical instrument which was designed specifically as a predictor of obstructive CAD and ACS.

At the present time, the SACS Score is in the process of scientic validation. The study is being conducted at St. Joseph's Hospital in Tampa, Florida.

For more information, please log onto the National Institutes of Health (NIH) website: www.clinicaltrials.gov In the SEARCH box, enter study ID number: NCT000947804.

For institutions interested in participating in the study, please contact Principal Investigator Wayne Ruppert at: wwruppert@aol.com

NOTE:

Until the SACS score is validated via appropriate scientific method, we do not advocate its use as an adjunct to clinical decision making.

ACCELERATED DIAGNOSTIC PROTOCOLS (ADPs) include the use of serial ECGs and cardiac markers to rule out ACS, usually over a 6 – 12 hour period. If serial ECGs and cardiac markers are negative, then a confirmatory evaluation is performed to rule out inducible ischemia.[38] Because the focus of this textbook is on *ECG evaluation*, we present Exercise Treadmill Testing (ETT) first, and include a case study which emphasizes the value of ETT. In clinical practice, other diagnostic procedures (e.g.: echocardiogram, coronary CT angiogram, and myocardial perfusion imaging) may be more appropriate for certain patients than ETT. To obtain additional information about the use of other diagnostic procedures employed in ADPs, we refer you to read the American Heart Association's Scientific Statement "Testing of Low-Risk Patients Presenting to the Emergency Department with Chest Pain,"[39] which has served as the basis for much of our information provided in this section.

EXERCISE TREADMILL TESTING

The first standardized Exercise Stress Test (EST) was used in 1929 by Arthur Master at Mt. Sinai Hospital in New York City. EST, now referred to as Exercise Treadmill Testing (ETT), is commonly used to identify patients whom are at increased risk for adverse coronary events, and is especially valuable in cases where the patient's resting ECG is normal or inconclusive for ischemic changes.

The underlying physiology behind ETT is simple and well established; in patients with obstructive CAD, coronary blood flow can not increase adequately to meet increased myocardial oxygen demands, resulting in ischemia.

☞ The end-points for ETT are: provocation of *typical* or *atypical ACS symptoms*, *ECG changes consistent with ischemia (0.10 mV or more of ST depression or elevation, dysrhythmias* and/or a decrease in blood pressure of 10 mm/Hg or more.[40] A negative ETT is when there are no exercise induced abnormalities at 85% of the patient's age-predicted maximum heart rate (MPHR). A non-diagnostic study is when the patient is unable to achieve 85% MPHR without abnormalities. [41] Chronotropic incompetence, abnormal heart rate recovery, and hypotension during ETT are also poor prognostic indicators.

Figures concerning the sensitivity and specificity of ETT vary based on which studies and academic papers are referenced. According to Newman et al, *in a general population of patients, sensitivity is reported as 71.4% and specificity 90.4%*[42]

Our practical experience with patients in the cath lab reveals that there is a higher incidence of false positive ETTs in female patients. Breast tissue and a low exercise tolerance are often factors. Regarding the higher incidence of false positive ETTs, we find it's much better to send patients home after a normal cardiac catheterization, with "good news, your stress test lied," as opposed to patients keeling over at home after being told "everything checked out just fine with your heart during your stress test."

Typically, ETT falls into the continuum of care, as indicated, when:

reasonable suspicion exists that coronary artery disease is present,
less invasive studies are negative or inconclusive for CAD, and
There are no contraindications present for conducting EST.

The case study presented on the next page emphasizes the value of EST. In this case, a 71 year old male presented to a physician's office with a complaint of exertional chest pressure, syncope, and dizziness. A resting ECG was obtained, with normal results. *Nuclear perfusion and 2-D/M Doppler echocardiogram revealed no discernable ischemia and normal heart function respectively.*

---

[38] Erza Amsterdam, MD et al, Circulation 2010;122:756-776
[39] ibid
[40] NJ Fortuin and JL Weiss, *Circulation* 1977;56:p699
[41] Erza Amsterdam, MD et al, Circulation 2010;122:756-776
[42] R Newman, et al, J of Am Board of Fam Med 2008;21:531-8

CASE STUDY: RELEVANCE OF STRESS TESTING

CHIEF COMPLAINT and SIGNIFICANT HISTORY:

71 y/o male presents to the cardiologist's office, c/o EXERTIONAL SUBSTERNAL CHEST PRESSURE and DIZZINESS.   PMHx of Hypertension, AV Nodal Reentrant Tachycardia and vertigo.

RISK FACTOR PROFILE:

☀ FAMILY HISTORY - both parents.
☑ PREVIOUS CIGARETTE SMOKER
☑ CHOLESTEROL - unknown.
☑ AGE - OVER 65
☑ HYPERTENSION

PHYSICAL EXAM: Patient alert, oriented x 3, skin warm, dry, color normal,
carotids 2+ bilaterally, no bruits, Lungs clear, HS S1, S2 normal, no murmurs/gallops/rubs.
Extremities: good distal pulses, no edema.

VITAL SIGNS: BP: 118/60, P: 74, R: 16, SAO2: 98%

LABS: CARDIAC MARKERS NEGATIVE.   BMP, CBC: WNL.

DIANOSTIC EVALUATIONS:

☞ 2-D/M-MODE DOPPLER ECHOCARDIOGRAM: NORMAL
      (LV size, Normal LV function, trace of mitral and tricuspid regurgitation).
☞ MYOCARDIAL PERFUSION STUDY: NORMAL.
      (LVEF = 60%, STRESS and REST TOMOGRAPHIC PERFUSION IMAGES = NORMAL).

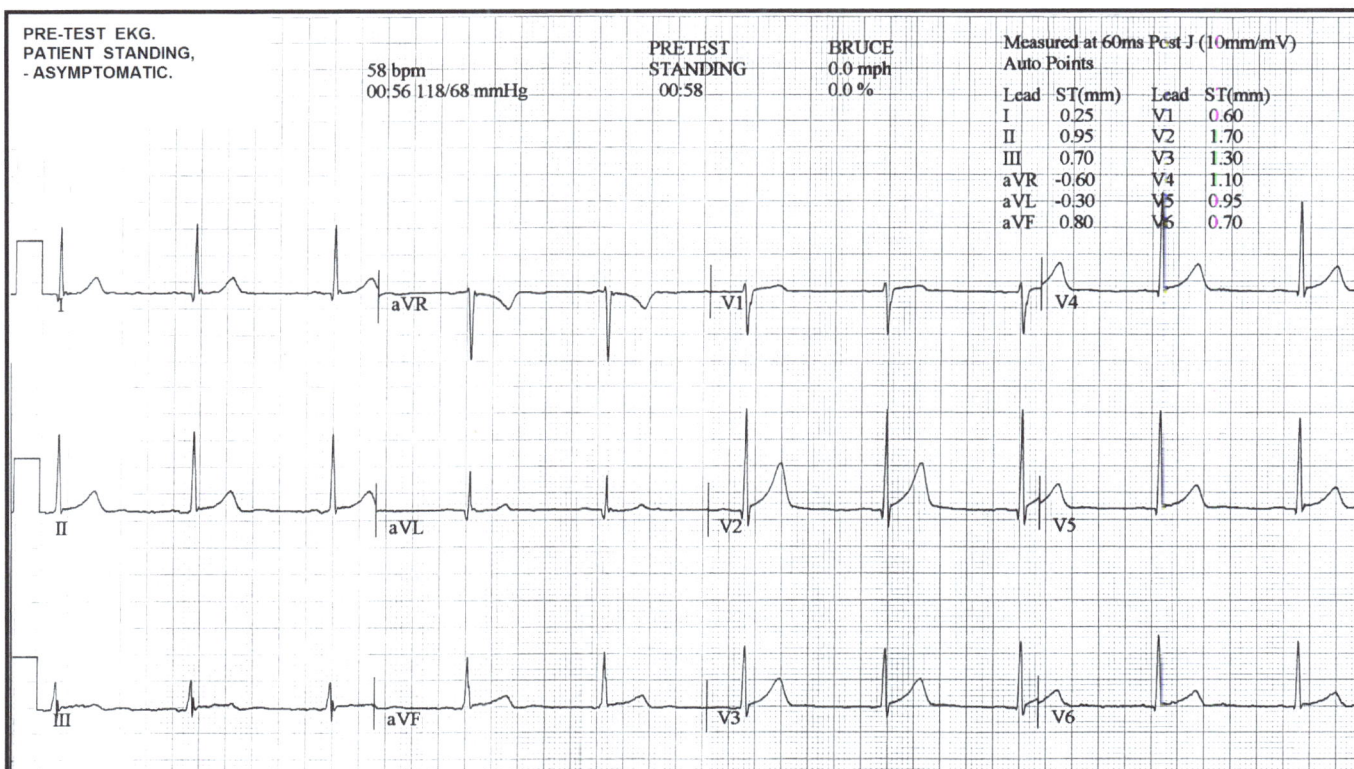

PRE-TEST EKG.
PATIENT STANDING,
- ASYMPTOMATIC.

58 bpm
00:56 118/68 mmHg

PRETEST
STANDING
00:58

BRUCE
0.0 mph
0.0 %

Measured at 60ms Post J (10mm/mV)
Auto Points

Lead	ST(mm)	Lead	ST(mm)
I	0.25	V1	0.60
II	0.95	V2	1.70
III	0.70	V3	1.30
aVR	-0.60	V4	1.10
aVL	-0.30	V5	0.95
aVF	0.80	V6	0.70

PEAK EXERCISE
- TEST ABORTED WHEN
  PATIENT REPORTED
  EXPERIENCING CHEST
  PRESSURE.

114 bpm

(PEAK EXERCISE)

EXERCISE
STAGE 2
05:01

BRUCE
2.5 mph
12.0 %

Measured at 60ms Post J (10mm/mV)
Auto Points

Lead	ST(mm)	Lead	ST(mm)
I	-1.20	V1	1.05
II	-1.70	V2	-1.40
III	-0.45	V3	-1.25
aVR	1.50	V4	-1.00
aVL	-0.35	V5	-1.05
aVF	-1.10	V6	-1.55

LATERAL-ANTERIOR WALL — CIRC.(OM) - or - LAD (DIAG) — I — 2 mm ST SEGMENT DEPRESSION

BASILAR SEPTUM — 2.5 mm ST SEGMENT ELEVATION — aVR — LMCA / 1st SEPTAL PERFORATOR

ANTERIOR - SEPTAL WALL — LAD — V1

ANTERIOR WALL — LAD — V4 — 2 mm ST SEGMENT DEPRESSION

INFERIOR WALL — RCA - or - CIRCUMFLEX — II — 3 mm ST SEGMENT DEPRESSION

LATERAL-ANTERIOR WALL — CIRC.(OM) - or - LAD (DIAG) — aVL

ANTERIOR - SEPTAL WALL — LAD — V2 — 2 mm ST SEGMENT DEPRESSION

LATERAL WALL — CIRCUMFLEX — V5 — 2.5mm ST SEGMENT DEPRESSION

INFERIOR WALL — RCA - or - CIRCUMFLEX — III — 2 mm ST SEGMENT DEPRESSION

INFERIOR WALL — RCA - or - CIRCUMFLEX — aVF — 2.5mm ST SEGMENT DEPRESSION

ANTERIOR WALL — LAD — V3 — 2.5mm ST SEGMENT DEPRESSION

LATERAL WALL — CIRCUMFLEX — V6 — 3 mm ST SEGMENT DEPRESSION

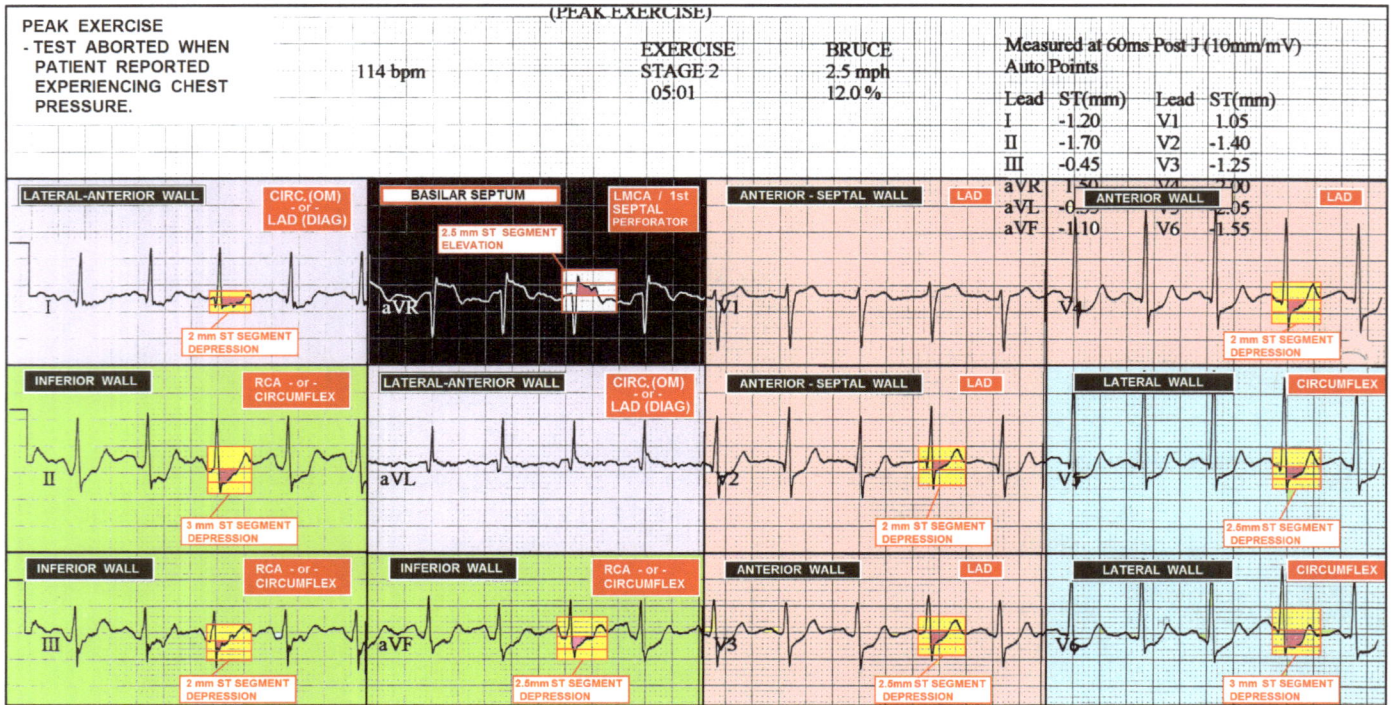

The ECG taken above was recorded during exercise just before the test was aborted due to the patient reporting chest pressure. Note significant J point depression with upsloping ST segments in every lead except aVL and V1. Also note lead aVR, which shows ST elevation. The significance of aVR elevation during EST is associated with high deree of LAD stenosis.[43] As depicted by our color-coding of each region of the myocardium based on arterial distribution, note that ischemic changes are visible in each of the three common arterial distributions: the *anterior wall* (fed by the *left anterior descending artery*), the *lateral wall* (fed by the *circumflex artery*), and the *inferior wall* (fed by the *right coronary artery* in 75-80% of the population and the *circumflex artery* in 10-15% of the population)

The patient's subsequent cardiac catheterization angiography is presented below:

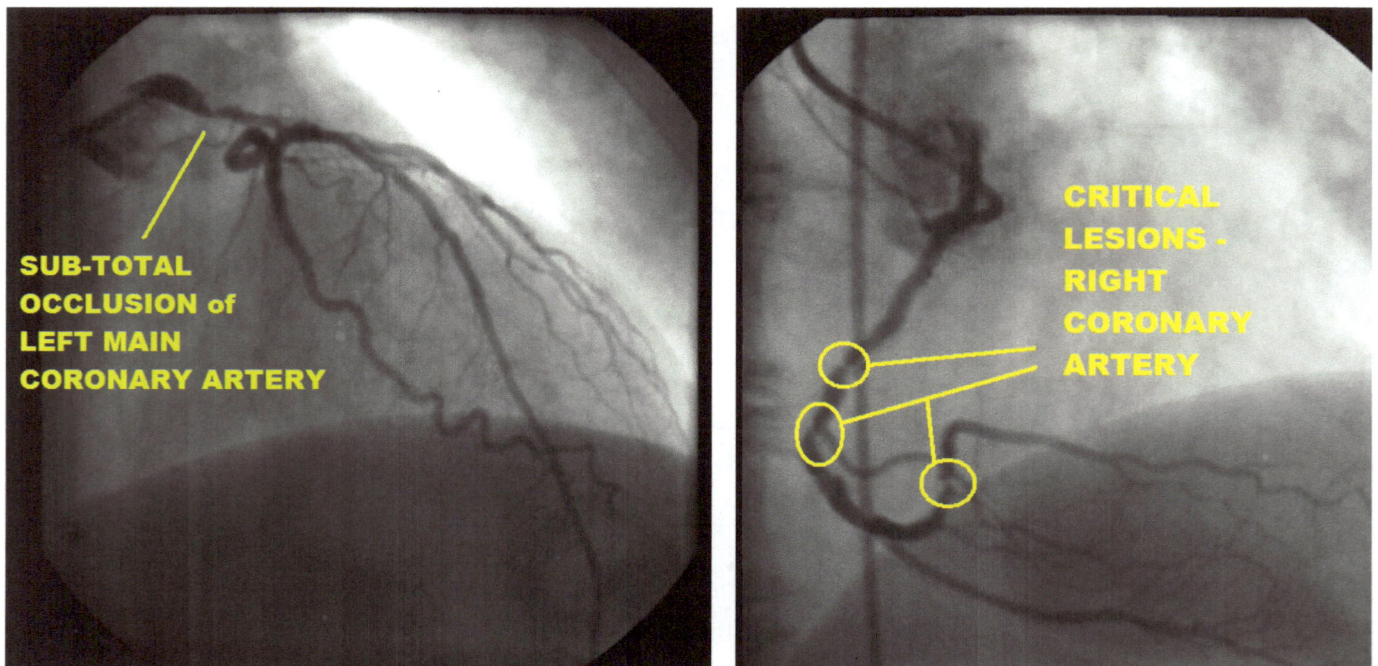

SUB-TOTAL OCCLUSION of LEFT MAIN CORONARY ARTERY

CRITICAL LESIONS - RIGHT CORONARY ARTERY

---

[43] J Neill et al, Eur J Nucl Med 2007;34(3):338-45

160

Instead of triple vessel disease, we discovered a sub-total occlusion of the LEFT MAIN coronary artery, which effectively jeopardizes the *left anterior descending* and *circumflex* distributions, and critical lesions of the *right coronary artery.* This patient underwent successful emergency coronary artery bypass graft surgery within 24 hours of cardiac catheterization.

☞ The clinician must be aware that there is a well-documented history of *decreased sensitivity of myocardial nuclear imaging with respect to cases of triple-vessel and left main coronary artery occlusions. The increase in false-negative results occurs in the absence of relative perfusion differences due to similar-grade stenosis in all vessels.* Although technological advances are improving the sensitivity and specificity of cardiac nuclear imaging, this case study, which occurred in 2008, underscores the absolute value of the clinician remaining vigilant with respect to a *patient's presenting symptoms* and *risk factor profile,* and pursuing every modality of diagnostic testing until a concrete and definitive diagnosis is obtained. When a patient's life depends on accurate diagnosis, *"every stone needs to be turned over until the truth is discovered."*

Case Study contributed by Xavier Prida, MD, FACC

---

* TABLE of EXERCISE STRESS TEST CONTRINDICATIONS:

Absolute Contraindications to Exercise Stress Testing:
- ☐ Acute myocardial infarction (within 2 days)
- ☐ High-risk unstable angina
- ☐ Uncontrolled cardiac arrhythmias
- ☐ Symptomatic severe aortic stenosis
- ☐ Uncontrolled symptomatic heart failure
- ☐ Acute pulmonary embolus / pulmonary infarction
- ☐ Acute myocarditis / Pericarditis
- ☐ Acute aortic dissection

Relative Contraindications to Exercise Stress Testing:
- ☐ Left main coronary stenosis
- ☐ Moderate stenotic valvular heart disease
- ☐ Electrolyte abnormalities
- ☐ Severe arterial hypertension (>200 systolic / 100 diastolic)
- ☐ Tachyarrhythmias / bradyarrhythmias
- ☐ Hypertrophic cardiomyopathy and other forms of outflow tract obstruction
- ☐ Mental / physical impairment leading to inability or unwillingness to exercise
- ☐ High-degree atrioventricular block

* R Newman, et al : J of American Board of Family Medicine 2008;21:531-8

For those wishing to review more detailed information about EST, we refer you to the following resources:

ACC/AHA 2002 Guideline Update for Exercise Testing Article: A Report of the American College of Cardiology/American Heart Association Task Force on Practice Guidelines. Raymond Gibbons, et al. Online version of article available at:
http://circ.ahajournals.org/cgi/content/full/106/14/1883
Update on Exercise Stress Testing, by Gerald Fletcher, et al., American Family Physician 2006;74:1749-54. Online access: http://www.aafp.org/afp
Predictive Value of Exercise Stress Testing in a Family Medicine Population, by Robert Newman, et al., Journal of the American Board of Family Medicine 2008;21:531-8. Online access: http://www.jabfm.org

ECHOCARDIOGRAPHIC STUDIES:

The value of echocardiographic (echo) studies in the evaluation of suspected ACS patients is the ability to detect resting wall motion abnormalities (RWMA) in resting studies, and inducible wall motion abnormalities in stress echocardiographic studies. Ischemia induced RWMAs are often detectable by echo almost immediately after the onset of symptoms, making this an effective and valuable tool for screening patients in the ED. Variables which determine the accuracy of the resting echo include size of ischemic zone (may not be detectable when there is less than 20% of transmural myocardial thickness), and timing of the study in relationship to the onset of symptoms. A recent study of patients admitted with suspected ACS symptoms gives the resting echocardiogram a 97% negative predictive value, and a 24% positive predictive value.[44] Stress echocardiography, performed using exercise or pharmacological agents, can be used to induce wall motion abnormalities in patients without resting wall motion abnormalities. Stress echo sensitivity is reported at 86%, and specificity 81%.[45] *An added benefit of an echocardiogram in the ED setting is the ascending aorta and aortic arch can be evaluated for abnormalities consistent with dissection!*

CORONARY CT ANGIOGRAPHY:

With the advent of the 64-slice multi-detector CT scanner, evaluation of an ED patient's coronary arteries can now be achieved with a spatial resolution approaching (but still inferior to) that of traditional coronary angiography. In two recent studies with a combined study population of 468 patients, the Coronary CT Angiographic study (CT Angio) produced a 100% negative predictability rate for ruling out obstructive coronary arterial lesions.[46] An added benefit of obtaining a CT study on ED chest pain patients is its capability of excluding the diagnoses of pulmonary embolus and aortic dissection. Disadvantages of the CT Angio is the radiation exposure to patients (equal to 250 - 500 chest X-rays, depending on patient body size), and the need to inject approximately 80ml of IV contrast solution.

MYOCARDIAL PERFUSION IMAGING:

Myocardial perfusion imaging (MPI), like echo studies, is often used in patients without evident AMI or ischemia. MPI can be administered at rest, or with stress induced by exercise or pharmacological agents. Sensitivity of stress MPI is reported at 87%, and specificity at 73%.[47] MPI is often preferred over ETT for patients with baseline ECG abnormalities.

---

[44] Amsterdam, E. et al, "AHA Scientific Statement- Testing of Low Risk Patients Presenting to the Emergency Department With Chest Pain:" Circulation 2010;122:756-776
[45] ibid
[46] ibid
[47] ibid

CASE STUDIES:

We begin each case study by presenting the patient's *chief complaint, significant history, physical exam, pertinent labs,* and *CAD risk factors.* Beneath this information is a "*Quadrad of ACS Checklist.*" On the opposite page is the patient's *12 lead ECG.*

The Quadrad of ACS Checklist is used to demonstrate the importance of factoring a patient's *symptoms, ECG findings, ACS risk factors* and *cardiac markers* into the clinical decision making process. In cases where the patient's ECG is normal, and/or symptoms are atypical, your ability to consider all of the pertinent findings in the "quadrad of ACS" is often critical to making an accurate diagnosis.

To *reinforce your knowledge of essential concepts* and *exercise your critical thinking skills*, we provide a *worksheet,* located just below the patient's ECG. We encourage you to take the role of the lead physician and complete this information:

- *Suspected DIAGNOSIS of the patient's condition*
- *ECG findings*
- *Suspected "Culprit Artery" (in cases of AMI)*
- *Suspected "Potential Complications" that you anticipate the patient may exhibit*
- *Immediate Care Plan (any additional diagnostic studies, treatment, etc).*

On the following pages, where applicable, you will find:

- *A color-coded ECG*, with the abnormalities highlighted, and computer-generated diagnosis
- *Angiography from the patient's cardiac catheterization.* Where applicable, this includes images *before* and *after* percutaneous coronary intervention (PCI).
- *computer generated images of the patient's coronary arteries*
- In STEMI case studies, we *list and illustrate the critical structure(s) of the heart that were adversely affected by the blockage – and present potential complications that clinicians should expect in the event these structures fail.*

We conclude each case study by providing the *patient's outcome*, along with a *case study summary* of *educational objectives* specific to the case.

NOTE: To be HIPAA compliant, we have eliminated every marker of patient identity:

- patient's name
- age (may have been altered +/- 5 years)
- sex (may have been altered, unless clinically relevant)
- date and year of occurrence (some cases have occurred up to 20 years ago)
- Hospital location (cases are from multiple hospitals in several states)

In a few cases, with appropriate endorsement, we identify the physician(s) who managed the patient's care.

ECG IDENTIFICATION of the INFARCT RELATED ARTERY

IN CASE STUDIES of 11 VARIATIONS of ACUTE MI in PATIENTS with TYPICAL CORONARY ARTERY ANATOMY

ST ELEVATION in LEADS:	ST DEPRESSION in LEADS:	REGION of MYOCARDIUM	"CULPRIT" ARTERY	STRUCTURES at RISK	POTENTIAL COMPLICATIONS *	THERAPEUTIC INTERVENTIONS to CONSIDER ** ***	SEE CASE STUDY
V1 - V4 + possibly V5 / V6	NONE	ANTERIOR SEPTAL	MID-LEFT ANTERIOR DESCENDING	• up to 45% LV MUSCLE MASS • BUNDLE BRANCHES	• LV PUMP FAILURE: • CARDIOGENIC SHOCK • PULMONARY EDEMA • HEART BLOCKS • BUNDLE BRANCH BLOCK	• INOTROPES • Intra-AORTIC BALLOON PUMP • ET INTUBATION • TRANSCUTANEOUS/ TRANSVENOUS PACING	1
V1 - V4 I and aVL + possibly V5/V6 aVR	II, III, and/or aVF	ANTERIOR SEPTAL LATERAL	PROXIMAL LEFT ANTERIOR DESCENDING	SAME as ABOVE, plus: • EXTENSION OF THROMBUS into L. MAIN CORONARY ARTERY	SAME AS ABOVE, BUT WITH HIGHER INCIDENCE / SEVERITY	SAME AS ABOVE	3
I, aVL	MAY or MAY NOT be present	LATERAL (ANTERO-LATERAL JUNCTION)	EITHER: -DIAGONAL -RAMUS -OBTUSE MARG.	• approx 25-35% of LV MUSCLE MASS	• MODERATE RISK of LV FAILURE	• INOTROPES vs. SMALL FL. CHALLENGE	2
I, aVL, aVR V1, V2 + possibly V3 - V6	II, III, aVF, + possibly V3 - V6	GLOBAL LV	LEFT MAIN CORONARY ARTERY	• 75-100% of LV MUSCLE • BUNDLE of HIS • BUNDLE BRANCHES	• PROFOUND LV FAILURE, • CARDIOGENIC SHOCK • PULMONARY EDEMA • HEART BLOCKS • HIGH RATE of MORTALITY	• INOTROPES • Intra-AORTIC BALLOON PUMP • ET INTUBATION • TRANSCUTANEOUS/TRANS- • VENOUS PACING	4
V5 - V6 + possibly I, aVL	NONE or II, III, and/or aVF	LATERAL	CIRCUMFLEX (non-DOMINANT)	• 20 - 30 % LV MUSCLE MASS • SINUS NODE (45% pop.)	• MODERATE RISK of LV FAILURE • SINUS NODE DYSFUNCTION (BRADY-ASYSTOLE)	• INOTROPES vs. SMALL FL. CHALLENGE • ATROPINE / PACING	5
II, III, aVF	I, aVL	INFERIOR	RCA (75-80% pop.) or CIRCUMFLEX (10-15% pop.)	• 15-25% LV MUSCLE MASS • SINUS NODE • AV NODE	• MODERATE RISK of LV FAIL • BRADYCARDIA - • HEART BLOCKS	• INOTROPES vs. SMALL FL. CHALLENGE • ATROPINE • TRANSCUTANEOUS PACING	6
II, III, aVF, + V3R - V6R	I, aVL	INFERIOR RIGHT-VENTRICULAR	DOMINANT RCA	• 15-25% LV MUSCLE MASS • RIGHT VENTRICLE • SINUS NODE • AV NODE	• MODERATE RISK of LV FAIL • EXTREME HYPOTENSION from NITRATES/VASODIL. • BRADYCARDIA - • HEART BLOCKS	• FLUID CHALLENGES (if NO Sx of PULMONARY EDEMA • INOTROPES (if Sx of LV PUMP FAILURE) • ATROPINE / PACING	7
II, III, aVF +	V1 - V3, + possibly V4, V5, V6	INFERIOR - POSTERIOR	"EXTREME" DOMINANT RCA or CIRCUMFLEX	• 25-45% LV MUSCLE MASS • SINUS NODE • AV NODE	• LV PUMP FAILURE / CARDIOGENIC SHOCK • BRADYCARDIA • HEART BLOCKS	• INOTROPES • Intra-AORTIC BALLOON PUMP • ET INTUBATION • ATROPINE / PACING	8
II, III, aVF, V5, V6 + possibly I, aVL	V1-V3, poss V4-V6	INFERIOR-POSTERIOR-LATERAL	PROXIMAL DOMINANT CIRCUMFLEX	• 35-55% LV MUSCLE MASS • SINUS NODE • AV NODE	• PROFOUND LV PUMP FAILURE / CARDIOGENIC SHOCK / PULM. EDEMA • BRADYCARDIA • HEART BLOCKS	• INOTROPES • Intra-AORTIC BALLOON PUMP • ET INTUBATION • TRANSCUTANEOUS/TRANS-VENOUS PACING	9
II, III, aVF V1-V4 + possibly I, aVL, V5, V6	aVR	ANTERIOR-SEPTAL-LATERAL-INFERIOR	TRANS-APICAL LEFT ANTERIOR DESCENDING	• 50-70% LV MUSCLE MASS • BUNDLE of HIS • BUNDLE BRANCHES	• PROFOUND LV PUMP FAILURE / CARDIOGENIC SHOCK / PULM. EDEMA • HEART BLOCKS	• INOTROPES • Intra-AORTIC BALLOON PUMP • ET INTUBATION • TRANSCUTANEOUS/TRANS-VENOUS PACING	10
NONE	V1-V3, + possibly V4-V6	POSTERIOR	POSTERIOR LATERAL VESSEL(S)	• 20-30% LV MUSCLE MASS • AV NODE	• MODERATE RISK of LV FAILURE • AV NODE DYSFUNCTION	• INOTROPES vs. SMALL FL. CHALLENGE • ATROPINE / PACING	12

* ALL PATIENTS experiencing AMI are at ELEVATED RISK for DEVELOPMENT of LETHAL CARDIAC DYSRHYTHMIAS / CARDIAC ARREST
** ALL AMI PATIENTS SHOULD BE CONSIDERED FOR STAT REPERFUSION THERAPY - FOLLOW AHA ACLS / INSTITUTIONAL PROTOCOL FOR SPECIFIC THERAPY
*** "TREATMENTS to CONSIDER" ARE POSSIBLE INTERVENTIONS which are commonly utilized. FOLLOW PHYSICIAN ORDERS, ACLS and/or INSTITUTIONAL PROTOCOLS for specific therapy.

The above table describes eleven common types of acute MI, classified by the zone of myocardial infarction. Our case studies have been chosen for their educational relevance; each is about as "typical" as we could find, in patients with common coronary arterial anatomy. The information conveyed in this section is consistent with our collective observations of acute MI patients in the cardiac catheterization lab, as well as information presented in current medical journals.

Beware that in your daily clinical practice, you will inevitably encounter patients who don't present the way those in our case studies have.   These may be patients with multiple cardiac abnormalities that alter the ECG, or may simply be patients with atypical coronary arterial anatomy (see bottom of page 28).   That's one of the things that makes medicine so interesting; there will be patients who present to you whose "hearts won't have read the book" -- they'll be the "atypical ones" who challenge you, and ultimately redefine much of what you have previously been taught!

STEMI CASE STUDIES:

This section features case studies of patients whom presented with symptoms of Acute Coronary Syndrome and ECGs with ST segment elevation. All were diagnosed with ST segment elevation myocardial infarction by cardiac catheterization.

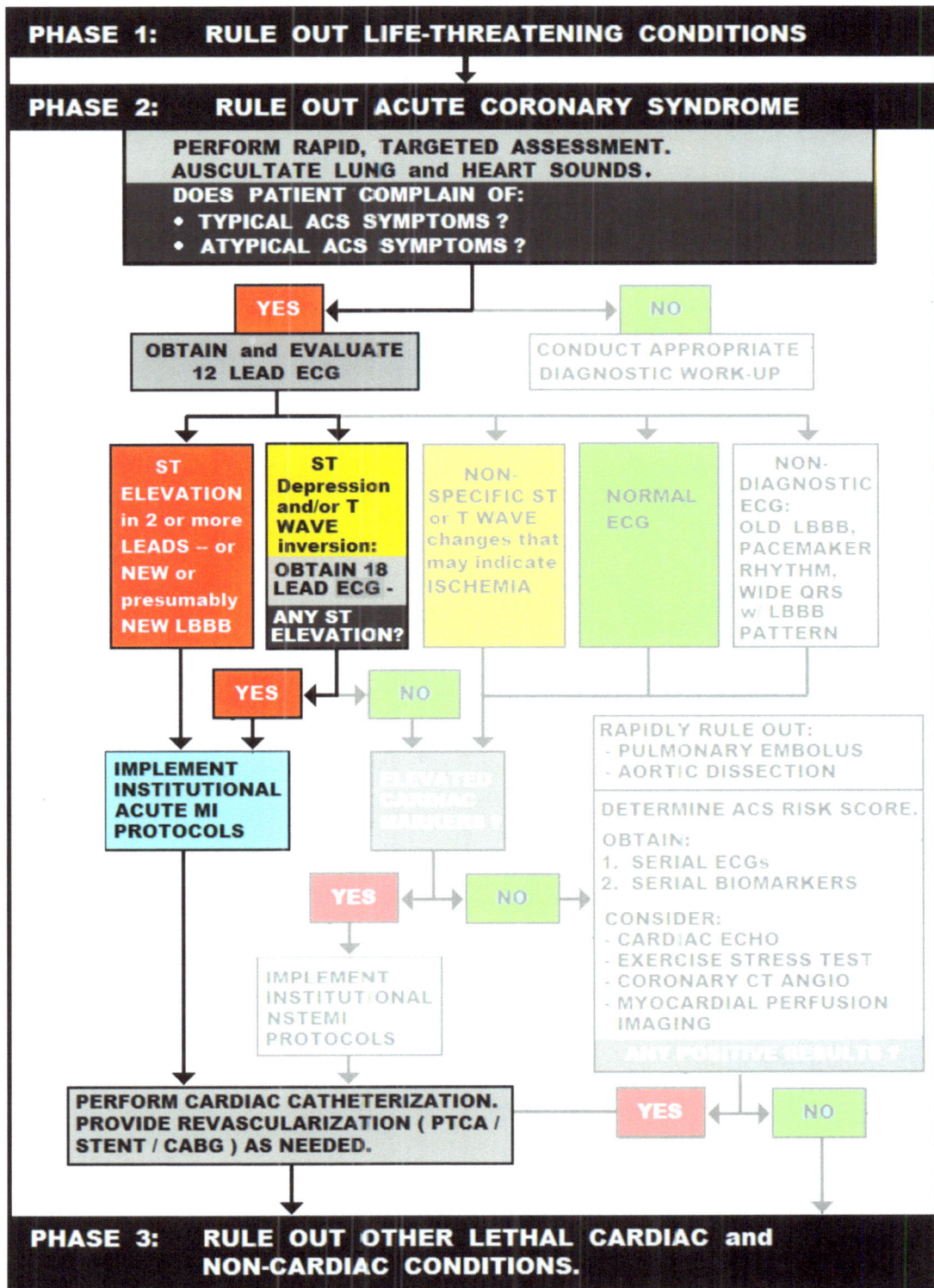

PHASE 1:   RULE OUT LIFE-THREATENING CONDITIONS

PHASE 2:   RULE OUT ACUTE CORONARY SYNDROME

PERFORM RAPID, TARGETED ASSESSMENT.
AUSCULTATE LUNG and HEART SOUNDS.
DOES PATIENT COMPLAIN OF:
- TYPICAL ACS SYMPTOMS ?
- ATYPICAL ACS SYMPTOMS ?

YES | NO

OBTAIN and EVALUATE 12 LEAD ECG | CONDUCT APPROPRIATE DIAGNOSTIC WORK-UP

ST ELEVATION in 2 or more LEADS -- or NEW or presumably NEW LBBB

ST Depression and/or T WAVE inversion: OBTAIN 18 LEAD ECG - ANY ST ELEVATION?

NON-SPECIFIC ST or T WAVE changes that may indicate ISCHEMIA

NORMAL ECG

NON-DIAGNOSTIC ECG: OLD LBBB, PACEMAKER RHYTHM, WIDE QRS w/ LBBB PATTERN

YES | NO

IMPLEMENT INSTITUTIONAL ACUTE MI PROTOCOLS

RAPIDLY RULE OUT:
- PULMONARY EMBOLUS
- AORTIC DISSECTION

DETERMINE ACS RISK SCORE.
OBTAIN:
1. SERIAL ECGs
2. SERIAL BIOMARKERS
CONSIDER:
- CARDIAC ECHO
- EXERCISE STRESS TEST
- CORONARY CT ANGIO
- MYOCARDIAL PERFUSION IMAGING

YES | NO

IMPLEMENT INSTITUTIONAL NSTEMI PROTOCOLS

PERFORM CARDIAC CATHETERIZATION. PROVIDE REVASCULARIZATION (PTCA / STENT / CABG) AS NEEDED.

YES | NO

PHASE 3:   RULE OUT OTHER LETHAL CARDIAC and NON-CARDIAC CONDITIONS.

CASE STUDY 1 - STEMI

CHIEF COMPLAINT and SIGNIFICANT HISTORY:

72 y/o male, c/o CHEST "HEAVINESS," started 20 minutes before calling 911. Pain is "8" on 1-10 scale, also c/o mild shortness of breath. Has had same pain "intermittently" x 2 weeks.

RISK FACTOR PROFILE:

- **FAMILY HISTORY** - father died of MI at age 77
- **FORMER CIGARETTE SMOKER** - smoked for 30 year - quit 27 years ago
- **DIABETES** - oral meds and diet controlled
- **HIGH CHOLESTEROL** - controlled with STATIN meds
- **AGE: OVER 65**

PHYSICAL EXAM: Patient calm, alert, oriented X 4, skin cool, dry, pale. No JVD, Lungs clear bilaterally. Heart sounds normal S1, S2. No peripheral edema.

VITAL SIGNS: BP: 100/64, P: 75, R: 20, SAO2: 94%

LABS: FIRST TROPONIN: 6.4

QUADRAD OF ACS CHECKLIST

☑ **SYMPTOMS of ACS**
- ◆ TYPICAL ACS - eg:
- ◆ ATYPICAL ACS - eg:

☑ **ECG ABNORMALITIES**
- ✔ ◆ ST ELEVATION (J POINT plus 40 ms)
- ◆ HYPERACUTE T WAVES - and/or -
- ◆ NEW or PRESUMABLY NEW LBBB
- ◆ ST DEPRESSION (>0.5 mm @ J POINT) and/or
- ◆ INVERTED or BIPHASIC T WAVES and/or
- ◆ DYNAMIC ST SEGMENT and/or T WAVE CHANGES IN SERIAL EKGs

☑ **RISK FACTORS - 3 or more**
- ✔ ◆ FAMILY HISTORY
- ✔ ◆ DIABETES
- ✔ ◆ ↑ LDL and/or ↓ HDL
- ◆ SMOKING
- ✔ ◆ AGE: 65 or MORE
- ◆ HYPERTENSION

☑ **CARDIAC MARKERS**
- ◆ ELEVATED TROPONIN and/or CK/MB

4 **TOTAL**

SUSPECTED ACUTE MI:

INITIAL MANAGEMENT

- **VITAL SIGNS**
- **"O.M.I."**
  - Oxygen
  - Monitor (ecg)
  - IV (plus draw lab samples)
- **12 LEAD ECG**
  Obtain and interpret within 10 minutes of patient's arrival.
- **"M.O.N.A."**
  - Morphine
  - Oxygen (if not already done)
  - Nitroglycerin
  - Aspirin
- **RAPID, FOCUSED ASSESSMENT**
- **HEART / LUNG SOUNDS**
- **SEND LAB SAMPLES:**
  - Cardiac Markers
  - Electrolytes
  - Coagulation Studies

72 yr Male	Caucasian		Vent. rate	75	BPM
Loc:3	Option:23		PR interval	162	ms
			QRS duration	98	ms
			QT/QTc	382/426	ms
			P-R-T axes	72 13	83

👉 **EVALUATE EKG for indicators of ACS:**

- ST SEGMENT ELEVATION / DEPRESSION
- HYPERACUTE T WAVES
- CONVEX ST SEGMENTS
- OTHER ST SEGMENT / T WAVE ABNORMALTIES

Leads: I, aVR, V1, V4, II, aVL, V2, V5, III, aVF, V3, V6

CASE STUDY QUESTIONS:

NOTE LEADS WITH ST ELEVATION:

NOTE LEADS WITH ST DEPRESSION:

WHAT IS THE SUSPECTED DIAGNOSIS ?

WHAT IS THE "CULPRIT ARTERY" -- if applicable ?

LIST ANY CRITICAL STRUCTURES COMPROMISED:

LIST ANY POTENTIAL COMPLICATIONS:

167

72 yr		Vent. rate	75	BPM	Normal sinus rhythm
Male	Caucasian	PR interval	162	ms	Anteroseptal infarct , possibly acute
		QRS duration	98	ms	*** ** ** ** * ACUTE MI ** ** ** ** **
		QT/QTc	382/426	ms	Abnormal ECG
Loc:	Option:2	P–R–T axes	72 13	83	

ST SEGMENT ELEVATION

LATERAL - ANTERIOR DIAG. (LAD) or OM (CIRC).	BASILAR SEPTUM	ANTERIOR - SEPTAL LAD	ANTERIOR LAD
I	aVR	V1	V4
INFERIOR DOMINANT RCA or CIRC.	LATERAL - ANTERIOR DIAG. (LAD) or OM (CIRC).	ANTERIOR - SEPTAL LAD	LATERAL CIRC. or LAD
II	aVL	V2	V5
INFERIOR DOMINANT RCA or CIRC.	INFERIOR DOMINANT RCA or CIRC.	ANTERIOR LAD	LATERAL CIRC. or LAD
III	aVF	V3	V6

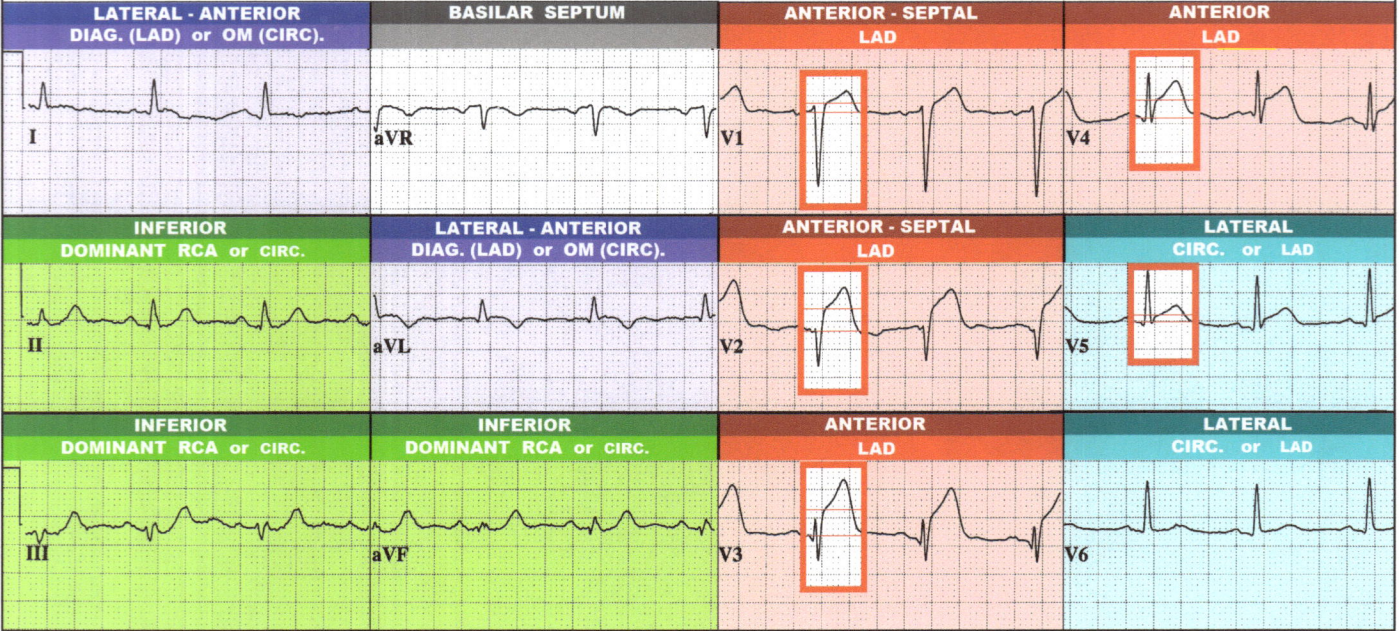

As illustrated in the diagram to the left, leads V1 – V4 "view" the anterior-septal aspects of the left ventricle. Therefore when ST elevation is seen in leads V1 – V4, we suspect anterior-septal STEMI.

It is not unusual to see anterior wall STEMI extending to the lateral region, with ST elevation noted in leads V5 and possibly V6. In this case, ST elevation is only seen in one lateral lead, V5, and therefore does not "qualify" as a lateral wall STEMI.

V1 - V4 VIEW THE ANTERIOR-SEPTAL WALL
of the LEFT VENTRICLE

V1, V2 - ANTERIOR / SEPTAL
V3, V4 - ANTERIOR

SPINE

RV   LV   V6

V5

ANTERIOR CHEST WALL

V1 V2 V3 V4

RUPPERT, WAYNE	ID: 7445683659	05-OCT-2006	JOHNS-HOPKINS UNIV.
38 Yrs	Vent. Rate: 68	NORMAL SINUS RHYTHM	
MALE	P-R Int.: 160 ms	Normal EKG	
	QRS: 100 ms	Very Healthy Athletic EKG !	

I	AVR	V1	V4
II	AVL	V2	V5
III	AVF	V3	V6

☞ **The ANTERIOR-SEPTAL WALL is fed by the LEFT ANTERIOR DESCENDING ARTERY.**

As a general guideline, *the LAD supplies between 40-50% of the LV muscle mass* in most people, which is illustrated in the diagram at the top of the next page.

BLOOD SUPPLY TO VENTRICLES:
COMMON ARTERIAL DISTRIBUTIONS

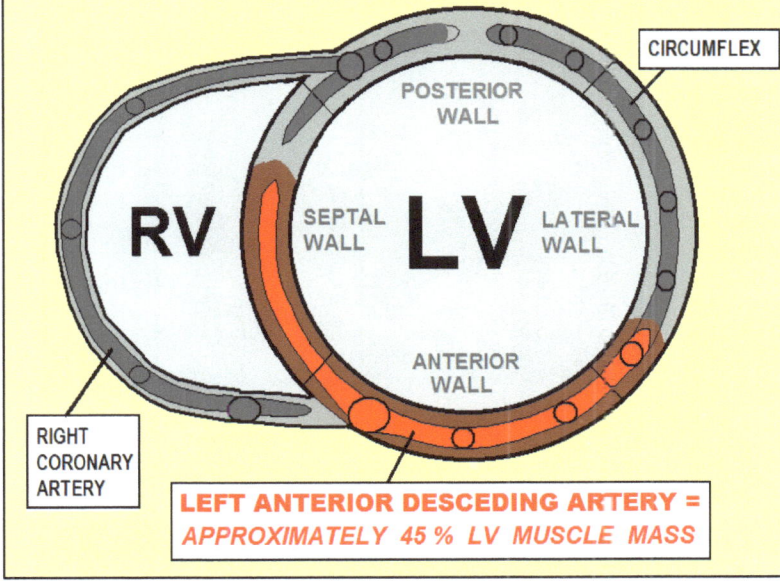

CIRCUMFLEX

POSTERIOR WALL

RV

SEPTAL WALL

LV

LATERAL WALL

ANTERIOR WALL

RIGHT CORONARY ARTERY

LEFT ANTERIOR DESCEDING ARTERY = APPROXIMATELY 45 % LV MUSCLE MASS

In the early stage of acute myocardial infarction, cells cut off from the supply of oxygen and glucose convert to *anaerobic metabolism*. In this phase, myocardial cell contraction becomes markedly diminished. While this physiological change serves to delay cell death, in cases of anterior wall MI, where up to 45% of the left ventricle stops contracting normally, it often results in *LV pump failure*, leading to *cardiogenic shock* and *pulmonary edema*.

TREATMENT OF CARDIOGENIC SHOCK: Traditional accepted pharmacological treatment for hypotension secondary to LV pump failure has been with Dopamine (2 – 20 mcg/kg/min IV) or Dobutamine (2 – 20 mcg/kg/min IV) for blood pressures between 70 - 100 mmHg, and Norepinephrine (0.5 – 30 mcg/min IV) for systolic pressures below 70 mmHg.

1. Although we have used Dopamine in the acute setting for many years with good results in the raising the patient's blood pressure, a recent study indicates that when used to treat cardiogenic shock, the complication rates (incidence of cardiac dysrhythmia and mortality within 28 days) for Dopamine are nearly twice that of Norepinephrine (207 events [24.1%] for Dopamine vs. 102 events [12.4%] for norepinephrine).[48]

CASE STUDY SUMMARY

NOTE LEADS WITH ST ELEVATION:	V1 - V5	NOTE LEADS WITH ST DEPRESSION:	NONE

SUSPECTED DIAGNOSIS: ACUTE ANTERIOR - SEPTAL STEMI

SUSPECTED "CULPRIT ARTERY" (if applicable): MID LEFT ANTERIOR DESCENDING ARTERY (LAD)

IMMEDIATE CONCERNS FOR ALL STEMI PATIENTS:

- BE PREPARED TO MANAGE SUDDEN CARDIAC ARREST (PRIMARY V - FIB / V- TACH, BRADYCARDIAS / HEART BLOCKS)
- STAT REPERFUSION THERAPY: THROMBOLYTICS vs. CARDIAC CATHETERIZATION and PCI
- CONSIDER NEEDS FOR ANTI-PLATELET and ANTI-COAGULATION THERAPY

CRITICAL STRUCTURES COMPROMISED:	POTENTIAL COMPLICATIONS:	POSSIBLE CRITICAL INTERVENTIONS:
40-50% of the LV MUSCLE MASS	LV PUMP FAILURE leading to: - CARDIOGENIC SHOCK - PULMONARY EDEMA	INOTROPIC AGENTS ET INTUBATION I.A.B.P. INSERTION
	VENTRICULAR DYSRHYTHMIAS (VT / VF)	DEFIBRILLATION / ANTIARRHYTHMIC AGENTS
Potential compromise of BLOOD SUPPLY to: - Bundle of His - Proximal Bundle Branches	HIGH-GRADE HEART BLOCKS (2nd - 3rd degree) BUNDLE BRANCH BLOCKS	TRANSCUTANEOUS or TRANSVENOUS PACING

[48] "Comparison of Dopamine vs. Norepinephrine in Treatment of Shock," D.DeBacker et. al. NEJM 2010;362:779-789

When ANTERIOR WALL MI is noted on the ECG, the clinician should evaluate for *reciprocal ST Depression* in the INFERIOR LEADS (II, III, and aVF):

- The presence of reciprocal depression in the Inferior Leads indicates the blockage is in the PROXIMAL segment of the LAD; an ominous finding in Anterior Wall STEMI!

- Absence of reciprocal depression (such as in this case study) is consistent with *mid-LAD occlusion*, distal to the take-off of the first Diagonal.[49],[50]

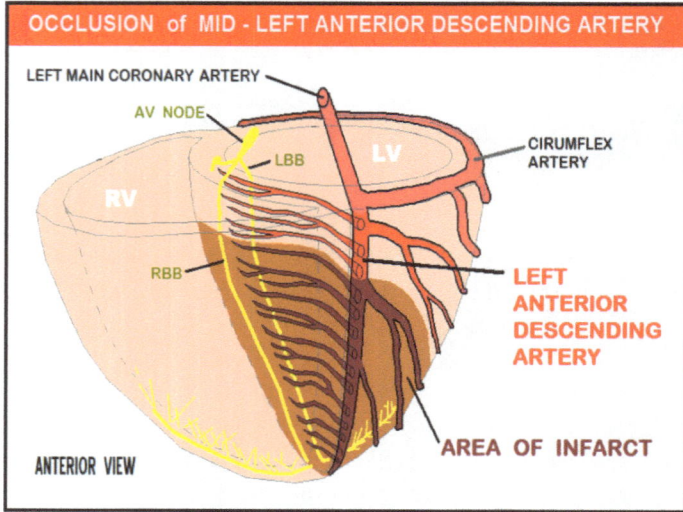

OCCLUSION of MID - LEFT ANTERIOR DESCENDING ARTERY

MID - LAD 100% OCCLUDED

RAO CRANIAL VIEW

The image to the left illustrates the area of infarct caused by an occlusion of the *mid-left anterior descending artery*. The bundle branches (seen in yellow) are potentially compromised. If high-grade heart block is seen with acute *anterior-septal MI*, atropine may not be effective, due to the cause of heart block being damage to the bundle branches; acetylcholine receptor sites are typically not found in the ventricles. Therefore, pacing would be a more effective way to increase ventricular heart rate.

This patient's LV gram, to the right, illustrates significant ANTERIOR WALL AKINESIS, with an Ejection Fraction of 42%.

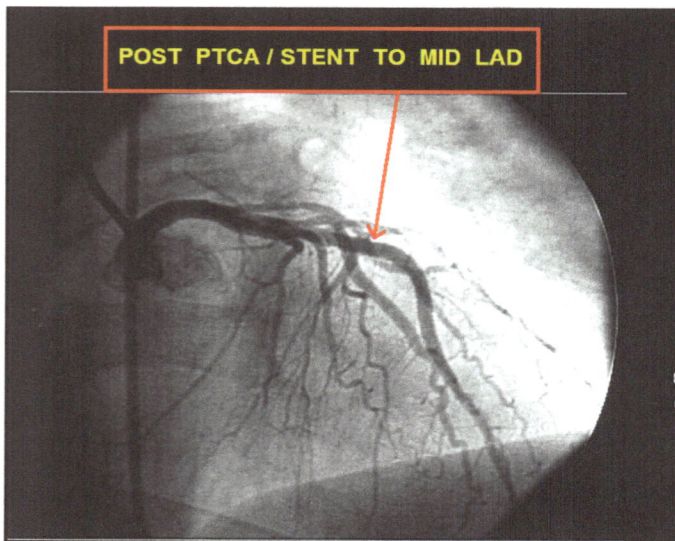

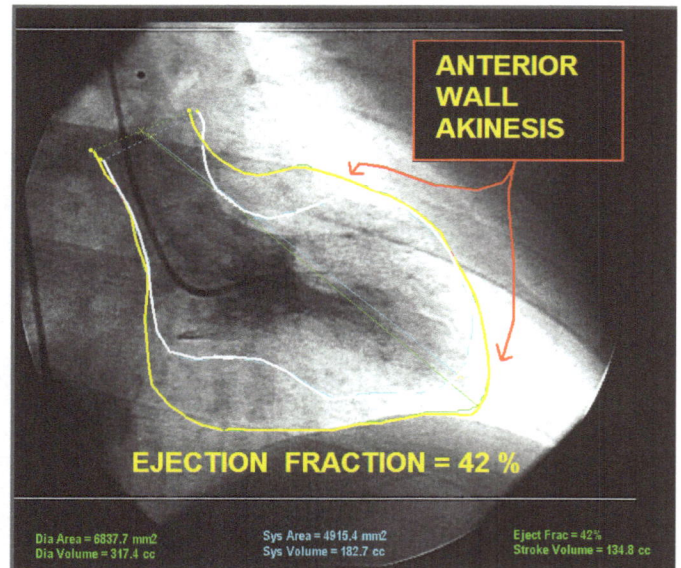

POST PTCA / STENT TO MID LAD

ANTERIOR WALL AKINESIS

EJECTION FRACTION = 42 %

Dia Area = 6837.7 mm2   Sys Area = 4915.4 mm2   Eject Frac = 42%
Dia Volume = 317.4 cc   Sys Volume = 182.7 cc   Stroke Volume = 134.8 cc

The image to the left shows the patient's LAD, post PTCA and placement of a drug-eluting stent.

[49] "Use of the Electrocardiogram in Acute Myocardial Infarction," Zimetbaum, et al, NEJM 348:933-940
[50] "Value of Electrocardiogram in Localizing Occlusion of LAD in Anterior MI," Engelen, et al, J Am Coll Cardiol 1999;34:389-95

CASE PROGRESSION:

During the Emergency Department phase, the patient did not exhibit significant hypotension. His relative hemodynamic stability could be due to his lesion being mid-LAD, as opposed to proximal LAD. His diagnosis of Acute Anterior Wall STEMI was made within ten minutes of his initial evaluation. He was taken to the cardiac catheterization suite without delay, where PTCA and placement of a Drug Eluting Stent (DES) were performed. His recovery was uncomplicated, and he was discharged three days later. As with all patients whom undergo DES placement, PLAVIX 75mg once daily for a minimum of one year was prescribed.

During a follow-up visit one year later, the patient reported he was "doing well," and has not had any significant episodes of angina. During this visit, the ECG shown below was recorded:

73 yr		Vent. rate	59	BPM	Sinus bradycardia	**This EKG recorded ONE YEAR post**
Male	Caucasian	PR interval	144	ms	Anterolateral infarct	**Anterior wall STEMI.**
		QRS duration	88	ms	Abnormal ECG	
Room:CCR		QT/QTc	416/411	ms		
Loc:7	Option:35	P–R–T axes	5 99	25		

Significant Q waves (QS complexes) are noted in the anterior leads, V1-V4, with no progression of R waves, a finding consistent with anterior wall necrosis. It is interesting to note that in this ECG, *significant Q waves (QS complexes) are noted in all four of the lateral leads (I, aVL, V5 and V6)* -- during the patient's acute event, no significant ST elevation was noted in the lateral leads.

☞ **A word about ANTERIOR-SEPTAL WALL MI and HIGH GRADE HEART BLOCKS:**

Although the LAD supplies blood to the *Bundle of His* and the *Proximal Bundle Branches* via the First Septal Performator Artery, high grade heart blocks (2nd and 3rd degree) occur infrequently in Anterior-Septal Wall STEMI. In a study where colored dyes were injected into the coronary arteries of cadaver hearts, it was discovered that the Bundle of His and the proximal Bundle Branches were DUALLY SUPPLIED with blood from the First Septal Performator Artery (originates from the LAD), and the AV Nodal Artery (originates from the RCA in right dominant systems, and the Circumflex in left dominant systems).[51] Having a "dual blood supply" to the Bundle of His and proximal bundle branches was noted in 9 of the 10 hearts used in the study. This explains why High Grade Heart Block is an infrequent complication in cases of Anterior-Septal STEMI. Health Care Professionals must none-the-less remain vigilant – when high grade heart blocks DO occur with Anterior-Septal STEMI, it usually requires immediate pacing.

---

[51] RJ Frink et al, Circulation: January 1973 p 8-18

CHIEF COMPLAINT and SIGNIFICANT HISTORY:

46 y/o Female walks into ED TRIAGE, with chief complaint of EPIGASTRIC PAIN, NAUSEA and WEAKNESS. Symptoms have been intermittent for last two days. She was awakened early this morning with the above symptoms, which are now PERSISTENT.

RISK FACTOR PROFILE:

⬥※ **FAMILY HISTORY** - father died of CAD, older brother had CABG, age 39
⬥※ **DIABETES** - diet controlled
⬥※ **HYPERTENSION**

PHYSICAL EXAM: Pt. CAOx4, anxious, SKIN cold, clammy, diaphoretic.   No JVD.
Lungs: clear, bilaterally.   Heart Sounds: Normal S1, S2.

VITAL SIGNS: BP: 168/98, P: 110, R: 24,   SAO2: 97% on O2 4 LPM via nasal canula

LABS: TROPONIN ultra = 2.8

QUADRAD OF ACS CHECKLIST

☑ **SYMPTOMS of ACS**

- ◆ TYPICAL ACS - eg:
- ✔ ◆ ATYPICAL ACS - eq:

☑ **ECG ABNORMALITIES**

- ✔ ◆ ST ELEVATION (J POINT plus 40 ms)
- ◆ HYPERACUTE T WAVES · and/or ·
- ◆ NEW or PRESUMABLY NEW LBBB
- ◆ ST DEPRESSION (>0.5 mm @ J POINT) and/or
- ◆ INVERTED or BIPHASIC T WAVES and/or
- ◆ DYNAMIC ST SEGMENT and/or T WAVE CHANGES IN SERIAL EKGs

☑ **RISK FACTORS - 3 or more**

- ✔ ◆ FAMILY HISTORY
- ✔ ◆ DIABETES
- ◆ ↑LDL and/or ↓HDL
- ◆ SMOKING
- ◆ AGE: 65 or MORE
- ✔ ◆ HYPERTENSION

☑ **CARDIAC MARKERS**

- ◆ ELEVATED TROPONIN and/or CK/MB

4 TOTAL

ACS RISK ASSESSMENT: *Determinng the probability that your patient suffers from Acute Coronary Syndrome.*

During the initial evaluation of patients presenting with ACS-like symptoms, clinicians must consider the findings in four major categories – which we referred to as "The Quadrad of ACS" (see page 98):

- **PRESENTING SYMPTOMS**,
- **ECG ABNORMALITIES**,
- **CARDIAC MARKERS**,
- **RISK FACTOR PROFILE**.

Careful analysis of this information will maximize your accuracy in diagnosing or ruling out ACS. Therefore, we advocate the use of ACS Risk assessment tools in order to assure consistency during your patient evaluation process. As such, we provide the a "QUADRAD OF ACS CHECKLIST" for case studies presented in this chapter.

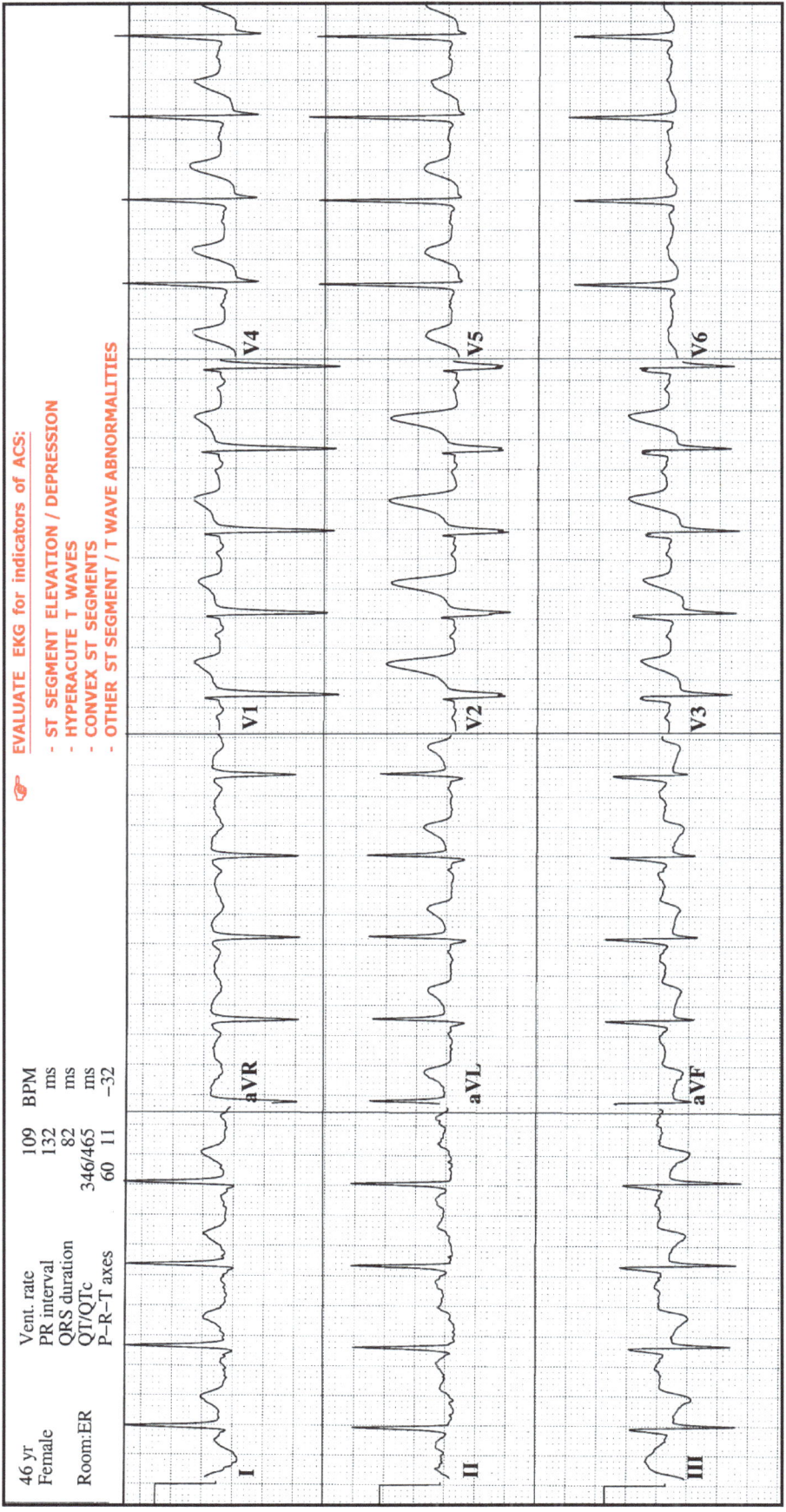

46 yr
Female

Room:ER

Vent. rate	109	BPM
PR interval	132	ms
QRS duration	82	ms
QT/QTc	346/465	ms
P–R–T axes	60 11	–32

☞ EVALUATE EKG for indicators of ACS:

- ST SEGMENT ELEVATION / DEPRESSION
- HYPERACUTE T WAVES
- CONVEX ST SEGMENTS
- OTHER ST SEGMENT / T WAVE ABNORMALITIES

I   aVR   V1   V4

II   aVL   V2   V5

III   aVF   V3   V6

CASE STUDY QUESTIONS:

NOTE LEADS WITH ST ELEVATION:

NOTE LEADS WITH ST DEPRESSION:

WHAT IS THE SUSPECTED DIAGNOSIS ?

WHAT IS THE "CULPRIT ARTERY" – if applicable ?

LIST ANY CRITICAL STRUCTURES COMPROMISED:

LIST ANY POTENTIAL COMPLICATIONS:

173

46 yr	Vent. rate	109	BPM	
Female	PR interval	132	ms	
	QRS duration	82	ms	
Room:ER	QT/QTc	346/465	ms	
	P–R–T axes	60 11 –32		

Sinus tachycardia
Left ventricular hypertrophy with repolarization abnormality
ST elevation consider lateral injury or acute infarct
*** ** ** ** * ACUTE MI ** ** ** **

ST SEGMENT ELEVATION

ST SEGMENT DEPRESSION

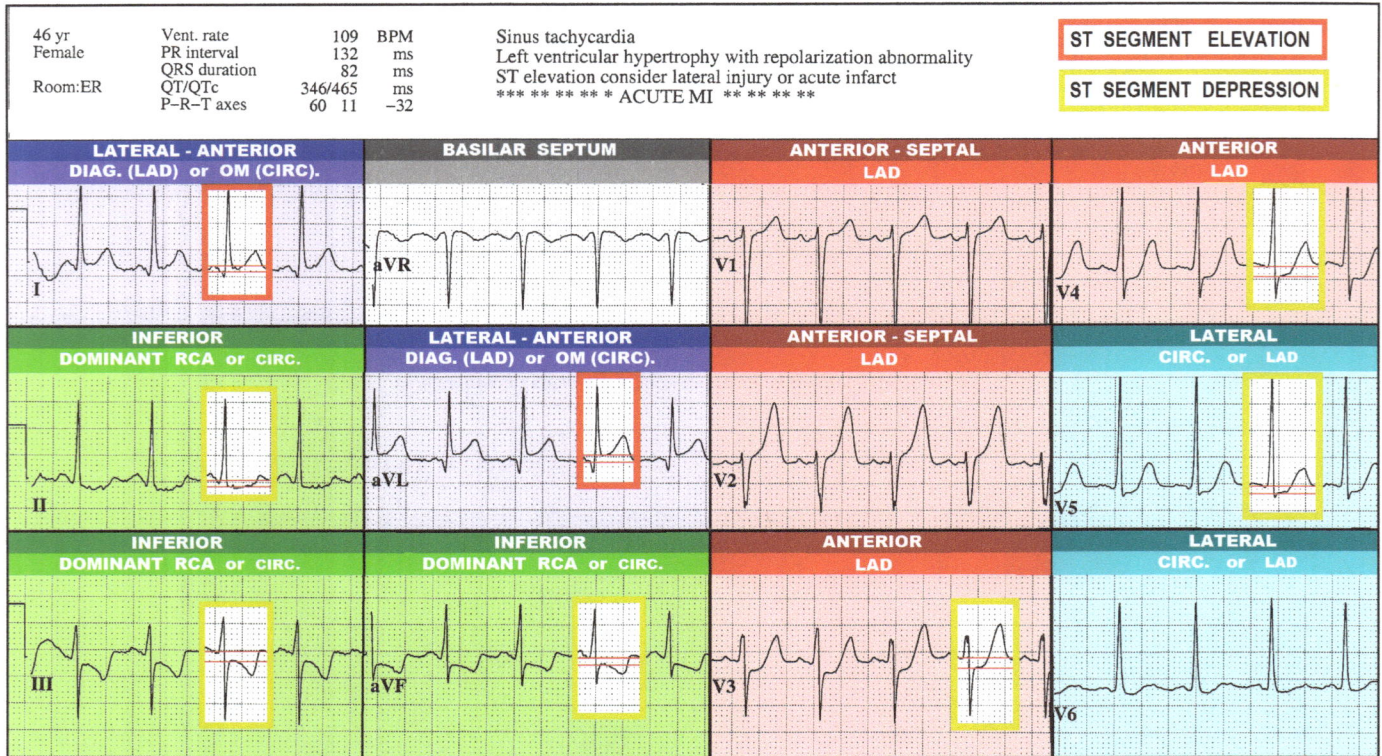

LATERAL - ANTERIOR DIAG. (LAD) or OM (CIRC).	BASILAR SEPTUM	ANTERIOR - SEPTAL LAD	ANTERIOR LAD
I	aVR	V1	V4
INFERIOR DOMINANT RCA or CIRC.	LATERAL - ANTERIOR DIAG. (LAD) or OM (CIRC).	ANTERIOR - SEPTAL LAD	LATERAL CIRC. or LAD
II	aVL	V2	V5
INFERIOR DOMINANT RCA or CIRC.	INFERIOR DOMINANT RCA or CIRC.	ANTERIOR LAD	LATERAL CIRC. or LAD
III	aVF	V3	V6

LEADS I and aVL view the ANTERIOR-LATERAL JUNCTION

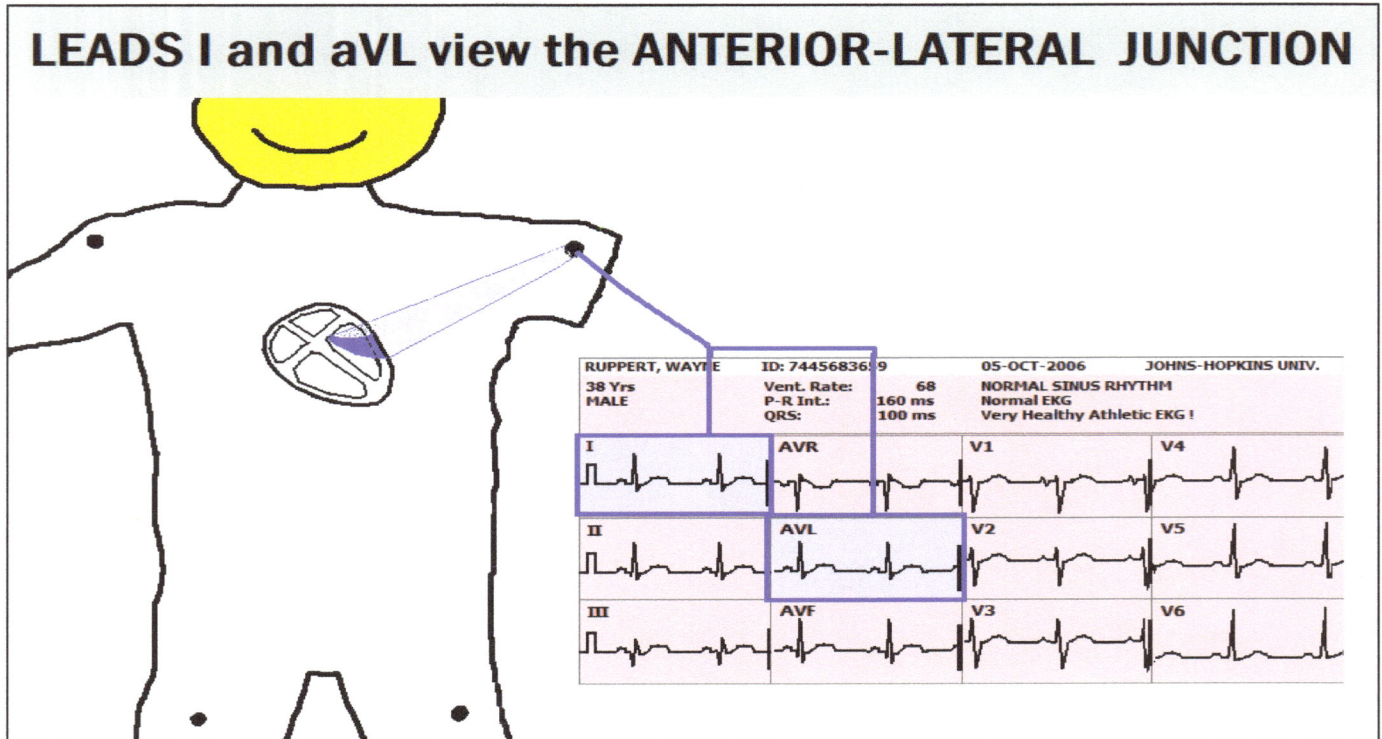

Leads I and aVL view a slice of the left ventricle which extends from the anterior to lateral surface, and is superiorly oriented, as shown in the image to the left.   I refer to this zone as the *"anterior-lateral junction,"* and think of it as a kind of "buffer zone" between the anterior and lateral surfaces of the left ventricle.   With respect to the ECG, ST changes can be seen in leads I and aVL during *anterior wall MI* resulting from an occlusion in the *proximal* aspect of the *left anterior descending artery*, and during *lateral wall MI* resulting from occlusion in the *proximal* aspect of the *circumflex artery*.   When the circumflex artery is dominant and supplies the inferior wall, an occlusion in its proximal aspect often results in inferior-posterior-lateral MI.

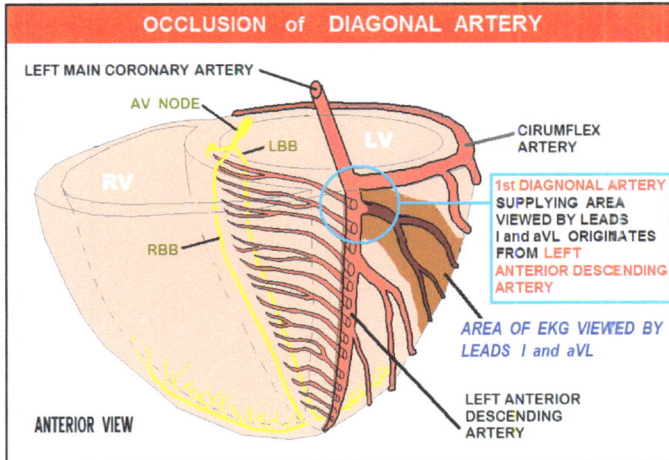

OCCLUSION of DIAGONAL ARTERY

In cases of ANTERIOR MI, when ST elevation is noted in Leads V1 – V4 + *Leads I and aVL*, it is suggestive of an obstructive in the PROXIMAL LAD (proximal to the takeoff of the FIRST DIAGONAL branch).[52] Diagonal arteries originate off of the proximal Left Anterior Descending, as seen in the diagram to the left. The patient in our case study has this anotomical configuration. Our patient's blockage involves ONLY the First Diagonal Artery, which is why ST elevation is seen ONLY in leads 1 and aVL. If the blockage had been in the proximal LAD, before the take-off of the 1st Diagonal Branch, ST elevation would have been seen in the Anterior Leads (V1 – V4), in addition to Leads I and aVL.

In cases of LATERAL MI, when ST elevation is noted in Leads V5 and V6 + *Leads I and aVL*, it is suggestive of an obstruction in the CIRCUMFLEX (proximal to the takeoff of the FIRST OBTUSE MARGINAL branch). [53] In patients with a non-dominant circumflex artery, an obstruction proximal to the first obtuse marginal branch (OM1) would result in ST elevation primarily in leads I, aVL, V5 and V6. In patients with a dominant circumflex artery, a lesion proximal to OM1 would result in ST elevation in leads I, aVL, V5, V6, II, III, and aVF.[54]

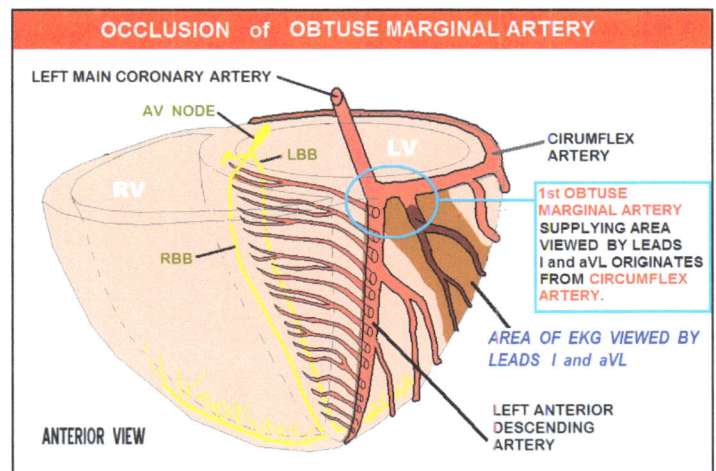

OCCLUSION of OBTUSE MARGINAL ARTERY

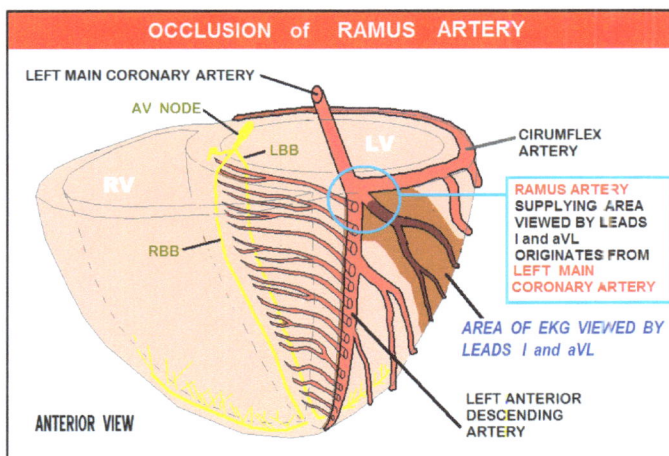

OCCLUSION of RAMUS ARTERY

In patients whom have a Ramus artery, it originates directly from the LEFT MAIN CORONARY ARTERY between the LAD and the Circumlex Arteries. It supplies the region of the heart viewed by leads I and aVL, as seen to the left.

---

[52] Birnbaum, et al, *Postgrad Med J* 2003;79:490–504
[53] Birnbaum, et al, *Postgrad Med J* 2003;79:490–504
[54] "Use of the Electrocardiogram in Acute Myocardial Infarction," Zimetbaum, et al, NEJM 348:933-940

CASE PROGRESSION: As the patient was being prepared for transport to the Cardiac Cath Lab, she experienced an episode of Ventricular Fibrillation. This was witnessed, and was treated with immediate defibrillation at 200 joules, which effectively restored sinus rhythm. A loading dose of 150mg. of Amiodarone was infused over ten minutes, followed by a maintenance infusion of 1mg/minute. She was transported to the Cath Lab without further episodes of electrical instability. The culprit artery, shown below, was the First Diagonal branch off of the LAD. As both the angiography of her coronary arteries and her Left Ventricular angiogram demonstrate, damage to her overall LV function was minimal. The fact that this patient's zone of infarction did not involve any critical structures of the heart's electrical conduction system, and did not involve a substantial amount of LV muscle mass emphases the reality that all patients experiencing AMI can experience sudden cardiac arrest, and that clinicians must remain vigilant and ready to provide immediate resuscitation at all times.

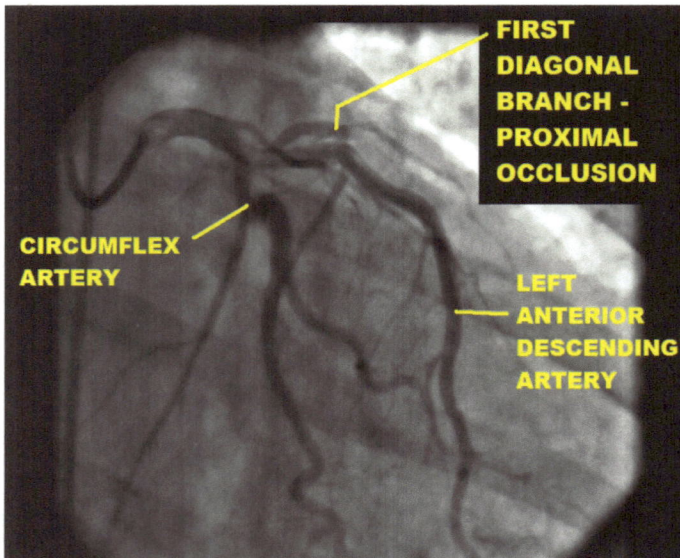

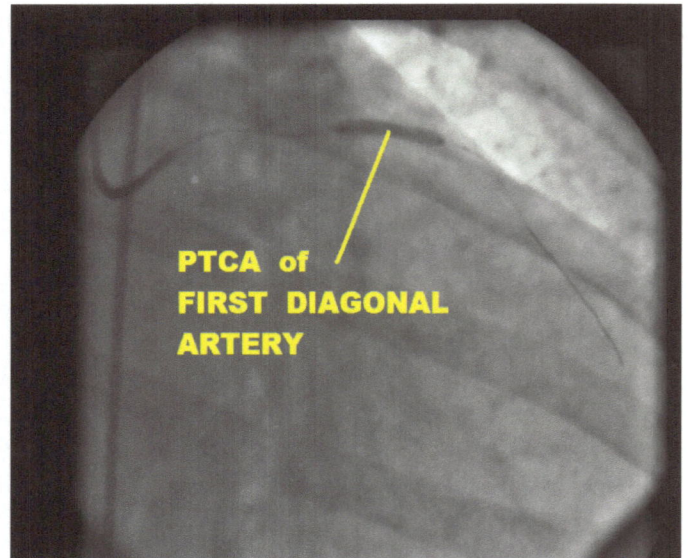

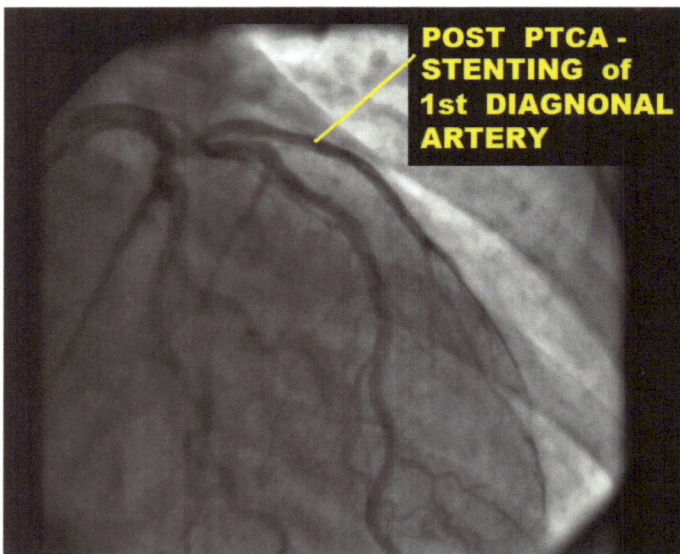

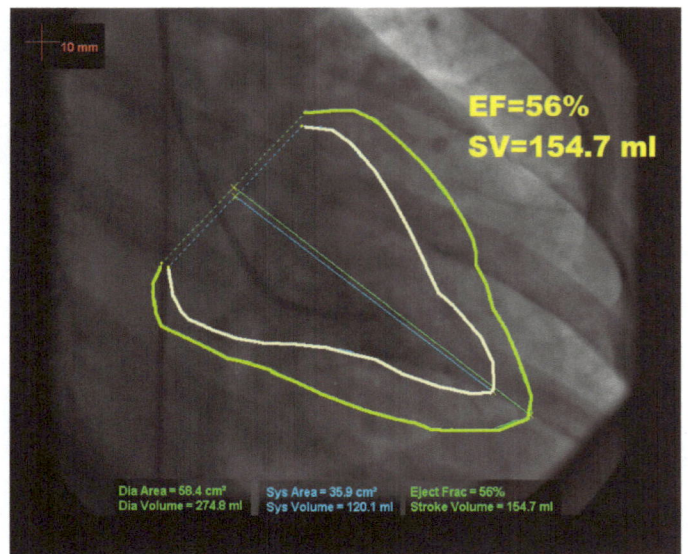

Based on the patient's Left Ventricular Angiogram (bottom right image), damage to the LV pump function has been minimal – her EF is calculated at 56%, which is just inside our normal range of 55-70%.

ST ELEVATION: I, aVL	ST DEPRESSION: II, III, aVF, V3 - V5

SUSPECTED DIAGNOSIS: ACUTE LATERAL WALL M.I.

SUSPECTED "CULPRIT ARTERY" (if applicable):

USUALLY ONE OF THE SMALLER SIDE-BRANCH ARTERIES:

1. DIAGONAL ARTERY. (This is a side-branch artery off of the LEFT ANTERIOR DESCENDING (LAD) artery.
2. OBTUSE MARGINAL ARTERY. (This is a side-branch artery off of the CIRCUMFLEX artery)
3. RAMUS ARTERY.

IMMEDIATE CONCERNS FOR ALL STEMI PATIENTS:

- BE PREPARED TO MANAGE SUDDEN CARDIAC ARREST (PRIMARY V - FIB / V- TACH, BRADYCARDIAS / HEART BLOCKS)
- STAT REPERFUSION THERAPY: THROMBOLYTICS vs. CARDIAC CATHETERIZATION and PCI
- CONSIDER NEEDS FOR ANTI-PLATELET and ANTI-COAGULATION THERAPY

CRITICAL STRUCTURES COMPROMISED:	POTENTIAL COMPLICATIONS:	POSSIBLE CRITICAL INTERVENTIONS:
15-30% of the LV MUSCLE MASS	POSSIBLE MODERATE LV PUMP FAILURE	INOTROPIC AGENTS ET INTUBATION I.A.B.P. INSERTION

CASE DISCUSSION: There are several essential teaching points that should be learned from this Case Study:

- This patient exhibited ATYPICAL SYMPTOMS in her initial presentation to the ED. At no time during her coronary event did she experience any form of chest pain or chest discomfort. She fits into the known category of female patients whom do not expereince typical symptoms during acute coronary events. Please refer to page 102 for a complete description of this phenonemon.

- ST Elevation was seen exclusively in leads I and aVL. Her AMI was caused by an occlusion in the first diagonal artery, which branches off of the LAD. It is a somewhat misleading belief that this area "belongs exclusively to the Lateral Wall,' and therefore is always fed by the Circumflex Artery. This region is commonly supplied by side-branch arteries originating off the LAD (Diagonal arteries) or the Circumflex (Obtuse Marginal arteries). In less-common scenarios, this region is supplied by a Ramus artery.

- When ST elevation is seen in ANTERIOR leads (V1-V4) along with leads I and aVL, it indicates the obstruction is most likely in the proximal segment of the LAD, with the zone of infarct including the First Diagonal artery, which causes ST elevation in I and aVL (SEE CASE STUDY 3, coming up next, which begins on page 178).

- When ST elevation is seen mainly in LATERAL leads (V5, V6), along with leads I and aVL, it is a good indicator that the occlusion is located in the proximal Circumflex artery, with the zone of infarct including the First Obtuse Marginal Artery. This type may or may not include ST elevation in the INFERIOR leads; this is determined by the patient's degree of RCA or Circumflex dominance.

- The patient in this case study suffered from SPONTANEOUS VENTRICULAR FIBRILLATION, making it clear that ANY form of myocardial infarction can cause a lethal cardiac dysrhthmia, regardless of the location and size of infarct. Everyone anticipates patients whom suffer from massive MI may develop cardiac arrest, as well as those with damage to critical structures, such as the SA and AV Nodes. THIS PATIENT'S area of infarct was relatively small, and did not include any critical structures – *yet she went into V-Fib*. *We must always remain vigilant for such episodes, regardless of the type and extent of MI.*

CASE STUDY 3: STEMI

CHIEF COMPLAINT and SIGNIFICANT HISTORY:

29 y/o male presents to the ER c/o "HEAVY CHEST PRESSURE" x 30 minutes. The patient states he was playing football with friends after eating a large meal. Pt. also c/o nausea. Denies DIB.

RISK FACTOR PROFILE:

- 💣☀ **FAMILY HISTORY** - father died of MI age 46
- 💣☀ **CURRENT CIGARETTE SMOKER**
- 💣☀ **"MILD" HYPERTENSION** - untreated
- ☑ **CHOLESTEROL** - unknown - "never had it checked."

PHYSICAL EXAM:
Patient alert, oriented X 4, skin cool, dry, pale. Patient restless. No JVD, Lungs clear bilaterally. Heart sounds normal S1, S2. No peripheral edema.

VITAL SIGNS:
BP: 104/78, P: 76, R: 20, SAO2: 96%

LABS:
INITIAL CARDIAC MARKERS - NEGATIVE

QUADRAD OF ACS CHECKLIST

☑ **SYMPTOMS of ACS**
- ✔ ◆ TYPICAL ACS - eg:
- ◆ ATYPICAL ACS - eg:

☑ **ECG ABNORMALITIES**
- ✔ ◆ ST ELEVATION (J POINT plus 40 ms)
- ◆ HYPERACUTE T WAVES - and/or -
- ◆ NEW or PRESUMABLY NEW LBBB
- ◆ ST DEPRESSION (>0.5 mm @ J POINT) and/or
- ◆ INVERTED or BIPHASIC T WAVES and/or
- ◆ DYNAMIC ST SEGMENT and/or T WAVE CHANGES IN SERIAL EKGs

☑ **RISK FACTORS - 3 or more**
- ✔ ◆ FAMILY HISTORY
- ✔ ◆ DIABETES
- ◆ ↑ LDL and/or ↓ HDL
- ✔ ◆ SMOKING
- ◆ AGE: 65 or MORE
- ◆ HYPERTENSION

☐ **CARDIAC MARKERS**
- ◆ ELEVATED TROPONIN and/or CK/MB

3 **TOTAL**

SUSPECTED ACUTE MI:

INITIAL MANAGEMENT

- **VITAL SIGNS**

- **"O.M.I."**
  - Oxygen
  - Monitor (ecg)
  - IV (plus draw lab samples)

- **12 LEAD ECG**
  Obtain and interpret within 10 minutes of patient's arrival.

- **"M.O.N.A."**
  - Morphine
  - Oxygen (if not already done)
  - Nitroglycerin
  - Aspirin

- **RAPID, FOCUSED ASSESSMENT**

- **HEART / LUNG SOUNDS**

- **SEND LAB SAMPLES:**
  - Cardiac Markers
  - Electrolytes
  - Coagulation Studies

29 yr
Male   Caucasian

Loc:3   Option:20

DOS::

Vent. rate	75	BPM
PR interval	176	ms
QRS duration	90	ms
QT/QTc	362/404	ms
P–R–T axes	70 50	–11

14:07 Hours

☞ **EVALUATE** the EKG for signs of ACS:
- ST SEGMENT ELEVATION / DEPRESSION
- HYPERACUTE T WAVES
- CONVEX / FLAT ST SEGMENTS
- OTHER ST - T WAVE ABNORMALITIES

I aVR V1 V4

II aVL V2 V5

III aVF V3 V6

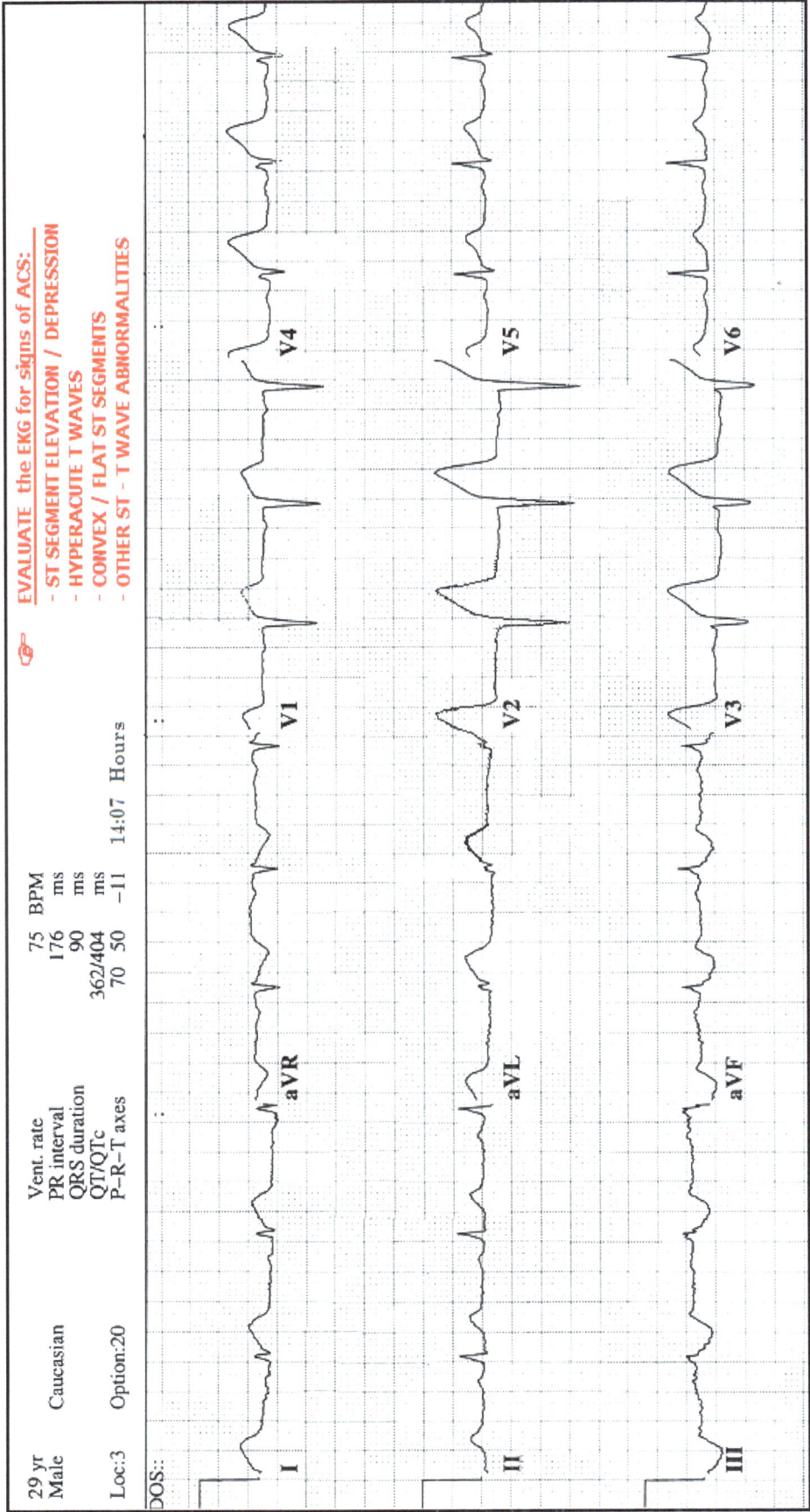

CASE STUDY QUESTIONS:

NOTE LEADS WITH ST ELEVATION:

NOTE LEADS WITH ST DEPRESSION:

WHAT IS THE SUSPECTED DIAGNOSIS ?

WHAT IS THE "CULPRIT ARTERY" -- if applicable ?

LIST ANY CRITICAL STRUCTURES COMPROMISED:

LIST ANY POTENTIAL COMPLICATIONS:

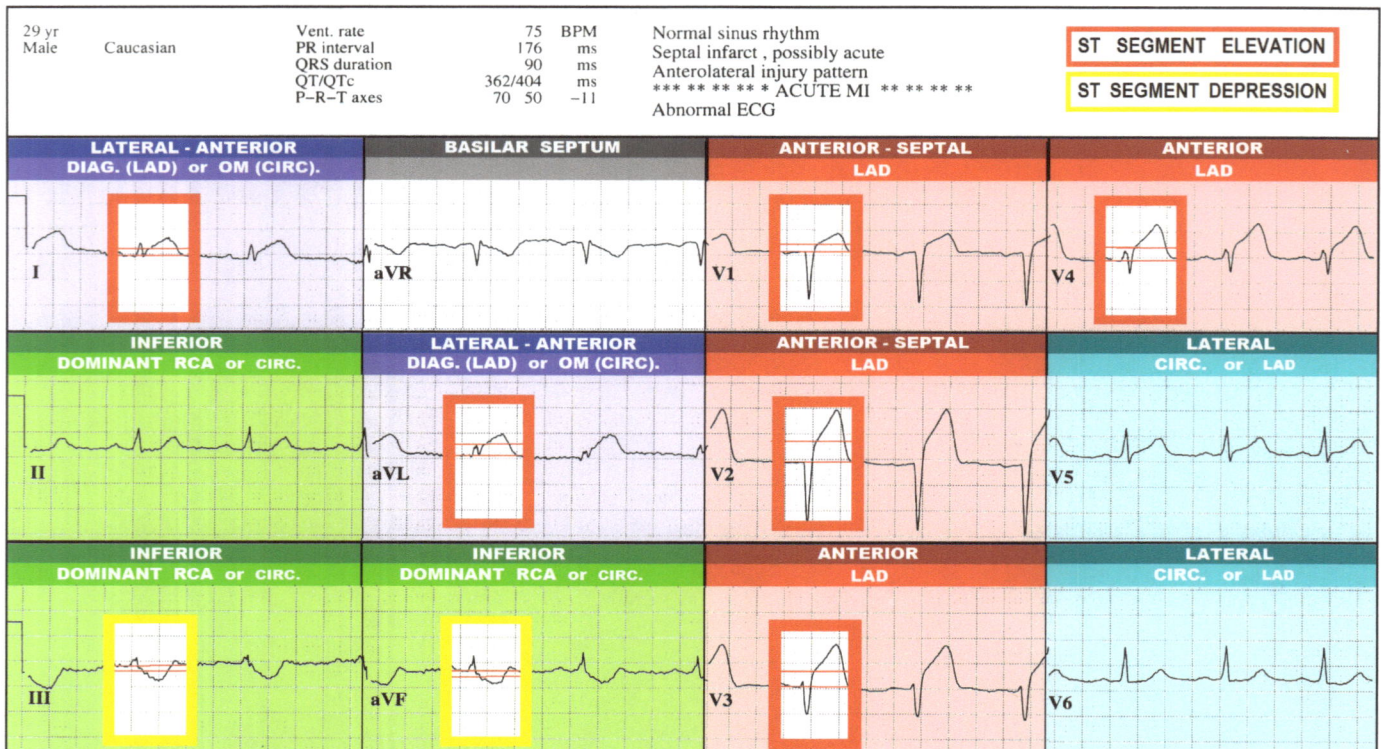

29 yr Male	Caucasian	Vent. rate	75	BPM	Normal sinus rhythm	ST SEGMENT ELEVATION

ECG report header:

29 yr Male	Caucasian		

Vent. rate 75 BPM
PR interval 176 ms
QRS duration 90 ms
QT/QTc 362/404 ms
P–R–T axes 70 50 –11

Normal sinus rhythm
Septal infarct , possibly acute
Anterolateral injury pattern
*** ** ** ** * ACUTE MI ** ** ** **
Abnormal ECG

ST SEGMENT ELEVATION

ST SEGMENT DEPRESSION

ECG 12-lead grid:

LATERAL - ANTERIOR DIAG. (LAD) or OM (CIRC).	BASILAR SEPTUM	ANTERIOR - SEPTAL LAD	ANTERIOR LAD
I	aVR	V1	V4
INFERIOR DOMINANT RCA or CIRC.	LATERAL - ANTERIOR DIAG. (LAD) or OM (CIRC).	ANTERIOR - SEPTAL LAD	LATERAL CIRC. or LAD
II	aVL	V2	V5
INFERIOR DOMINANT RCA or CIRC.	INFERIOR DOMINANT RCA or CIRC.	ANTERIOR LAD	LATERAL CIRC. or LAD
III	aVF	V3	V6

☞ THERE ARE TWO IMPORTANT CLUES that the patient's BLOCKAGE is in the ***PROXIMAL*** LEFT ANTERIOR DESCENDING ARTERY:

1. When ST elevation is noted in leads I and aVL in cases of ANTERIOR WALL STEMI, it is a good indicator that the FIRST DIAGONAL BRANCH is included in the zone of infarction.
2. RECIPROCAL ST DEPRESSION in the INFERIOR LEADS (II, III, and/or aVF) is an indication that the LAD is blocked proximal to the FIRST DIAGONAL BRANCH.[55]

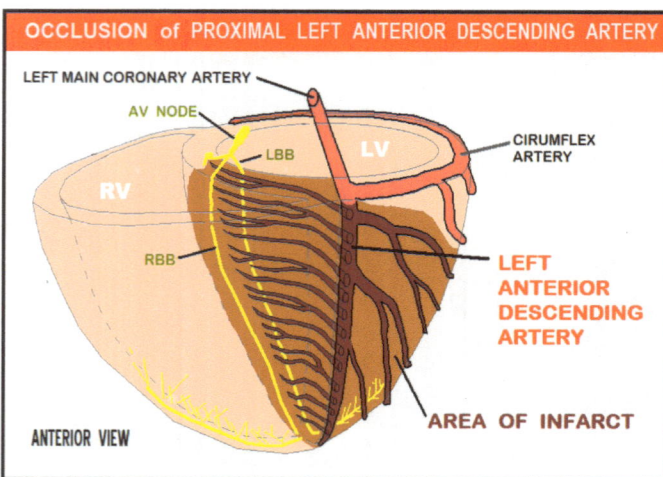

OCCLUSION of PROXIMAL LEFT ANTERIOR DESCENDING ARTERY

LEFT MAIN CORONARY ARTERY
AV NODE
LBB
LV
CIRUMFLEX ARTERY
RV
RBB
LEFT ANTERIOR DESCENDING ARTERY
AREA OF INFARCT
ANTERIOR VIEW

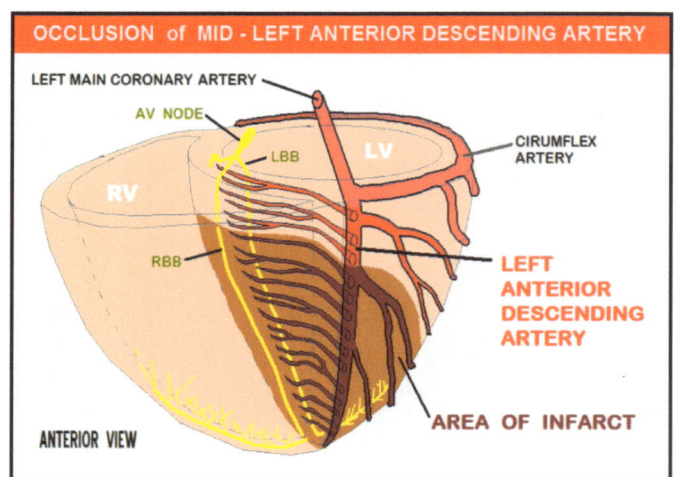

OCCLUSION of MID - LEFT ANTERIOR DESCENDING ARTERY

LEFT MAIN CORONARY ARTERY
AV NODE
LBB
LV
CIRUMFLEX ARTERY
RV
RBB
LEFT ANTERIOR DESCENDING ARTERY
AREA OF INFARCT
ANTERIOR VIEW

The distinction between ***mid-LAD*** and ***proximal LAD*** lesions is important to note because proximal LAD lesions tend to **have higher incidence of:**

- **LV pump failure.** In mid-LAD lesions, LV function of the superior aspect of the anterior wall often remains intact, as seen in Case Study 1. Proximal LAD lesions usually result in dysfunction of the entire anterior-septal wall. The two images seen above illustrate this difference.

---

[55] "Use of the Electrocardiogram in Acute Myocardial Infarction," Zimetbaum, et al, NEJM 348:933-940

When this happens, *rapid hemodynamic decompensation, dysrhythmia, cardiac arrest* and *death* often result. Case Study 4 on page 183 provides an example of this.

CASE PROGRESSION:

Within ten minutes of his arrival in the Emergency Department, the patient was diagnosed as having an Acute Anterior-Septal-Lateral Wall STEMI. The Cardiac Cath Lab Team was paged. The patient was placed on O2 at 4 liters per minute via nasal canula, and an IV of NS was initiated at a KVO rate. One 325 mg. aspirin po, was administered. At 14:48 hours (29 minutes after the first ECG was obtained), the patient complained of increased chest pressure, shortness of breath, and nausea. He became notably more restless, with skin cooler, more ashen and diaphoretic than before. A second ECG was obtained, shown below:

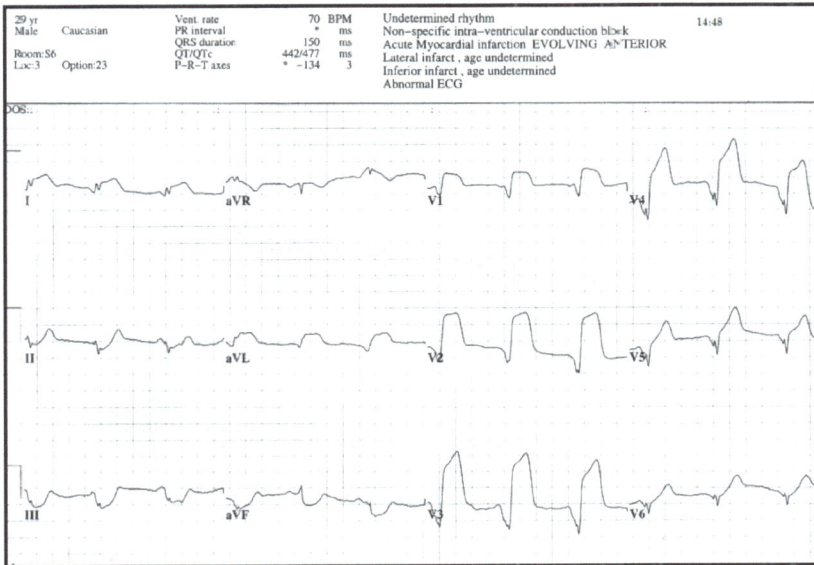

Repeat vital signs indicated his blood pressure dropped to 66/40, pulse rate 70, respirations 24, and SAO2 88% . Lung sounds revealed fine crackles bilaterally in the lower and mid-fields. His oxygen was increased to 15 LPM via non-rebreather. A Dopamine drip at 10mcg/kg/minute was initiated. At this point, the Cardiac Cath Team arrived and began transporting the patient to the Cath Lab. While being wheeled to the Cath Lab, his blood pressure continued to drop. His Dopamine drip was titrated upward until 20mcg/kg/minute was reached. The patient reported his breathing was becoming more difficult, and stated to the cath lab team, "I am going to die." A STAT page was placed to Anesthesia for possible intubation as the interventional cardiologist accessed the patient's right femoral artery. The following image was obtained after the left main coronary artery was canulated:

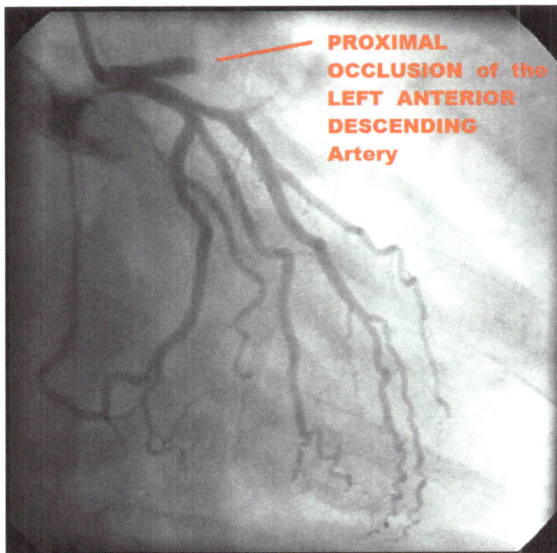

PROXIMAL OCCLUSION of the LEFT ANTERIOR DESCENDING Artery

A .014 guidewire was placed across the lesion, which was then opened with a monorail PTCA balloon. After stent placement, TIMI III blood flow was restored. The image below was taken immediately after stent deployment in the proximal LAD:

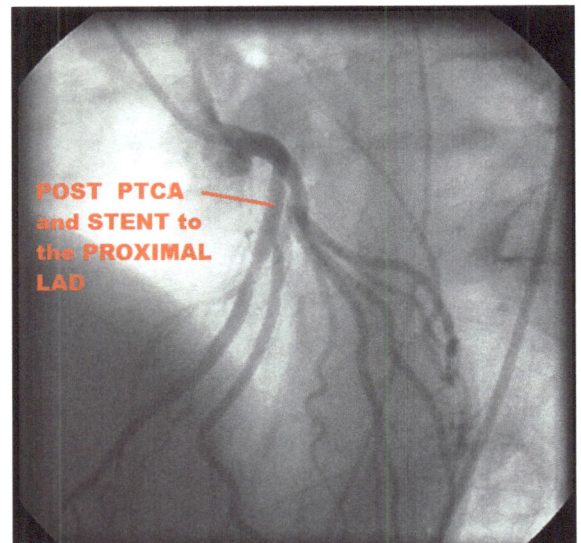

POST PTCA and STENT to the PROXIMAL LAD

Within approximately twenty minutes post stent placement, the patient reported his pain as a "3" on a 1-10 scale, and his breathing markedly improved.

By the time the patient left the Cath Lab, his Dopamine drip had been discontinued, and his blood pressure was stable at 110/66.   The ECG below was recorded in the Coronary Care Unit just after the patient arrived from the Cath Lab.

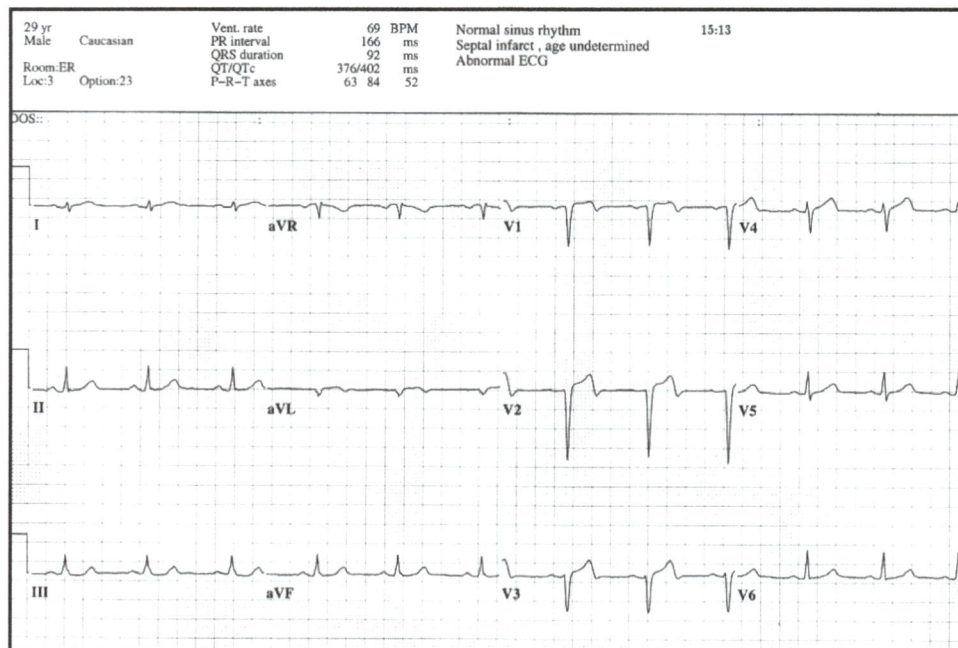

29 yr   Caucasian   Vent. rate   69   BPM   Normal sinus rhythm   15:13
Male   PR interval   166   ms   Septal infarct , age undetermined
                            QRS duration   92   ms   Abnormal ECG
Room:ER   QT/QTc   376/402   ms
Loc:3   Option:23   P–R–T axes   63 84   52

DOS::

I   aVR   V1   V4

II   aVL   V2   V5

III   aVF   V3   V6

QS complexes are noted in leads V1 – V3, consistent with anterior wall necrosis.   R wave progression is slightly delayed, with transition between V4 and V5.   Lead aVL is the only lateral lead displaying the significant Q waves (QS complexes).

The patient's recovery was uncomplicated.   He was discharged three days later.

In the several years since his AMI, this patient remains under the care of his cardiologist.   His medications include: Lipitor, a beta blocker, antiplatelet therapy and ASA 81 mg. per day.   He has been symptom-free since.

His decision to go straight to the hospital when his symptoms began no doubt saved his life – and helped to preserve his LV function. A recent echocardiogram showed his EF as 55%, with near-normal anterior wall function.

CASE STUDY SUMMARY

ST ELEVATION: V1 - V5, I, aVL	ST DEPRESSION: III, aVF

SUSPECTED DIAGNOSIS: ACUTE ANTERIOR - SEPTAL STEMI

SUSPECTED "CULPRIT ARTERY" (if applicable): PROXIMAL LEFT ANTERIOR DESCENDING ARTERY (LAD)

IMMEDIATE CONCERNS FOR ALL STEMI PATIENTS:

- BE PREPARED TO MANAGE SUDDEN CARDIAC ARREST (PRIMARY V - FIB / V- TACH, BRADYCARDIAS / HEART BLOCKS)
- STAT REPERFUSION THERAPY: THROMBOLYTICS vs. CARDIAC CATHETERIZATION and PCI
- CONSIDER NEEDS FOR ANTI-PLATELET and ANTI-COAGULATION THERAPY

CRITICAL STRUCTURES COMPROMISED:	POTENTIAL COMPLICATIONS:	POSSIBLE CRITICAL INTERVENTIONS:
40-50% of the LV MUSCLE MASS	LV PUMP FAILURE leading to: - CARDIOGENIC SHOCK - PULMONARY EDEMA	INOTROPIC AGENTS ET INTUBATION I.A.B.P. INSERTION
	VENTRICULAR DYSRHYTHMIAS (VT / VF)	DEFIBRILLATION / ANTIARRHYTHMIC AGENTS
Potential compromise of BLOOD SUPPLY to: - Bundle of His - Proximal Bundle Branches	HIGH-GRADE HEART BLOCKS (2nd - 3rd degree) BUNDLE BRANCH BLOCKS	TRANSCUTANEOUS or TRANSVENOUS PACING

CASE STUDY 4: CRITICAL DECISIONS SCENARIO

As per current AHA recommendations, your hospital's policy is to send every STEMI patient to the Cardiac Catheterization Lab for emergency PCI.

You are the ranking medical officer on duty in the ED when two acute STEMI patients arrive, ten minutes apart.   The Cath Lab has one lab open, and can take ONE patient immediately.
Both patients duration of symptoms and state of hemodynamic stability are similar.

QUESTION 1: WHICH PATIENT WOULD YOU SEND TO SEND TO THE CATH LAB, STAT?

PATIENT A:
44 y/o MALE, CHEST PAIN x 1 HOUR,
BP: 78/46,   P: 70,   R: 28.   CARDIAC MARKERS: NEGATIVE

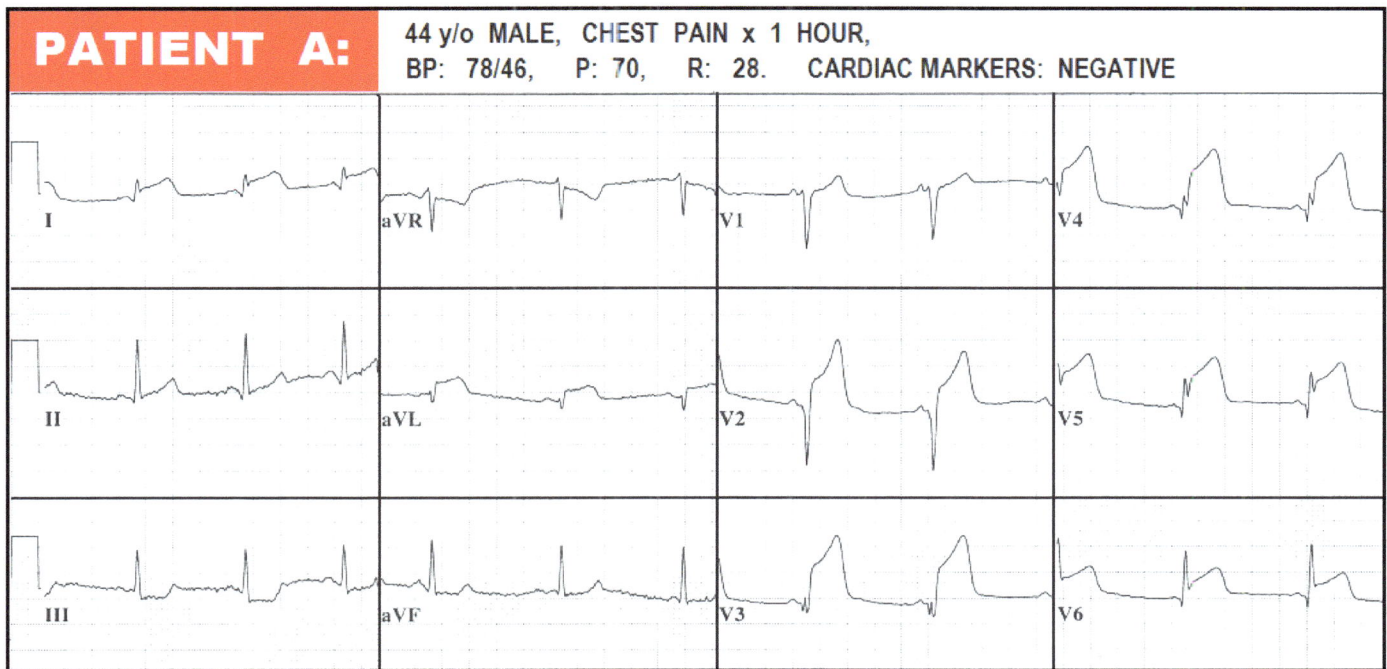

--------------------OR--------------------

PATIENT B:
36 y/o MALE, CHEST PAIN x 1 HOUR,
BP: 80/48,   P: 120,   R: 28   CARDIAC MARKERS: NEGATIVE

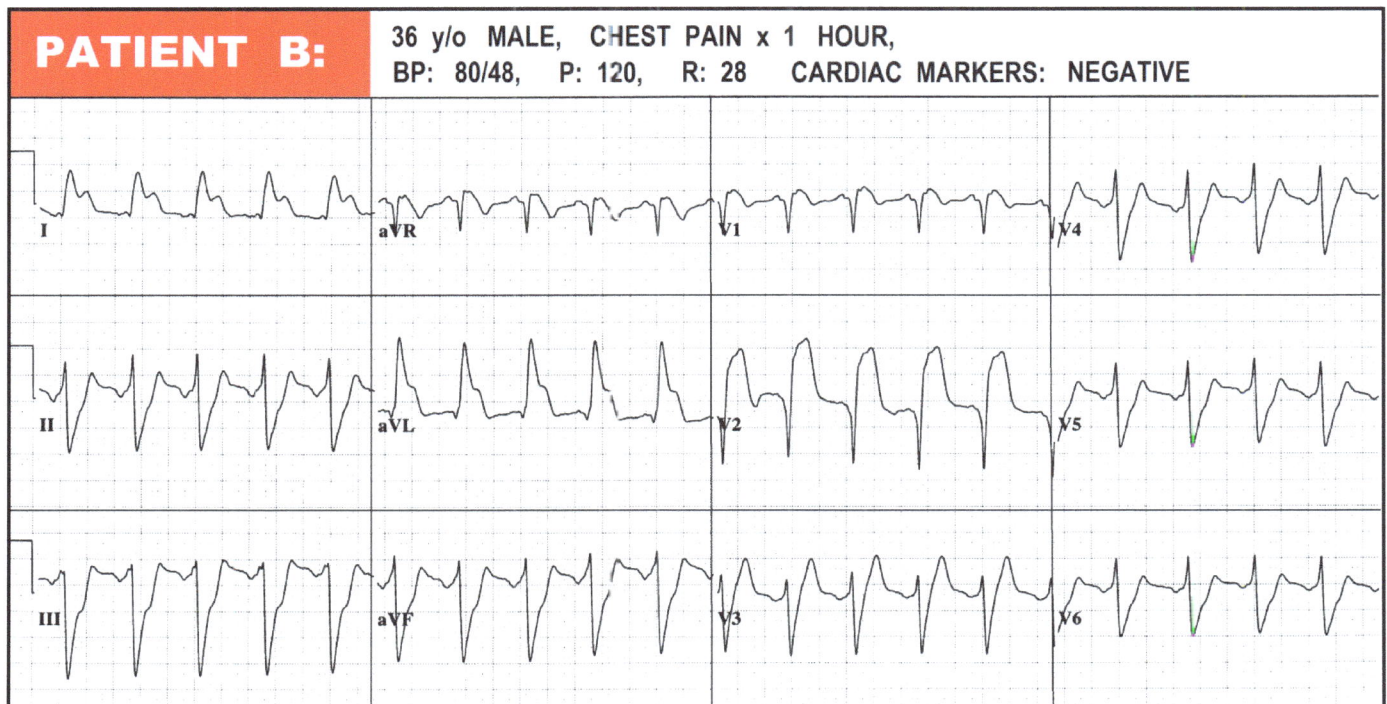

The Cath Lab Coordinator advises you they won't be able to accommodate the second patient until they've finished with the first. She informs you this will take at least *one hour, probably longer*.

QUESTION 2:   WHAT WILL YOU DO WITH THE PATIENT WHO DOES NOT GO TO THE CATH LAB FIRST?

A.   **Wait for the Cath Lab to finish the first patient, then send the second patient, while managing the patient's hemodynamic stability in the ED**
B.   **Administer thrombolytic therapy STAT in the ED, if the patient has no absolute contraindications**
C.   **Transfer the patient to another facility that is PCI capable.**

ANSWER to QUESTION I: *PATIENT B should be sent to the Cath Lab FIRST.*

Rationale: Based on the 12 Lead ECGs, both patients are suffering from *acute Anterior-Lateral Wall STEMI*. However the markers for *identifying the culprit artery*, present on each ECG, indicate:

- **PATIENT A has a proximal occlusion of the LEFT ANTERIOR DESCENDING ARTERY (LAD). The LAD supplies approximately 40-50% of the Left Ventricular Muscle Mass.**

- **PATIENT B has a total occlusion of the LEFT MAIN CORONARY ARTERY (LMCA). The LMCA supplies up to 75% of the LV Muscle Mass in RIGHT DOMINANT Coronary artery systems, and up to 100% of the LV Muscle Mass in LEFT DOMINANT Coronary artery systems.**

Total LMCA obstructions involve occlusions of both the LAD and Circumflex arterial distributions, and are approximately three times more likely to result in cardiogenic shock and death than an isolated LAD occlusion. Angiography for both patients is shown below:

PATIENT A – (LAD Occlusion):

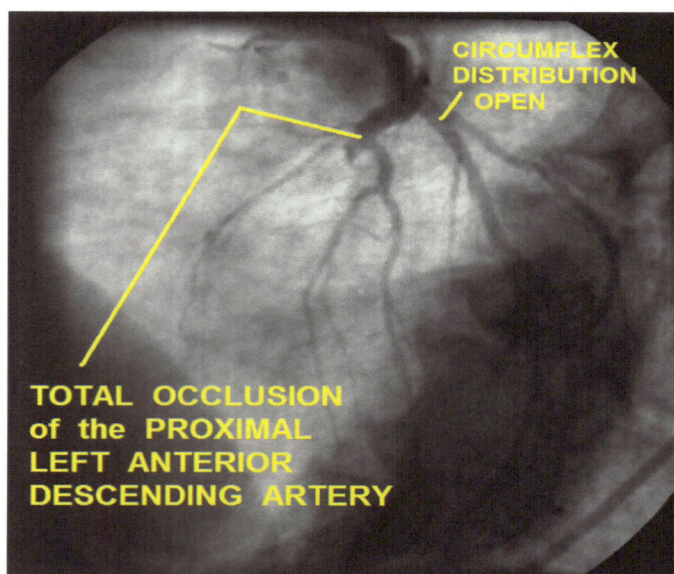

CIRCUMFLEX DISTRIBUTION / OPEN

TOTAL OCCLUSION of the PROXIMAL LEFT ANTERIOR DESCENDING ARTERY

PATIENT B – (LMCA Occlusion):

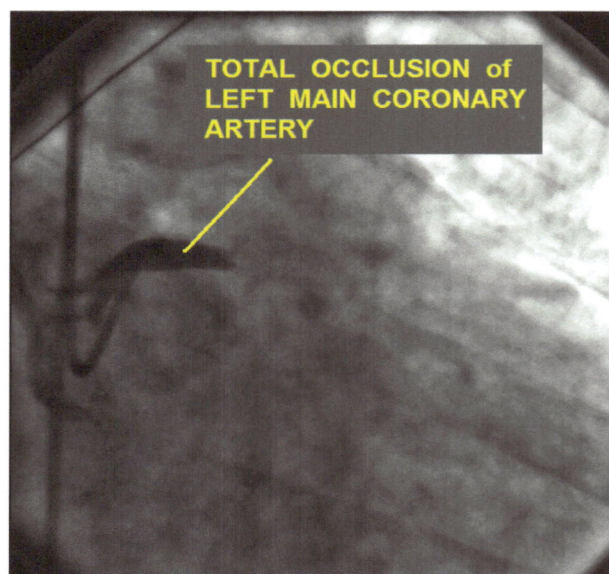

TOTAL OCCLUSION of LEFT MAIN CORONARY ARTERY

The images below illustrate the differences between proximal LAD and LMCA occlusions:

PATIENT A - (LAD occlusion):

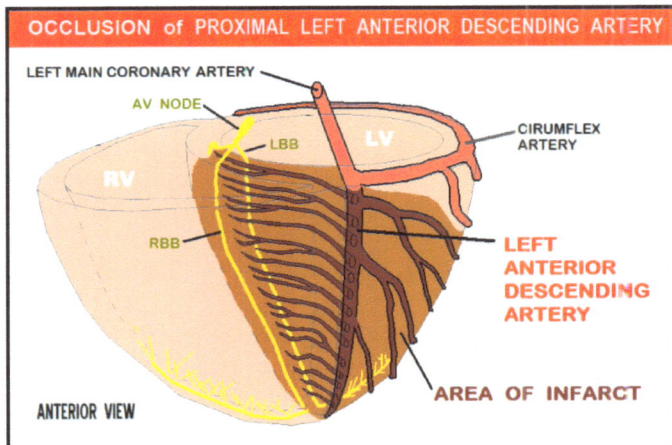

OCCLUSION of PROXIMAL LEFT ANTERIOR DESCENDING ARTERY

ANTERIOR VIEW

The LEFT ANTERIOR DESCENDING ARTERY

SUPPLIES 40 - 50 % OF THE LEFT VENTRICULAR MUSCLE MASS

LEFT ANTERIOR DESCEDING ARTERY = APPROXIMATELY 45 % LV MUSCLE MASS

PATIENT B - (LMCA occlusion):

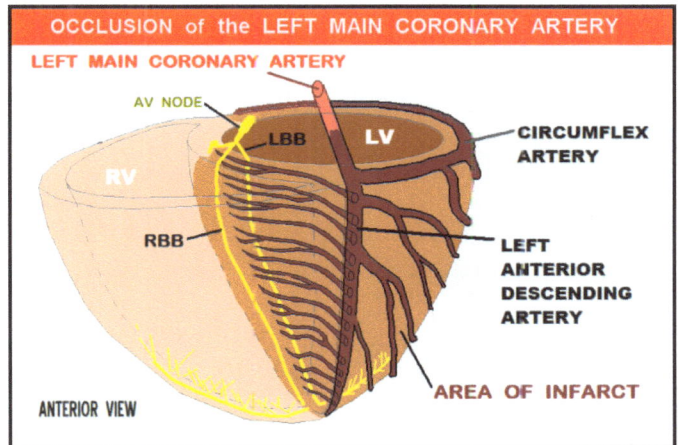

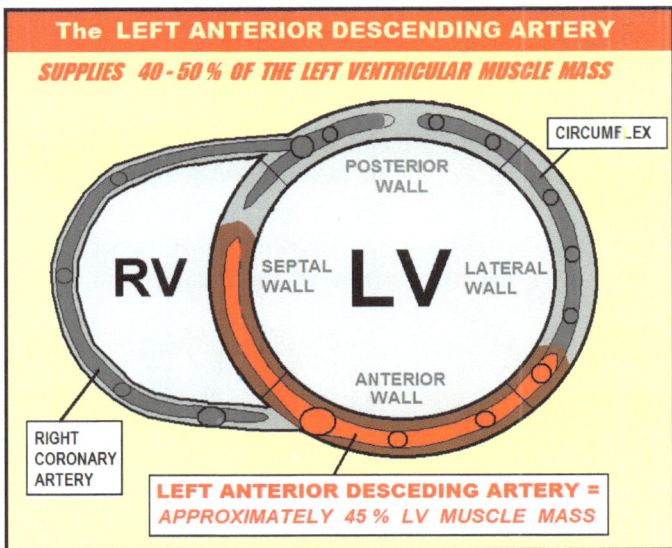

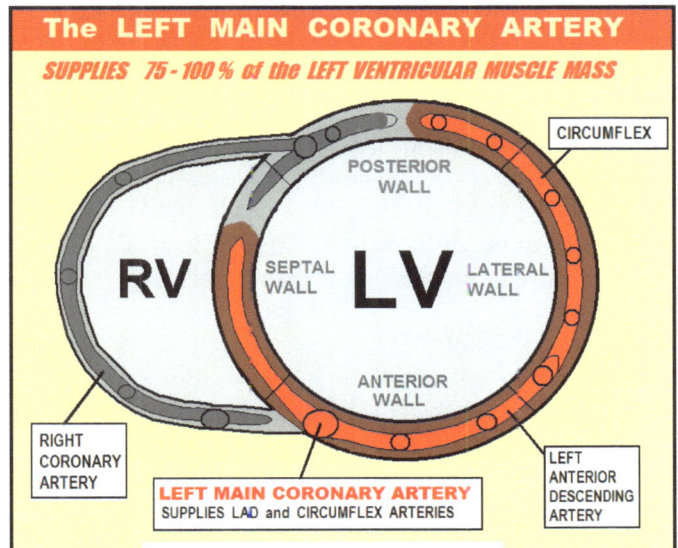

OCCLUSION of the LEFT MAIN CORONARY ARTERY

ANTERIOR VIEW

The LEFT MAIN CORONARY ARTERY

SUPPLIES 75 - 100 % of the LEFT VENTRICULAR MUSCLE MASS

LEFT MAIN CORONARY ARTERY SUPPLIES LAD and CIRCUMFLEX ARTERIES

STEMI caused by LMCA occlusion is rare, and for obvious reasons, carries a high mortality rate. Most patients who survive total LMCA occlusions fit into one or both of the following categories:

- Have developed *collateral circulation* from the RCA to the LAD and CX arterial distributions, or have underwent previous coronary artery bypass surgery (CABG), and have patent bypass grafts around the native LMCA
- Are "Right Dominant," with large RCA distributions, whom are in close proximity to a medical center where rapid diagnosis of STEMI and reperfusion can be achieved.

☞ If you had chosen to send PATIENT A to the Cath Lab first, you fall into the category of nearly every health care professional who was surveyed! Most chose PATIENT A over PATIENT B, because the 12 lead ECGs of acute proximal LAD occlusions are more impressive; they usually display *significantly more ST elevation* than the ECGs of total LMCA occlusions.

Next, we'll take a look at some specific ECG indicators of STEMI caused by LMCA occlusion.

ECG Clues...
for IDENTIFYING STEMI CAUSED BY LEFT MAIN CORONARY ARTERY occlusion:

- ☑ ST ELEVATION in ANTERIOR LEADS (V1 - V4) and LATERAL LEADS (V5 & V6)
- ☑ ST DEPRESSION or ISOELCTRIC J POINTS may be seen in V LEADS .... mainly V2 and/or V3 *caused by COMPETING FORCES of ANTERIOR vs. POSTERIOR WALL MI.* *+
  → NOTE: it is very unusual to see ST DEPRESSION in V LEADS with isolated ANTERIOR WALL MI when caused by occluded LAD.
- ☑ ST ELEVATION in AVR is GREATER THAN ST ELEVATION in V1 *+
- ☑ ST ELEVATION in AVR GREATER THAN 0.5 mm
- ☑ ST ELEVATION in LEAD I and AVL (caused by NO FLOW to DIAGONAL / OBTUSE MARGINAL BRANCHES) *
- ☑ ST DEPRESSION in LEADS II, III, and AVF. (in cases of LMCA occlusion of DOMINANT CIRCUMFLEX, leads II, III, and AVF may show ST ELEVATION or ISOELECTRIC J POINTS) *+
- ☑ NEW / PRESUMABLY NEW RBBB, and/or LEFT ANTERIOR FASICULAR BLOCK *+

---

* Kurisu et al, HEART 2004, SEPTEMBER: 90 (9): 1059-1060
+ Yamaji et al, JACC vol. 38, No. 5, 2001, November 1, 2001:1348-54

A few comments on the information provided in the table shown above:

- The precordial leads can show ST elevation, ST depression, a combination of ST elevation and ST depression, or isoelectric ST segements. This is due to the competing forces of ANTERIOR WALL INFARCTION (ST elevation) vs. POSTERIOR WALL INFARCTION (ST depression).
- ST elevation of at least 0.5mm in lead aVR is reported in over 63% of the cases of acute LMCA occlusion described in current medical journals. ST elevation in lead aVR is due to ischemia of the basilar ventricular septum.
- In the ECGs of STEMI caused by LMCA occlusion that we present in this book, we note the pattern of Left Anterior Fascicular Block in every case.
- ALSO NOTE that in every one of our LEFT MAIN occlusion STEMI ECGs, there is either significant ST elevation or depression in EACH of the 12 leads.

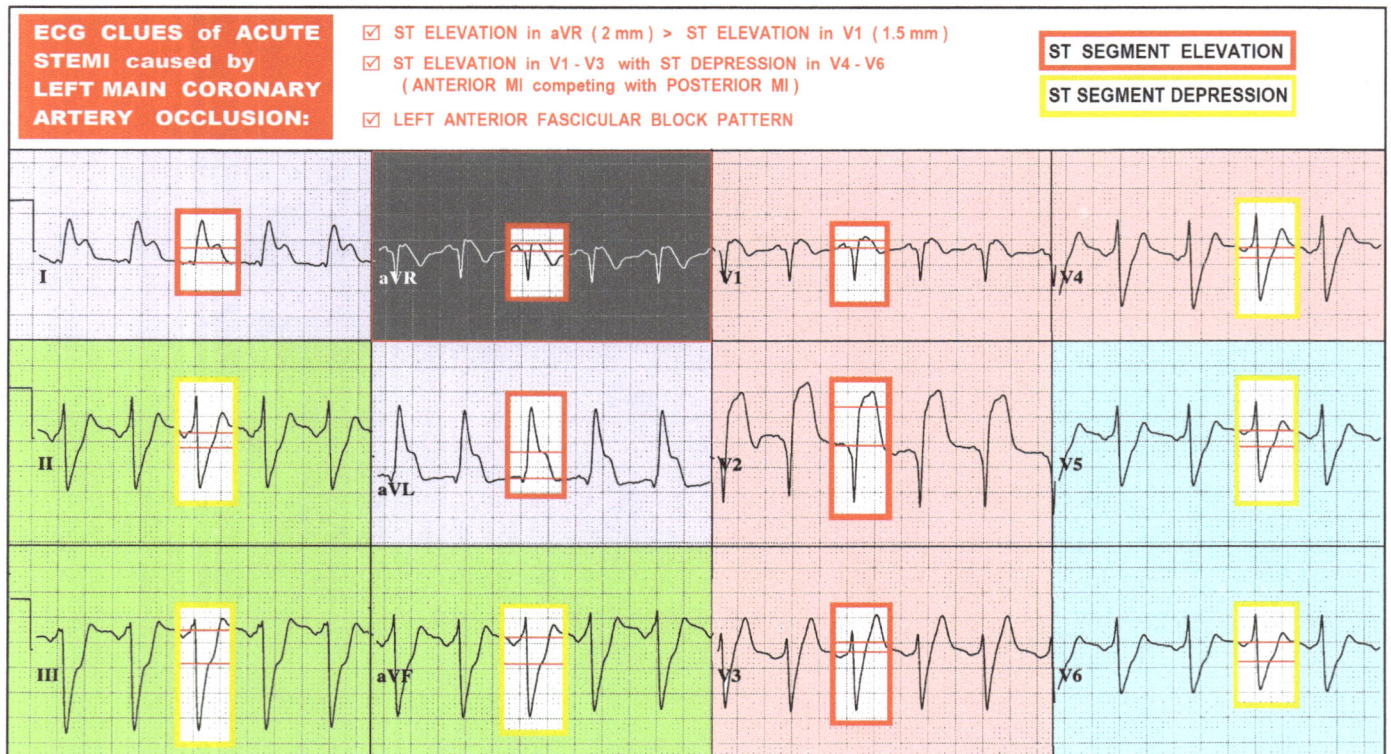

ECG CLUES of ACUTE STEMI caused by LEFT MAIN CORONARY ARTERY OCCLUSION:
- ☑ ST ELEVATION in aVR (2 mm) > ST ELEVATION in V1 (1.5 mm)
- ☑ ST ELEVATION in V1 - V3 with ST DEPRESSION in V4 - V6 (ANTERIOR MI competing with POSTERIOR MI)
- ☑ LEFT ANTERIOR FASCICULAR BLOCK PATTERN

ST SEGMENT ELEVATION
ST SEGMENT DEPRESSION

☞ Notice the similarities of the four ECGs shown below and on the next page. All are from FOUR DIFFERENT STEMI patients found to have total Left Main Coronary Artery occlusions in the Cardiac Cath Lab. *Commit these findings to memory, as your ability to rapidly identify and initiate reperfusion therapy in a patient suffering from STEMI caused by LMCA occlusion may have a significant impact on the patient's outcome.*

36 yr		Vent. rate	123	BPM
Male	Caucasian	PR interval	96	ms
		QRS duration	130	ms
Room:C-		QT/QTc	310/443	ms
Loc:3		P–R–T axes	* –53	43

Sinus tachycardia with short PR
Left ventricular hypertrophy with QRS widening
Cannot rule out Septal infarct , age undetermined
Lateral injury pattern
=** ** ** ** * ACUTE MI ** ** ** **

ACUTE STEMI caused by LEFT MAIN CORONARY ARTERY OCCLUSION

ECG CLUES of ACUTE STEMI caused by LEFT MAIN CORONARY ARTERY OCCLUSION:

☑ ST ELEVATION in leads I and aVL
☑ INCONSISTENCY of ST SEGEMENT in leads V1 - V6 : V1 - V3 ST ELEVATION, V4 - V6 ST DEPRESSION
   (COMPETING FORCES of ANTERIOR vs. POSTERIOR M.I.)
☑ PATTERN of LEFT ANTERIOR FASCICULAR BLOCK (POS. QRS lead I; NEG rS leads II, III)
☑ ST ELEVATION in lead aVR > 0.5 mm

43 yr	Vent. rate	183	BPM
Male	PR interval	*	ms
	QRS duration	106	ms
	QT/QTc	240/418	ms
	P–R–T axes	* –34	–18

Atrial fibrillation with rapid ventricular response
with premature ventricular or aberrantly conducted complexes
Left axis deviation
ST elevation consider anterolateral injury or acute infarct
** ** ** ** * ACUTE MI * ** ** ** **

ACUTE STEMI caused by LEFT MAIN CORONARY ARTERY OCCLUSION

ECG CLUES of ACUTE STEMI caused by LEFT MAIN CORONARY ARTERY OCCLUSION:

☑ ST ELEVATION in leads I and aVL
☑ INCONSISTENCY of ST SEGEMENT in leads V1 - V6 : V1 - V2 ST ELEVATION, V3 - V6 ST DEPRESSION
   (COMPETING FORCES of ANTERIOR vs. POSTERIOR M.I.)
☑ PATTERN of LEFT ANTERIOR FASCICULAR BLOCK (POS. QRS lead I; NEG rS leads II, III)

Vent. rate	155	BPM
PR interval	*	ms
QRS duration	110	ms
QT/QTc	300/482	ms
P–R–T axes	* −83	−34

ACUTE STEMI caused by LEFT MAIN CORONARY ARTERY OCCLUSION

(Leads: I, aVR, V1, V4, II, aVL, V2, V5, III, aVF, V3, V6)

ECG CLUES of ACUTE STEMI caused by LEFT MAIN CORONARY ARTERY OCCLUSION:

- ☑ ST ELEVATION in LEADS I, aVL, V1 - V2, V4 - V6 with ST DEPRESSION in V3: (COMPETING FORCES of ANTERIOR vs. POSTERIOR M.I.)
- ☑ RIGHT BUNDLE BRANCH BLOCK PATTERN, with
- ☑ LEFT ANTERIOR FASCICULAR BLOCK PATTERN

Name:
ID:
Patient ID:
Incident:
Age 37   Sex:

12-Lead 4	HR 107 bpm	
06 Oct 87	12:44:13	
PR 0.154s	QRS 0.182s	
QT/QTc	0.332s/0.443s	
P-QRS-T Axes	89° -62° 44°	

- *** ACUTE MI SUSPECTED ***
- Abnormal ECG **Unconfirmed**
- Sinus tachycardia
- Left anterior fascicular block
- Cannot rule out Anteroseptal infarct,

ACUTE STEMI caused by LEFT MAIN CORONARY ARTERY OCCLUSION

x1.0 .05-40Hz 25mm/sec

MEDTRONIC Pt

ECG CLUES of ACUTE STEMI caused by LEFT MAIN CORONARY ARTERY OCCLUSION:

- ☑ ST ELEVATION in LEADS I, aVL, V1 - V6
- ☑ ST ELEVATION in aVR GREATER THAN 0.5 mm
- ☑ ST ELEVATION in aVR GREATER THAN LEAD V1
- ☑ LEFT ANTERIOR FASCICULAR BLOCK PATTERN

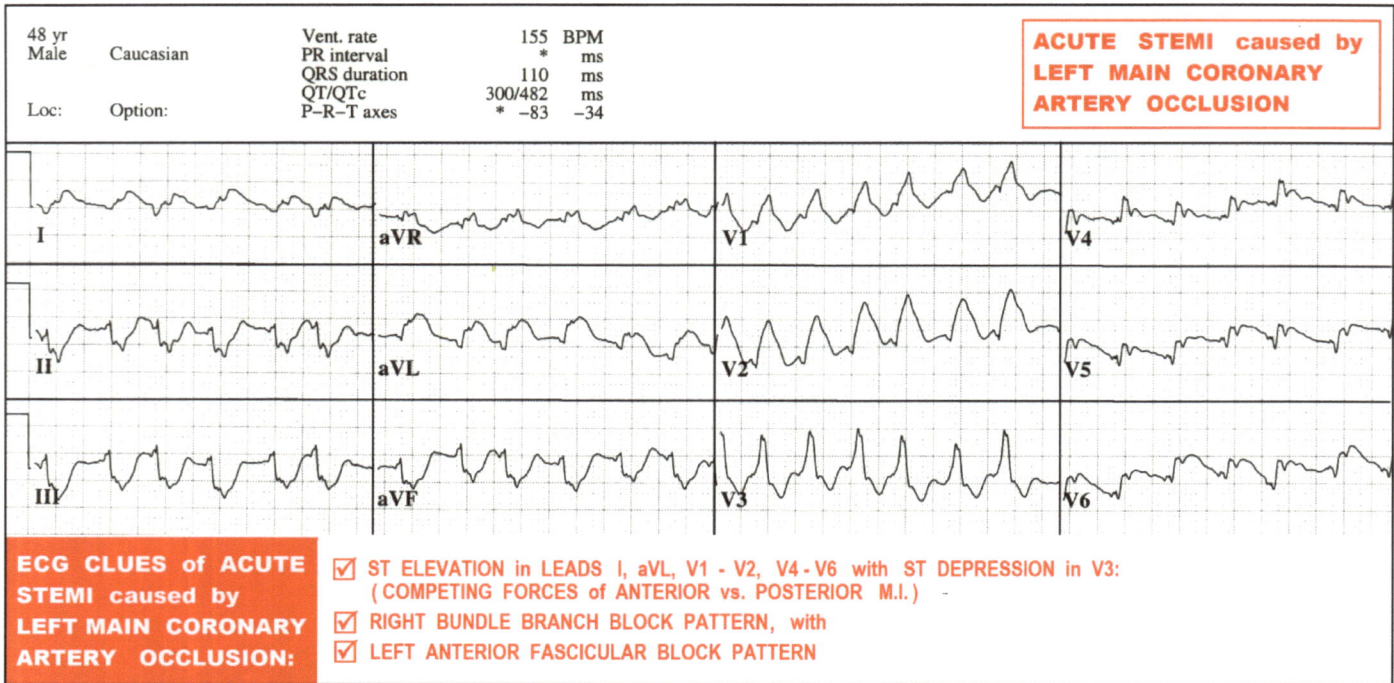

In the ECGs on this page, significant ST elevation is noted throughout the precordial leads. Both patients had large RCA distributions, which protected much of their posterior walls, leaving the ***ST segment elevating forces*** of Anterior Wall MI unopposed.

Conversely, in the ECGs on the previous page, ST elevation is noted only in leads V1 and V2. In leads V3 – V6, there is J point depression, with upsloping ST segments. ECGs on the previous page are examples of the "competing forces of concurrent ANTERIOR and POSTERIOR wall MI" -- both patients had large circumflex distributions supplying their posterior walls.

CONCLUSIONS:

QUESTION 1:   WHICH PATIENT SHOULD BE TAKEN FIRST FOR IMMEDIATE CARDIAC
CATHETERIZATION for EMERGENCY PCI ?

ANSWER: PATIENT B was taken emergently to the Cardiac Cath Lab - both the ED physician
and the Interventional Cardiologist correctly identified the EKG patterns
of LMCA occlusion.

QUESTION 2:   WHAT COURSE OF ACTION SHOULD BE TAKEN WITH THE PATIENT NOT CHOSEN
TO BE SENT TO THE CATH LAB FIRST?

ANSWER: PATIENT A received thrombolytic therapy in the ED. It was determined that
THROMBOLYTIC THERAPY would achieve the FASTEST ROUTE to REPERFUSION --
-- by at least 60 minutes.

PATIENT B underwent emergency thrombectomy, PTCA and stenting of his Left Main Coronary Artery with a drug-eluting stent in the Cardiac Catheterization Lab. His angiography is shown below:

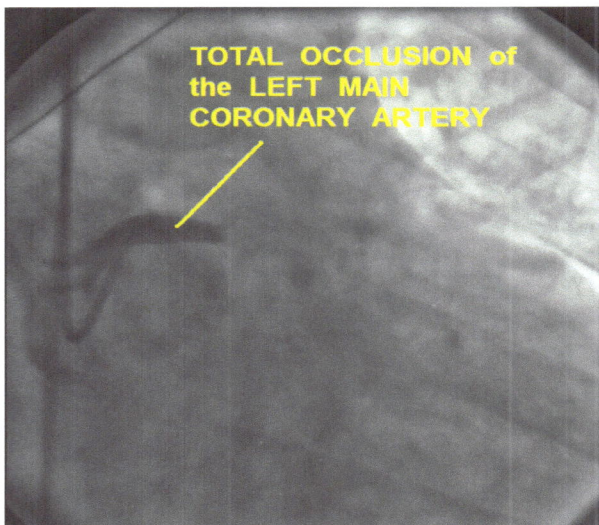

TOTAL OCCLUSION of the LEFT MAIN CORONARY ARTERY

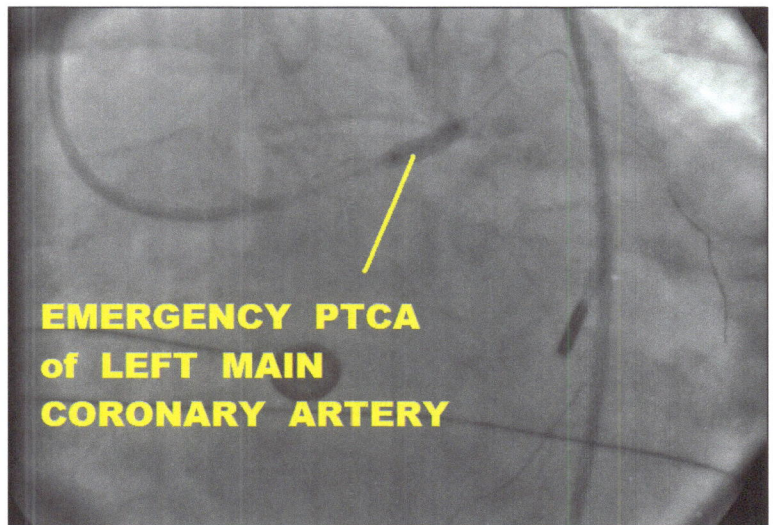

EMERGENCY PTCA of LEFT MAIN CORONARY ARTERY

Despite the dismal mortality rate associated with STEMI from total LMCA occlusion, this patient survived and was later discharged. His EF is estimated at approximately 30%. He received an ICD, and is currently stable.

His survival of this ordeal is no doubt attributed to his quick arrival in the ED after his symptoms started, the rapid diagnosis of his condition, and his expedient triage to the cardiac catheterization lab for emergency PCI.

Case contributed by Humberto Coto, MD, FACC

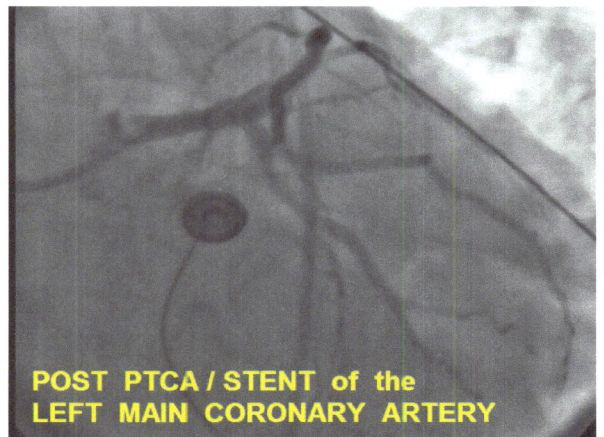

POST PTCA / STENT of the LEFT MAIN CORONARY ARTERY

CASE STUDY 5 - STEMI

CHIEF COMPLAINT and SIGNIFICANT HISTORY:

51 y/o MALE reports to ED c/o intermittent CHEST PRESSURE, substernal w radiation to neck and jaw. Pain is currently present, "4" on 1-10 scale. Patient given one ASA 325mg by EMS prior to arrival.

RISK FACTOR PROFILE:

- 💣✳ **FAMILY HISTORY** - Mother and maternal uncle both have CAD.
- 💣✳ **CURRENT CIGARETTE SMOKER**
- 💣✳ **CHOLESTEROL** - LDL elevated, patient currently on Statin medication

PHYSICAL EXAM: Patient alert, oriented X 4, skin cool, dry, pale. Patient restless. No JVD, Lungs clear bilaterally. Heart sounds normal S1, S2. No peripheral edema.

VITAL SIGNS: BP: 162/94   P: 84   R: 20   SAO2: 98% on 4 LPM O2

LABS: TROPONIN: 5.9

QUADRAD OF ACS CHECKLIST

☑ **SYMPTOMS of ACS**
- ✔ ◆ TYPICAL ACS - eg:
- ◆ ATYPICAL ACS - eg:

☑ **ECG ABNORMALITIES**
- ◆ ST ELEVATION (J POINT plus 40 ms)
- ✔ ◆ HYPERACUTE T WAVES - and/or -
- ◆ NEW or PRESUMABLY NEW LBBB
- ◆ ST DEPRESSION (>0.5 mm @ J POINT) and/or
- ◆ INVERTED or BIPHASIC T WAVES and/or
- ◆ DYNAMIC ST SEGMENT and/or T WAVE CHANGES IN SERIAL EKGs

☑ **RISK FACTORS - 3 or more**
- ✔ ◆ FAMILY HISTORY
- ◆ DIABETES
- ✔ ◆ ↑ LDL and/or ↓ HDL
- ✔ ◆ SMOKING
- ◆ AGE: 65 or MORE
- ◆ HYPERTENSION

☑ **CARDIAC MARKERS**
- ◆ ELEVATED TROPONIN and/or CK/MB

4 **TOTAL**

SUSPECTED ACUTE MI:

INITIAL MANAGEMENT

- **VITAL SIGNS**

- **"O.M.I."**
  - Oxygen
  - Monitor (ecg)
  - IV (plus draw lab samples)

- **12 LEAD ECG**
  Obtain and interpret within 10 minutes of patient's arrival.

- **"M.O.N.A."**
  - Morphine
  - Oxygen (if not already done)
  - Nitroglycerin
  - Aspirin

- **RAPID, FOCUSED ASSESSMENT**

- **HEART / LUNG SOUNDS**

- **SEND LAB SAMPLES:**
  - Cardiac Markers
  - Electrolytes
  - Coagulation Studies

51 yr
Male Caucasian

Room:ER
Loc:3 Option:23

Vent. rate	86	BPM
PR interval	150	ms
QRS duration	94	ms
QT/QTc	364/435	
P–R–T axes	79 56	28

☞ EVALUATE EKG for indicators of ACS:

- ST SEGMENT ELEVATION / DEPRESSION
- HYPERACUTE T WAVES
- CONVEX ST SEGMENTS
- OTHER ST SEGMENT / T WAVE ABNORMALITIES

I aVR V1 V4

II aVL V2 V5

III aVF V3 V6

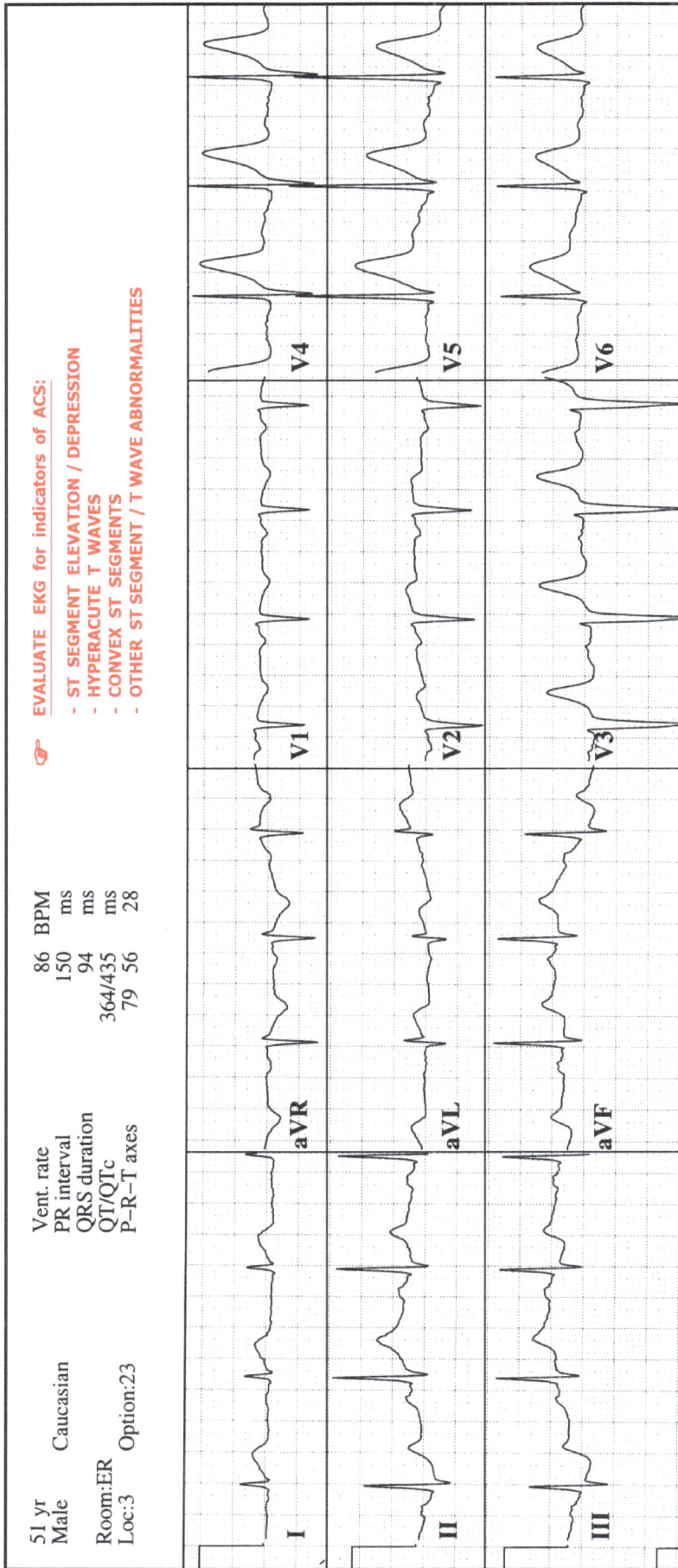

CASE STUDY QUESTIONS:

NOTE LEADS WITH ST ELEVATION:

NOTE LEADS WITH ST DEPRESSION:

WHAT IS THE SUSPECTED DIAGNOSIS ?

WHAT IS THE "CULPRIT ARTERY" -- if applicable ?

LIST ANY CRITICAL STRUCTURES COMPROMISED:

LIST ANY POTENTIAL COMPLICATIONS:

51 yr		Vent. rate		86	BPM	Normal sinus rhythm
Male	Caucasian	PR interval		150	ms	ST elevation consider lateral injury or acute infarct
		QRS duration		94	ms	* ** ** ** * ACUTE MI * ** ** ** **
Room:ER		QT/QTc		364/435	ms	Abnormal ECG
Loc:3	Option:23	P–R–T axes		79 56	28	

ST SEGMENT ELEVATION

ST SEGMENT DEPRESSION

LATERAL - ANTERIOR DIAG. (LAD) or OM (CIRC).	BASILAR SEPTUM	ANTERIOR - SEPTAL LAD	ANTERIOR LAD
I	aVR	V1	V4
INFERIOR DOMINANT RCA or CIRC.	LATERAL - ANTERIOR DIAG. (LAD) or OM (CIRC).	ANTERIOR - SEPTAL LAD	LATERAL CIRC. or LAD
II	aVL	V2	V5
INFERIOR DOMINANT RCA or CIRC.	INFERIOR DOMINANT RCA or CIRC.	ANTERIOR LAD	LATERAL CIRC. or LAD
III	aVF	V3	V6

Primary ST elevation is seen in leads V4, V5, and V6. In lead I, the J Point is isoelectric; however the J-T APEX is FLAT, and when the ST segment is measured 40ms beyond the J point, there is approximately 1.5mm of ST elevation, enough to enough to be condsidered "positive" for STEMI. In aVL, there is ST elevation at the J point of approximately 1mm. The findings of ST elevation primarily in V5 and V6 indicate this is a LATERAL WALL MI, and the culprit artery is most likely the CIRCUMFLEX. When ST elevation is also seen in leads I and aVL, the lesion is most likely in the proximal aspect, before the takeoff of the first obtuse marginal branch. Absence of ST elevation in leads II, III, and aVF along with NO ST depression in V1 – V3 indicate the BLOCKED CIRCUMFLEX ARTERY is most likely small and non-dominant. Since all but lead V4 are considered lateral leads, this is a Lateral Wall STEMI, with some "spill-over" of the zone of infarct into the anterior wall.

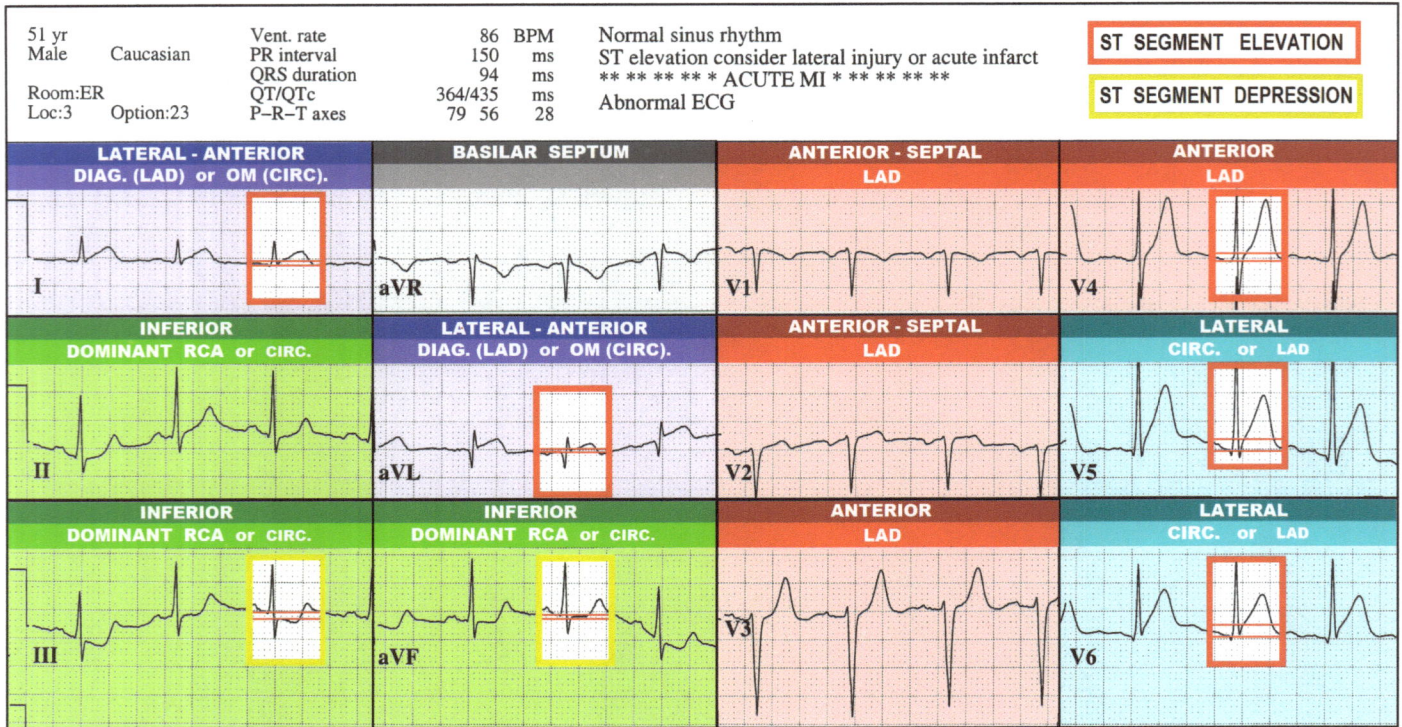

V5 - V6 VIEW THE LATERAL WALL
of the LEFT VENTRICLE

As illustrated in the diagram to the left, leads V5 and V6 "view" the lateral aspect of the left ventricle. Therefore when ST elevation is seen in leads V5 and V6, we suspect LATERAL WALL STEMI.

It is not unusual to see lateral wall STEMI extending to the anterior region, with ST elevation noted in lead V4. In this case, ST elevation is seen in lead V4, but since it is seen in only ONE of the four contiguous anterior leads, we typically don't say there is "anterior involvement."

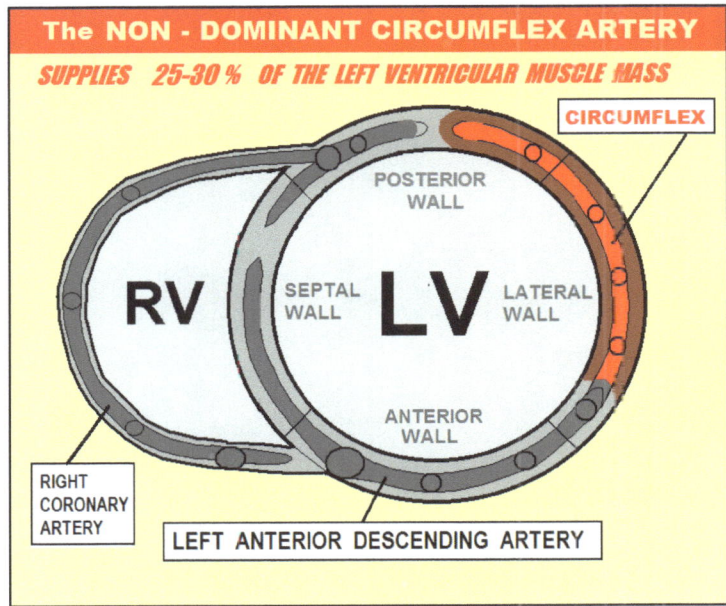

The **NON - DOMINANT CIRCUMFLEX ARTERY**
SUPPLIES 25-30 % OF THE LEFT VENTRICULAR MUSCLE MASS

In approximately 75% of the population, the Circumflex artery is small and non-dominant. In these patients, the RIGHT CORONARY ARTERY is DOMINANT. (The term "dominant," when describing coronary artery anatomy, refers to the artery that feeds the INFERIOR WALL of the Left Ventricle: RCA vs. CIRCUMFLEX).

Lateral Wall STEMI caused by blockage of a non-dominant Circumflex typically results in a small-to-moderate amount of damage to LV function, since a non-dominant Circumflex supplies 25-30% of the LV muscle mass. That is the case with our patient in this case study; there was no discernable compromise to hemodynamic stability.

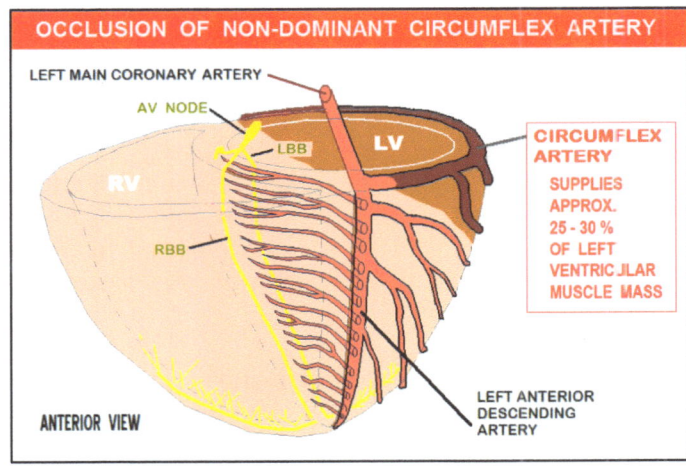

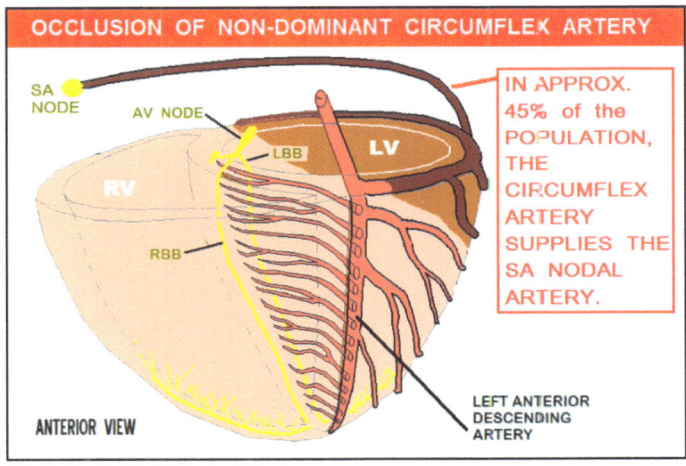

In addition to the possibility of mild – moderate hypotension, dysfunction of the SINUS (SA) NODE may be observed. In Approximately 45 percent of the population, the SA Node receives its blood supply from the Circumflex artery, with the remainder of the population (55%), the SA Node is supplied by the Right Cornary Artery. *Note that being "right or left dominant" poses no bearing on whether the SA Nodal artery originates from the RCA or the Circumflex.* "Right and Left Dominance" refers to "which artery gives rise to the POSTERIOR DESCENDING ARTERY, which supplies the INFERIOR WALL."

When the SA Node is compromised, expect to see SINUS BRADYCARDIA, SINUS ARREST (with a possible Junctional Escape or Accelerated Idioventricular Rhythm), or ASYSTOLE. Be prepared to manage SA Node dysfunction with ATROPINE, PACING (transcutaneous or transvenous), and/or CPR, in cases of asystole.

LAD - NO OBSTRUCTIONS

TOTAL OBSTRUCTION - MID CIRCUMFLEX

SMALL, NON-DOMINANT CIRCUMFLEX ARTERY - NOW OPEN AFTER PTCA

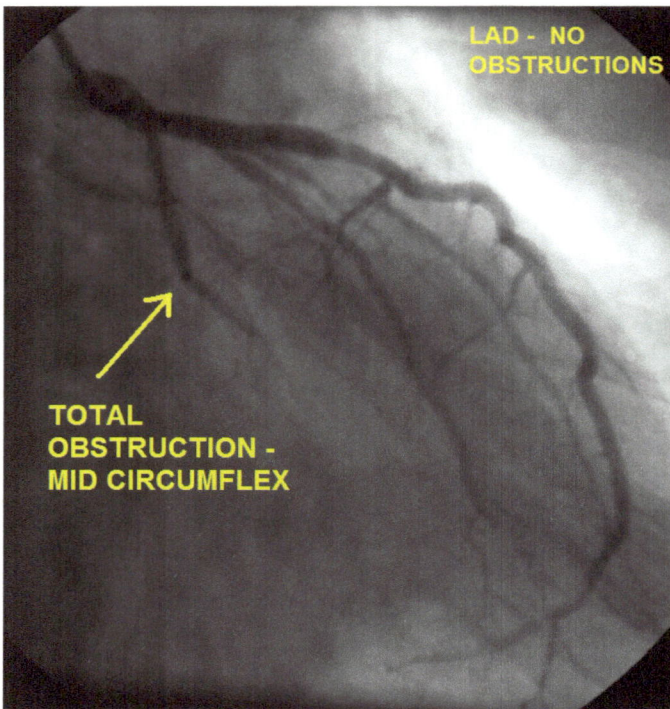

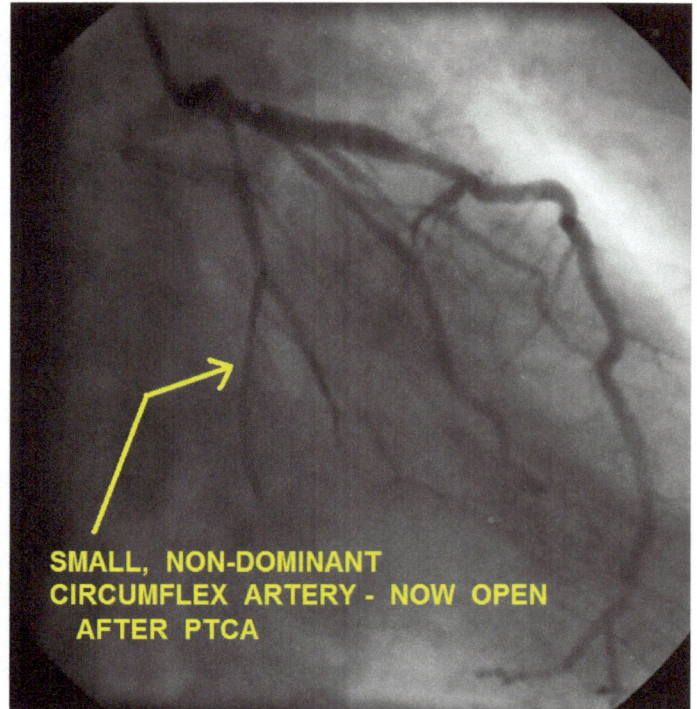

As we expected to see, angiography in the Cath Lab revealed obstruction of a small, non-dominant Circumflex artery. The above images are pre- and post-emergency PTCA of the Circumflex artery.

DOMINANT RIGHT CORONARY ARTERY

Since our patient had a small, non-dominant Circumflex artery, his Right Coronary Artery was dominant; it gave rise to the Posteior Desending Artery (PDA). Angiography of his RCA revealed diffuse plaquing throughout, with no obstructive lesions.

This patient's coronary artery configuration is "typical" – approximately 75% of the population have RIGHT DOMINANT systems.

Approximately 15% have LEFT DOMINANT systems, where the CIRCUMFLEX gives rise to the PDA.

The remaining 10% of the populus have varying degrees of COMBINED RIGHT and LEFT DOMINANCE, as will be illustrated by the next several case studies.

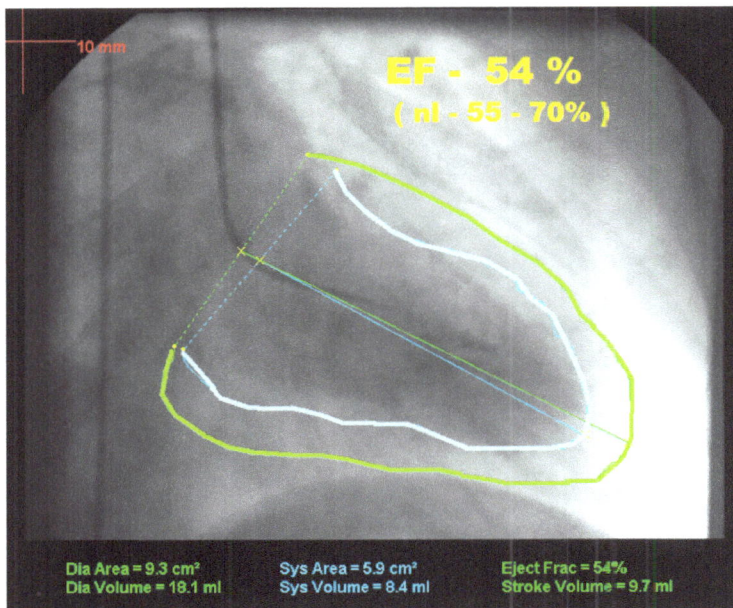

EF - 54 %
(nl - 55 - 70%)

Dia Area = 9.3 cm²
Dia Volume = 18.1 ml

Sys Area = 5.9 cm²
Sys Volume = 8.4 ml

Eject Frac = 54%
Stroke Volume = 9.7 ml

Fortunately, a Non-Dominant Circumflex artery does not supply a large area of Left Ventricular Muscle Mass. As witnessed in the current case study, there was no significant drop in systolic blood pressure. As is typical for this type of STEMI, our patient suffered minimal damage to his LV function; his LV Ejection Fraction is 54%.

The NORMAL RANGE for LV EJECTION FRACTION is 55 – 70%.

CASE STUDY SUMMARY

ST ELEVATION:	ST DEPRESSION:
I, aVL, V4, V5, V6	III, aVF

SUSPECTED DIAGNOSIS: ACUTE LATERAL WALL M.I.

SUSPECTED "CULPRIT ARTERY" (if applicable):

CIRCUMFLEX ARTERY, small - non dominant.

IMMEDIATE CONCERNS FOR ALL STEMI PATIENTS:

- BE PREPARED TO MANAGE SUDDEN CARDIAC ARREST (PRIMARY V - FIB / V- TACH, BRADYCARDIAS / HEART BLOCKS)
- STAT REPERFUSION THERAPY: THROMBOLYTICS vs. CARDIAC CATHETERIZATION and PCI
- CONSIDER NEEDS FOR ANTI-PLATELET and ANTI-COAGULATION THERAPY

CRITICAL STRUCTURES COMPROMISED:	POTENTIAL COMPLICATIONS:	POSSIBLE CRITICAL INTERVENTIONS:
15-30% OF THE LV MUSCLE MASS	SLIGHT POSSIBILITY OF LV PUMP FAILURE.	INOTROPIC AGENTS
THE SINUS NODE BLOOD SUPPLY IS FROM THE CIRCUMFLEX ARTERY IN APPROX. 45% of POPULATION.	SA NODE DYSFUNCTION: - BRADYCARDIA - JUNCTIONAL RHYTHM - ASYSTOLE	- ATROPINE - TRANSCUTANEOUS PACING - CPR

CHIEF COMPLAINT and SIGNIFICANT HISTORY:

40 y/o male arrived in the ER after having "heavy chest pressure" for 20 minutes. He states pressure is sub-sternal, without radiation, and is constant. No SOB, nausea, or light-headedness.

RISK FACTOR PROFILE:

🔥 **FAMILY HISTORY** - Grandfather (maternal) AMI age 46 *

🔥 **FORMER CIGARETTE SMOKER** (smoked 15 years, quit 2 years ago) **

🔥 **CHOLESTEROL** - LDL elevated, patient currently on Statin medication

PHYSICAL EXAM: Patient is alert & oriented x 4, skin warm, dry, color normal. He is mildly anxious. Lungs clear, heart sounds normal S1, S2. No peripheral edema or JVD noted.

VITAL SIGNS: BP: 144/88   P: 70   R: 16   SAO2: 99% on 4 LPM O2

LABS: TROPONIN: < .04

* some risk factor assessment tools only accept nuclear family

** some risk factor assessment tools state smoke-free >1year = non-smoker

QUADRAD OF ACS CHECKLIST

☑ **SYMPTOMS of ACS**
- ✔ ◆ TYPICAL ACS - eg:
- ◆ ATYPICAL ACS - eg:

☑ **ECG ABNORMALITIES**
- ✔ ◆ ST ELEVATION (J POINT plus 40 ms)
- ◆ HYPERACUTE T WAVES - and/or -
- ◆ NEW or PRESUMABLY NEW LBBB
- ◆ ST DEPRESSION (>0.5 mm @ J POINT) and/or
- ◆ INVERTED or BIPHASIC T WAVES and/or
- ◆ DYNAMIC ST SEGMENT and/or T WAVE CHANGES IN SERIAL EKGs

☐ **RISK FACTORS - 3 or more**
- ✔ ◆ FAMILY HISTORY
- ◆ DIABETES
- ✔ ◆ ↑ LDL and/or ↓ HDL
- ✔ ◆ SMOKING
- ◆ AGE: 65 or MORE
- ◆ HYPERTENSION

☐ **CARDIAC MARKERS**
- ◆ ELEVATED TROPONIN and/or CK/MB

2 **TOTAL**

NOTE: We did not include family history and cigarette smoking in this patient's "Quadrad of ACS Checklist." These items were not included as factors in the Quadrad checklist because according to **TIMI guidelines:**

- *family history*[56] only includes the "nuclear" family: *parents, siblings*, and *children* of the patient. Grandparents, aunts, uncles, etc. are not considered when assesing family history.

- *tobacco use* is considered "active" only if the patient has engaged in tobacco use within the past month, and a "former smoker" is described as one whom has smoked within the past one year.

---

[56] "TIMI Definitions for Commonly Used Terms in Clinical Trials," www.TIMI.org

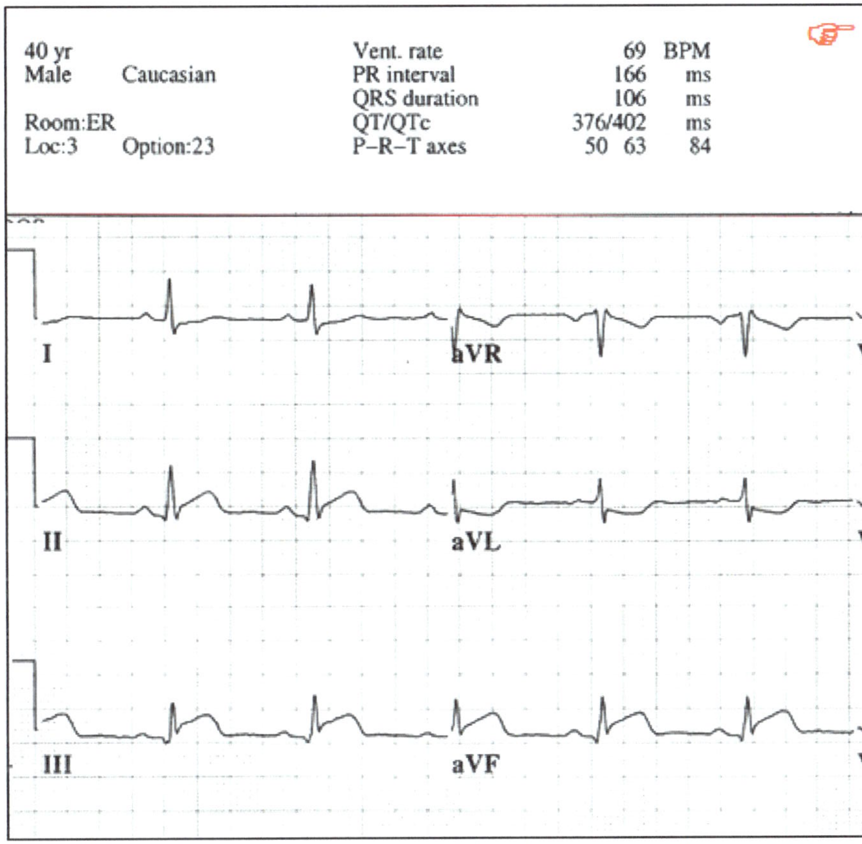

40 yr
Male Caucasian

Room:ER
Loc:3 Option:23

Vent. rate	69	BPM
PR interval	166	ms
QRS duration	106	ms
QT/QTc	376/402	ms
P–R–T axes	50 63	84

Leads: I, aVR, V1, V4 — II, aVL, V2, V5 — III, aVF, V3, V6

☞ **EVALUATE EKG for indicators of ACS:**
- **ST SEGMENT ELEVATION / DEPRESSION**
- **HYPERACUTE T WAVES**
- **CONVEX ST SEGMENTS**
- **OTHER ST SEGMENT / T WAVE ABNORMALITIES**

CASE STUDY QUESTIONS:

NOTE LEADS WITH ST ELEVATION:	NOTE LEADS WITH ST DEPRESSION:
WHAT IS THE SUSPECTED DIAGNOSIS ?	
WHAT IS THE "CULPRIT ARTERY" -- if applicable ?	
LIST ANY CRITICAL STRUCTURES COMPROMISED:	**LIST ANY POTENTIAL COMPLICATIONS:**

197

40 yr		Vent. rate	69	BPM	Normal sinus rhythm
Male	Caucasian	PR interval	166	ms	Inferior infarct , possibly acute
		QRS duration	106	ms	** ** ** ** * ACUTE MI * ** ** ** **
Room:ER		QT/QTc	376/402	ms	Abnormal ECG
Loc:	Option:	P–R–T axes	50 63 84		No previous ECGs available

ST SEGMENT ELEVATION

ST SEGMENT DEPRESSION

LATERAL - ANTERIOR DIAG (LAD) or OM (CIRC)	BASILAR SEPTAL 1st SEPTAL PERF.	ANTERIOR SEPTAL LAD	ANTERIOR LAD
I	aVR	V1	V4
INFERIOR RCA or CIRC.	LATERAL - ANTERIOR DIAG (LAD) or OM (CIRC)	ANTERIOR SEPTAL LAD	LATERAL CIRC. or LAD
II	aVL	V2	V5
INFERIOR RCA or CIRC.	**INFERIOR RCA or CIRC.**	ANTERIOR LAD	LATERAL CIRC. or LAD
III	aVF	V3	V6

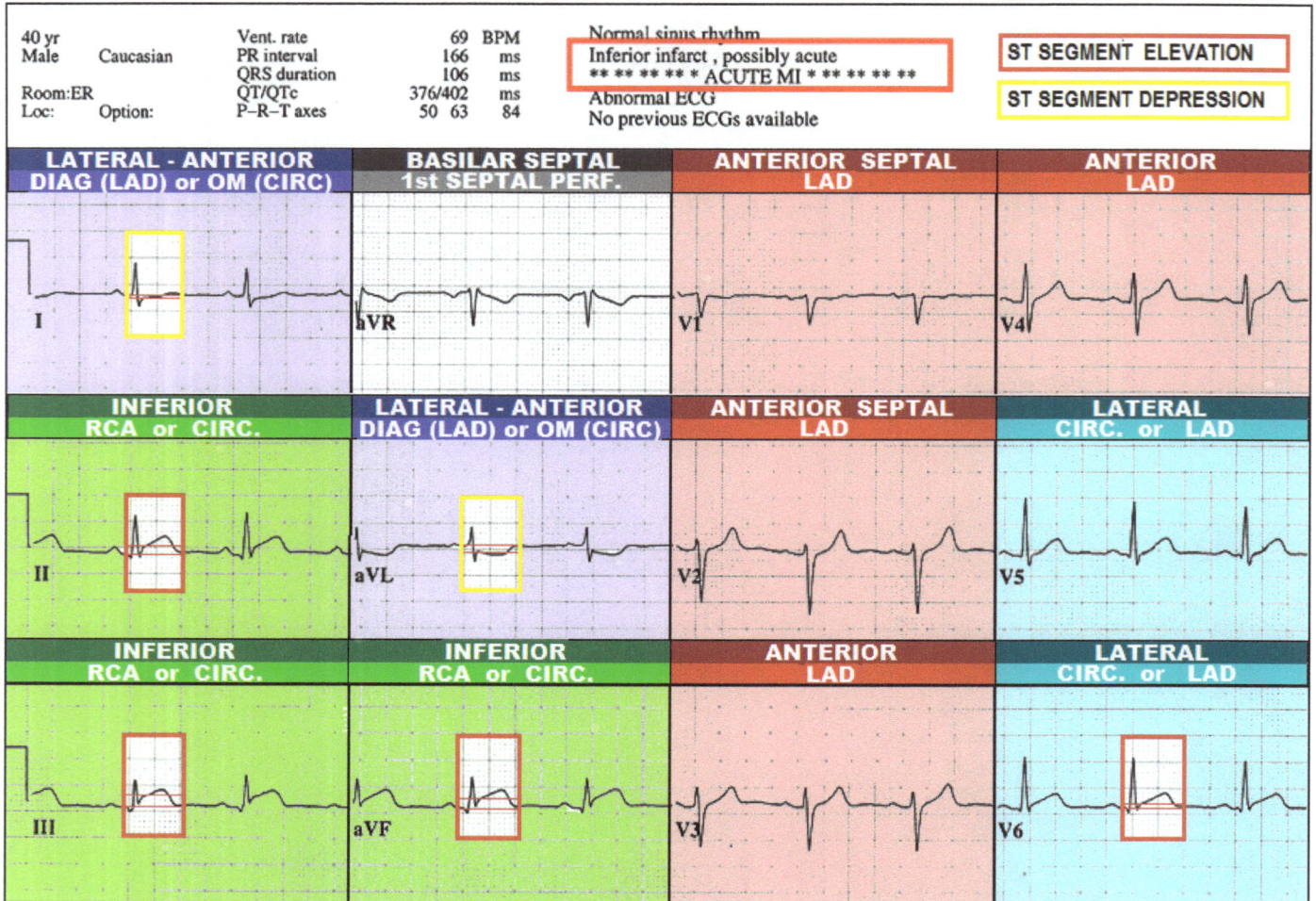

Leads II, III, an aVF view the inferior wall of the left ventricle.

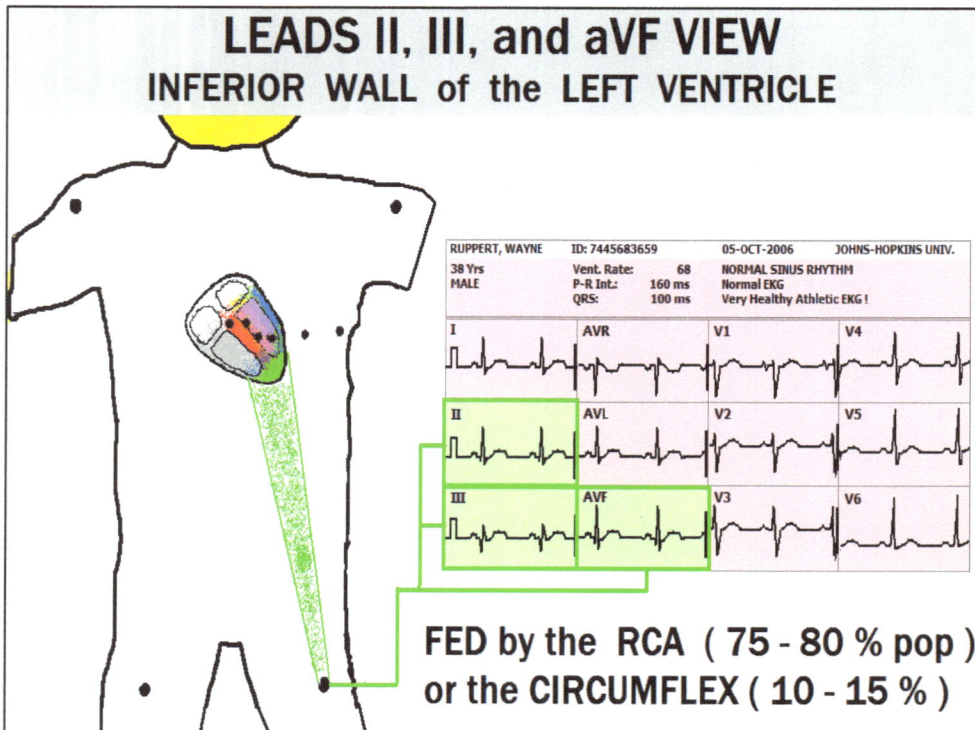

LEADS II, III, and aVF VIEW
INFERIOR WALL of the LEFT VENTRICLE

RUPPERT, WAYNE	ID: 7445683659	05-OCT-2006	JOHNS-HOPKINS UNIV.
38 Yrs	Vent. Rate: 68	NORMAL SINUS RHYTHM	
MALE	P-R Int.: 160 ms	Normal EKG	
	QRS: 100 ms	Very Healthy Athletic EKG !	

I   AVR   V1   V4

II   AVL   V2   V5

III   AVF   V3   V6

FED by the RCA (75 - 80 % pop)
or the CIRCUMFLEX (10 - 15 %)

Patients suffering from *inferior wall MI* present with varying degrees of hemodynamic stability. Many patients will present in a normal hemodynamic state: normal vital signs, alert and oriented and in minimal distress. Other patients with inferior wall MI will present with bradycardia and heart block. Yet others will present in *profound cardiogenic shock*. The wide variation in hemodynamic stability of patients with acute inferior wall MI is due to the multiple arterial configurations which supply blood to the inferior wall, and can vary significantly from one patient to the next.

(See pages 25-28 to view several common variations in coronary artery anatomy with respect to the *inferior wall blood supply*). Because there are multiple anatomical variations in how the inferior wall receives its blood supply, *inferior wall MIs* fall into several categories, with some listed in the table to the right.

In 75-80% of the population, the *Right Coronary Artery* (RCA) supplies the inferior wall of the left ventricle. Since a majority of the population has this arterial configuration, most inferior wall MIs fall into the top two categories listed in the table to the right: *Inferior* or *Inferior-Right Ventricular (RV) MI.*

As the infarct size increases to include multiple zones of the myocardium, the patient's degree of hemodynamic stability is likely to decrease.

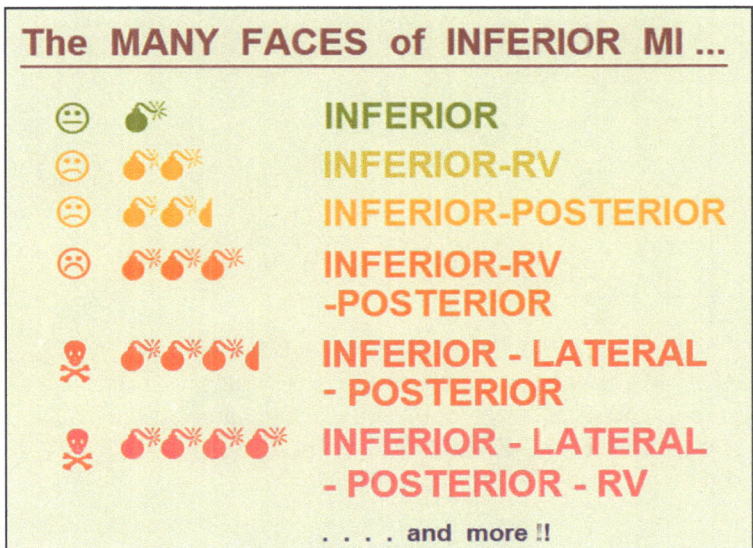

The MANY FACES of INFERIOR MI ...

☺	☀	**INFERIOR**
☹	☀☀	**INFERIOR-RV**
☹	☀☀	**INFERIOR-POSTERIOR**
☹	☀☀☀	**INFERIOR-RV -POSTERIOR**
☠	☀☀☀☀	**INFERIOR - LATERAL - POSTERIOR**
☠	☀☀☀☀☀	**INFERIOR - LATERAL - POSTERIOR - RV**

. . . . and more !!

CASE STUDY SUMMARY

ST ELEVATION:	ST DEPRESSION:
II, III, aVF	**I, aVL**

SUSPECTED DIAGNOSIS: **ACUTE INFERIOR WALL M.I.**

SUSPECTED "CULPRIT ARTERY" (if applicable):

RIGHT CORONARY ARTERY - DOMINANT

IMMEDIATE CONCERNS FOR ALL STEMI PATIENTS:

- BE PREPARED TO MANAGE SUDDEN CARDIAC ARREST (PRIMARY V - FIB / V- TACH, BRADYCARDIAS / HEART BLOCKS)
- STAT REPERFUSION THERAPY: THROMBOLYTICS vs. CARDIAC CATHETERIZATION and PCI
- CONSIDER NEEDS FOR ANTI-PLATELET and ANTI-COAGULATION THERAPY

CRITICAL STRUCTURES COMPROMISED:	POTENTIAL COMPLICATIONS:	POSSIBLE CRITICAL INTERVENTIONS:
15-25% OF THE LV MUSCLE MASS	SLIGHT POSSIBILITY OF MILD LV FAILURE.	FLUID CHALLENGE INOTROPIC AGENTS
100% OF THE RIGHT VENTRICLE	EXTREME SENSITIVITY TO NITRATES AND OPIATES	FLUID BOLUSES
SINUS NODE ARTERY SUPPLIED BY RCA 55% of Pop.	BRADYCARDIA ASYSTOLE	ATROPINE TRANSCUTANEOUS PACING
AV NODAL ARTERY SUPPLIED BY DOMINANT ARTERY (RCA or Circ) IN MOST PATIENTS	AV NODAL BLOCKS: - 1 DEGREE - 2nd DEGREE type I, II - 3rd DEGREE	ATROPINE TRANSCUTANEOUS PACING

The patient in our case study has one electrocardiographic indicator of *Inferior Wall MI* (IWMI) due to occlusion of a *dominant Right Coronary Artery (RCA).* ECG indicators of IWMA caused by RCA occlusion are[57]:
- ST elevation in Lead III is greater than ST Elevation I Lead II. Conversely, occlusion of the Circumflex artery often results in ST elevation in Lead II being equal to or greater than that of Lead III.

---

[57] "Use of the Electrocardiogram in Acute Myocardial Infarction," Zimetbaum, et al, NEJM 348:933-940

The table to the left reflects my direct observation of the frequency of occurrence of several variations of inferior wall MI as seen in the cardiac cath lab at St. Joseph's Hospital over an eleven year span. (1999-2010)   I have observed a higher incidence of *inferior* and *inferior-right ventricular MIs* than the other types of MI listed in the table to the left, an observation which is consistent with the fact that 75-80% of the population have a *dominant right coronary artery* which supplies blood to the inferior wall and the right ventricle.

For the 75-80% of the population with a dominant RCA, the *posterior wall* of the left ventricle is jointly supplied by both the *RCA* and the *circumflex artery*, as illustrated in the image to the right.

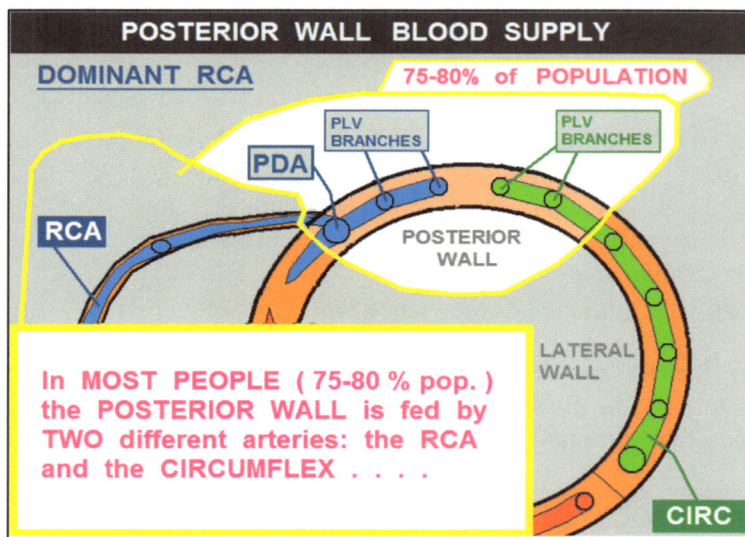

When patients with a dominant RCA experience inferior wall MI, *posterior wall involvement* is usually limited due to the fact that the posterior wall receives its blood supply jointly from both the RCA and the Circumflex arteries.

The larger area, "*multi-site*" inferior wall MIs usually result when a *dominant circumflex artery* (10-15% population) or an "*extreme dominant*" RCA (3-5% population) become occluded. The first two images below depict how a *dominant circumflex artery* supplies blood to the entire posterior and inferior regions:

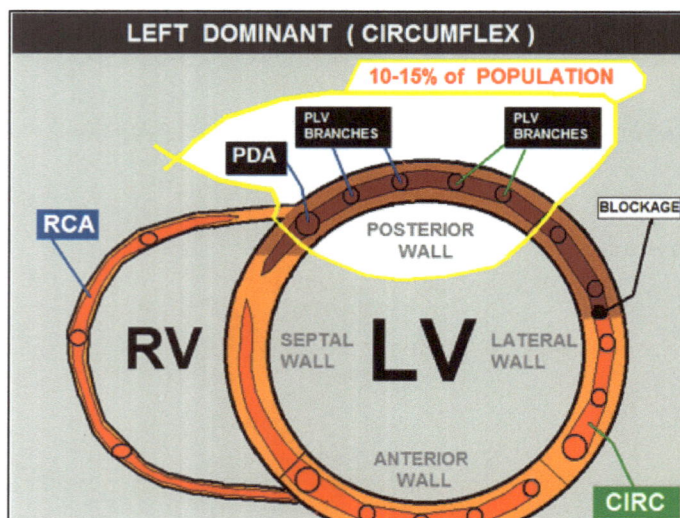

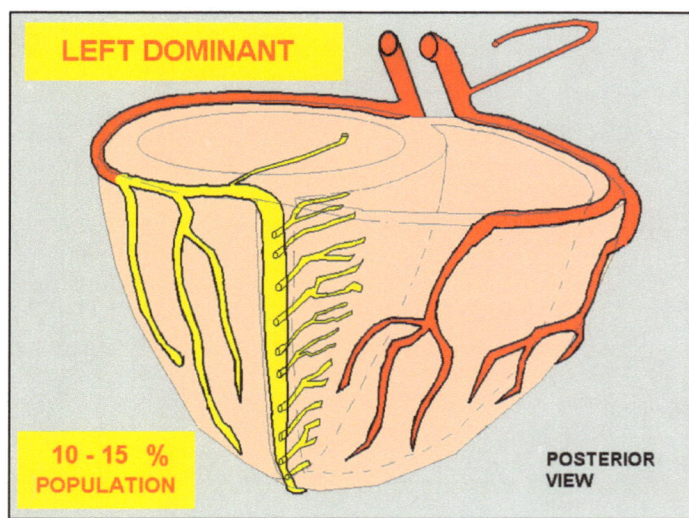

The top left image shows a "cutaway" view of the ventricles. We placed a "blockage" in the circumflex artery to illustrate how a blockage would cut off the blood flow to the *lateral wall, posterior wall*, and *inferior wall*.   The above right image, which shows a 3-dimensional view of the left and right ventricles, shows the distal circumflex branch (in yellow). As you can see, the entire posterior wall, and the inferior wall, is served by a dominant circumflex artery. (See Case Study 9 on page 218).

At the top of the next page, we show two images which illustrate how an *extreme dominant RCA* supplies blood to all of the posterior wall, and the inferior wall.

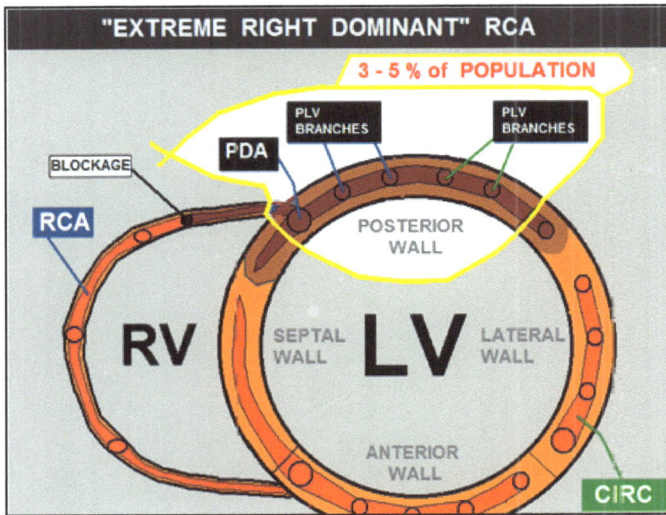

"EXTREME RIGHT DOMINANT" RCA

3 - 5 % of POPULATION

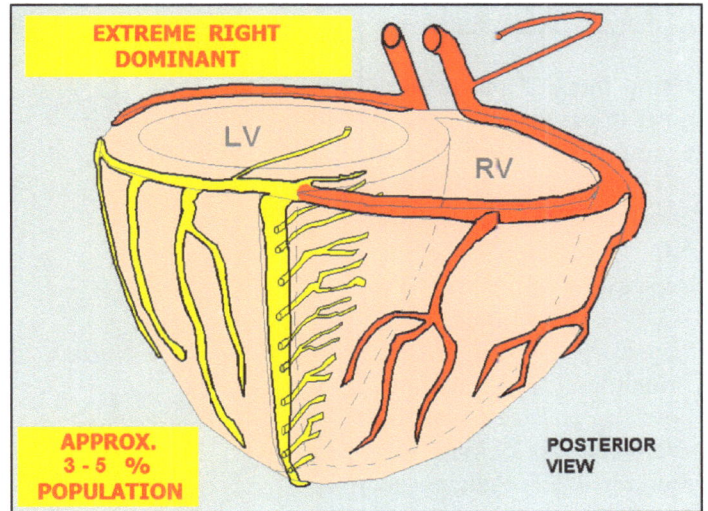

EXTREME RIGHT DOMINANT

APPROX. 3 - 5 % POPULATION

POSTERIOR VIEW

We've placed a "blockage" in the distal RCA (top left image), to illustrate how this could affect the entire posterior wall in patients who have an "abnormally large" RCA (see Case Study 8, page 212). In the above right image, you can appreciate how this "abnormally dominant" RCA (shaded yellow) supplies blood to nearly *all* of the *inferior* and *posterior* surfaces.

Hopefully we have provided an adequate explanation of how different coronary artery anatomical variations can lead to inferior wall MI presenting with so many variations. Our next goal is to demonstrate how you can quickly determine "which type" of inferior wall MI your patient is presenting with. Being able to determine your patient's zone-of-infarct is important. This information will assist you with anticipating complications your patient may experience throughout the course of his/her care, and can aid you in determining the most appropriate course of therapy.

To quickly determine the extent of injury in patients presenting with inferior wall MI, you should implement the "3 Step Process," described in the diagram below:

The 3 Step Process involves carefully scrutinizing the ECG for:

- *Reciprocal ST depression* in leads **V1-V3** signifies Posterior Wall MI
- *ST elevation in leads I, aVL, V5-V6* indicates Lateral Wall MI. ST elevation in Leads I and aVL favors occlusion in the circumflex artery.
- *ST elevation in leads V4R, V5R, and V6R*. These leads are not part of the 12 Lead ECG. You must reposition the ECG leads on the right side of the patient's chest, as shown on page 43. ST elevation in these leads signifies Right Ventricular MI, and is consistent with occlusion in the Right Coronary Artery.

The MANY FACES of INFERIOR MI ...

☞ WHEN YOU OBSERVE AN INFERIOR WALL MI (S-T ELVATION LEADS II, III, and AVF) ... ALWAYS LOOK FOR THE FOLLOWING INDICATORS TO ASSESS THE EXTENT OF THE MI:

INDICATOR	COMPLICATION
1. S-T DEPRESSION IN THE V-LEADS (PREDOMINANTLY V1 - V3)	➡ POSTERIOR WALL MI
2. S-T ELEVATION IN LEADS V5, V6, LEAD I, and AVL	➡ LATERAL WALL MI
3. S-T ELEVATION in LEADS V3r - V6r (RIGHT-SIDED EKG)	➡ R. VENTRICULAR MI

Instead of implementing the "3 Step Process" described above, you can obtain an 18 lead ECG, as shown on page 44. In addition to providing the information that the 3 Step Process does, the 18 Lead ECG supplies you with Posterior Leads (V7-V9), which directly view the posterior wall. ST elevation in leads V7 – V9 indicates Posterior Wall MI.

STEP 1:

Using the ECG from our current case study as an example, we first rule out Posterior Wall MI by confirming that there is NO reciprocal ST depression in Leads V1-V3. (See page 41, "Basic 12 Lead ECG Principles," to review how the posterior wall is evaluated by looking for reciprocal ST changes in Leads V1 – V3)

In this case study, the lack of ST Depression rules out posterior wall involvement – at least at the current time.

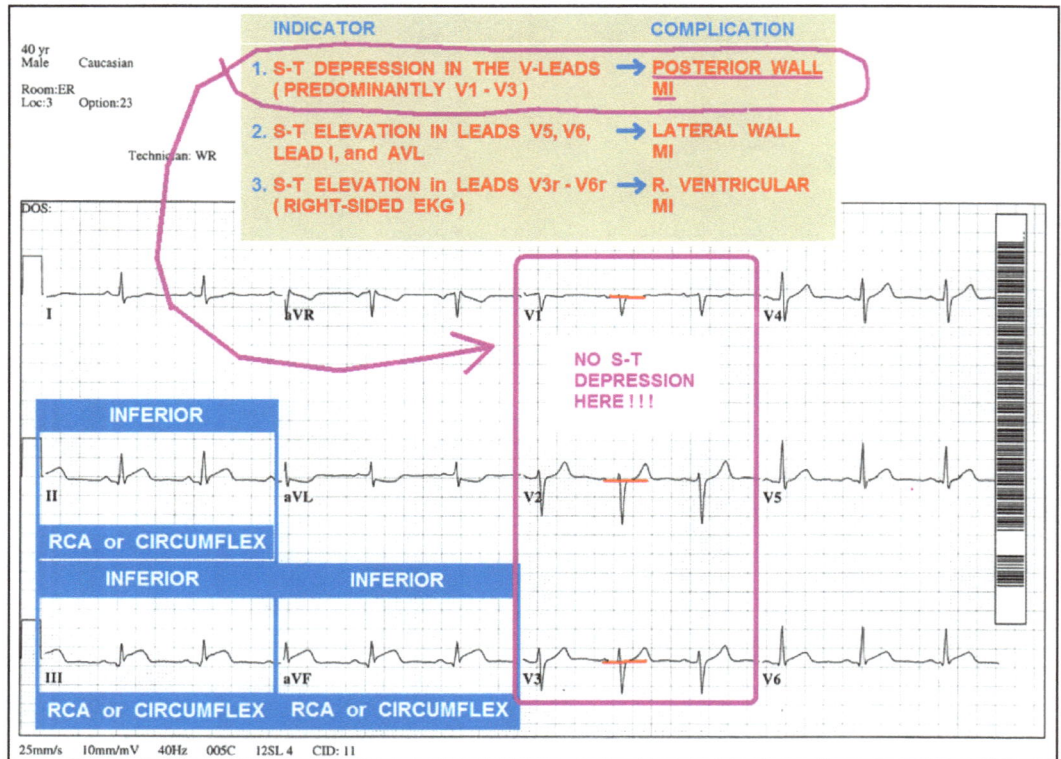

Be sure to obtain **serial ECGs**; as is true of any acute MI, the zone of infarction could extend. Subsequent ECGs could show the development of ST depression in the precordial leads, which would indicate that our patient's MI has extended to the posterior wall.

STEP 2:

When we evaluate leads I, aVL, V5 and V6, we note ST elevation in V6 only.

Since ST elevation is noted in only one of the four contiguous lateral leads, it is not "considered positive" for lateral MI.

In this ECG, we see ST Depression in Leads I and aVL.

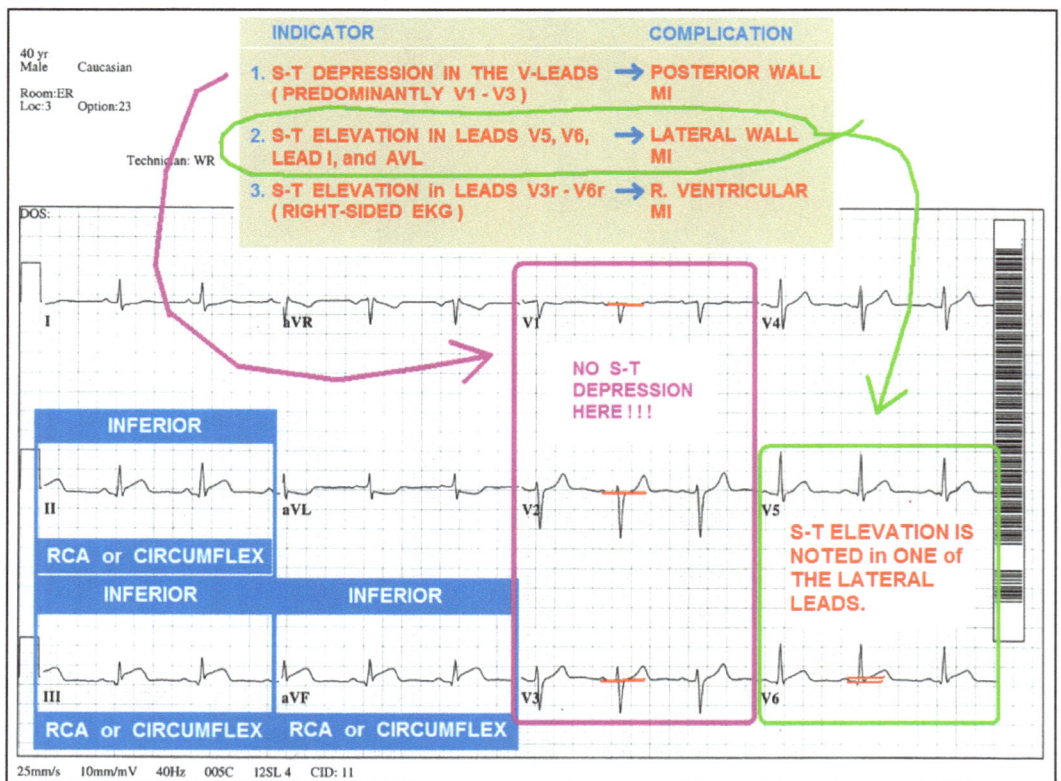

STEP 3:

Step 3 is to record a right sided ECG. In this case, a right sided ECG was obtained, but not saved. The right-sided ECG did not show any ST elevation in the right ventricular leads, therefore ruling out right ventricular MI.

Based on the findings of our 3 Step Process, we have ruled out Posterior, Lateral, and Right Ventricular Wall MI. This patient was taken to the Cath Lab, where the following images were obtained:

99 % OCCLUSION of MID - DOMINANT RIGHT CORONARY ARTERY

The image to the left shows the location of the patient's lesion, located in the mid-right coronary artery. As you can see, the blockage resulted in a sub-total occlusion. In this case, the patient was treated with thrombolytic, antiplatelet and anticoagulation therapy prior to being transferred to a hospital capable of PCI. Medication therapy resolved the patient's symptoms and ST elevation. Cardiac catheterization was performed the following day.

The patient's left coronary artery system is shown to the right. His arteries are unusually small, with diffuse plaque build-up throughout.

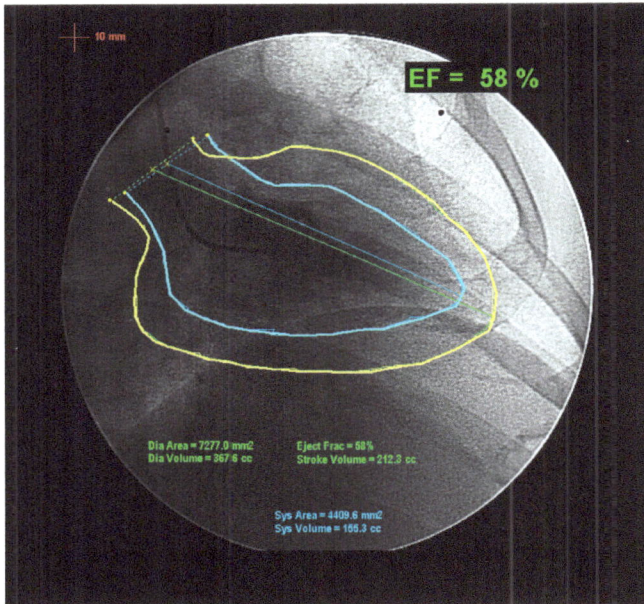

LEFT CORONARY ARTERY VASCULATURE: DIFFUSE PLAQUE, NO FOCAL LESIONS

EF = 58 %

Dia Area = 7277.0 mm2
Dia Volume = 367.6 cc
Eject Frac = 58%
Stroke Volume = 212.3 cc
Sys Area = 4409.6 mm2
Sys Volume = 155.3 cc

The patient's left ventricular angiogram shows his ejection fraction (EF) is preserved, at 58%. The normal range is 55-70%.

Case Study contribution by John Toole, MD, FACC

CASE STUDY 7 - STEMI

CHIEF COMPLAINT and SIGNIFICANT HISTORY:

46 yr. old MALE arrives in ER, C/O SUDDEN ONSET OF CHEST PRESSURE 45 MINUTES AGO. PAIN IS CONSTANT, PRESSURE-LIKE, AND NOT EFFECTED BY POSITION, MOVEMENT or DEEP INSPIRATION. ALSO C/O D.I.B.

RISK FACTOR PROFILE:

- 💣 **CURRENT CIGARTTE SMOKER x 18 YEARS**
- 💣 **HYPERTENSION**
- 💣 **HIGH LDL CHOLESTEROL**

PHYSICAL EXAM: Patient is alert & oriented x 4, skin warm, dry, color normal. Non-anxious
Lungs clear, normal S1, S2. No JVD, No ankle edema.

VITAL SIGNS: BP: 136/88   P: 88   R: 20   SAO2: 100% on 4 LPM O2

LABS: TROPONIN: < .04

QUADRAD OF ACS CHECKLIST

- ☑ **SYMPTOMS of ACS**
  - ✔ ◆ TYPICAL ACS - eg:
  - ◆ ATYPICAL ACS - eg:
- ☑ **ECG ABNORMALITIES**
  - ✔ ◆ ST ELEVATION (J POINT plus 40 ms)
  - ◆ HYPERACUTE T WAVES - and/or -
  - ◆ NEW or PRESUMABLY NEW LBBB
  - ◆ ST DEPRESSION (>0.5 mm @ J POINT) and/or
  - ◆ INVERTED or BIPHASIC T WAVES and/or
  - ◆ DYNAMIC ST SEGMENT and/or T WAVE CHANGES IN SERIAL EKGs
- ☑ **RISK FACTORS - 3 or more**
  - ◆ FAMILY HISTORY
  - ◆ DIABETES
  - ✔ ◆ ↑ LDL and/or ↓ HDL
  - ✔ ◆ SMOKING
  - ◆ AGE: 65 or MORE
  - ✔ ◆ HYPERTENSION
- ☐ **CARDIAC MARKERS**
  - ◆ ELEVATED TROPONIN and/or CK/MB

3 **TOTAL**

SUSPECTED ACUTE MI:

INITIAL MANAGEMENT

- **VITAL SIGNS**

- **"O.M.I."**
  - Oxygen
  - Monitor (ecg)
  - IV   (plus draw lab samples)

- **12 LEAD ECG**
  Obtain and interpret within 10 minutes of patient's arrival.

- **"M.O.N.A."**
  - Morphine
  - Oxygen (if not already done)
  - Nitroglycerin
  - Aspirin

- **RAPID, FOCUSED ASSESSMENT**

- **HEART / LUNG SOUNDS**

- **SEND LAB SAMPLES:**
  - Cardiac Markers
  - Electrolytes
  - Coagulation Studies

46 yr		Vent. rate	82	BPM
Male	Caucasian	PR interval	168	ms
		QRS duration	96	ms
		QT/QTc	384/448	ms
Loc:3	Option:23	P–R–T axes	76 81	88

☞ EVALUATE EKG for indicators of ACS:

- ST SEGMENT ELEVATION / DEPRESSION
- HYPERACUTE T WAVES
- CONVEX ST SEGMENTS
- OTHER ST SEGMENT / T WAVE ABNORMALITIES

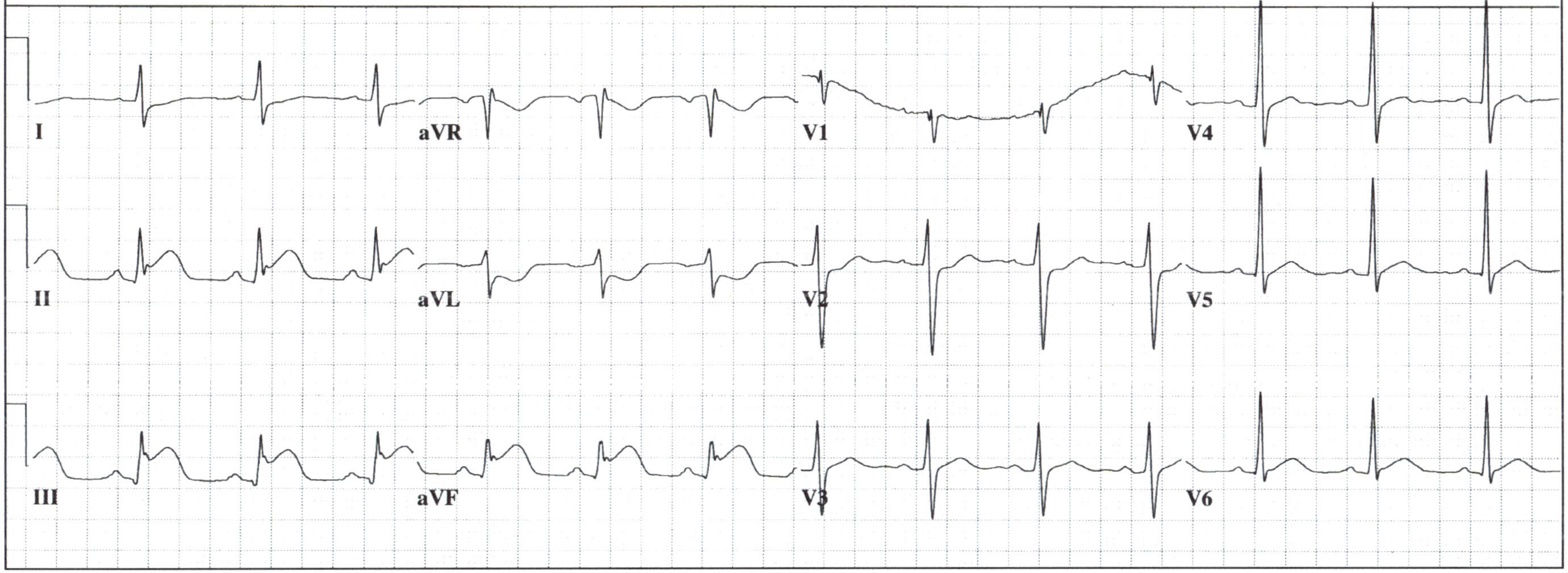

I   aVR   V1   V4
II   aVL   V2   V5
III   aVF   V3   V6

CASE STUDY QUESTIONS:

NOTE LEADS WITH ST ELEVATION:

NOTE LEADS WITH ST DEPRESSION:

WHAT IS THE SUSPECTED DIAGNOSIS ?

WHAT IS THE "CULPRIT ARTERY" – if applicable ?

LIST ANY CRITICAL STRUCTURES COMPROMISED:

LIST ANY POTENTIAL COMPLICATIONS:

Like the previous case study, primary ST segment elevation is noted in the INFERIOR leads, II, III, and aVF.

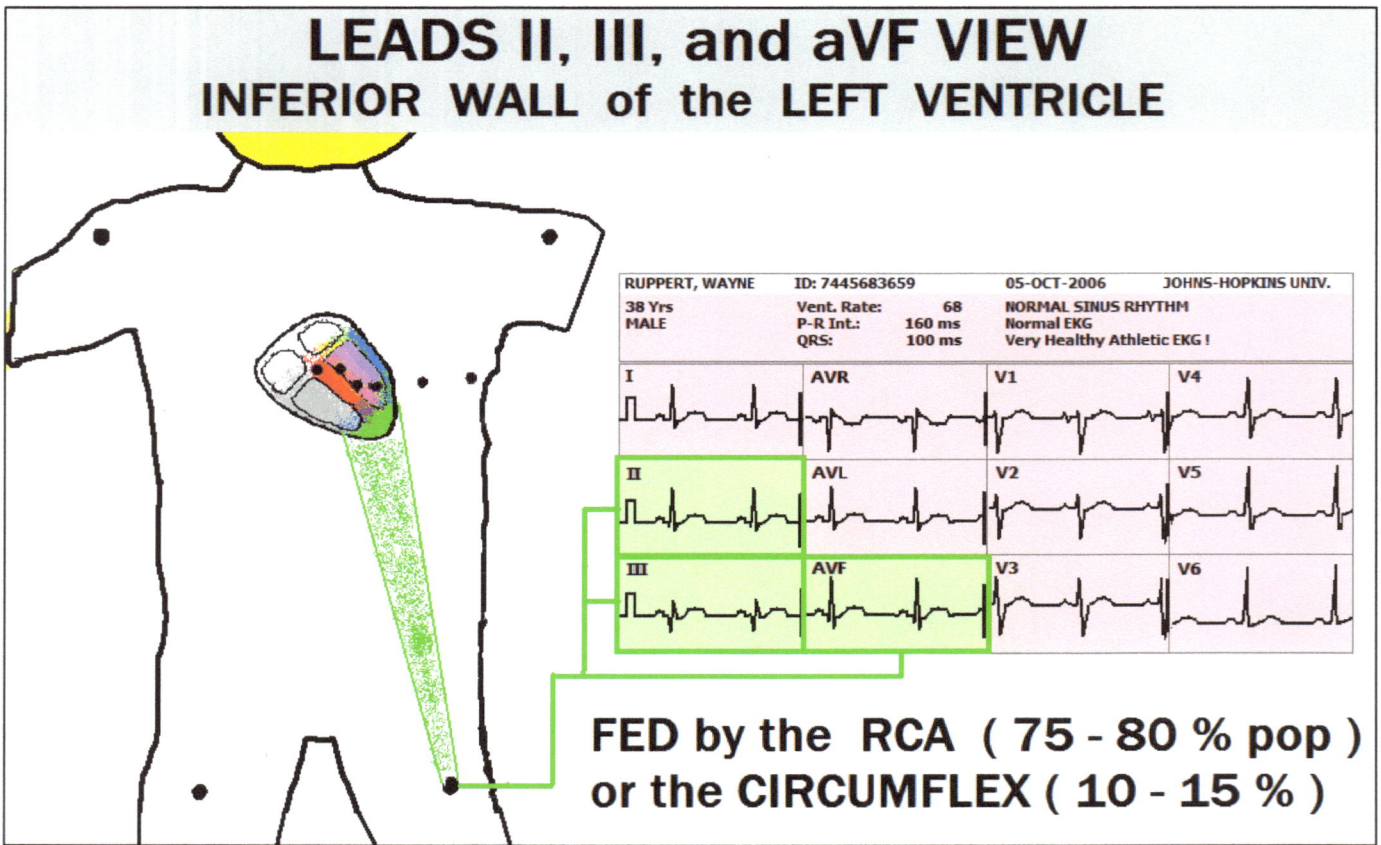

LEADS II, III, and aVF VIEW
INFERIOR WALL of the LEFT VENTRICLE

| RUPPERT, WAYNE | ID: 7445683659 | 05-OCT-2006 | JOHNS-HOPKINS UNIV. |

38 Yrs
MALE

Vent. Rate: 68
P-R Int.: 160 ms
QRS: 100 ms

NORMAL SINUS RHYTHM
Normal EKG
Very Healthy Athletic EKG !

FED by the RCA (75 - 80 % pop)
or the CIRCUMFLEX (10 - 15 %)

Our next priority regarding the ECG is to rule out *posterior, lateral,* and *right ventricular infarction.*

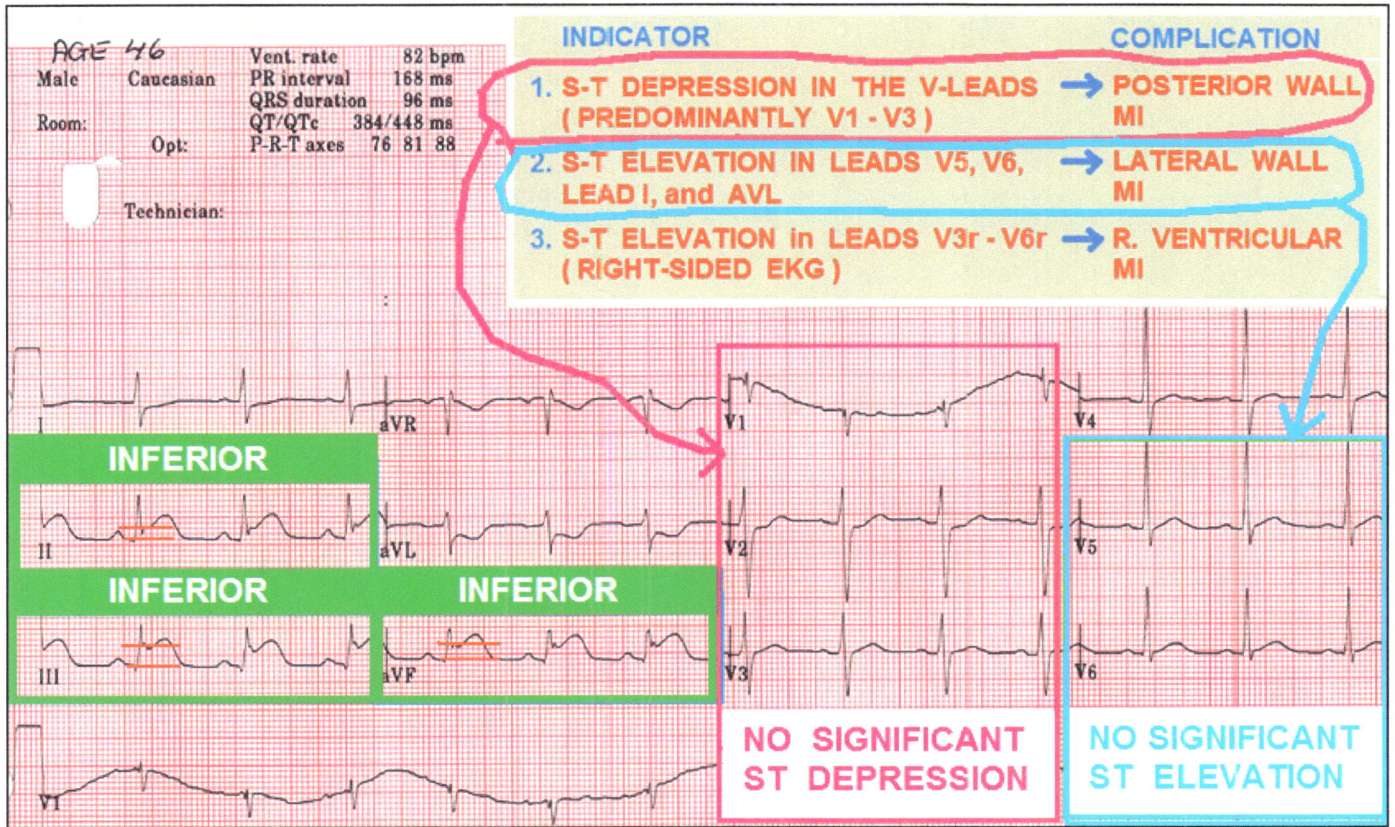

Based on the above ECG findings, neither *posterior* nor *lateral* wall infarction are present. The next priority is to obtain a right sided ECG to rule out *right ventricular infarction*.

TO OBTAIN A RIGHT-SIDED ECG:

To evaluate the right ventricle for signs of ACS, simply move leads V4, V5, and V6 from their position on the left chest wall to the "mirror-opposite" location on the right chest wall. The image to the right depicts the appropriate lead placement. Lead V4r is located at the 5th intercostal space at the mid-clavicular line. V5r is located on the same plane as V4r, only at the anterior axillary line, and V6r on the same plane, at the mid-axillary line.

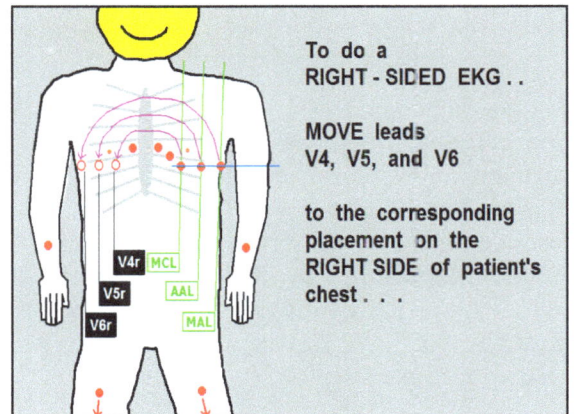

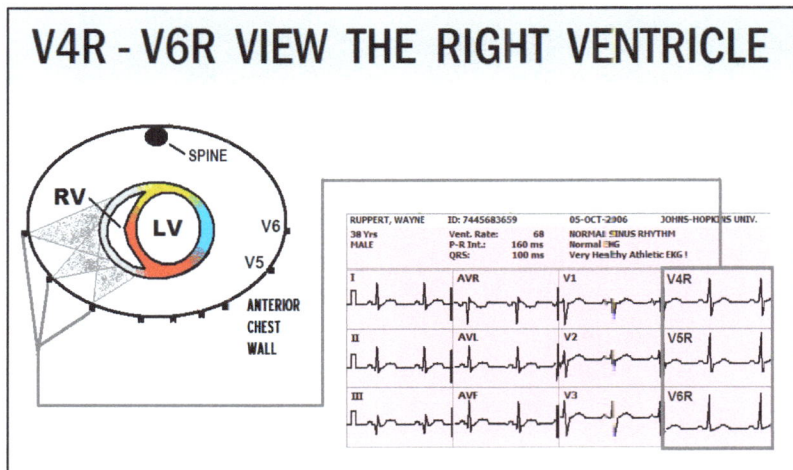

The image to the left illustrates how the right ventricular leads "see" the right ventricle.

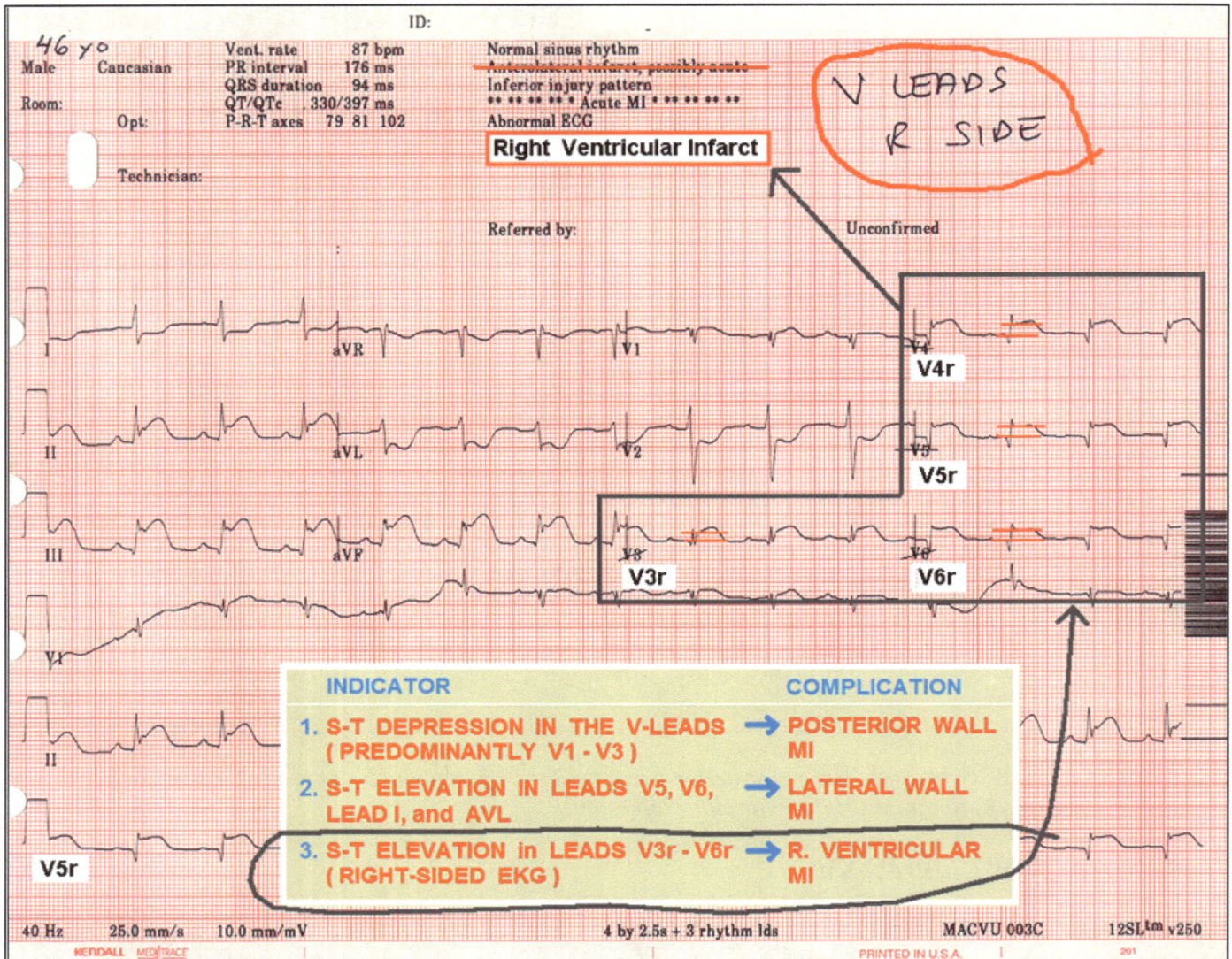

ECG printout annotations:

ID:

46 yo
Male   Caucasian
Room:
Opt:
Technician:

Vent. rate   87 bpm
PR interval   176 ms
QRS duration   94 ms
QT/QTc   330/397 ms
P-R-T axes   79 81 102

Normal sinus rhythm
Anterolateral infarct, possibly acute
Inferior injury pattern
** ** ** ** * Acute MI * ** ** ** **
Abnormal ECG

Right Ventricular Infarct

Referred by: Unconfirmed

V LEADS R SIDE

V4r
V5r
V3r   V6r

V5r

INDICATOR		COMPLICATION
1. S-T DEPRESSION IN THE V-LEADS (PREDOMINANTLY V1 - V3)	→	POSTERIOR WALL MI
2. S-T ELEVATION IN LEADS V5, V6, LEAD I, and AVL	→	LATERAL WALL MI
3. S-T ELEVATION in LEADS V3r - V6r (RIGHT-SIDED EKG)	→	R. VENTRICULAR MI

40 Hz   25.0 mm/s   10.0 mm/mV   4 by 2.5s + 3 rhythm lds   MACVU 003C   12SL™ v250

KENDALL MEDITRACE   PRINTED IN U.S.A.   201

For our right-sided ECG, I elected to include V3R. As you can see, V3R through V6R show profound ST segment elevation, indicating **Right Ventricular Myocardial Infarction** (RVMI). Note the computer printout says: "Anterior-Lateral Infarct, Possibly Acute." I had to cross it out, and write "Right Sided ECG" at the top of the page, and re-label leads V3R through V6R. *The ECG machine does not know we've repositioned the leads!*

Inferior-right ventricular MI is almost exclusively caused by an obstruction in the *proximal right coronary artery,* as shown in the illustration to the right.[58]

This information proved extremely valuable for those us caring for this patient in the emergency department: as is true with most RVMI patients, he experienced the typical sensitivity to nitrates. His initial blood pressure was 136/88. Less than one minute after the administration of ONE squirt of gr. 1/150th nitroglycerin spray, his blood pressure dropped to 60/38, pulse rate 110. His skin became pale, cool and diaphoretic, and he began to vomit.

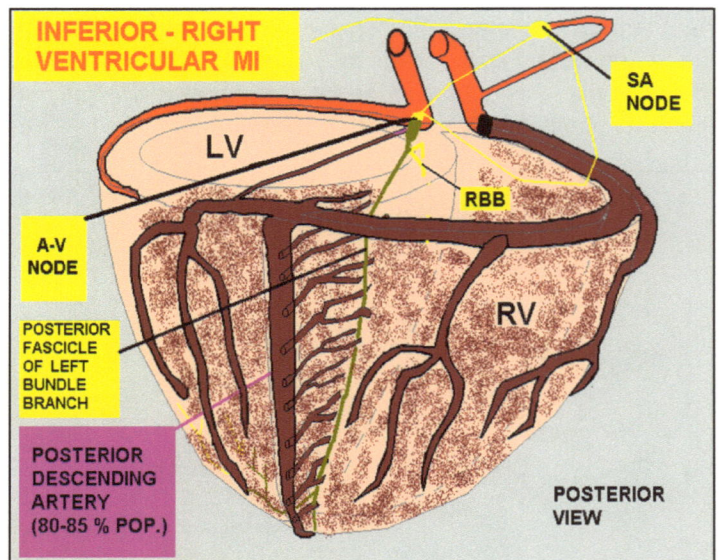

INFERIOR - RIGHT VENTRICULAR MI
SA NODE
LV
RBB
A-V NODE
POSTERIOR FASCICLE OF LEFT BUNDLE BRANCH
RV
POSTERIOR DESCENDING ARTERY (80-85 % POP.)
POSTERIOR VIEW

---

[58] Wung, et. al., from the University of Arizona, published in the Journal of Electrocardiography, Volume 39, Issue 3, pp 275 – 281

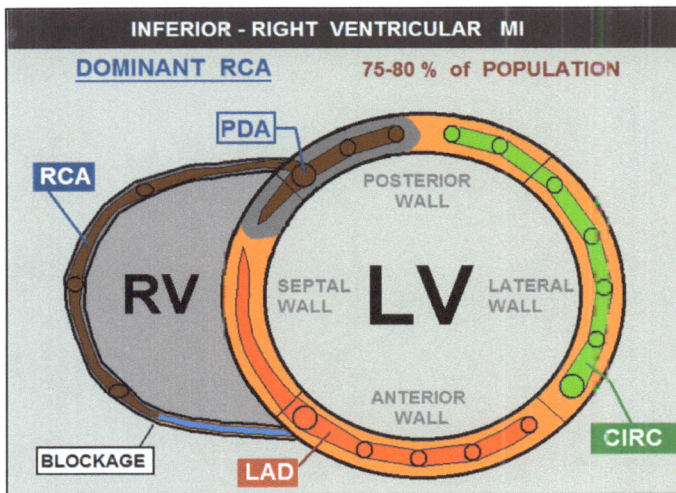

INFERIOR - RIGHT VENTRICULAR MI

DOMINANT RCA   75-80 % of POPULATION

RCA · PDA · POSTERIOR WALL · RV · LV · SEPTAL WALL · LATERAL WALL · ANTERIOR WALL · CIRC · BLOCKAGE · LAD

In typical cases of Inferior-Right Ventricular MI, the patient's LV function is usually normal or near-normal. The sudden drop in cardiac output after the administration of vasodilators is caused by a combination of venous pooling plus failure of the right ventricle to pump blood adequately to the lungs. In RVMI, nearly all of the right ventricle's blood supply has been cutoff, while only a relatively small section of the left ventricle is affected, as shown in the illustration to the left. Recall that when oxygen and glucose supplies are cut off from cardiac muscle cells, they respond by converting to anaerobic metabolism, and stop contracting.

When a large region of the right ventricle stops contracting effectively, blood is no longer being pumped to the lungs; only "backpressure" from left ventricular outflow keeps blood moving through the venous system and back to the heart. So when vasodilators such as nitroglycerin or morphine are given, veins suddenly dilate, resulting in a decrease in blood returning to the right side of the heart. It's a vicious cause-and-effect cycle: less blood getting to the lungs means less blood coming back to the left side of the heart which results in decreased left ventricular filling, which leads to a drop in left ventricular output. And suddenly you have a patient who is hypotensive and in shock.

Treatment for hypotension in patients with Inferior-RVMI, especially when resulting from administration of a vasodilator, is IV fluid administration. As seen in the algorithm to the right, when hypotension is seen in acute MI, you must first determine if pulmonary edema is present. Ideally this is done by chest X-ray, but in the acute MI setting, auscultation of lung sounds should provide sufficient information.

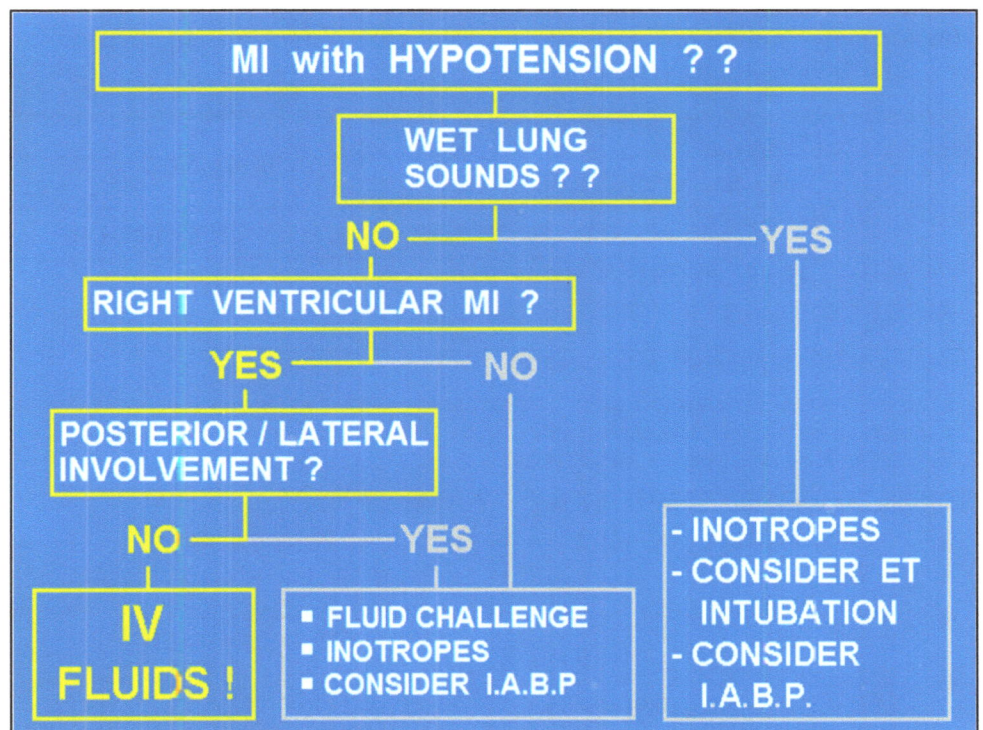

MI with HYPOTENSION ? ?

WET LUNG SOUNDS ? ?

NO ———— YES

RIGHT VENTRICULAR MI ?

YES ——— NO

POSTERIOR / LATERAL INVOLVEMENT ?

NO ——— YES

IV FLUIDS !

- FLUID CHALLENGE
- INOTROPES
- CONSIDER I.A.B.P

- INOTROPES
- CONSIDER ET INTUBATION
- CONSIDER I.A.B.P.

In cases of Inferior-RVMI, there is usually good LV function and pulmonary edema is not an issue. In these cases, IV fluid challenges, such as with Normal Saline (0.9% solution) is indicated and very effective in restoring adequate blood pressure.

It's a good practice to always evaluate lung sounds to rule out pulmonary edema prior to administering IV fluid boluses. In our case study, our patient was given a 300cc rapid fluid bolus of intravenous normal saline. His vital signs were reassessed: his blood pressure had risen to 88/42, pulse rate 96; still not acceptable. His lung sounds were reevaluated, and found to be clear. An additional IV fluid bolus of 200cc of NS was given. Repeat vital signs revealed his BP had risen to 110/60, with his pulse rate 86. At that point, he was taken to the cath lab, where the images on the next page were obtained:

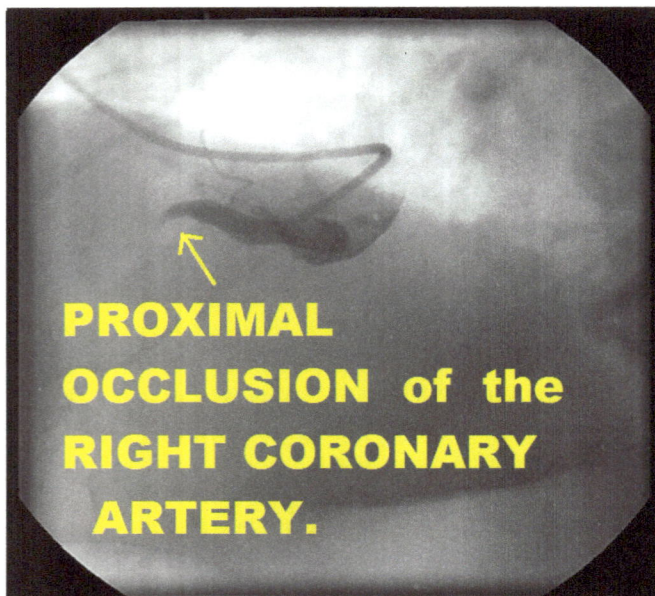

PROXIMAL OCCLUSION of the RIGHT CORONARY ARTERY.

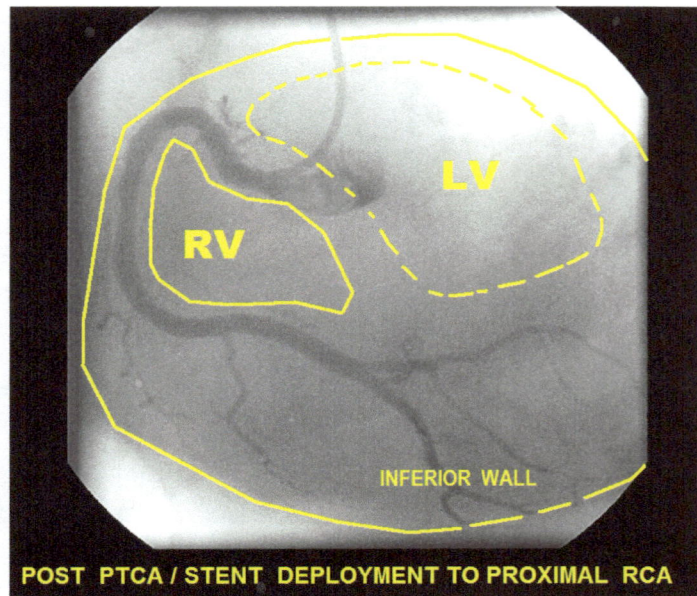

LV

RV

INFERIOR WALL

POST PTCA / STENT DEPLOYMENT TO PROXIMAL RCA

The above images show pre- and post-PTCA and stent deployment to the proximal right coronary artery. As these images illustrate, the arterial occlusion affected nearly the entire right ventricle, with only a small region of left ventricular involvement. This patient's RCA is a typical dominant right coronary artery that is found in approximately 75-80% of the population. His clinical presentation, response to medical therapy, and outcome are typical for Inferior-Right Ventricular MI.

CASE STUDY SUMMARY

ST ELEVATION: II, III, aVF , V4R - V6R	ST DEPRESSION: I, aVL

SUSPECTED DIAGNOSIS: ACUTE INFERIOR - RIGHT VENTRICULAR WALL MI

SUSPECTED "CULPRIT ARTERY" (if applicable):

RIGHT CORONARY ARTERY - DOMINANT

IMMEDIATE CONCERNS FOR ALL STEMI PATIENTS:

- BE PREPARED TO MANAGE SUDDEN CARDIAC ARREST (PRIMARY V - FIB / V- TACH, BRADYCARDIAS / HEART BLOCKS)
- STAT REPERFUSION THERAPY: THROMBOLYTICS vs. CARDIAC CATHETERIZATION and PCI
- CONSIDER NEEDS FOR ANTI-PLATELET and ANTI-COAGULATION THERAPY

CRITICAL STRUCTURES COMPROMISED:	POTENTIAL COMPLICATIONS:	POSSIBLE CRITICAL INTERVENTIONS:
15-25% OF THE LV MUSCLE MASS	SLIGHT POSSIBILITY OF MILD LV FAILURE.	FLUID CHALLENGE INOTROPIC AGENTS
100% OF THE RIGHT VENTRICLE	EXTREME SENSITIVITY TO NITRATES AND OPIATES	FLUID BOLUSES
SINUS NODE ARTERY SUPPLIED BY RCA 55% of Pop.	BRADYCARDIA ASYSTOLE	ATROPINE TRANSCUTANEOUS PACING
AV NODAL ARTERY SUPPLIED BY DOMINANT ARTERY (RCA or Circ) IN MOST PATIENTS	AV NODAL BLOCKS: - 1 DEGREE - 2nd DEGREE type I, II - 3rd DEGREE	ATROPINE TRANSCUTANEOUS PACING

Case Study contribution by James Irwin, MD, FACC and Matthew Glover, MD, FACC

EVOLVING RIGHT VENTRICULAR MI results in development of Q waves recorded in the right precordial leads.[59] The ECG below is that of a 64 year old male who presented to the ED after 36 hours of continuous chest pain and dyspnea.

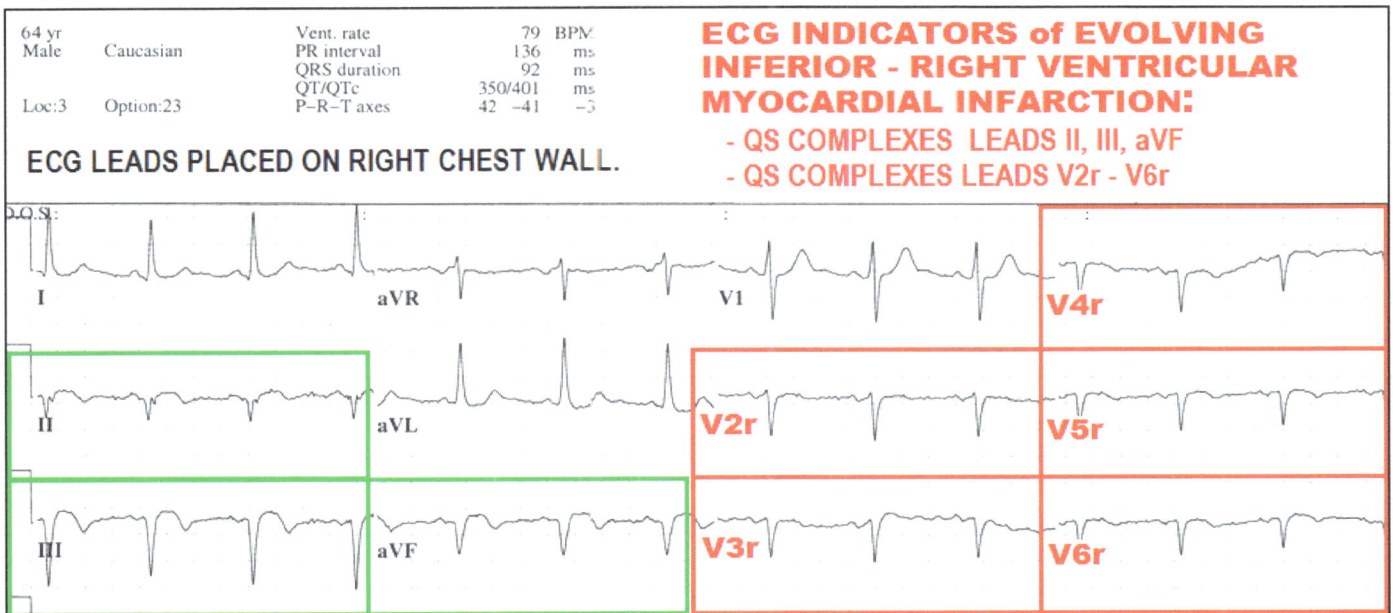

64 yr		Vent. rate	79	BPM
Male	Caucasian	PR interval	136	ms
		QRS duration	92	ms
		QT/QTc	350/401	ms
Loc:3	Option:23	P–R–T axes	42 –41	–3

ECG LEADS PLACED ON RIGHT CHEST WALL.

ECG INDICATORS of EVOLVING INFERIOR - RIGHT VENTRICULAR MYOCARDIAL INFARCTION:
- QS COMPLEXES LEADS II, III, aVF
- QS COMPLEXES LEADS V2r - V6r

This patient decided to come to the emergency department when his dyspnea became "unbearable." Upon arrival in the ED, his blood pressure was 113/74, pulse rate 80, respiratory rate 28 per minute, with an oxygen saturation of 91%.

His initial ECG showed an almost fully evolved inferior wall MI: QS complexes in leads II, III, and aVF, with residual ST segment elevation. We then obtained the above "right-sided ECG," which demonstrated QS complexes throughout the right ventricle. As is true of most RVMI patients, his BP dropped precipitously when nitroglycerin was administered (BP dropped from 113/74 to 56/32). After clear lungs were auscultated, 700cc of normal saline were required to stabilize his blood pressure.

He was taken to the cardiac catheterization lab where a proximal occlusion of his right coronary artery was discovered. Reperfusion was achieved with PTCA and STENT placement.

☞ *HELPFUL TIP in cases of SUSPECTED AMI:*

DURING EMERGENCY PATIENT EVALUATION with a BEDSIDE ECG MONITOR, USE LEAD MCL-4-R (Modified Chest Lead 4 – Right Precordium) before administration of vasodilator medications:

This is especially true when you implement bedside ECG monitoring using lead II, and ST elevation is observed, an indicator of Inferior Wall STEMI. In events where it is important to rapidly identify the presence of right ventricular MI, you may obtain an ECG tracing of lead V4r. This can be accomplished very quickly in the ED or prehospital setting with a bedside or crash-cart ECG monitor by placing the positive electrode in the V4r position (5th intercostal space, mid-clavicular line on the patient's right precordium), and switching the lead selector to the "lead III" position. This gives you a modified chest lead (MCL) V4r. I have found this technique especially helpful prior to administering the first nitroglycerin tablet. If ST elevation is observed in lead MCL4-R, it indicates the presence of right ventricular MI. As our right ventricular MI case study describes on pages 208 and 209, patients with RVMI suffer precipitous drops in blood pressure when vasodilators are administered.

---

[59] Zehender, M et. al., NEJM 1993; 14: 328: 981-988: "Right Ventricular Infarction as Predictor of Prognosis after AMI"

CASE STUDY 8 - STEMI

CHIEF COMPLAINT and SIGNIFICANT HISTORY:

A 74 y/o MALE arrives via EMS. He complains of "CRUSHING" SUB-STERNAL CHEST PRESSURE with radiation to the SHOULDERS, NECK, and RIGHT ARM.

RISK FACTOR PROFILE:

- 💣 OVER 65 YEARS of AGE
- 💣 HYPERTENSION
- 💣 HIGH LDL CHOLESTEROL

PHYSICAL EXAM: Patient is alert & oriented x 4, ANXIOUS, with COOL, PALE, DIAPHORETIC SKIN. Lung Sounds are CLEAR bilaterally.

VITAL SIGNS: BP: 73/48   P: 70   R: 24   SAO2: 94% on 4 LPM O2

LABS: TROPONIN: < .04

QUADRAD OF ACS CHECKLIST

☑ **SYMPTOMS of ACS**
- ✔️ TYPICAL ACS - eg:
- ◆ ATYPICAL ACS - eg:

☑ **ECG ABNORMALITIES**
- ✔️ ST ELEVATION (J POINT plus 40 ms)
- ◆ HYPERACUTE T WAVES - and/or -
- ◆ NEW or PRESUMABLY NEW LBBB
- ✔️ ST DEPRESSION (>0.5 mm @ J POINT) and/or
- ◆ INVERTED or BIPHASIC T WAVES and/or
- ◆ DYNAMIC ST SEGMENT and/or T WAVE CHANGES IN SERIAL EKGs

☑ **RISK FACTORS - 3 or more**
- ◆ FAMILY HISTORY
- ◆ DIABETES
- ✔️ ↑ LDL and/or ↓ HDL
- ◆ SMOKING
- ✔️ AGE: 65 or MORE
- ✔️ HYPERTENSION

☐ **CARDIAC MARKERS**
- ◆ ELEVATED TROPONIN and/or CK/MB

3 **TOTAL**

During the first few seconds of patient contact, it was evident the patient was in shock: he had cool, pale, diaphoretic skin and was anxious. When patients present in this state of hemodynamic compromise, we must rapidly determine the cause. When patients are conscious and able to answer questions, this makes our job easier: by just asking the right questions, patients will usually tell us what the problem is.

Based on the case study information above, we suspect a cardiac component to our patient's shock-like presentation.

We quickly placed the patient on O2, obtained a 12 Lead ECG, vital signs, started an IV and obtained an initial set of labs.

SHOCK ASSESSMENT

LOC:	ANXIOUS RESTLESS LETHARGIC UNCONSCIOUS	AWAKE ALERT & ORIENTED
SKIN:	PALE / ASHEN CYANOTIC COOL DIAPHORETIC	NORMAL HUE WARM DRY
BREATHING:	TACHYPNEA	NORMAL
PULSE:	WEAK / THREADY TOO FAST or SLOW	STRONG
STATUS:	💣 SHOCK 💣	NORMAL

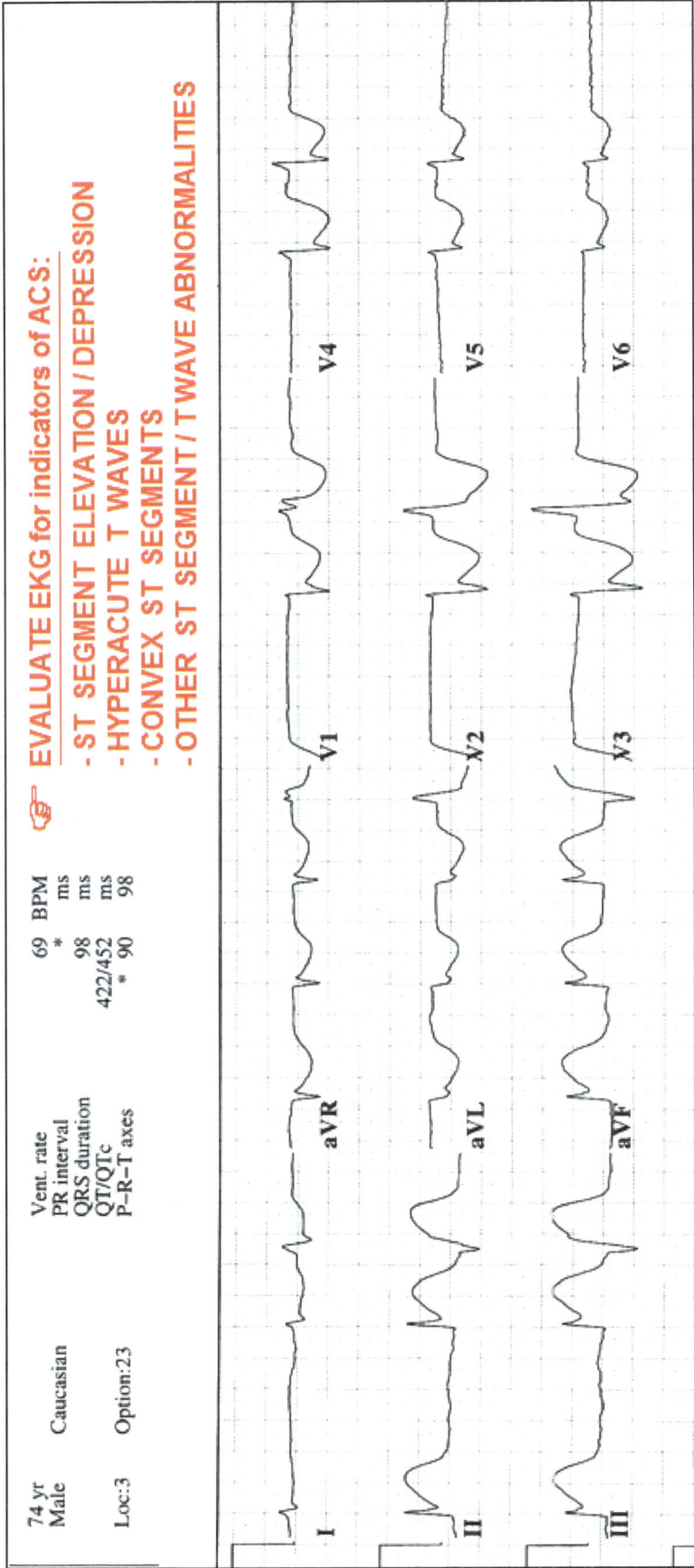

74 yr Male	Caucasian		Vent. rate	69	BPM
			PR interval	*	ms
Loc:3	Option:23		QRS duration	98	ms
			QT/QTc	422/452	ms
			P–R–T axes	* 90	98

☞ EVALUATE EKG for indicators of ACS:

- ST SEGMENT ELEVATION / DEPRESSION
- HYPERACUTE T WAVES
- CONVEX ST SEGMENTS
- OTHER ST SEGMENT / T WAVE ABNORMALITIES

Leads: I, aVR, V1, V4 / II, aVL, V2, V5 / III, aVF, V3, V6

CASE STUDY QUESTIONS:

NOTE LEADS WITH ST ELEVATION: NOTE LEADS WITH ST DEPRESSION:

WHAT IS THE SUSPECTED DIAGNOSIS ?

WHAT IS THE "CULPRIT ARTERY" -- if applicable ?

LIST ANY CRITICAL STRUCTURES COMPROMISED: LIST ANY POTENTIAL COMPLICATIONS:

213

74 yr
Male   Caucasian

Loc:3   Option:23

Vent. rate   69   BPM
PR interval   *   ms
QRS duration   98   ms
QT/QTc   422/452   ms
P–R–T axes   * 90   98

*** Acute MI ***
INFERIOR-POSTERIOR injury pattern

ST SEGMENT ELEVATION
ST SEGMENT DEPRESSION

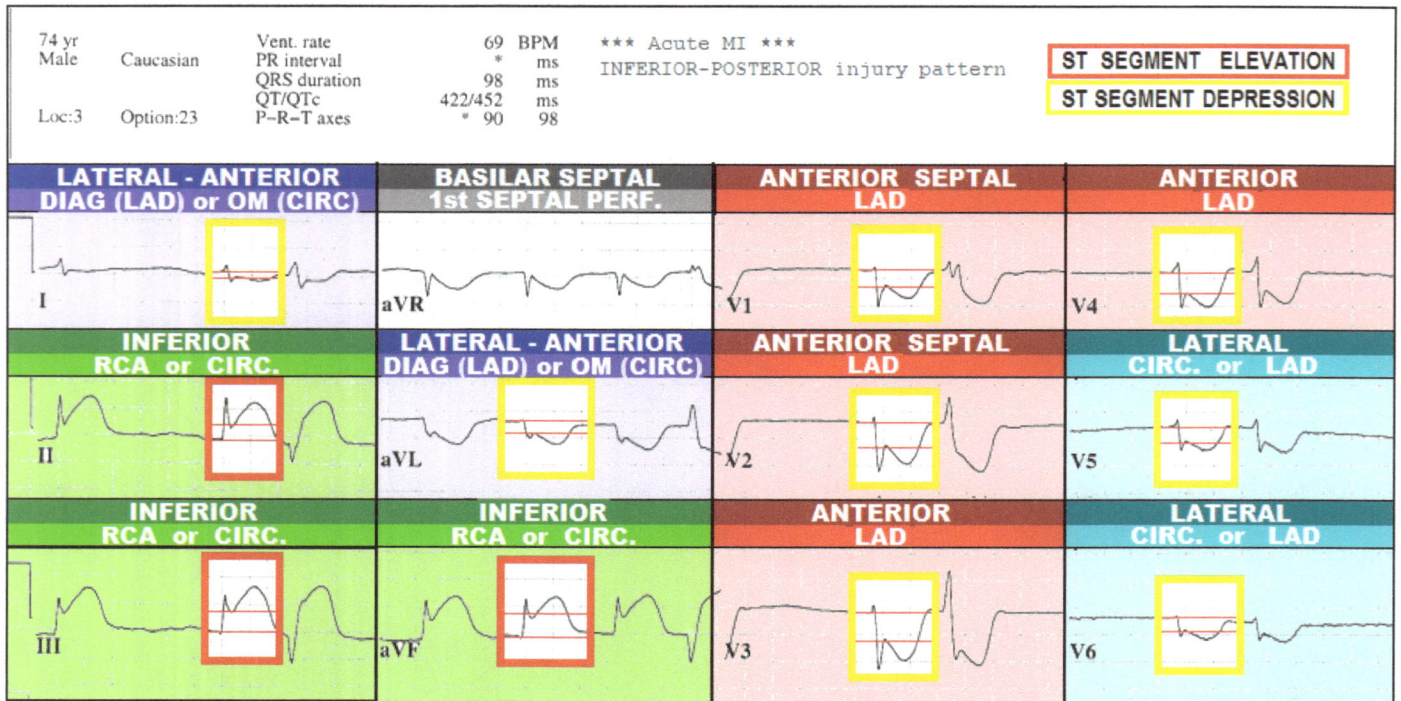

LATERAL - ANTERIOR DIAG (LAD) or OM (CIRC)	BASILAR SEPTAL 1st SEPTAL PERF.	ANTERIOR SEPTAL LAD	ANTERIOR LAD
INFERIOR RCA or CIRC.	LATERAL - ANTERIOR DIAG (LAD) or OM (CIRC)	ANTERIOR SEPTAL LAD	LATERAL CIRC. or LAD
INFERIOR RCA or CIRC.	INFERIOR RCA or CIRC.	ANTERIOR LAD	LATERAL CIRC. or LAD

Significant ST segment elevation is noted in leads II, III, and aVF, which view the inferior wall of the left ventricle.

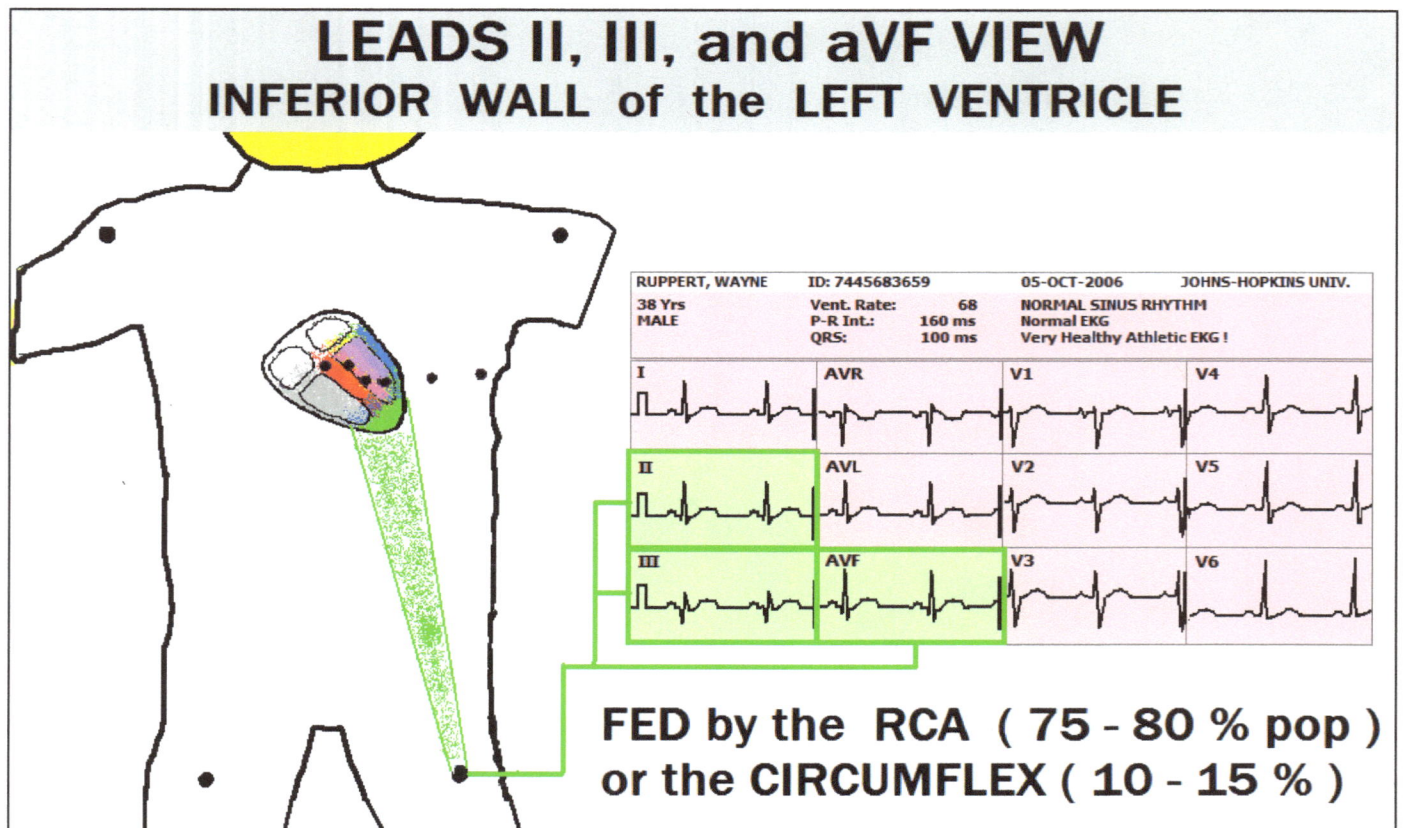

LEADS II, III, and aVF VIEW
INFERIOR WALL of the LEFT VENTRICLE

RUPPERT, WAYNE   ID: 7445683659   05-OCT-2006   JOHNS-HOPKINS UNIV.
38 Yrs   Vent. Rate: 68   NORMAL SINUS RHYTHM
MALE   P-R Int.:   160 ms   Normal EKG
QRS: 100 ms   Very Healthy Athletic EKG !

FED by the RCA (75 - 80 % pop)
or the CIRCUMFLEX (10 - 15 %)

Due to the presence of ST elevation in leads II, III, and aVF, acute inferior wall MI is suspected. As we have previously stated, when acute inferior wall MI is noted on the ECG, our next priority is to rule out *posterior, lateral,* and ***right ventricular MI.*** To do this, we will implement the "3 Step Process" utilized in the two previous case studies.

74 yr		Vent. rate	69	BPM
Male	Caucasian	PR interval	*	ms
		QRS duration	98	ms
		QT/QTc	422/452	ms
Loc:3	Option:23	P–R–T axes	* 90	98

R SIDED EKG was obtained, NO ST ELEVATION was noted in RV Leads

INDICATOR		COMPLICATION
1. S-T DEPRESSION IN THE V-LEADS (PREDOMINANTLY V1 - V3)	→	POSTERIOR WALL MI
2. S-T ELEVATION IN LEADS V5, V6, LEAD I, and AVL	→	LATERAL WALL MI
3. S-T ELEVATION in LEADS V3r - V6r (RIGHT-SIDED EKG)	→	R. VENTRICULAR MI

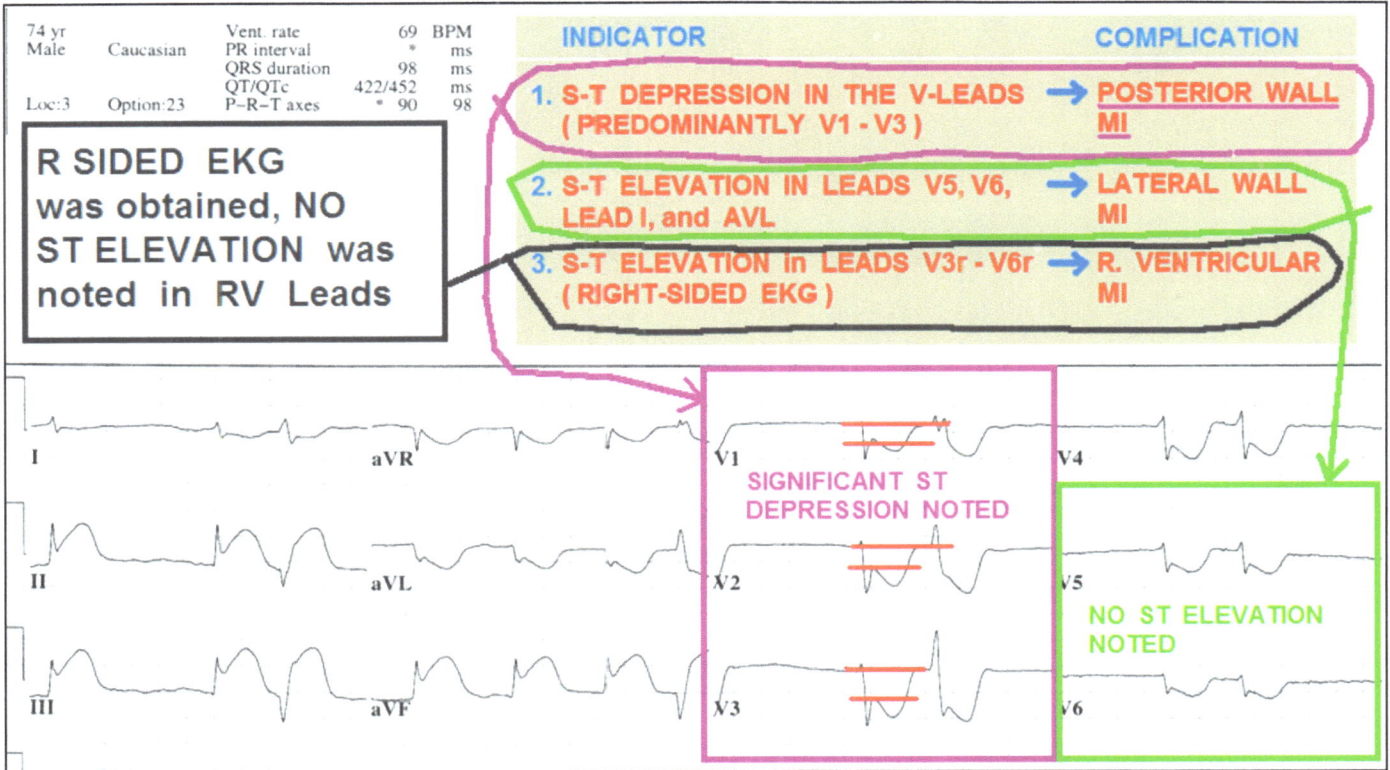

I aVR V1 V4

SIGNIFICANT ST DEPRESSION NOTED

II aVL V2 V5

NO ST ELEVATION NOTED

III aVF V3 V6

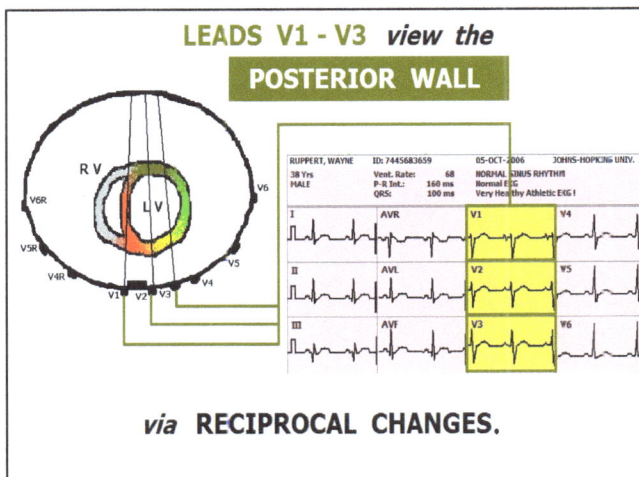

LEADS V1 - V3 *view the* **POSTERIOR WALL**

via **RECIPROCAL CHANGES.**

Based on the results of our 3 Step Process, we have identified our patient's ECG diagnosis as "inferior-posterior wall MI."

Recall from our "Basic 12 Lead ECG Concepts" chapter, on page 41, that leads V1 – V3 "see" the posterior wall via reciprocal changes.

Inferior-Posterior MI affects approximately 25-45% of the LV muscle mass, and often causes more *left ventricular dysfunction* than incidents of isolated Inferior Wall MI. With a greater region of LV muscle impairment, patients are more likely to exhibit *hypotension* and *pulmonary edema*. The patient in this case study presented with hypotension, a typical finding in patients experiencing Posterior Wall MI.

Significant Posterior Wall MI often results from the occlusion of either a *dominant circumflex artery* (above left), or an *"extreme dominant" RCA* (above right). As is depicted in the above images, occlusion of either a dominant circumflex or extreme dominant RCA can affect enough LV muscle to result in *clinically significant LV pump failure*.

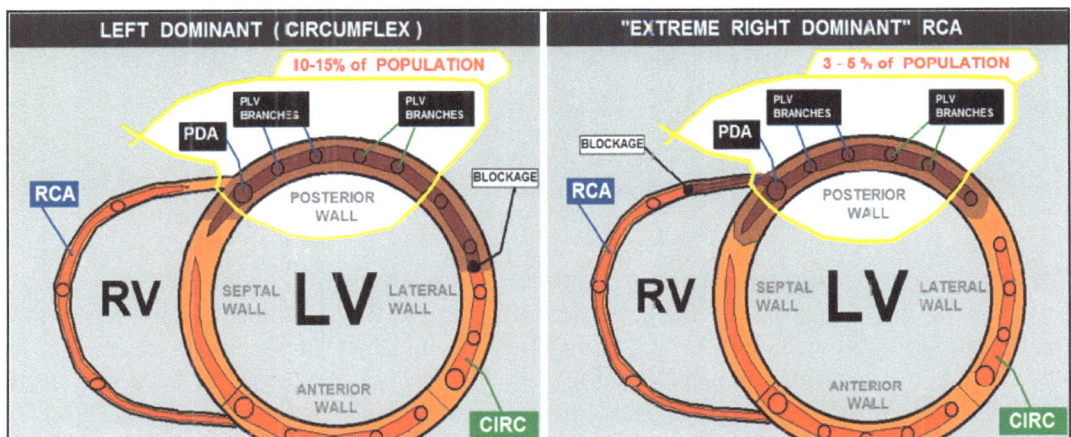

Another relevant point in this case study is the presence of either sinus node and/or AV node failure. As seen in the patient's rhythm strip, there are frequent "skipped beats" noted. Without discernable P waves, it is difficult to determine if we're looking at a 2nd Degree type I heart block (Wenchebach), Sinus Arrest with irregular junctional escape complexes, or an accelerated junctional rhythm with AV nodal block.

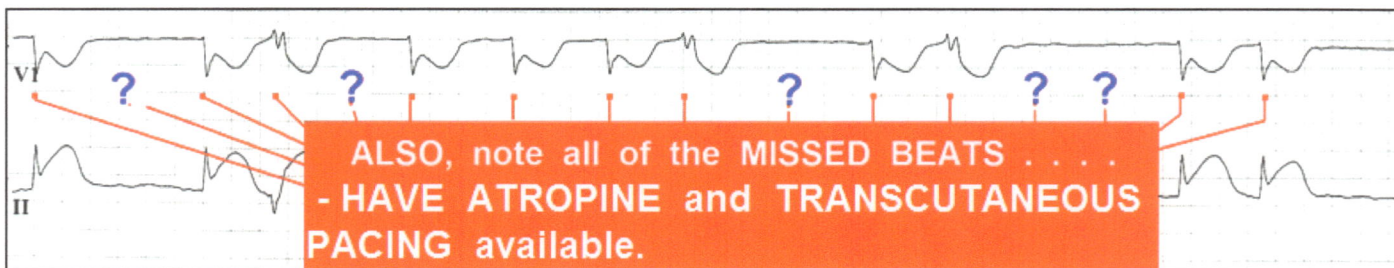

ALSO, note all of the MISSED BEATS . . . . - HAVE ATROPINE and TRANSCUTANEOUS PACING available.

The following points must be emphasized when managing patients with acute Inferior Wall MI:
- Both sinus node and AV node dysfunction are known complications associated with Inferior Wall MI.
- Sinus node and AV node dysfunction can result in clinically significant bradycardias and ventricular asystole.
- Clinicians must be prepared to manage high grade heart blocks, bradycardias and ventricular asystole.

CASE PROGRESSION: After confirming the absence of pulmonary edema by auscultation of the patient's lungs, a 250cc IV fluid bolus of normal saline was administered. Repeat vital signs showed the blood pressure had risen to 80/53, with a pulse rate 70. At that point, the decision was made to administer a Dopamine infusion at 7mcg/kg/minute. Ten minutes after the Dopmaine infusion was initiatied, a repeat blood pressure was obtained: 94/70. The patient was transported to the cardiac cath lab, where the following images were obtained:

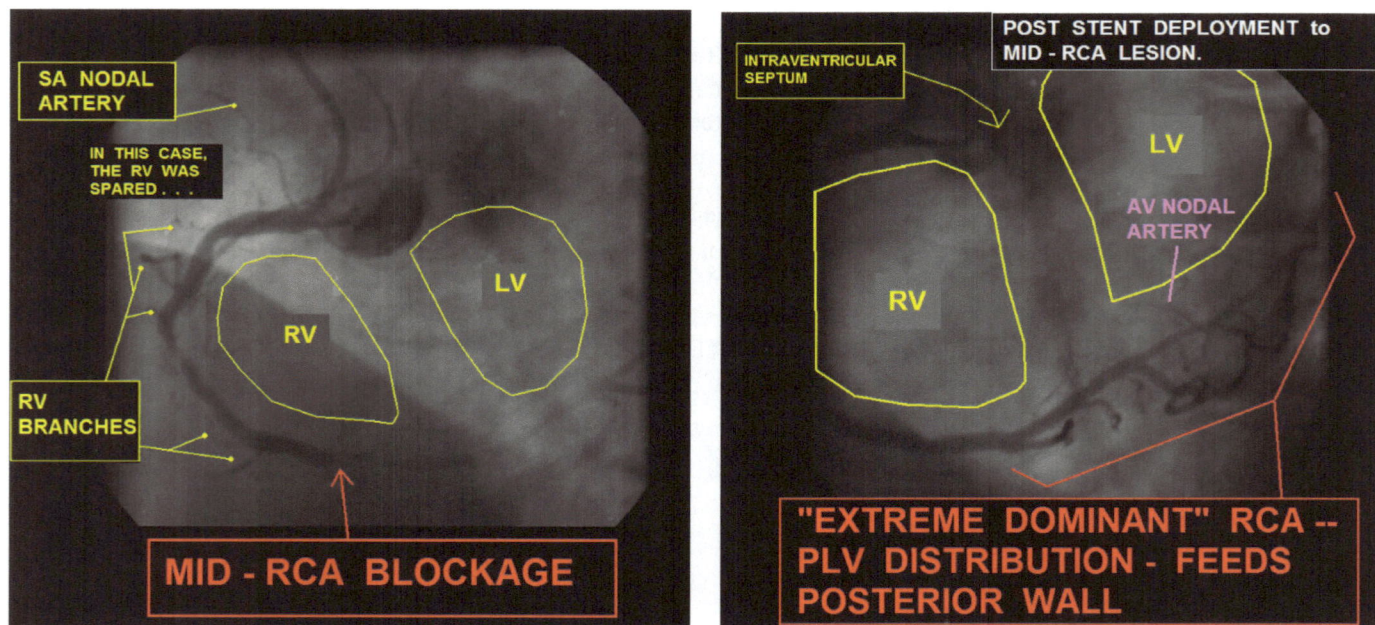

The results of cardiac catheterization confirm the patient's MI resulted from a total obstruction of an "extreme dominant RCA." Because the blockage was *distal* to the Right Ventricular branches, the patient did not incur Right Ventricular MI. Note that if the patient's blockage had been proximal to the right ventricular branch, the patient would have incurred inferior-posterior-right ventricular MI. In the pre-intervention image (above left), the SA nodal artery is noted, which arises in the proximal RCA. In the post-intervention image (above right), the AV Nodal artery is noted. Since only the AV node was affected by the MI, it is likely that the irregular rhythm we observed resulted from occlusion of the AV nodal artery during the course of the acute event.

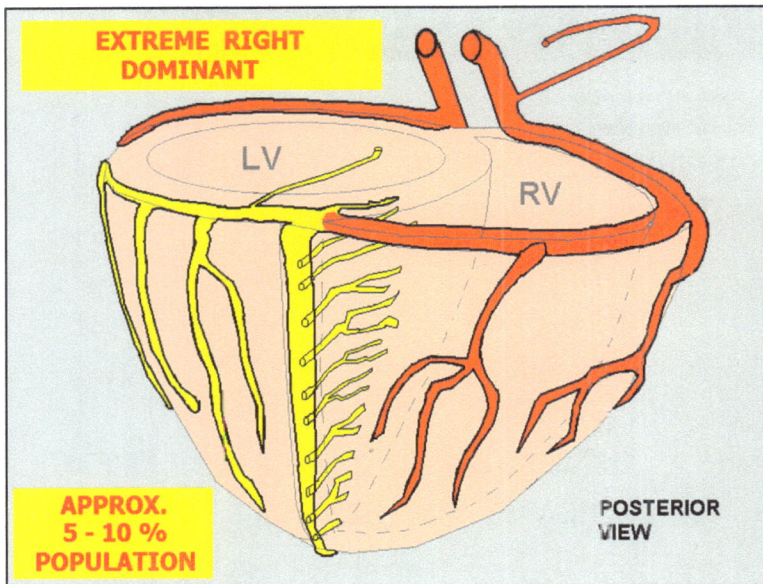

EXTREME RIGHT DOMINANT

LV

RV

APPROX. 5 - 10 % POPULATION

POSTERIOR VIEW

Our patient's coronary artery anatomy closely resembles that seen in the image to the left. Note that an "extreme dominant RCA" supplies blood to most of the posterior wall.

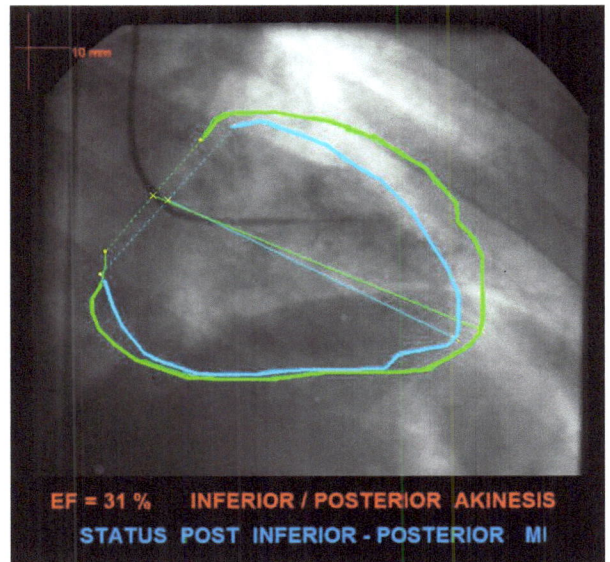

EF = 31%   INFERIOR / POSTERIOR AKINESIS
STATUS POST INFERIOR - POSTERIOR MI

As a result of inferior-posterior MI, the patient's left ventricular ejection fraction is significantly impaired, at 31%. Recall the normal range for LVEF is 55-70%. This amount of LV dysfunction is common with Inferior-Posterior MI.

CASE STUDY SUMMARY

ST ELEVATION: **II, III, aVF**	ST DEPRESSION: **V1 - V3**

SUSPECTED DIAGNOSIS: ACUTE INFERIOR - POSTERIOR WALL MI

SUSPECTED "CULPRIT ARTERY" (if applicable):

"EXTREME" DOMINANT RIGHT CORONARY ARTERY

IMMEDIATE CONCERNS FOR ALL STEMI PATIENTS:

- BE PREPARED TO MANAGE SUDDEN CARDIAC ARREST (PRIMARY V - FIB / V- TACH, BRADYCARDIAS / HEART BLOCKS)
- STAT REPERFUSION THERAPY: THROMBOLYTICS vs. CARDIAC CATHETERIZATION and PCI
- CONSIDER NEEDS FOR ANTI-PLATELET and ANTI-COAGULATION THERAPY

CRITICAL STRUCTURES COMPROMISED:	POTENTIAL COMPLICATIONS:	POSSIBLE CRITICAL INTERVENTIONS:
25 - 45% OF THE LV MUSCLE MASS	LV PUMP FAILURE: HYPOTENSION, PULMONARY EDEMA	SMALL FLUID BOLUS (in absence of PULMONARY EDEMA) INOTROPIC AGENTS
SINUS NODE ARTERY SUPPLIED BY RCA 55% of Pop.	BRADYCARDIA ASYSTOLE	ATROPINE TRANSCUTANEOUS PACING
AV NODAL ARTERY SUPPLIED BY DOMINANT ARTERY (RCA or Circ) IN MOST PATIENTS	AV NODAL BLOCKS: - 1 DEGREE - 2nd DEGREE type I, II - 3rd DEGREE	ATROPINE TRANSCUTANEOUS PACING

CASE STUDY 9 - STEMI

CHIEF COMPLAINT and SIGNIFICANT HISTORY:

42 y/o MALE arrived via EMS, c/o "HEAVY CHEST PRESSURE," SHORTNESS of BREATH X 40 min. He has experienced V-FIB and been DEFIBRILLATED multiple times

RISK FACTOR PROFILE:

- CIGARETTE SMOKER
- HYPERTENSION
- HIGH LDL CHOLESTEROL

PHYSICAL EXAM: Patient is alert & oriented x 4, ANXIOUS, with COOL, PALE, DIAPHORETIC SKIN. C/O NAUSEA, and is VOMITING. LUNG SOUNDS: COARSE CRACKLES, BASES, bilaterally

VITAL SIGNS: BP: 80/40   P: 70   R: 32   SAO2: 92 % on 15 LPM O2

LABS: TROPONIN: < .04

QUADRAD OF ACS CHECKLIST

- ☑ SYMPTOMS of ACS
  - ✓ TYPICAL ACS - eg:
  - ATYPICAL ACS - eg:
- ☑ ECG ABNORMALITIES
  - ✓ ST ELEVATION (J POINT plus 40 ms)
  - HYPERACUTE T WAVES - and/or -
  - NEW or PRESUMABLY NEW LBBB
  - ST DEPRESSION (>0.5 mm @ J POINT) and/or
  - INVERTED or BIPHASIC T WAVES and/or
  - DYNAMIC ST SEGMENT and/or T WAVE CHANGES IN SERIAL EKGs
- ☑ RISK FACTORS - 3 or more
  - FAMILY HISTORY
  - DIABETES
  - ✓ ↑ LDL and/or ↓ HDL
  - ✓ SMOKING
  - AGE: 65 or MORE
  - ✓ HYPERTENSION
- ☐ CARDIAC MARKERS
  - ELEVATED TROPONIN and/or CK/MB
- ☐ TOTAL

SHOCK ASSESSMENT

LOC:	ANXIOUS RESTLESS LETHARGIC UNCONSCIOUS	AWAKE ALERT & ORIENTED
SKIN:	PALE / ASHEN CYANOTIC COOL DIAPHORETIC	NORMAL HUE WARM DRY
BREATHING:	TACHYPNEA	NORMAL
PULSE:	WEAK / THREADY TOO FAST or SLOW	STRONG
STATUS:	SHOCK	NORMAL

The presence of cool, diaphoretic skin, anxiety, tachypnea, and hypotension indicate the patient is in shock. The presence of pulmonary edema indicates a component of LV failure.

Initial treatment should include:
- oxygen
- IV access / labs drawn and sent
- aspirin

In this case study, nitroglycerin and morphine were withheld due to the patient's hypotension. As per American Heart Association guidelines, nitroglycerin is contraindicated if systolic BP is less than 90mmhg.[60]

---

[60] "Handbook of Emergency Cardiovascular Care," American Heart Association 2006: p28

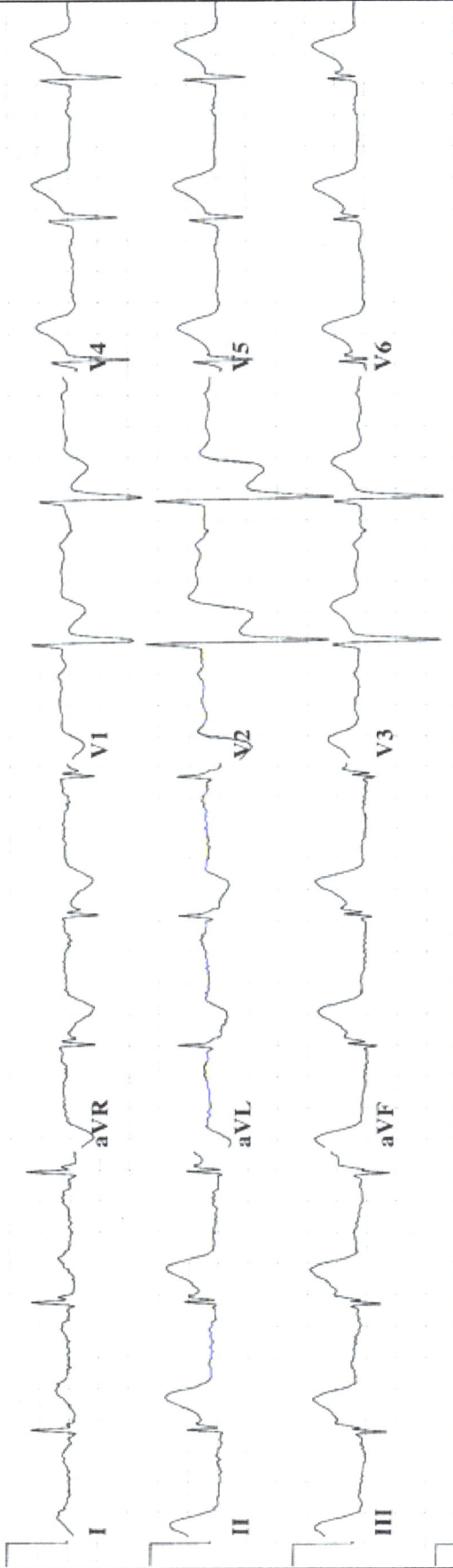

42 yr
Male
Caucasian

Loc:3   Option:23

Vent. rate	69	BPM
PR interval	196	ms
QRS duration	98	ms
QT/QTc	388/415	ms
P–R–T axes	14 28	81

☞ EVALUATE EKG for indicators of ACS:

- ST SEGMENT ELEVATION / DEPRESSION
- HYPERACUTE T WAVES
- CONVEX ST SEGMENTS
- OTHER ST SEGMENT / T WAVE ABNORMALITIES

I   aVR   V1   V4

II   aVL   V2   V5

III aVF   V3   V6

CASE STUDY QUESTIONS:

NOTE LEADS WITH ST ELEVATION:

NOTE LEADS WITH ST DEPRESSION:

WHAT IS THE SUSPECTED DIAGNOSIS ?

WHAT IS THE "CULPRIT ARTERY" -- if applicable ?

LIST ANY CRITICAL STRUCTURES COMPROMISED:

LIST ANY POTENTIAL COMPLICATIONS:

219

42 yr
Male   Caucasian

Loc:3   Option:23

Vent. rate   69 BPM
PR interval   196 ms
QRS duration   98 ms
QT/QTc   388/415 ms
P–R–T axes   14 28   81

*** Acute MI ***
Inferior-Posterior-Lateral Injury Pattern

ST SEGMENT ELEVATION
ST SEGMENT DEPRESSION

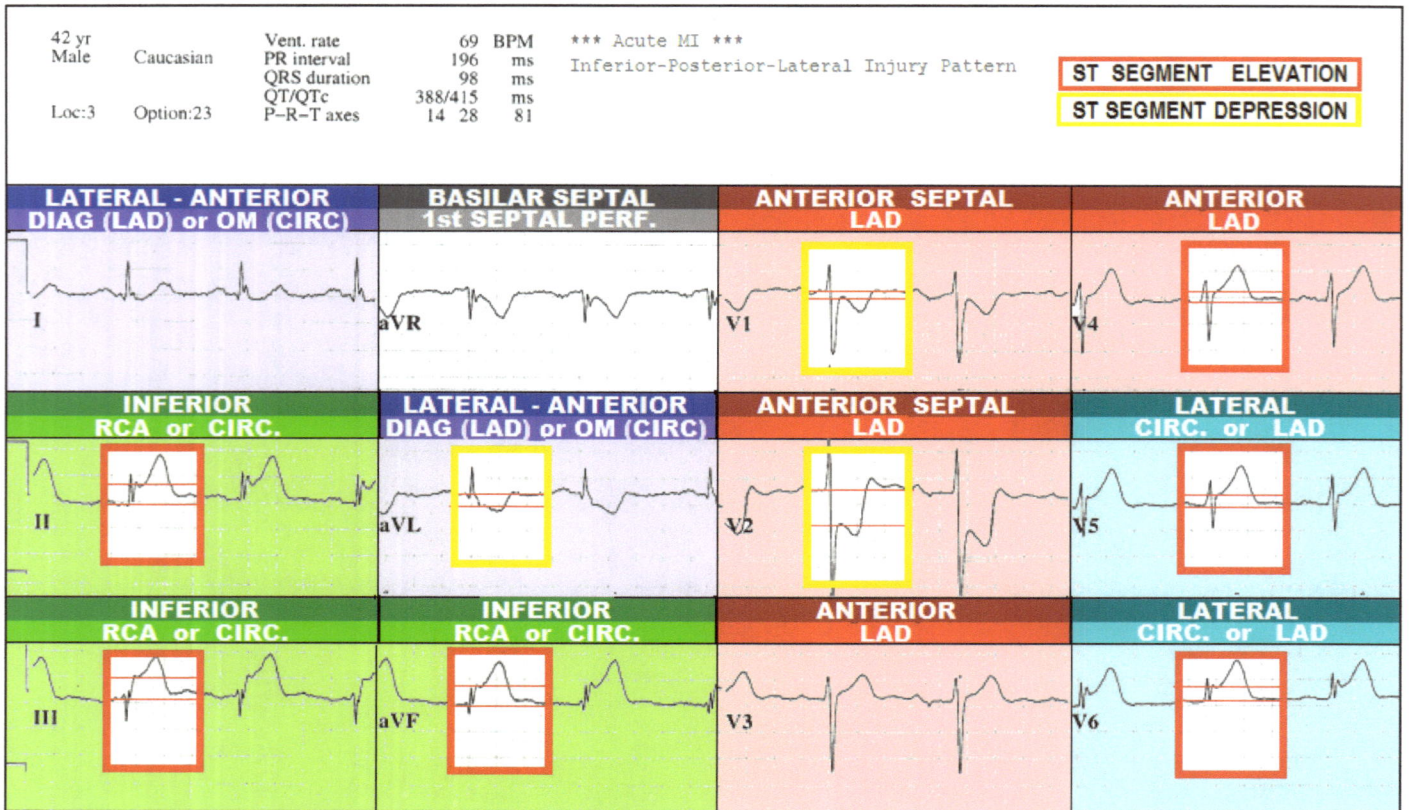

LATERAL - ANTERIOR DIAG (LAD) or OM (CIRC)	BASILAR SEPTAL 1st SEPTAL PERF.	ANTERIOR SEPTAL LAD	ANTERIOR LAD
I	aVR	V1	V4
INFERIOR RCA or CIRC.	**LATERAL - ANTERIOR DIAG (LAD) or OM (CIRC)**	**ANTERIOR SEPTAL LAD**	**LATERAL CIRC. or LAD**
II	aVL	V2	V5
INFERIOR RCA or CIRC.	**INFERIOR RCA or CIRC.**	**ANTERIOR LAD**	**LATERAL CIRC. or LAD**
III	aVF	V3	V6

The above ECG demonstrates ST segment elevation in inferior leads II, III, aVF, anterior lead V4, and lateral leads V5 and V6.   Regarding our "3 Step Process" for ECG evaluation when inferior wall MI is noted, we conclude this patient is experiencing acute inferior-posterior-lateral wall MI, as demonstrated by the image below:

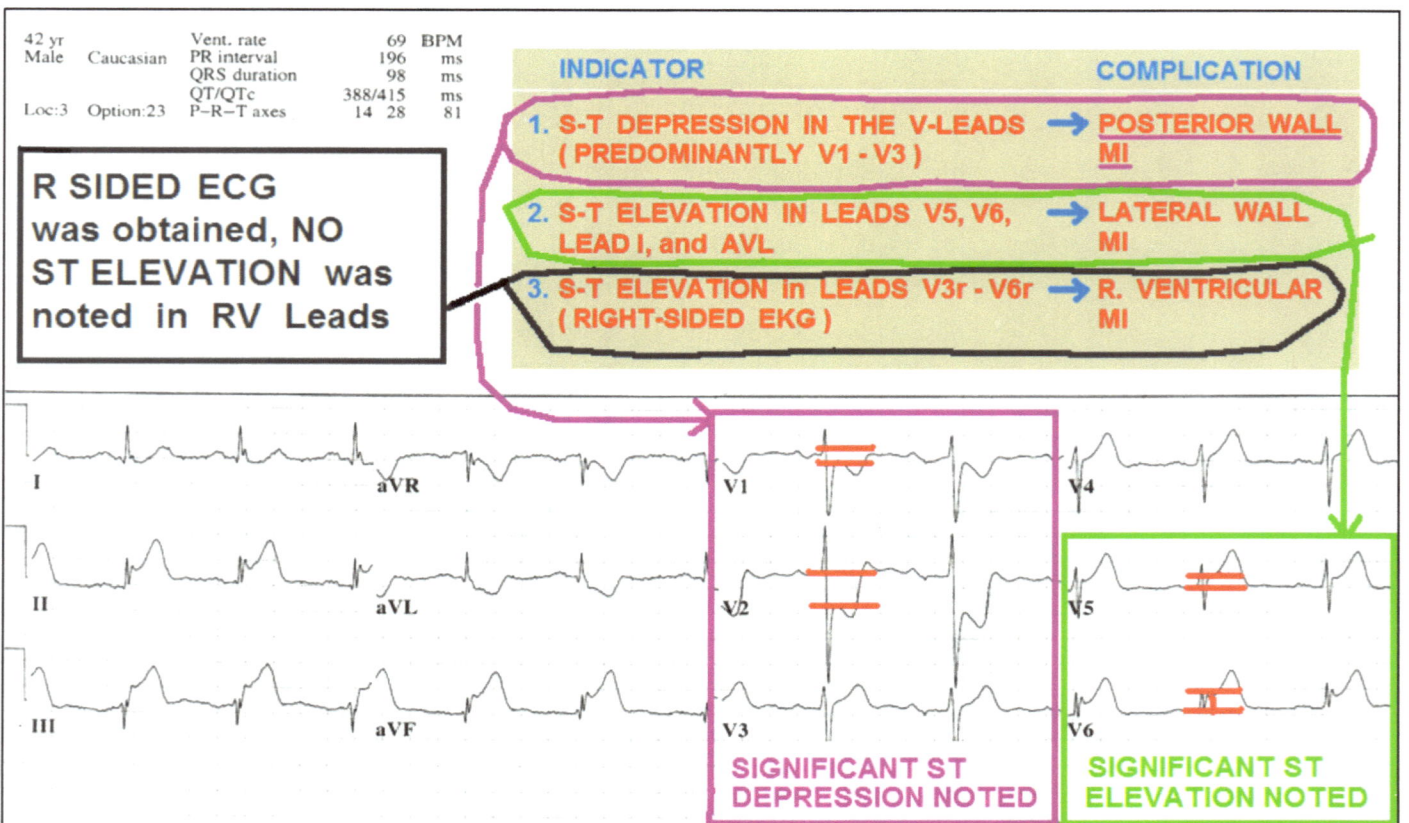

42 yr
Male   Caucasian

Loc:3   Option:23

Vent. rate   69 BPM
PR interval   196 ms
QRS duration   98 ms
QT/QTc   388/415 ms
P–R–T axes   14 28   81

R SIDED ECG was obtained, NO ST ELEVATION was noted in RV Leads

INDICATOR   COMPLICATION

1. S-T DEPRESSION IN THE V-LEADS → POSTERIOR WALL
   (PREDOMINANTLY V1 - V3)   MI

2. S-T ELEVATION IN LEADS V5, V6, → LATERAL WALL
   LEAD I, and AVL   MI

3. S-T ELEVATION in LEADS V3r - V6r → R. VENTRICULAR
   (RIGHT-SIDED EKG)   MI

SIGNIFICANT ST DEPRESSION NOTED

SIGNIFICANT ST ELEVATION NOTED

Regarding the ST segment elevation in lead V4, since ST elevation is seen in only one anterior lead, we don't classify this as an MI with anterior involvement. ==ST elevation must be present in two or more contiguous leads (those which view a specific region of the myocardium) in order to classify the MI as involving that specific region.==

Our ECG diagnosis of inferior-lateral-posterior MI is based on the following criteria:

- ST segment elevation in *inferior leads* II, III, and aVF (image to right)
- ST segment elevation in *lateral leads* V5 and V6. (image below, left)
- ST segment depression in leads V1-V2, which view the *posterior wall* via reciprocal changes in leads V1 – V3. (image below, right).

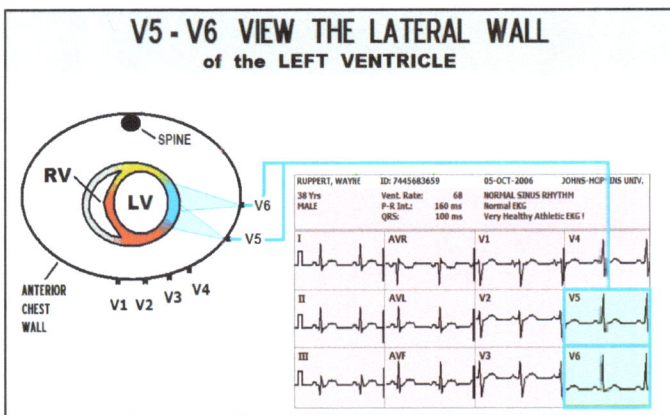

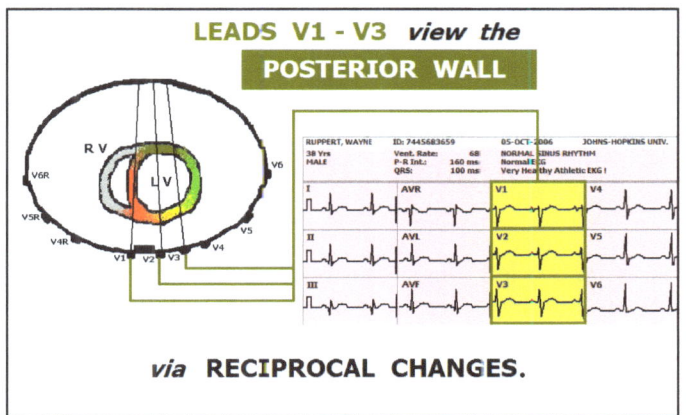

LEADS II, III, and aVF VIEW
INFERIOR WALL of the LEFT VENTRICLE

FED by the RCA (75 - 80 % pop)
or the CIRCUMFLEX (10 - 15 %)

V5 - V6 VIEW THE LATERAL WALL
of the LEFT VENTRICLE

LEADS V1 - V3 *view the*
POSTERIOR WALL

via RECIPROCAL CHANGES.

As we observed in the last case study, inferior-posterior wall MI is usually caused by blockage of either a dominant circumflex artery (below left image), or an "extreme dominant right" coronary artery (below right image).

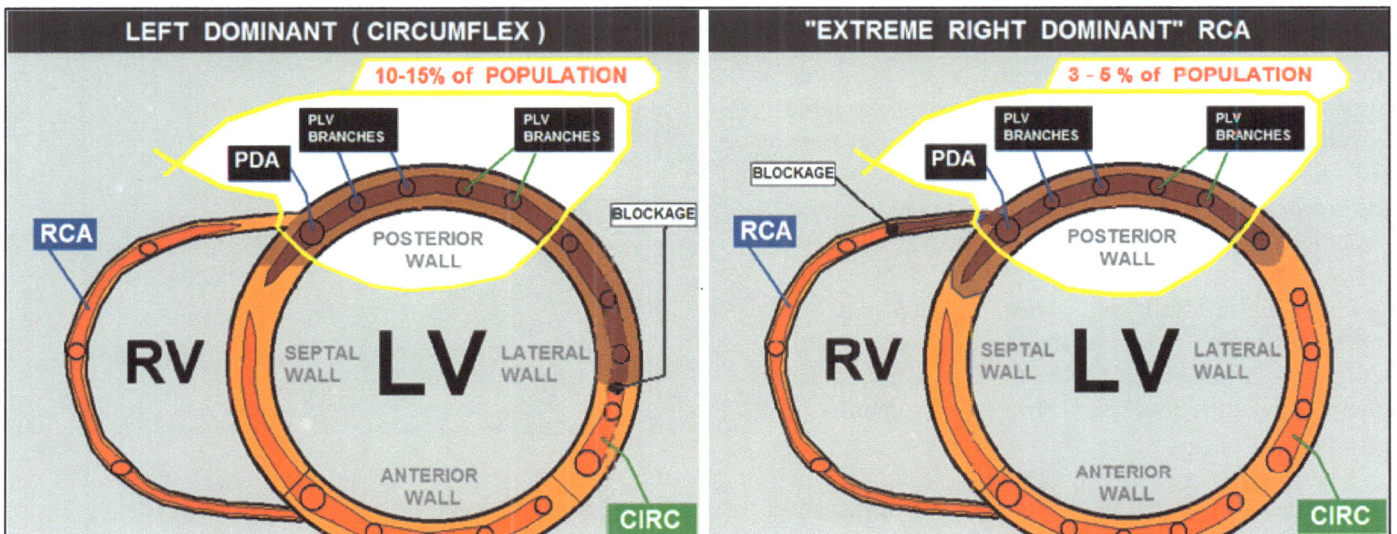

LEFT DOMINANT (CIRCUMFLEX)
10-15% of POPULATION

"EXTREME RIGHT DOMINANT" RCA
3 - 5 % of POPULATION

Since the circumflex artery usually supplies most of the lateral wall, ==when *inferior-posterior-lateral* wall MI is seen, the culprit artery is most likely a dominant circumflex artery with a proximal occlusion.==

In cases of lateral wall MI, the presence of ST elevation in leads I and aVL indicate a lesion in the ***proximal aspect*** of the circumflex artery, before the first obtuse marginal branch.   A general rule is: ***the more proximal the lesion, the larger the area of infarct***.

A dominant circumflex artery often supplies up to 55% of the LV muscle mass, as opposed to a non-dominant circumflex, which usually supplies between 25 and 30%, as illustrated below:

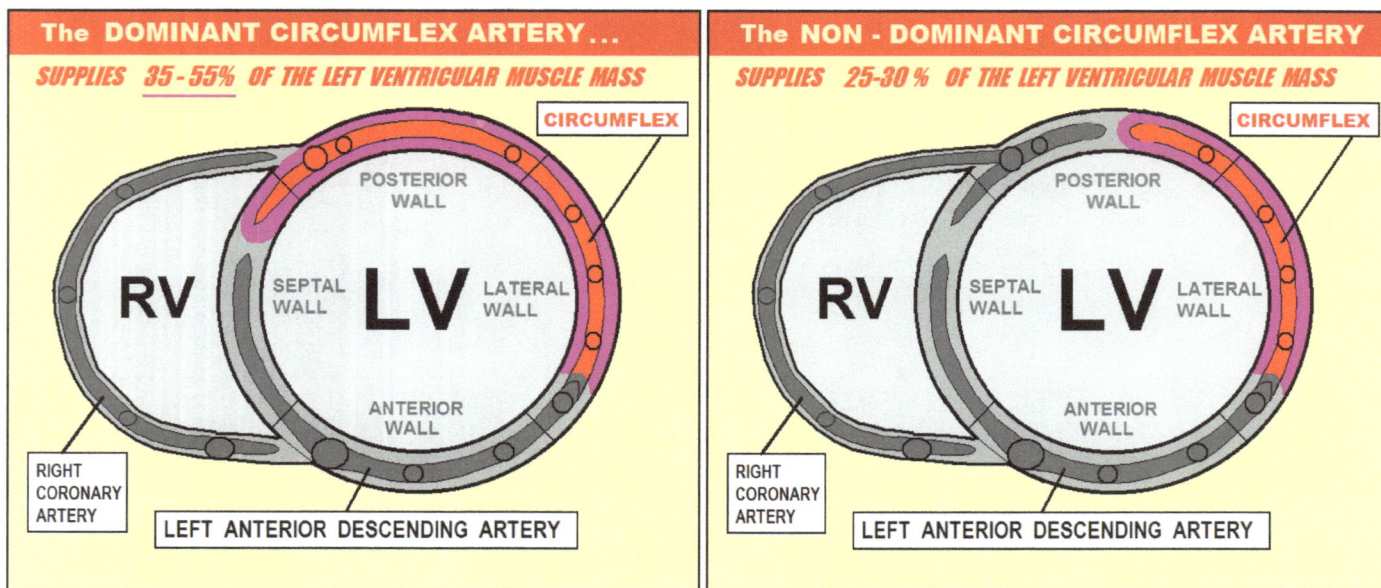

As the above left image illustrates, a dominant circumflex artery can supply more blood to the LV muscle mass than the left anterior descending artery.   A proximal occlusion of a dominant circumflex artery can result in devastating LV pump failure.

In our current case study, the lack of ST elevation in leads I and aVL favors a blockage ***after*** the origin of the first obtuse marginal branch.

Within fifteen minutes of arrival in the ED, our patient's condition rapidly deteriorated.   He became increasingly anxious, complained of increased shortness of breath, and exhibited profound diaphoresis.   Repeat vital signs revealed his BP dropped to 57/42, pulse 110, respirations 40, and SAO2 94% on O2 at 15 LPM via non-rebreather mask.   Lung sounds reveled coarse crackles throughout all fields bilaterally.

A dopamine infusion was initiated at 7 mcg/kg/minute and titrated upward until 20mcg/kg/minute was reached.   The patient's BP increased to 88/48, with improvement of symptoms.

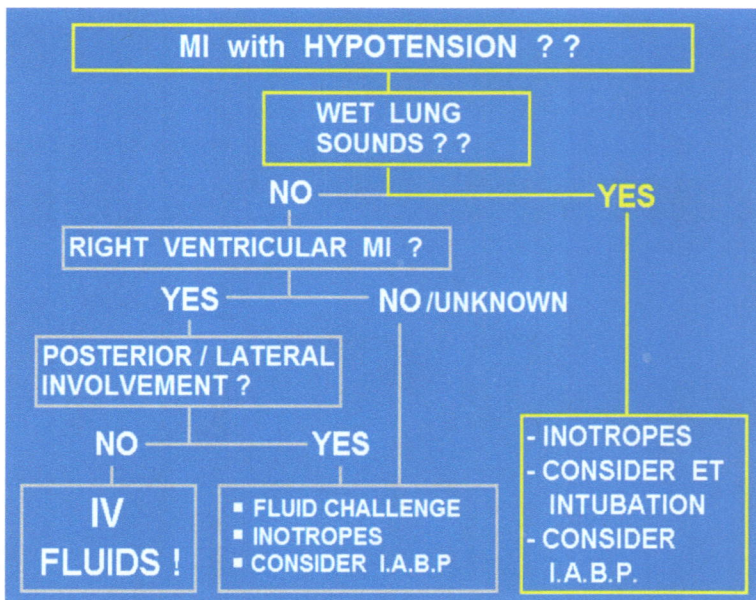

The patient was taken to the cardiac catheterization suite where the images on the next page were obtained.

CIRCUMFLEX ARTERY OCCLUDED with significant THROMBUS.

PTCA of CIRCUMFLEX ARTERY.

DOMINANT CIRCUMFLEX ARTERY OPEN POST THROMBECTOMY with STENT DEPLOYMENT.

LVEF = 43%

Dia Area = 11.8 cm²   Sys Area = 8.7 cm²   Eject Frac = 43%
Dia Volume = 27.7 ml   Sys Volume = 15.8 ml   Stroke Volume = 11.9 ml

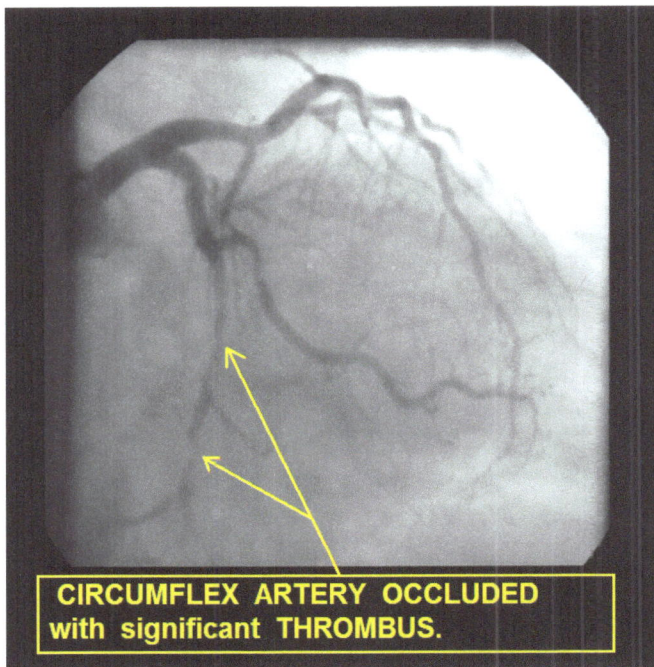

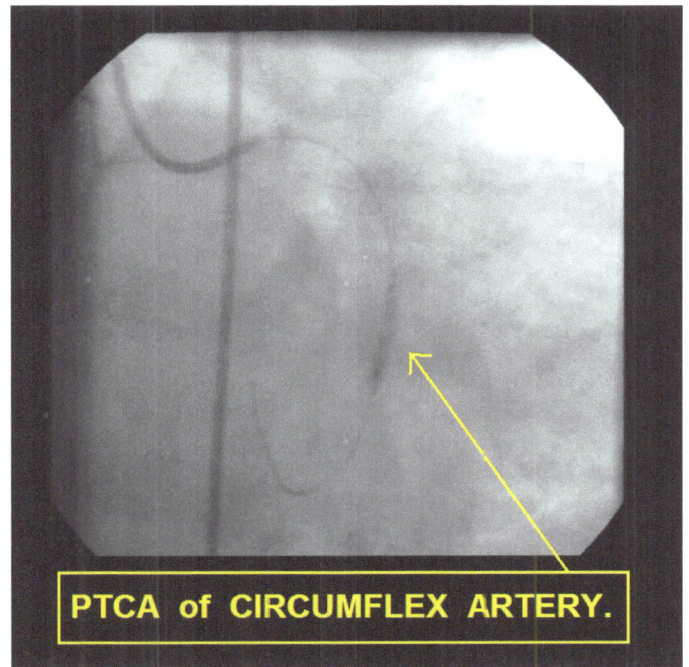

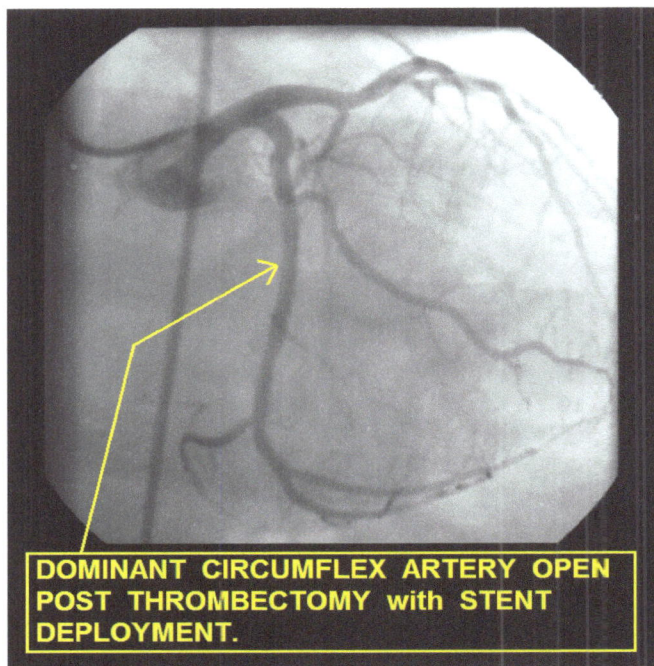

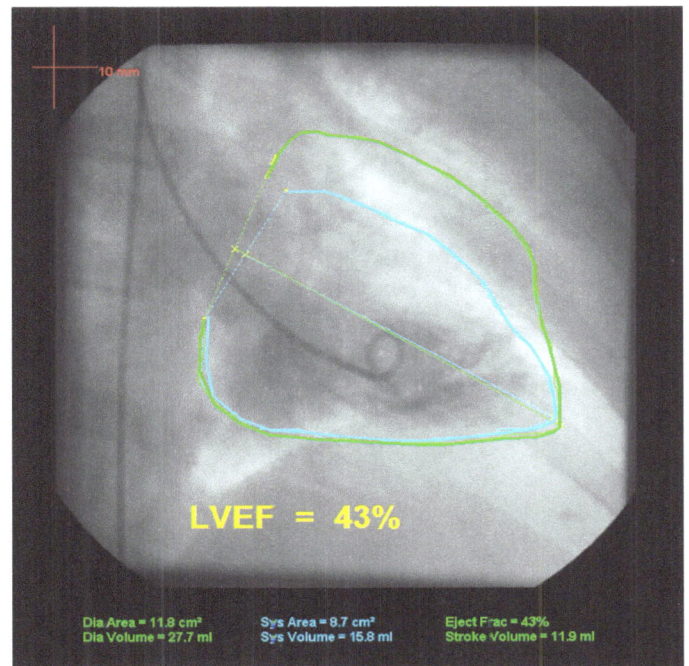

Our patient's post-MI left ventricular angiogram, taken in the RAO projection, demonstrates inferior-posterior akinesis. This finding, with an LVEF of 43%, is typical for inferior-posterior MI. To appreciate lateral wall function, an image would have to be obtained in the LAO projection, which was not done in order to minimize the patient's total amount of IV dye injection.

A complication to be aware of in multi-region MI is acute papillary muscle tear, which causes acute mitral valve regurgitation, a life-threatening disorder which is sometimes seen 7 – 10 days post MI.

CASE STUDY SUMMARY

ST ELEVATION:	ST DEPRESSION:
II, III, aVF, V5, V6	V1 - V3, POSSIBLY I and aVL

SUSPECTED DIAGNOSIS: ACUTE INFERIOR - POSTERIOR - LATERAL MI

SUSPECTED "CULPRIT ARTERY" (if applicable):

OCCLUSION of DOMINANT CIRCUMFLEX ARTERY

IMMEDIATE CONCERNS FOR ALL STEMI PATIENTS:

- BE PREPARED TO MANAGE SUDDEN CARDIAC ARREST (PRIMARY V - FIB / V- TACH, BRADYCARDIAS / HEART BLOCKS)
- STAT REPERFUSION THERAPY: THROMBOLYTICS vs. CARDIAC CATHETERIZATION and PCI
- CONSIDER NEEDS FOR ANTI-PLATELET and ANTI-COAGULATION THERAPY

CRITICAL STRUCTURES COMPROMISED:	POTENTIAL COMPLICATIONS:	POSSIBLE CRITICAL INTERVENTIONS:
30 - 55% of LV MUSCLE MASS	POSSIBLE SEVERE LV PUMP FAILURE	INOTROPIC AGENTS ET INTUBATION I.A.B.P. INSERTION
SA NODE	SINUS BRADYCARDIA / SINUS ARREST	ATROPINE TRANSCUTANEOUS PACING
AV NODE	HEART BLOCKS	ATROPINE TRANSCUTANEOUS PACING
SIGNIFICANT AMOUNT of PAPILLARY MUSCLE INSERTION to BASE of LV	ACUTE PAPILLARY MUSCLE TEAR and MITRAL VALVE REGURGITATION (7 - 10 DAYS)	INOTROPIC AGENTS DIEURETICS EMERGENCY SURGERY

224

HELPFUL HINT:

Think of LEADS I and aVL as "MULTIPLIERS" of the infarction zone in cases of STEMI.

When ST ELEVATION is noted in **leads I** and **aVL** during:

INFERIOR WALL STEMI (primary ST elevation in leads II, III, and/or aVF): it is usually indicative of a proximal occlusion of a dominant CIRCUMFLEX artery, involving the first Obtuse Marginal artery. Leads V5 and/or V6 may or may not be elevated. ST elevation of lead II may be higher than that of lead III. AMI caused by proximal obstruction of a dominant Circumflex artery can compromise up to 55% of the left ventricular muscle mass, with LV pump failure, cardiogenic shock and pulmonary edema as possible complications to anticipate, along with complications of inferior wall MI, which are AV node failure; 1st, 2nd, and 3rd degree heart blocks.

LACK OF ST elevation in leads I and aVL does not rule out proximal obstruction of a dominant circumflex artery. In some patients, the region of the heart viewed by leads I and aVL are supplied by a ramus artery, or the first diagonal branch of the LAD.

ANTERIOR WALL STEMI (primary ST elevation in leads V1 – V4): it is usually indicative of a proximal occlusion of the LEFT ANTERIOR DESCENDING artery, proximal to the origin of the FIRST DIAGONAL branch. Occlusion of the proximal LAD also results in ST depression in leads II, III, and aVF. When leads I and aVL are elevated along with V1 – V4, it is indicative of ANTERIOR-LATERAL STEMI, which can compromise up to 45% of the LV muscle mass, resulting in possible LV pump failure, cardiogenic shock and pulmonary edema.

LATERAL WALL STEMI (primary ST elevation in leads V5, V6): it is usually indicative of a proximal occlusion of a CIRCUMFLEX artery. When no ST elevation is noted in the inferior leads, the occluded circumflex artery is often non-dominant. This arterial distribution commonly supplies approximately 20-30% of the LV muscle mass, and in 45% of the population, the sinus node artery is perfused by the circumflex.

IN SUMMARY, when leads I and aVL present with ST elevation in cases of inferior, anterior and/or lateral MI, it usually indicates the lesion is located more proximally, compromises more LV muscle mass and results in higher incidence of LV pump failure and hypotension.

Reference sources:

Birnbaum, Y, Wagner, GS, Am J Cardiol 1999;83 143-48
Escola, MJ Int J Cardiol 2009; 131:3:378-83
Birnbaum, Y Postgrad Med J 2003;79:490-504
Zimetbaum, NEJM 2003; 348:933-940

CASE STUDY 10 - STEMI

CHIEF COMPLAINT and SIGNIFICANT HISTORY:

48 y/o FEMALE arrives via EMS, c/o "EXCRUCIATING HEAVINESS" in center of chest, X 1 hour. She also c/o nausea (vomited several times). Per EMS, she experienced 4 episodes of V-Fib, was defibrillated successfully each time. Amiodarone drip is running @ 1mg/min.

RISK FACTOR PROFILE:

- CIGARETTE SMOKER
- HYPERTENSION
- BROTHER HAD AMI AT AGE 44

PHYSICAL EXAM: CAO x 4, anxious, SKIN cool, pale, diaphoretic. Lung sounds: clear Heart Sounds normal S1, S2,

VITAL SIGNS: BP: 78/56   P: 100   R: 28   SAO2: 94% on 4 LPM O2

LABS: TROPONIN: < .04

QUADRAD OF ACS CHECKLIST

☑ SYMPTOMS of ACS
- ✔ TYPICAL ACS - eg:
- ◆ ATYPICAL ACS - eq:

☑ ECG ABNORMALITIES
- ✔ ST ELEVATION (J POINT plus 40 ms)
- ◆ HYPERACUTE T WAVES · and/or ·
- ◆ NEW or PRESUMABLY NEW LBBB
- ◆ ST DEPRESSION (>0.5 mm @ J POINT) and/or
- ◆ INVERTED or BIPHASIC T WAVES and/or
- ◆ DYNAMIC ST SEGMENT and/or T WAVE CHANGES IN SERIAL EKGs

☑ RISK FACTORS - 3 or more
- ✔ FAMILY HISTORY
- ◆ DIABETES
- ◆ ↑LDL and/or ↓HDL
- ✔ SMOKING
- ◆ AGE: 65 or MORE
- ✔ HYPERTENSION

☐ CARDIAC MARKERS
- ◆ ELEVATED TROPONIN and/or CK/MB

3 TOTAL

In the pre-hospital setting, the patient was given a total of 3 mg per kilogram of Lidocaine, yet continued to experience ventricular fibrillation. After the administration of Amiodarone 150mg, there were no recurrent episodes of V-fib.

As per the above algorithm, the patient received a 200cc fluid challenge of normal saline along with a dopamine infusion at 7mcg/kg/min. After this therapy was initiated, the patient's blood pressure increased to 113/68.

A right-sided ECG revealed normal ST segments, indicating no right-ventricular infarction.

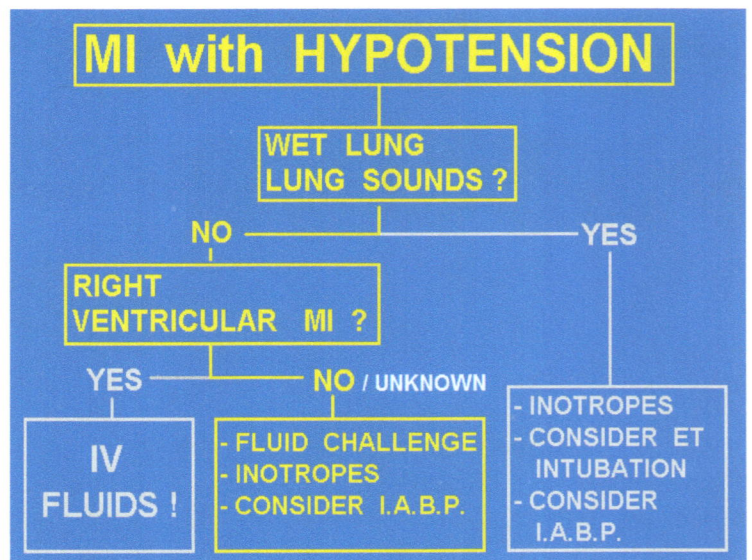

MI with HYPOTENSION algorithm — WET LUNG LUNG SOUNDS? NO → RIGHT VENTRICULAR MI? YES → IV FLUIDS! / NO/UNKNOWN → FLUID CHALLENGE, INOTROPES, CONSIDER I.A.B.P. YES → INOTROPES, CONSIDER ET INTUBATION, CONSIDER I.A.B.P.

48 yr
Female   Caucasian

Loc:3   Option:23

Vent. rate	98	BPM
PR interval	*	ms
QRS duration	112	ms
QT/QTc	354/451	ms
P–R–T axes	* 74	64

I aVR V1 V4

II aVL V2 V5

III aVF V3 V6

DOS:

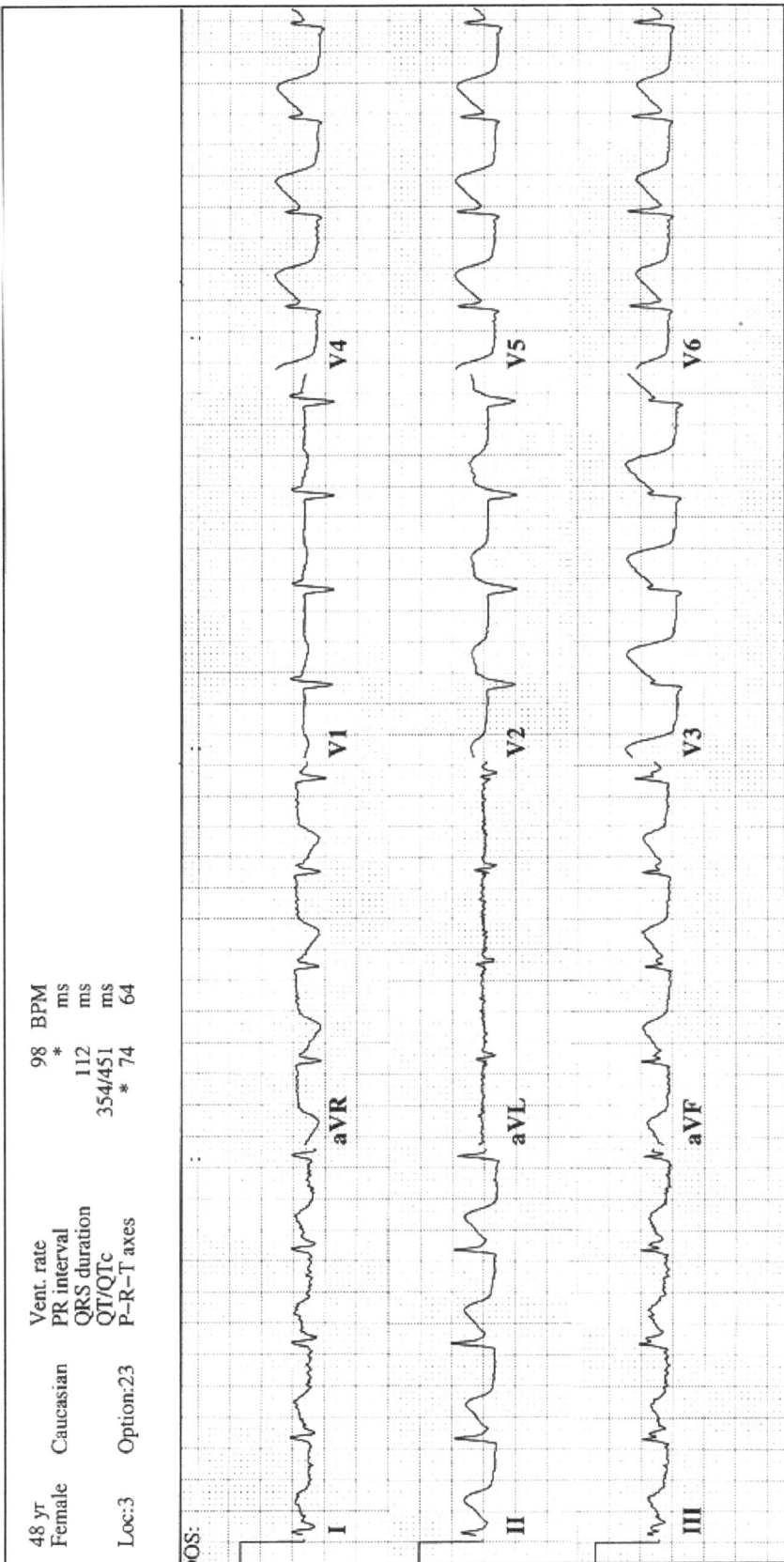

CASE STUDY QUESTIONS:

NOTE LEADS WITH ST ELEVATION:

NOTE LEADS WITH ST DEPRESSION:

WHAT IS THE SUSPECTED DIAGNOSIS ?

WHAT IS THE "CULPRIT ARTERY" – if applicable ?

LIST ANY CRITICAL STRUCTURES COMPROMISED:

LIST ANY POTENTIAL COMPLICATIONS:

48 yr		Vent. rate	98	BPM	Undetermined rhythm
Female	Caucasian	PR interval	*	ms	Low voltage QRS
		QRS duration	112	ms	Cannot rule out Anteroseptal infarct
		QT/QTc	354/451	ms	Inferolateral injury pattern
Loc:3	Option:23	P-R-T axes	* 74	64	** ** ** ** * ACUTE MI * ** ** ** **
					ACUTE APRICAL MI
					Abnormal ECG

ST SEGMENT ELEVATION

ST SEGMENT DEPRESSION

SO.... WHICH ARTERY IS IT ?

LAD ?

CIRC ?

BOTH LAD and DOMINANT CIRC ?

RCA ?

LEFT MAIN ?

ANOMOLOUS ?

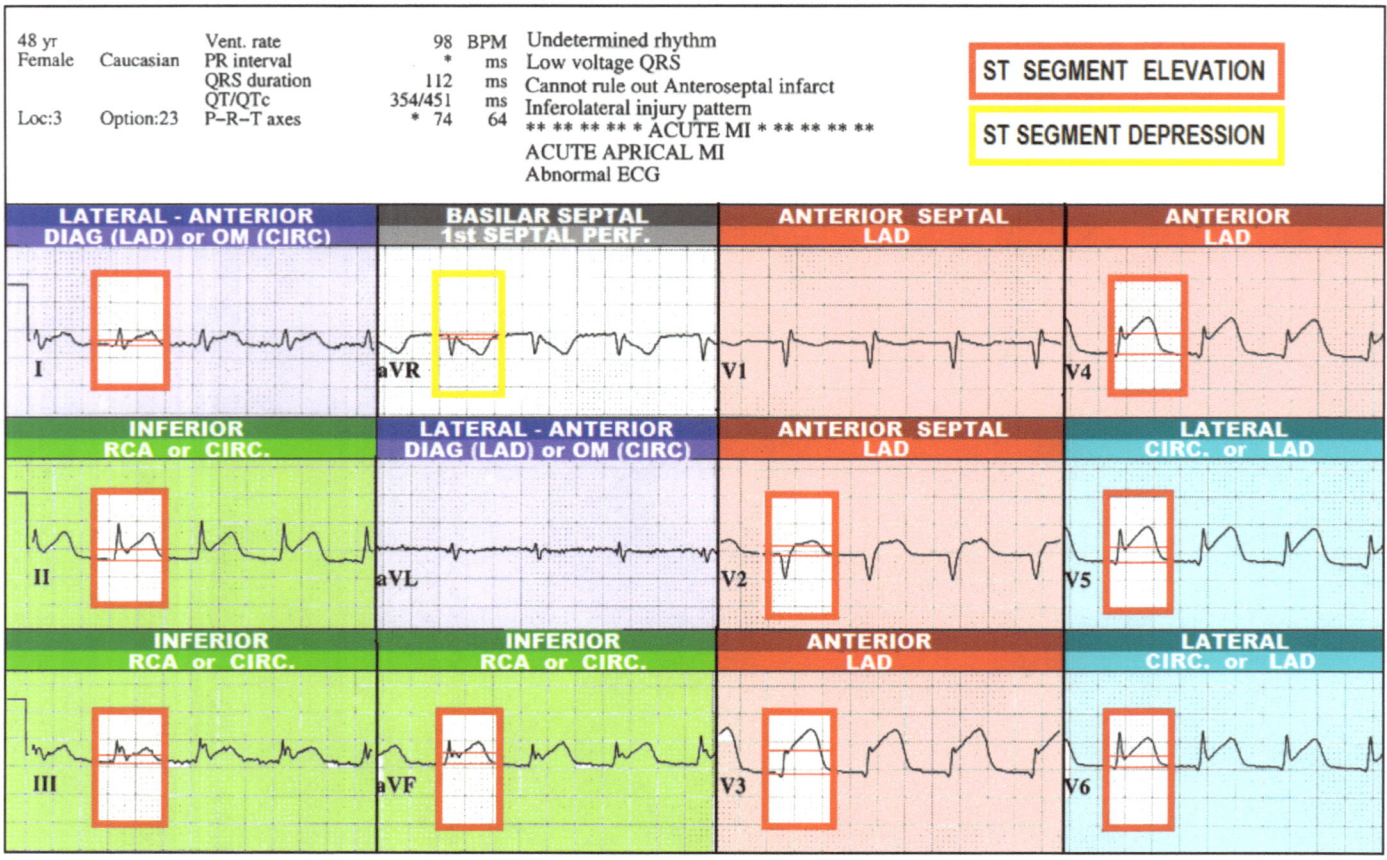

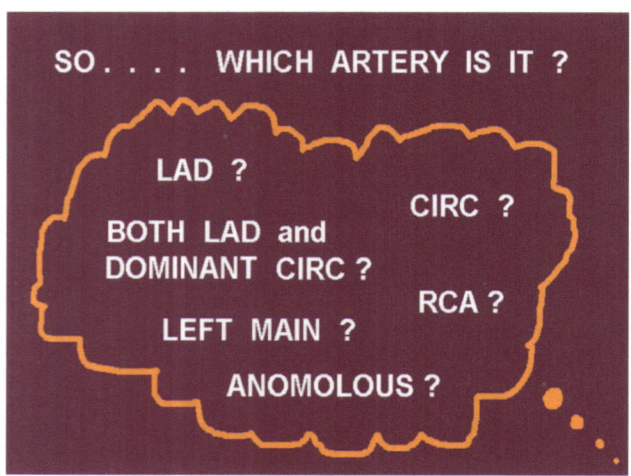

Based on the above ECG, this patient's diagnosis is ANTERIOR-LATERAL-INFERIOR MI. There is significant ST segment elevation in nine leads; 3 anterior, 3 lateral, and 3 inferior.

In the 90 – 95% of the population with common coronary artery anatomy, having this type of MI is not possible, unless the patient is unfortunate enough to develop blockages in the LAD and RCA or Circumflex arteries simultaneously.

On page 27 in the Essential Cardiac Anatomy and Physiology Chapter, we presented some of the less common anatomical variations. One such variation is known as the "trans-apical LAD," which is seen in approximately 5% of the population. As its name implies, the trans-apical LAD wraps around the apex of the heart to supply blood to the inferior wall, as seen in the image to the right.

Unless a source of collateral blood supply has developed, obstruction of a trans-apical LAD results in anterior-inferior wall MI. In our case study, the LAD also supplies some of the lateral wall.

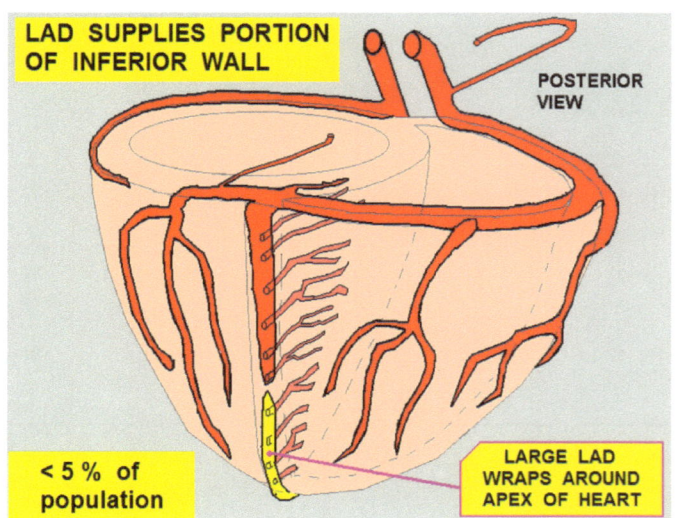

LAD SUPPLIES PORTION OF INFERIOR WALL

POSTERIOR VIEW

< 5 % of population

LARGE LAD WRAPS AROUND APEX OF HEART

The patient was taken to the cardiac cath lab, where the following images were obtained:

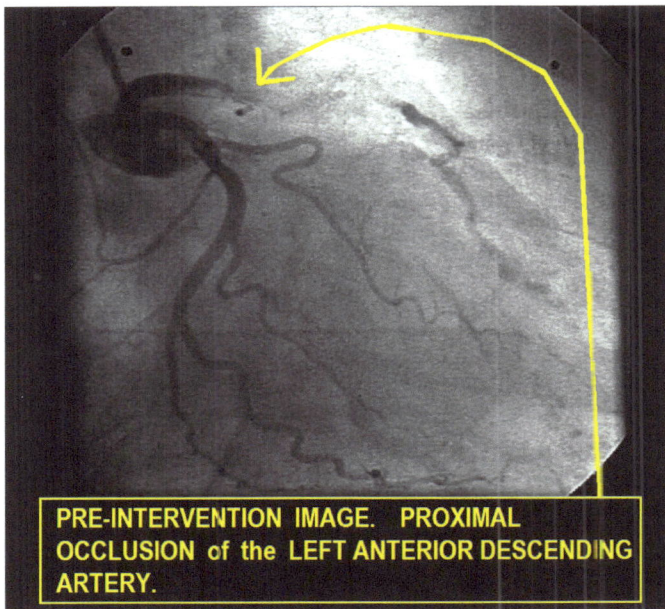

PRE-INTERVENTION IMAGE. PROXIMAL OCCLUSION of the LEFT ANTERIOR DESCENDING ARTERY.

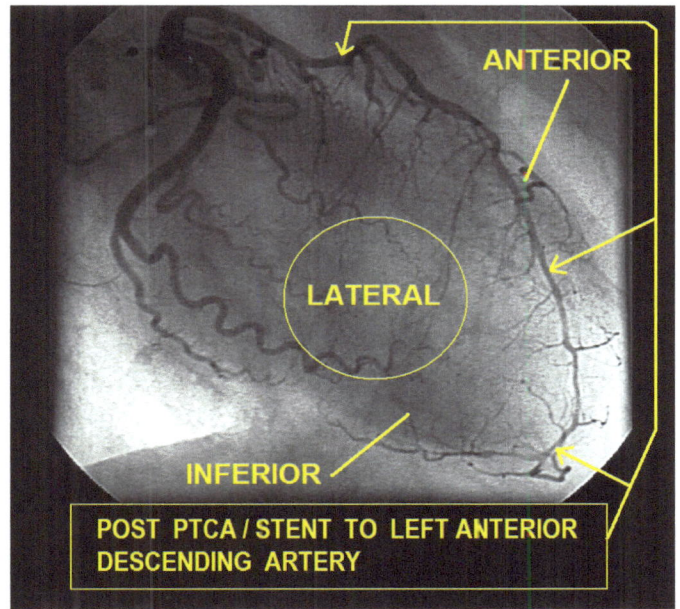

POST PTCA / STENT TO LEFT ANTERIOR DESCENDING ARTERY

Once the above angiographic images are viewed, one can appreciate how the ECG accurately displayed the patient's areas of infarct: *anterior, lateral* and *inferior.* Because the patient's left anterior descending artery supplies most of the inferior wall, her right coronary artery was small, and supplied blood to the right atrium and right ventricle.

Fortunately, this anatomical variation is not common. Our patient's pre-interventional left ventricular angiogram revealed an ejection fraction of 33%, which is consistent with the amount of sustained myocardial damage.

From a clinical standpoint, the patient did well. Because she arrived in the ED within one hour of the onset of symptoms, her LV function recovered quickly. By the end of the day, we were able to discontinue her Dopamine drip. Her recovery was uncomplicated, and she was discharged two days later.

CASE STUDY SUMMARY

ST ELEVATION: I, II, III, aVF, V2, V3, V4, V5, V6	ST DEPRESSION: aVR

SUSPECTED DIAGNOSIS: ACUTE ANTERIOR - INFERIOR - LATERAL MI

SUSPECTED "CULPRIT ARTERY" (if applicable):

OCCLUSION of TRANS-APICAL LEFT ANTERIOR DESCENDING ARTERY

IMMEDIATE CONCERNS FOR ALL STEMI PATIENTS:

- BE PREPARED TO MANAGE SUDDEN CARDIAC ARREST (PRIMARY V - FIB / V- TACH, BRADYCARDIAS / HEART BLOCKS)
- STAT REPERFUSION THERAPY: THROMBOLYTICS vs. CARDIAC CATHETERIZATION and PCI
- CONSIDER NEEDS FOR ANTI-PLATELET and ANTI-COAGULATION THERAPY

CRITICAL STRUCTURES COMPROMISED:	POTENTIAL COMPLICATIONS:	POSSIBLE CRITICAL INTERVENTIONS:
50-70% of the LEFT VENTRICULAR MUSCLE MASS	POSSIBLE SEVERE LV PUMP FAILURE	INOTROPIC AGENTS ET INTUBATION I.A.B.P. INSERTION
BUNDLE of HIS and BUNDLE BRANCHES	HIGH GRADE (2nd, 3rd DEGREE) HEART BLOCKS BUNDLE BRANCH BLOCKS	TRANSCUTANEOUS PACING

☞ REVIEW QUESTIONS:

REINFORCE YOUR KNOWLEDGE OF ESSENTIAL CONCEPTS:

ST Segment Elevation Myocardial Infarction (STEMI)

For questions 61 - 67, refer to PRACTICE ECG 6

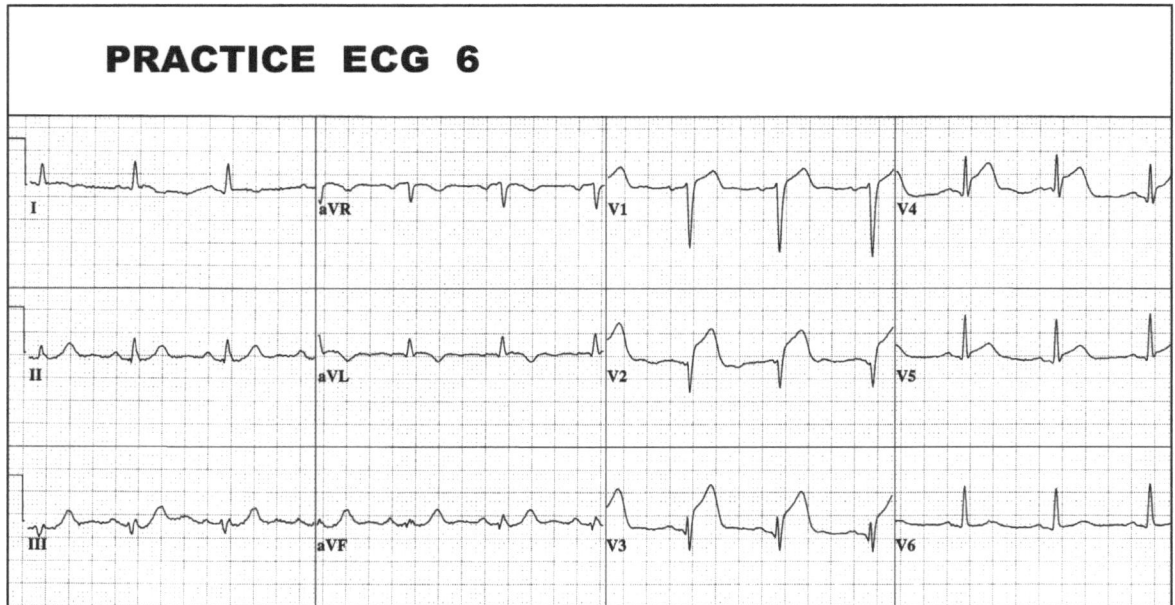

PRACTICE ECG 6

61. (p. 168) ST segment elevation is noted most prominently in leads _____.
    a. II, III, aVF
    b. V1 – V4
    c. V1 – V6, and I, aVL
    d. I, aVL

62. (p. 168) ST segment depression is noted in leads _____.
    a. I, aVL
    b. II, III, aVF
    c. V1 – V3
    d. No significant ST depression is noted in any leads

63. (p. 168) The above ECG indicates an acute _____ wall STEMI may be in progress.
    a. inferior
    b. anterior
    c. anterior-lateral
    d. lateral

64. (p. 168) This patient's coronary arterial blockage is most likely located in the _____.
    a. right coronary artery
    b. left anterior descending artery
    c. left main coronary artery
    d. circumflex artery

65. (p. 168) Occlusion of the left anterior descending artery compromises blood flow to approximately _____% of the left ventricular muscle mass.
   a. 5 - 10
   b. 20 - 30
   c. 20 - 70
   d. 40 - 50

66. (p. 169) Potential complications of anterior wall MI include LV pump failure, ventricular dysrhythmias, bundle branch blocks and _____.
   a. high grade (2nd, 3rd degree) heart blocks
   b. mental blocks
   c. writer's blocks
   d. H&R Blocks

67. (p. 169) Interventions you should be prepared for in cases of anterior wall STEMI include:
   a. manage cardiogenic shock
   b. perform transcutaneous pacing
   c. treat lethal dysrhythmias
   d. all of the above

For questions 68 - 70, refer to PRACTICE ECG 7

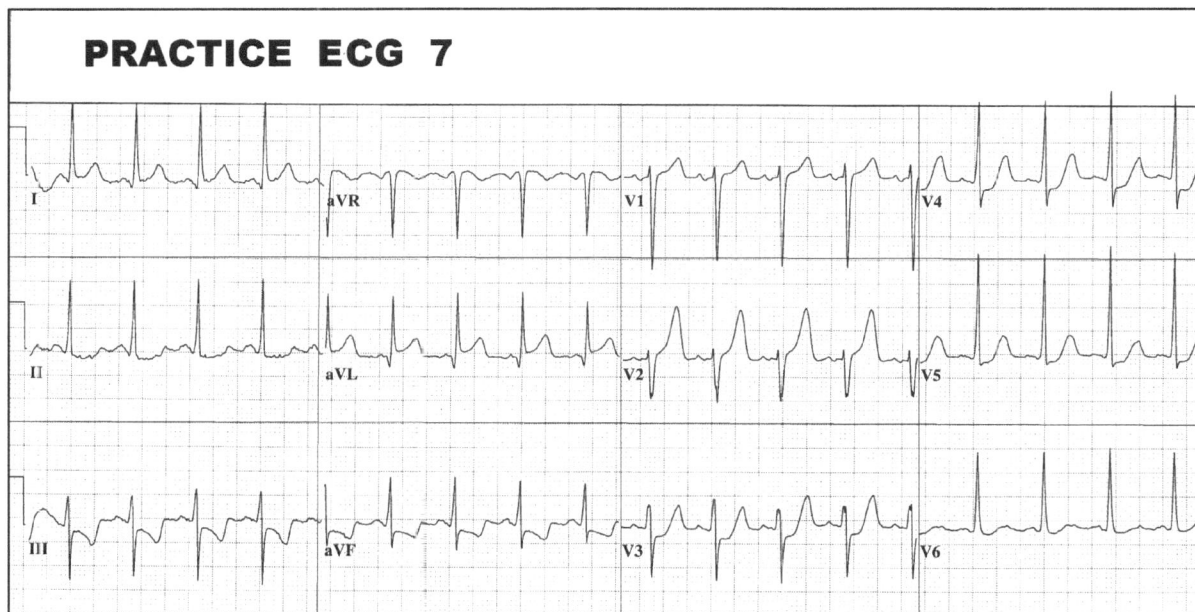

PRACTICE ECG 7

68. (p. 174) ST segment elevation is noted most prominently in leads:
   a. II, III, aVF
   b. V1 – V4
   c. V1 – V6, and I, aVL
   d. I, aVL

69. (p. 174) The above ECG reflects an acute _____ wall STEMI.
   a. inferior
   b. anterior
   c. anterior-lateral junction
   d. posterior

70. (p. 175) In cases of STEMI with ST segment elevation in leads I and aVL, the coronary arterial blockage could be located in the:
   a. proximal left anterior descending artery
   b. ramus artery
   c. proximal circumflex artery
   d. any of the above

71. (p. 176) Any patient suffering AMI can experience lethal dysrhythmias at any time, regardless of the size and location of the infarction.
   a. True
   b. False

For questions 72 - 77, refer to PRACTICE ECG 8

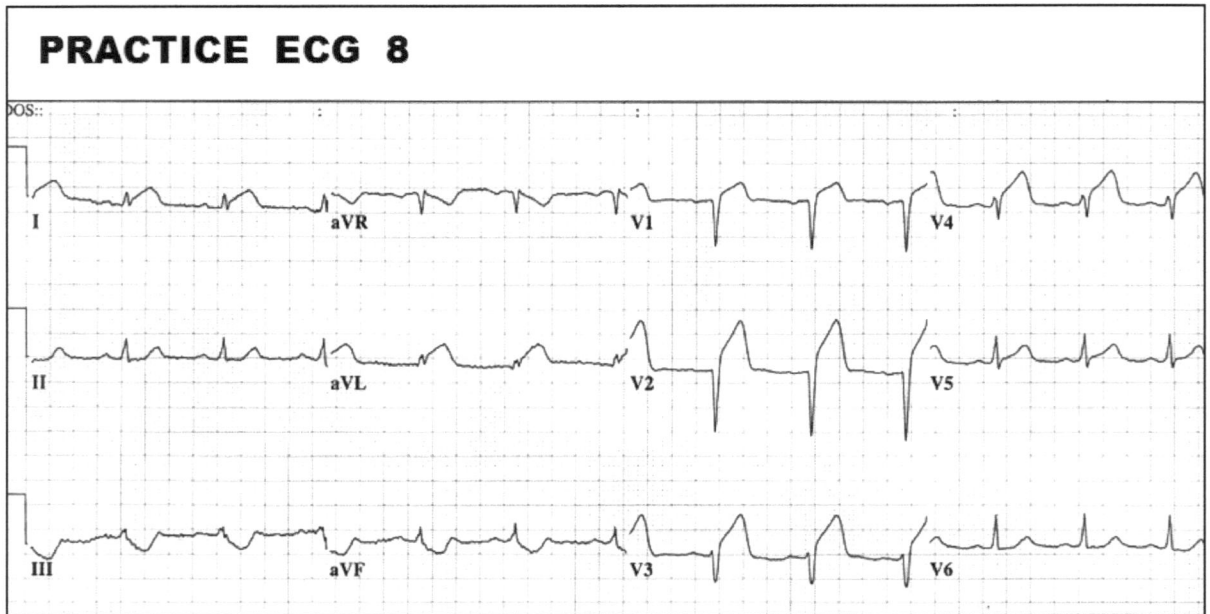

PRACTICE ECG 8

72. (p. 180) ST segment elevation is noted most prominently in leads:
   a. II, III, aVF
   b. V1 – V4
   c. V1 – V4, and I, aVL
   d. I, aVL

73. (p. 180) ST segment depression is noted in leads:
   a. I, aVL
   b. II, III, aVF
   c. V1 – V3
   d. No significant ST depression is noted in any leads

74. (p. 180) The above ECG is indicative of acute _____ wall STEMI.
   a. inferior
   b. anterior
   c. anterior-lateral
   d. lateral

232

75. (p. 180) This patient's coronary arterial blockage is most likely located in the _____.
   a. right coronary artery
   b. *proximal* left anterior descending artery
   c. left main coronary artery
   d. circumflex artery

76. (p. 180) Two important ECG clues that the occlusion is in the proximal vs. mid left anterior descending artery are:
   a. ST segment elevation is noted in leads I and aVL
   b. the patient casually informs you of this during the assessment interview
   c. there is reciprocal ST depression noted in the inferior leads (II, III, and/or aVF).
   d. both a and c

77. (p. 180,181) In cases of anterior wall MI caused by occlusion of the proximal vs. mid left anterior descending artery, there is a higher incidence of:
   a. LV pump failure and cardiogenic shock
   b. high grade (2nd and 3rd degree) heart block
   c. extension of the thrombus load into the left main and circumflex arteries.
   d. all of the above

For questions 78 - 80, refer to PRACTICE ECG 9

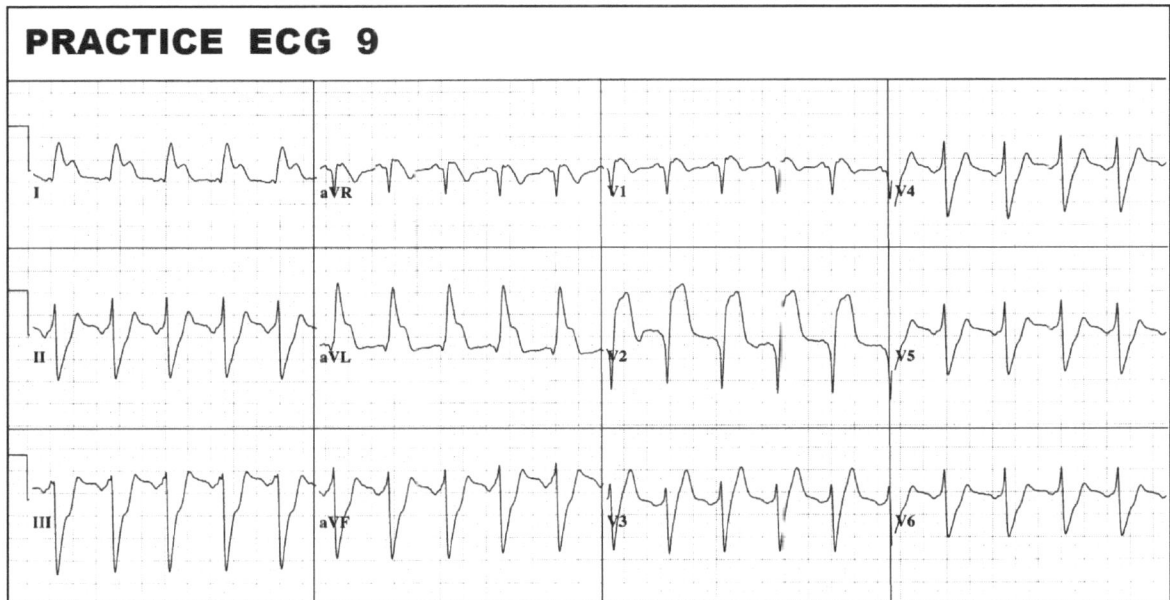

PRACTICE ECG 9

78. (p. 186) The above ECG is a "classic" example of STEMI caused by occlusion of the:
   a. dominant right coronary artery
   b. dominant circumflex artery
   c. mid left anterior descending artery
   d. left main coronary artery

79. (p. 186) Important clues that this patient is suffering from AMI caused by an obstruction of the left main coronary artery are:
   a. there is ST elevation in lead aVR which is equal to or greater than that in lead V1.
   b. ST elevation and ST depression are seen in the precordial leads, evidence of "competing forces of ANTERIOR vs. POSTERIOR wall MI.
   c. Left Anterior Fascicular Block pattern is present in leads I, II, and III.
   d. all of the above.

80. (p. 26) In patients with AMI caused by occlusion of the left main coronary artery whom have non-dominant circumflex arteries, approximately 55-75% of their LV muscle mass is affected. In patients with dominant circumflex arteries, approximately _____% of their LV muscle mass is affected.
   a. 20-30
   b. 40-50
   c. 60-70
   d. 90-100

For questions 81 - 87, refer to PRACTICE ECG 10

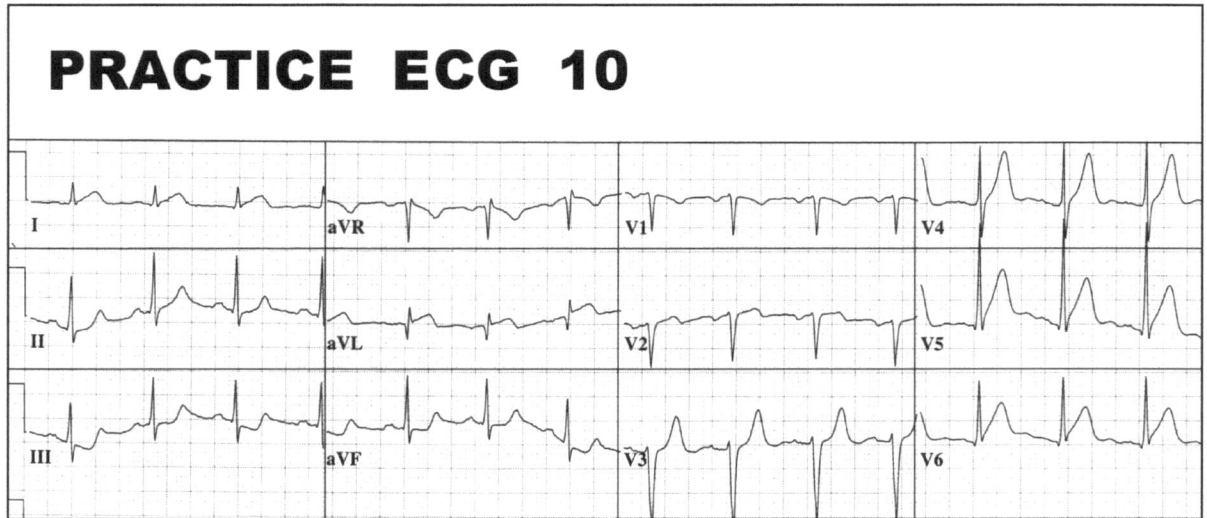

PRACTICE ECG 10

81. (p. 192) ST segment elevation is noted most prominently in leads:
   a. II, III, aVF
   b. V1 – V4
   c. V5 – V6, and I, aVL
   d. I, aVL

82. (p. 192) ST segment depression is noted in leads:
   a. I, aVL
   b. III, aVF
   c. V1 – V3
   d. No significant ST depression is noted in any leads

83. (p. 192) The above ECG indicates an acute _____ wall STEMI may be in progress.
   a. inferior
   b. anterior
   c. anterior-lateral
   d. lateral

84. (p. 192) In cases of lateral wall STEMI, the patient's occlusion is most likely located in the:
   a. left anterior descending artery
   b. circumflex artery
   c. right coronary artery
   d. left main coronary artery

85. (p. 192) Because there is no ST elevation noted in the inferior leads (II, III, and/or aVF) with this lateral wall STEMI, the patient most likely has occluded a *small, non-dominant* circumflex artery.
   a. True
   b. False

86. (p. 193) Occlusion of a non-dominant artery compromises blood flow to approximately _____% of the left ventricular muscle mass.
   a. 5 - 10
   b. 25 - 30
   c. 20 - 70
   d. 40 - 50

87. (p. 193) In most cases, lateral wall STEMI caused by the occlusion of a small, non-dominant circumflex artery usually results in LV pump failure with severe cardiogenic shock.
   a. true
   b. false

For questions 88- 98 refer to PRACTICE ECG 11

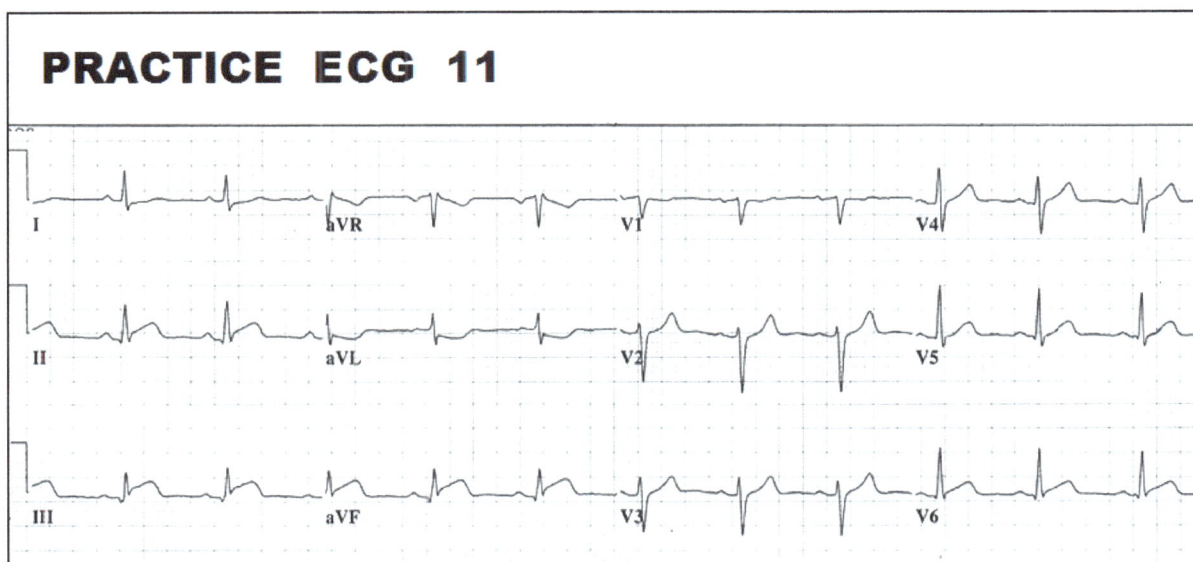

PRACTICE ECG 11

88. (p. 198) ST segment elevation is noted most prominently in leads:
   a. II, III, aVF
   b. V1 – V4
   c. V5 – V6, and I, aVL
   d. I, aVL

89. (p. 198) ST segment depression is noted in leads:
   a. I, aVL
   b. III, aVF
   c. V1 – V3
   d. No significant ST depression is noted in any leads

90. (p. 198) The above ECG indicates an acute _____ wall STEMI may be in progress.
   a. inferior
   b. anterior
   c. anterior-lateral
   d. lateral

91. (p. 199) In cases of inferior wall STEMI, the coronary artery most likely occluded is the:
    a. left anterior descending artery
    b. circumflex artery
    c. right coronary artery
    d. left main coronary artery

92. (p. 199) The inferior wall receives its blood supply from the right coronary artery in _____% of the population.
    a. 15-20
    b. 20-30
    c. 35-45
    d. 75-80

93. (p. 199) Occlusion of a dominant right coronary artery compromises blood flow to approximately _____% of the left ventricular muscle mass.
    a. 3 - 5
    b. 15 - 25
    c. 60 - 70
    d. 80 – 90

94. (p. 199) Since 75 – 80% of the population have a dominant right coronary artery that supplies blood to the inferior wall of the left ventricle, inferior and inferior-right ventricular MI are the most common forms of inferior wall STEMI.
    a. true
    b. false

95. (p. 199) The right coronary artery usually supplies blood to:
    a. sinus node
    b. right ventricle
    c. AV node
    d. all of the above

96. (p. 199) Potential complications of inferior wall MI include:
    a. bradycardia
    b. right ventricular infarction
    c. heart blocks (1st, 2nd, and 3rd degree)
    d. all of the above

97. (p. 201) When inferior wall MI is noted on the ECG, clinicians should remember to look for extension of the zone of infarct to the following region(s) of the heart:
    a. posterior wall
    b. right ventricle
    c. lateral wall
    d. all of the above

98. (p. 201, 202) In this book, we advocate performing the "3 Step Process" for ruling out posterior, right ventricular and lateral wall involvement in cases of inferior wall STEMI. The 3 Step Process consists of:
    a. evaluating leads V1 – V3 for reciprocal ST segment depression
    b. performing a right ventricular ECG
    c. evaluating leads V5 and V6 for ST segment elevation
    d. all of the above

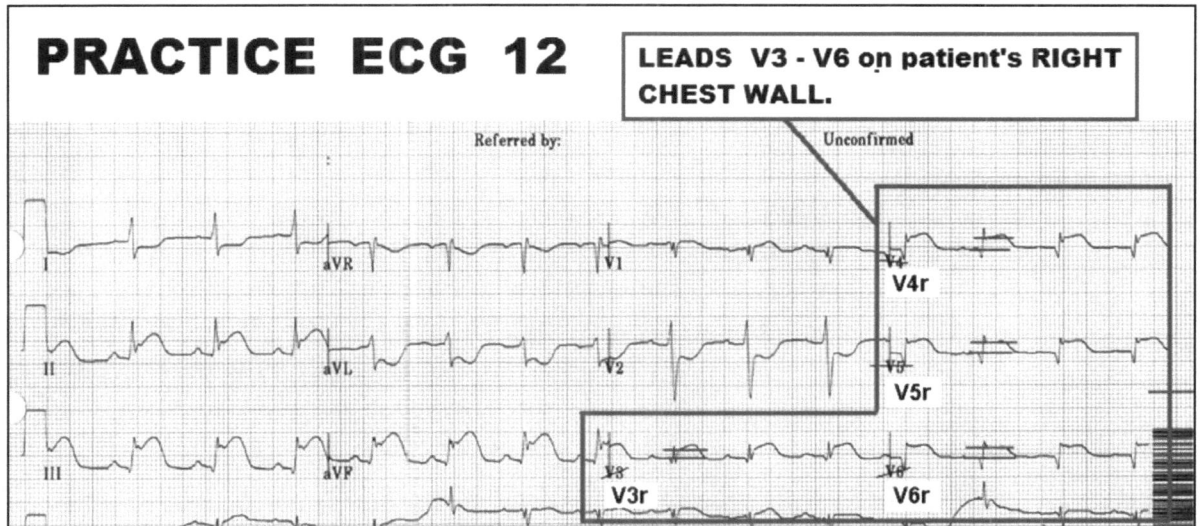

PRACTICE ECG 12

LEADS V3 - V6 on patient's RIGHT CHEST WALL.

Referred by: Unconfirmed

99. (p. 208) ST segment elevation is noted in leads:
   a. I, aVL
   b. II, III, and aVF
   c. V3r-V6r
   d. b and c

100. (p. 208) Based on the ECG, this patient is suffering from acute _____ MI.
   a. inferior-right ventricular
   b. anterior-lateral
   c. lateral
   d. inferior

101. (p. 208) Inferior-right ventricular MI is almost always caused by an occlusion of the:
   a. proximal left anterior descending artery
   b. proximal circumflex artery
   c. left main coronary artery
   d. proximal right coronary artery

102. (p. 208, 209) It's important to know about the presence of right ventricular MI at the bedside because the patient will:
   a. be extremely sensitive to nitrates, opiates and other vasodilators
   b. most likely suffer precipitous drop in blood pressure when nitroglycerin is given
   c. require IV fluids to correct hypotension caused by vasodilator medications
   d. all of the above

237

PRACTICE EKG 13

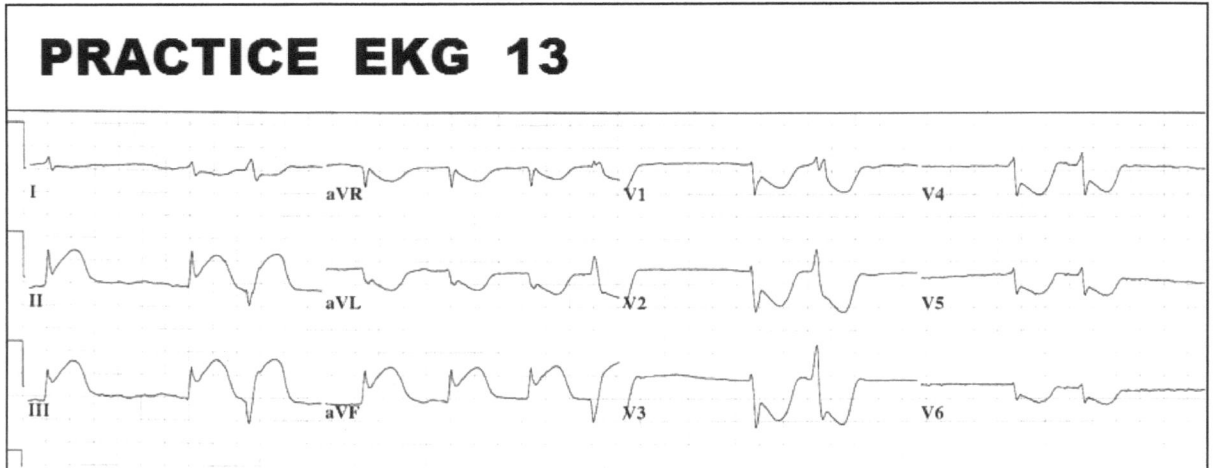

103. (p. 215) In the above ECG, there is ST segment elevation seen in leads:
    a. I and aVL
    b. II, III, and aVF
    c. II, III, aVF, and leads V1-V6
    d. V1-V4

104. (p. 215) In the above ECG, reciprocal ST segment depression is seen in leads:
    a. V1-V6
    b. II, III, aVF
    c. I and aVL
    d. No ST depression is noted on the ECG

105. (p. 215) This patient is most likely suffering from acute _____ MI.
    a. inferior-posterior
    b. inferior-lateral-right ventricular
    c. lateral
    d. anterior-septal

106. (p. 215) The zone-of-infarct in inferior-posterior MI can affect approximately _____% of the LV muscle mass.
    a. 15-25
    b. 20-35
    c. 25-45
    d. 90-95

107. (p. 217) In cases of inferior-posterior MI, clinicians should be prepared to manage:
    a. hypotension/cardiogenic shock
    b. sinus node dysfunction
    c. AV node dysfunction
    d. all of the above

108. (p. 216) In addition to ST changes, what other abnormality is seen on the 12 lead ECG?
    a. atrial flutter
    b. ventricular fibrillation
    c. skipped beats which could be caused by sinus node failure or 2nd degree type I heart block (Wenchebach)
    d. ventricular tachycardia

109. (p. 215) Inferior-posterior wall MI is usually caused by occlusion of a:
   a. dominant circumflex artery
   b. "extreme" dominant right coronary artery
   c. left anterior descending artery
   d. a and b

For questions 110 – 115, refer to PRACTICE ECG 14

PRACTICE EKG 14

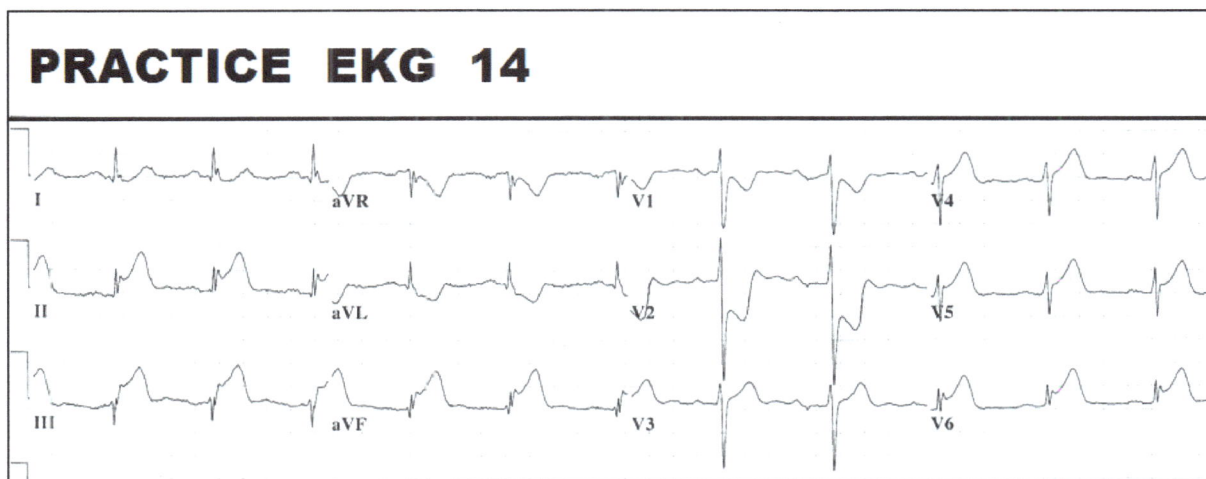

110. (p. 220, 221) Significant ST segment elevation is noted in leads:
   a. I, aVL, V1, V2
   b. II, III, aVF
   c. II, III, aVF, V4 – V6
   d. V4 – V6

111. (p. 220, 221) Significant ST depression is noted in leads:
   a. aVL, V1, V2
   b. II, III, aVF
   c. V4 – V6
   d. I, V3

112. (p. 221) This patient is most likely experiencing acute _____ STEMI.
   a. interior-posterior-lateral
   b. anterior-lateral
   c. posterior
   d. anterior-septal

113. (p. 221) In cases of inferior-posterior-lateral MI, the most likely cause is an occlusion in the:
   a. (dominant) circumflex artery
   b. mid left anterior descending artery
   c. proximal non-dominant right coronary artery
   d. mid non-dominant circumflex artery

114. (p. 222) The zone-of-infarction in cases of inferior-posterior-lateral MI usually affects approximately _____% of the LV muscle mass.
   a. 15-20
   b. 35-55
   c. 80-90
   d. 90-100

115. (p. 222) It is unusual for inferior-posterior-lateral MI to cause profound LV pump failure with cardiogenic shock.
   a. true
   b. false

For questions 116 - 119, refer to PRACTICE ECG 15.

PRACTICE EKG 15

116. (p. 227) ST segment elevation is noted in leads:
   a. II, III, aVF
   b. V1-V4
   c. aVR, aVL
   d. I, II, III, aVF, V2 – V6

117. (p. 227) This patient is most likely experiencing acute _____ wall STEMI.
   a. anterior-lateral-inferior
   b. posterior-lateral
   c. inferior-posterior-lateral
   d. anterior-septal

118. (p. 227) This type of MI is most likely caused by a proximal occlusion in a (an):
   a. dominant circumflex artery
   b. abnormally large transapical left anterior descending artery
   c. small, non-dominant right coronary artery
   d. ramus artery

119. (p. 228) Potential complications clinicians should anticipate in this type of MI include:
   a. profound cardiogenic shock: hypotension, pulmonary edema
   b. ventricular dysrhythmias (e.g. ventricular tachycardia, ventricular fibrillation)
   c. high grade heart blocks (2nd, 3rd degree)
   d. all of the above

NSTEMI CASE STUDIES:

Non-ST Segment Elevation Myocardial Infarction (NSTEMI) is an acute myocardial infarction which *does not* present with typical S-T segment elevation. There is often *S-T segment depression* from sub-endocardial (non Q wave producing) myocardial infarction. Occasionally, isolated *posterior wall infarction* will present with reciprocal ST segment depression in the anterior precordial leads. *Patients usually exhibit cardiac symptoms* (typical or atypical), and *cardiac markers* are abnormally elevated.

Previous medical terminology used to describe this phenomenon includes *Subendocardial Myocardial Infarction* and *Non-Q Wave Myocardial Infarction*. As its name implies, subendocardial MI involves injury to the subendocardium, and does not result in transmural necrosis. Because the necrotic region does not extend through the full thickness of LV muscle, the patient's LV function is often preserved or incurs minimal impairment. A more recent term for subendocardial MI is "non-Q wave myocardial infarction." Once again, as its name implies, the non-Q wave MI does not result in formation of abnormal Q waves on the 12 lead ECG.

As the flow chart to the left indicates, in cases of NSTEMI, the 12 Lead ECG may demonstrate *ST segment depression, subtle abnormal ST segment changes,* or may be entirely *normal*.

Acute posterior wall MI and *right ventricular MI* are often diagnosed as NSTEMI, but the area of myocardial injury is *transmural.* The right ventricle and posterior wall are missed by the 12 lead ECG because there are no ECG leads placed over the right chest wall or the patient's back which would pick up on indicative ST elevation.

Because the right ventricle and posterior wall are in two "blind spots" of the 12 lead ECG, when patients present with symptoms suspicious for ACS and no ST elevation on their 12 lead ECG, an 18 lead ECG should be obtained. This is especially true when the initial 12 lead ECG shows ST segment depression in leads V1-V4. As demonstrated in Case Study 12 on page 246, ST depression in the anterior leads may be reciprocal changes of acute posterior wall MI. If either posterior or right ventricular wall MI is diagnosed, the patient should be treated as an acute STEMI patient.

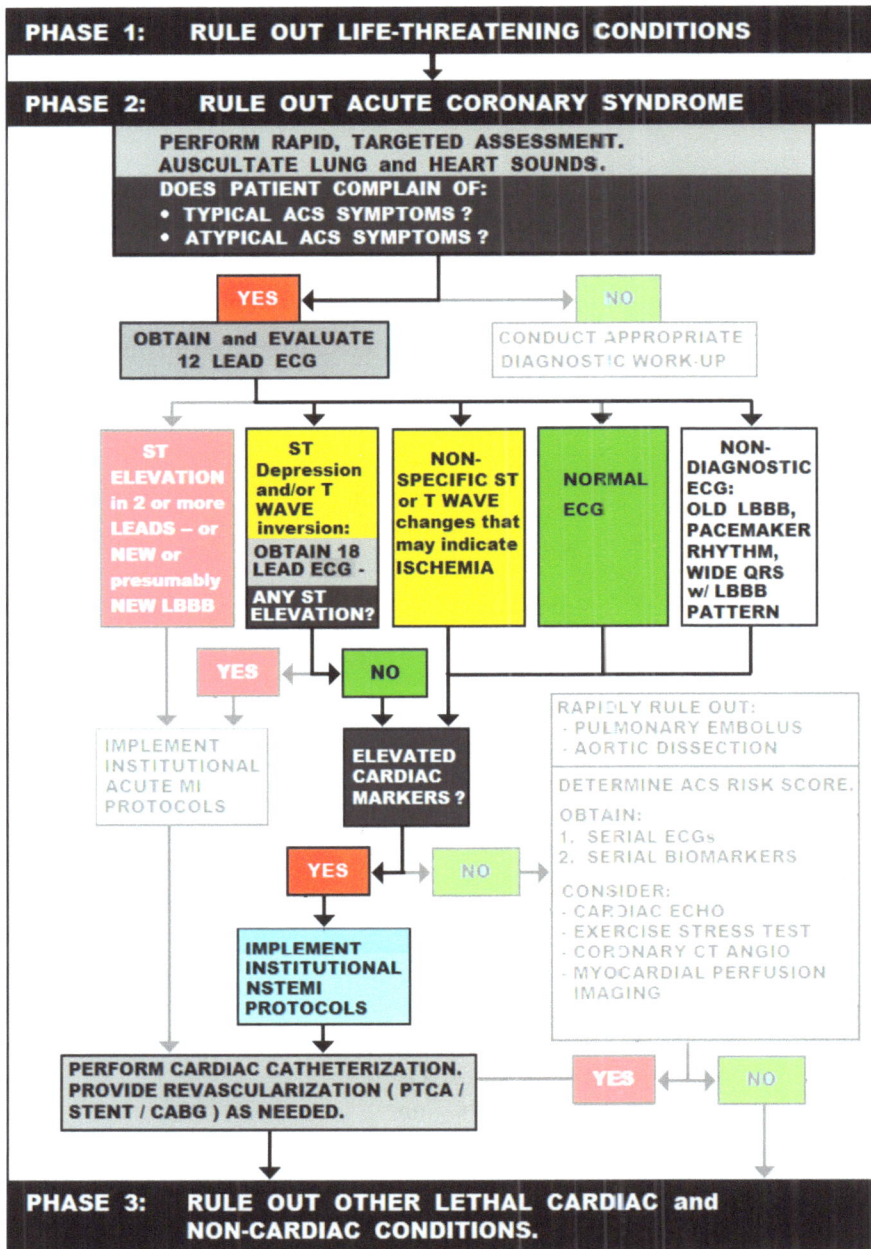

PHASE 1: RULE OUT LIFE-THREATENING CONDITIONS

PHASE 2: RULE OUT ACUTE CORONARY SYNDROME

PERFORM RAPID, TARGETED ASSESSMENT. AUSCULTATE LUNG and HEART SOUNDS.

DOES PATIENT COMPLAIN OF:
- TYPICAL ACS SYMPTOMS ?
- ATYPICAL ACS SYMPTOMS ?

YES / NO

OBTAIN and EVALUATE 12 LEAD ECG

CONDUCT APPROPRIATE DIAGNOSTIC WORK-UP

ST ELEVATION in 2 or more LEADS – or NEW or presumably NEW LBBB

ST Depression and/or T WAVE inversion: OBTAIN 18 LEAD ECG - ANY ST ELEVATION?

NON-SPECIFIC ST or T WAVE changes that may indicate ISCHEMIA

NORMAL ECG

NON-DIAGNOSTIC ECG: OLD LBBB, PACEMAKER RHYTHM, WIDE QRS w/ LBBB PATTERN

YES / NO

IMPLEMENT INSTITUTIONAL ACUTE MI PROTOCOLS

ELEVATED CARDIAC MARKERS ?

RAPIDLY RULE OUT:
- PULMONARY EMBOLUS
- AORTIC DISSECTION

DETERMINE ACS RISK SCORE.

OBTAIN:
1. SERIAL ECGs
2. SERIAL BIOMARKERS

CONSIDER:
- CARDIAC ECHO
- EXERCISE STRESS TEST
- CORONARY CT ANGIO
- MYOCARDIAL PERFUSION IMAGING

YES / NO

IMPLEMENT INSTITUTIONAL NSTEMI PROTOCOLS

PERFORM CARDIAC CATHETERIZATION. PROVIDE REVASCULARIZATION (PTCA / STENT / CABG) AS NEEDED.

YES / NO

PHASE 3: RULE OUT OTHER LETHAL CARDIAC and NON-CARDIAC CONDITIONS.

CHIEF COMPLAINT and SIGNIFICANT HISTORY:

42 y/o MALE in ED c/o INTERMITTENT SUBSTERNAL CHEST PAIN x 9 HOURS, "8" on 1-10 scale, pain does not radiate, not effected by position/deep inspiration. Denies DIB.
Pt. given NTG 0.4mg SL without releif of CHEST PAIN.

RISK FACTOR PROFILE:

💣 ELEVATED LDL CHOLESTEROL, LOW HDL CHOLESTEROL
✔ PATIENT DENIES SMOKING, FAMILY HISTORY, HYPERTENSION

PHYSICAL EXAM: CAOx4, SKIN WARM, DRY, COLOR NORMAL, NON-ANXIOUS,
LUNGS CLEAR, HEART SOUNDS NORMAL S1, S2, NO JVD, NO ANKLE EDEMA

VITAL SIGNS: BP: 122/76   P: 86   R: 16   SAO2: 98% on 2 LPM O2

LABS: TROPONIN: >500   CK: 4,410   CK MB: 224.1   CK INDEX: 5.1

QUADRAD OF ACS CHECKLIST

☑ **SYMPTOMS of ACS**
   - ✔ ◆ TYPICAL ACS - eg:
   - ◆ ATYPICAL ACS - eg:

☐ **ECG ABNORMALITIES**
   - ◆ ST ELEVATION (J POINT plus 40 ms)
   - ◆ HYPERACUTE T WAVES - and/or -
   - ◆ NEW or PRESUMABLY NEW LBBB
   - ◆ ST DEPRESSION (>0.5 mm @ J POINT) and/or
   - ◆ INVERTED or BIPHASIC T WAVES and/or
   - ◆ DYNAMIC ST SEGMENT and/or T WAVE CHANGES IN SERIAL EKGs

☐ **RISK FACTORS - 3 or more**
   - ◆ FAMILY HISTORY
   - ◆ DIABETES
   - ✔ ↑ LDL and/or ↓ HDL
   - ◆ SMOKING
   - ◆ AGE: 65 or MORE
   - ◆ HYPERTENSION

☑ **CARDIAC MARKERS**
   - ✔ ◆ ELEVATED TROPONIN and/or CK/MB ✔

2 **TOTAL**

This patient presented to the triage desk in the Emergency Department complaining a "dull aching sensation" in the center of his chest, and shortness of breath. At the time of triage, he stated the pain was a "8" on a 1 – 10 scale. He did not exhibit any signs of shock, nor did he appear to be in any distress.

He was given 325mg of aspirin, a STAT ECG was obtained, an IV of normal saline was started at a KVO rate, and a STAT ECG was recorded, as seen on the next page. The patient was given a total of 3 nitroglycerin 0.4mg tablets SL without change in symptoms. Blood specimens were drawn and sent to the lab for cardiac markers, electrolytes, complete blood count, and coagulation studies. He reported his pain decreased to a "2" after Morphine 4mg IV was administered.

Due to his typical ACS type symptoms and family history, serial ECGs were obtained. All four ECGs were normal, with no changes from the first.

SUSPECTED ACUTE MI:
INITIAL MANAGEMENT

- VITAL SIGNS
- "O.M.I."
  - Oxygen
  - Monitor (ecg)
  - IV (plus draw lab samples)
- 12 LEAD ECG
  Obtain and interpret within 10 minutes of patient's arrival.
- "M.O.N.A."
  - Morphine
  - Oxygen (if not already done)
  - Nitroglycerin
  - Aspirin
- RAPID, FOCUSED ASSESSMENT
- HEART / LUNG SOUNDS
- SEND LAB SAMPLES:
  - Cardiac Markers
  - Electrolytes
  - Coagulation Studies

42 yr
Male   Hispanic

Room:ED
Loc:3   Option:23

Vent. rate	67	BPM
PR interval	148	ms
QRS duration	94	ms
QT/QTc	400/422	ms
P–R–T axes	–5 34	59

"**unedited copy: report is computer generated only, without physician interpretation".
Normal sinus rhythm
Nonspecific ST abnormality
Abnormal ECG
No previous ECGs available

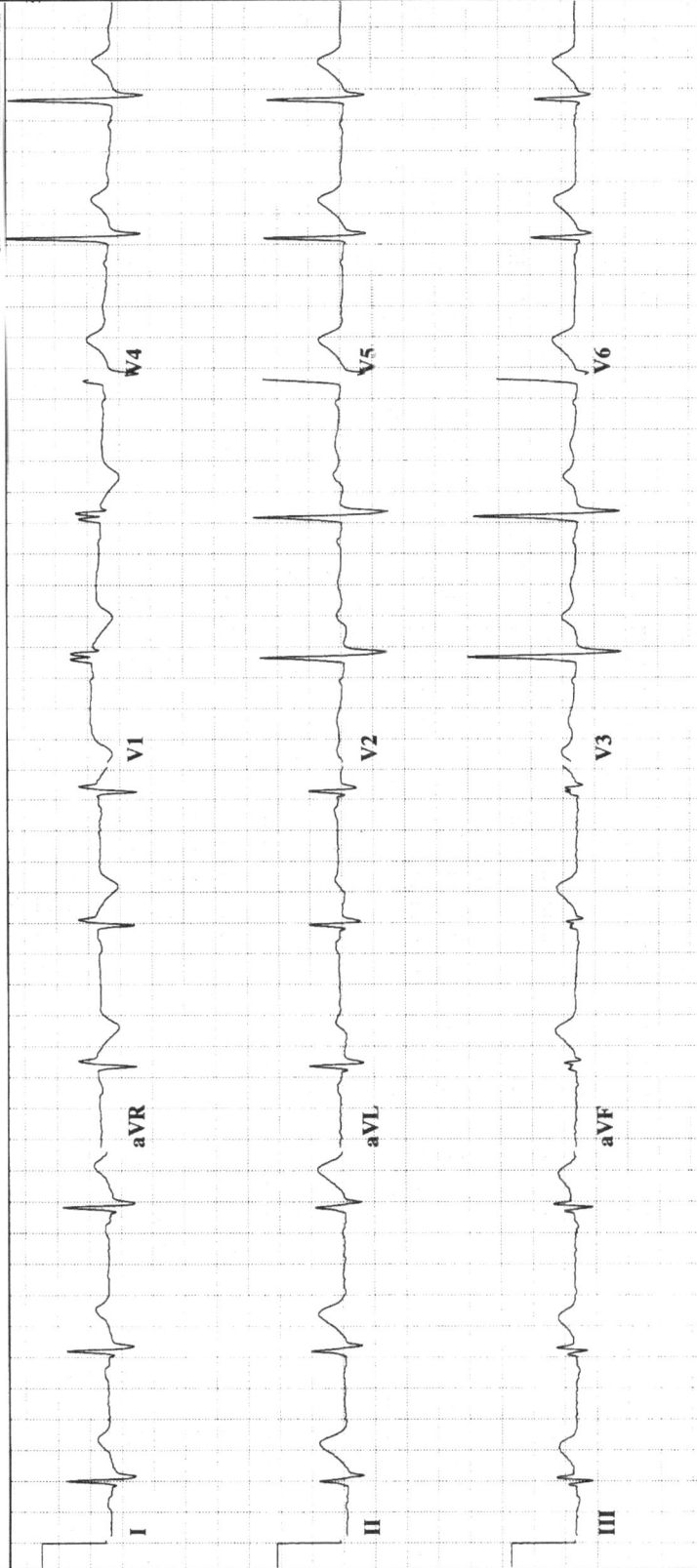

I   aVR   V1   V4

II   aVL   V2   V5

III   aVF   V3   V6

CASE STUDY QUESTIONS:

NOTE LEADS WITH ST ELEVATION:	NOTE LEADS WITH ST DEPRESSION:
WHAT IS THE SUSPECTED DIAGNOSIS ?	
WHAT IS THE "CULPRIT ARTERY" – if applicable ?	
LIST ANY CRITICAL STRUCTURES COMPROMISED:	LIST ANY POTENTIAL COMPLICATIONS:

243

In this case study, we intentionally left the ECG computer generated diagnosis in place. As you can see, the computer detects "Non-specific ST abnormality." It **does not** specify which leads the abnormality is in, nor does it attempt to render a specific diagnosis, such as "consider ischemia" or "acute myocardial infarction." An astute clinician would detect the ***flattening of the J-T Apex Segments*** in leads II, III, aVF, V5 and V6. Remember that flat and/or convex J-T Apex Segments are abnormal, and are associated with the early phase of acute MI. (See "ECG Diagnosis of Acute MI" on pages 116-117). Although these findings are arguably subtle, when you combine them with his classic ACS symptoms and Troponin value of >500, the flat J-T Apex Segments should become ***red flags***. In this case study, based on the patient's duration of symptoms and elevation of Troponin and CK, this MI is not in the early phase; it is most likely 12-24 hours in duration.

What is atypical about this case is the lack of significant ST segment elevation (only lead III has J point elevation), and the lack of significant Q waves. Note that transition is early; V1 and V2 are positive, although an argument could be made that early transition is due to an incomplete right bundle branch block based on the the RR' notching in V1.

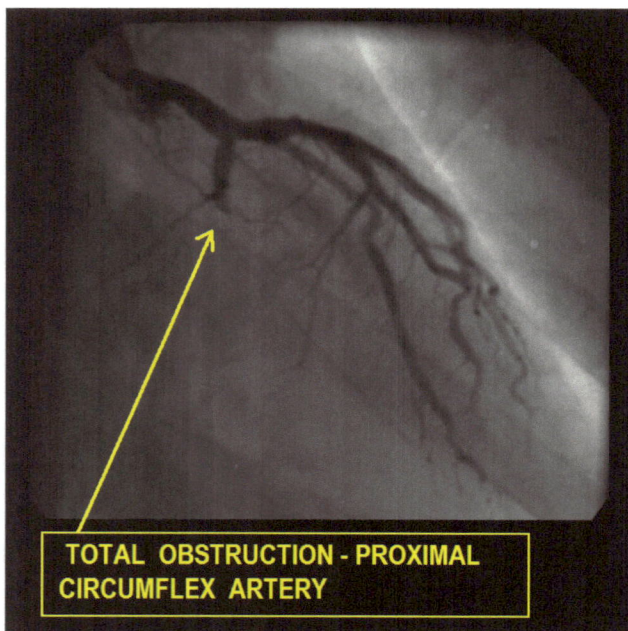

TOTAL OBSTRUCTION - PROXIMAL CIRCUMFLEX ARTERY

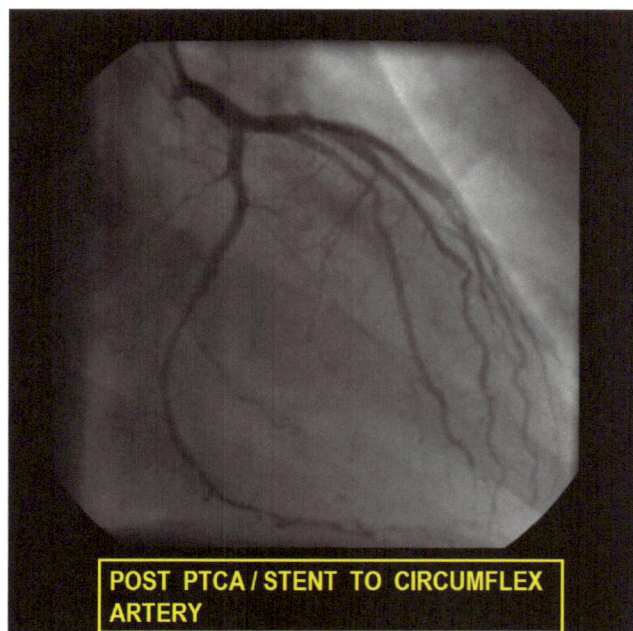

POST PTCA / STENT TO CIRCUMFLEX ARTERY

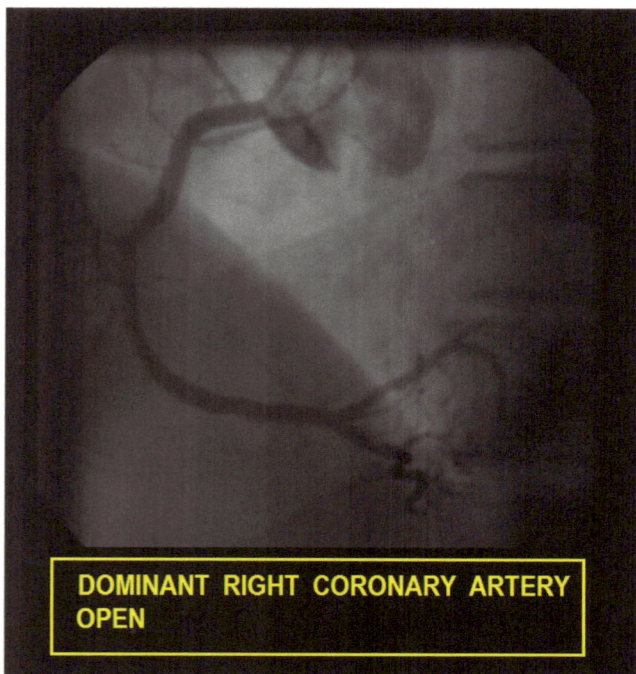

DOMINANT RIGHT CORONARY ARTERY OPEN

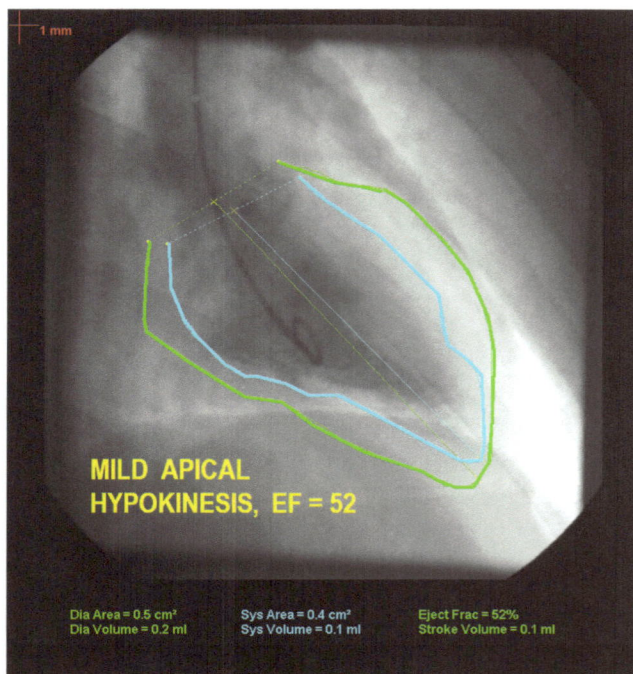

MILD APICAL HYPOKINESIS, EF = 52

| Dia Area = 0.5 cm² | Sys Area = 0.4 cm² | Eject Frac = 52% |
| Dia Volume = 0.2 ml | Sys Volume = 0.1 ml | Stroke Volume = 0.1 ml |

This case study should reinforce the concept that clinicians must remember to consider each of the four assessment components of the Quadrad of ACS in the clinical decision making process. As this case study demonstrates, *it is possible for patients to incur acute transmural MI secondary to total occlusion of a coronary artery without resultant ST segment elevation or depression on the 12 lead ECG.*

Experience with acute MI patients in the cath lab has taught us *if a patient has 2 or more "positives" in the "Quadrad of ACS" present, it is imperative that ACS aggressively be ruled out*. In this case study, the patient had two of the Quadrad of ACS present: *symptoms of ACS*, and *elevated cardiac markers*.

In the cath lab, we have noticed acute blockages of non-dominant or split-dominant circumflex arteries appear to cause most of the MIs that present without ST segment elevation on the 12 lead ECG; hence we've coined the term "silent circ." As this case study demonstrates, the name "silent circ" is well deserved!

CASE STUDY SUMMARY

ST ELEVATION:	ST DEPRESSION:
III	NONE.

SUSPECTED DIAGNOSIS: ACUTE NSTEMI - BASED ON SYMPTOMS & ELEVATED MARKERS

SUSPECTED "CULPRIT ARTERY" (if applicable):
UNABLE TO DETERMINE BASED ON 12 LEAD EKG PRESENTATION.

IMMEDIATE CONCERNS FOR ALL ACUTE MI PATIENTS:

- BE PREPARED TO MANAGE SUDDEN CARDIAC ARREST (PRIMARY V - FIB / V- TACH, BRADYCARDIAS / HEART BLOCKS)
- STAT REPERFUSION THERAPY: THROMBOLYTICS vs. CARDIAC CATHETERIZATION and PCI
- CONSIDER NEEDS FOR ANTI-PLATELET and ANTI-COAGULATION THERAPY

CRITICAL STRUCTURES COMPROMISED:	POTENTIAL COMPLICATIONS:	POSSIBLE CRITICAL INTERVENTIONS:
20 - 30% of LV MUSCLE MASS	POSSIBLE MINOR - MODERATE LV FAILURE.	SMALL FLUID CHALLENGE INOTROPIC AGENTS
45% of POPULATION HAS SINUS NODE SUPPLIED BY CIRCUMFLEX ARTERY	SINUS BRADYCARDIA SINUS ARREST	ATROPINE TRANSCUTANEOUS PACING

In this case study, we've noted the patient had unusually high troponin and CK values. Since *both* markers are extremely high, it is unlikely that an error occurred during lab processing. The degree of cardiac marker elevation is more consistent with a massive multi-site infarction than with a small region of the lateral wall. As is sometimes seen in medicine, the out-of-proportion cardiac marker elevation is one of those occurrences that falls outside the realm of typical expectations.

Case study contributed by Ben Mendoza, MD, FACC

CASE STUDY 12 - NSTEMI

CHIEF COMPLAINT and SIGNIFICANT HISTORY:

63 y/o MALE in ED complaining of continuous PRESSURE in both SHOULDERS, with radiation down the RIGHT ARM to the elbow x approx. 6 hours. He took Motrin 800mg. without relief. Also c/o intermittent NAUSEA. ==He DENIES CHEST PRESSURE / DISCOMFORT== and DIB.

RISK FACTOR PROFILE:

💣 **ELEVATED TRIGLYCERIDES and LOW HDL**
✔ SMOKER FOR 30+ YEARS, QUIT 6 YEARS AGO

PHYSICAL EXAM: CAOx4, SKIN WARM, DRY, COLOR PALE. PUPILS PERLA, NO JVD, LUNGS CLEAR, HEART SOUNDS NORMAL S1, S2. NO ANKLE EDEMA

VITAL SIGNS: BP: 106/50   P: 90   R: 20   SAO2: 96% on 4 LPM O2

LABS: TROPONIN: 66.3   CK: 187   CK MB: 4.2

QUADRAD OF ACS CHECKLIST

☑ **SYMPTOMS of ACS**
- ◆ TYPICAL ACS - eg:
- ✔◆ ATYPICAL ACS - eg:

☑ **ECG ABNORMALITIES**
- ◆ ST ELEVATION (J POINT plus 40 ms)
- ◆ HYPERACUTE T WAVES - and/or -
- ◆ NEW or PRESUMABLY NEW LBBB
- ✔◆ ST DEPRESSION (>0.5 mm @ J POINT) and/or
- ◆ INVERTED or BIPHASIC T WAVES and/or
- ◆ DYNAMIC ST SEGMENT and/or T WAVE CHANGES IN SERIAL EKGs

☐ **RISK FACTORS - 3 or more**
- ◆ FAMILY HISTORY
- ◆ DIABETES
- ◆ ↑ LDL and/or ↓ HDL
- ◆ SMOKING
- ◆ AGE: 65 or MORE
- ◆ HYPERTENSION

☑ **CARDIAC MARKERS**
- ✔◆ ELEVATED TROPONIN and/or ~~CK/MB~~

3 **TOTAL**

As is true of many NSTEMI cases, accurate diagnosis requires the clinician to be aware of atypical ACS symptoms, to have a high index of suspicion, and to consistently and aggressively rule out ACS.

In this case, the patient stated that at first, he thought he must have pulled a muscle in his shoulders or "pinched a nerve" in his upper back. He attributed the right arm pressure, which he also described as "numbness," to being neurological in nature, resulting from his pulled muscle. When it did not respond to 800mg of Motrin, and he became nauseous, his wife urged him to "go to the ER because it might be heart pain."

Upon his initial exam in the ED, his score on the Quadrad of ACS was a two: symptoms of ACS (atypical) and ECG abnormalities (ST segment depression).

Recall that when a patient has TWO or more positive values of the Quadrad of ACS, ACS should aggressively be ruled out. In this case, the ED physician ordered STAT cardiac markers, which revealed elevation of Troponin I.

The patient was taken directly to the cardiac catheterization lab, where the images on page 248 were obtained.

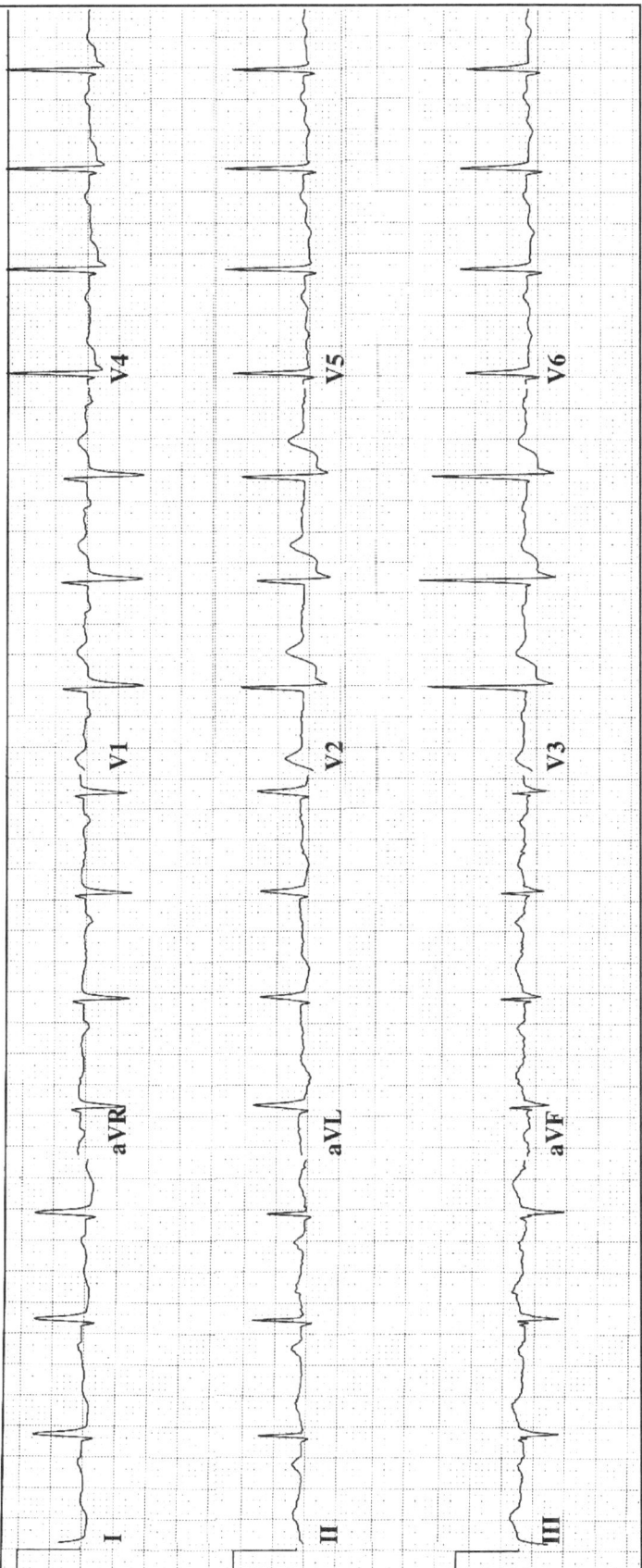

63 yr
Male   Hispanic

Room:VAM
Loc:3   Option:23

Vent. rate	88	BPM
PR interval	200	ms
QRS duration	94	ms
QT/QTc	352/425	ms
P–R–T axes	63 2	118

I   aVR   V1   V4

II   aVL   V2   V5

III   aVF   V3   V6

CASE STUDY QUESTIONS:

NOTE LEADS WITH ST ELEVATION:

NOTE LEADS WITH ST DEPRESSION:

WHAT IS THE SUSPECTED DIAGNOSIS ?

WHAT IS THE "CULPRIT ARTERY" – if applicable ?

LIST ANY CRITICAL STRUCTURES COMPROMISED:

LIST ANY POTENTIAL COMPLICATIONS:

247

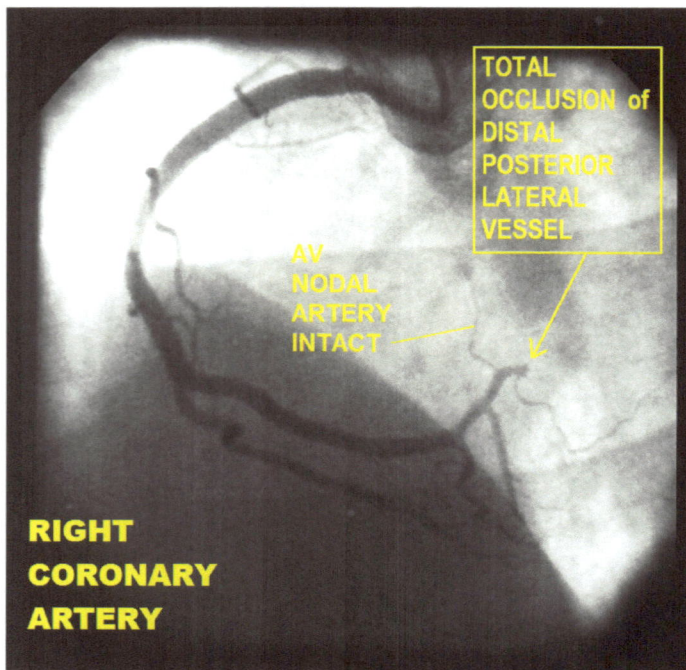

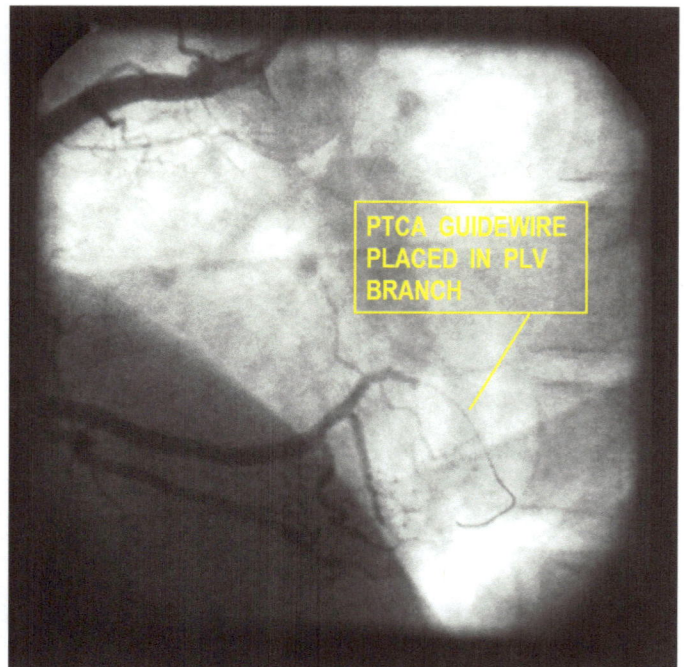

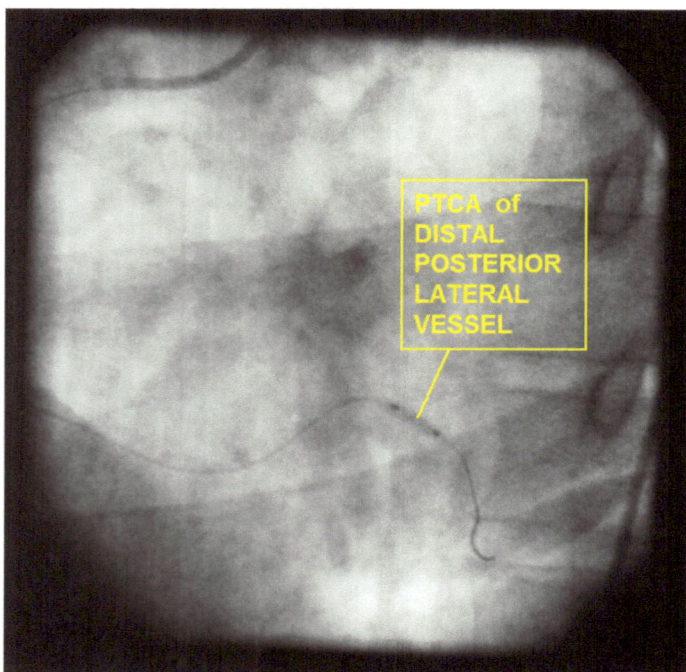

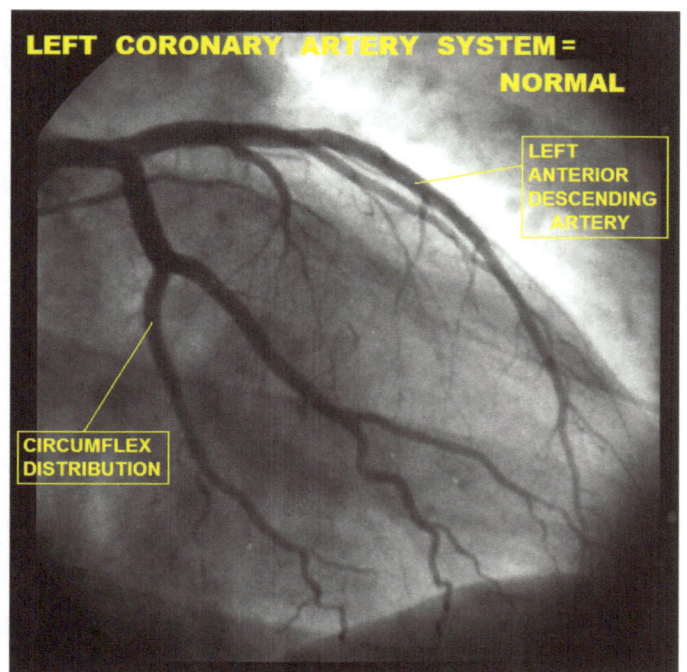

Coronary artery angiography revealed an obstructed distal posterior lateral vessel (PLV). As the above images demonstrate, PTCA was performed to open this vessel. The proximal and mid segment of the patient's right coronary artery, as well as his left coronary artery system were free of disease.

Obstruction of one or more of the posterior lateral vessels will result in infarction of the posterior wall of the left ventricle. In this case, one posterior lateral vessel was occluded, resulting in isolated posterior wall MI.

Since the 12 lead ECG does not have any leads that directly view the posterior wall, it will typically not display any ST segment elevation, as shown in the diagram to the right.

Typical 12 lead ECG findings of posterior wall MI are reciprocal ST depression in the anterior leads V1 – V3, and development of tall R waves in V1 through V3 (think of them as "reciprocal Q waves"). Although isolated posterior wall MI is classified as an "NSTEMI" because of the lack of ST elevation on the 12 lead ECG, the patient in this case study has incurred acute transmural myocardial injury.

Put in simpler terms, *"maybe we shouldn't discriminate against posterior wall MI and treat it differently than STEMI just because the 12 lead ECG doesn't adequately cover the entire myocardium."*

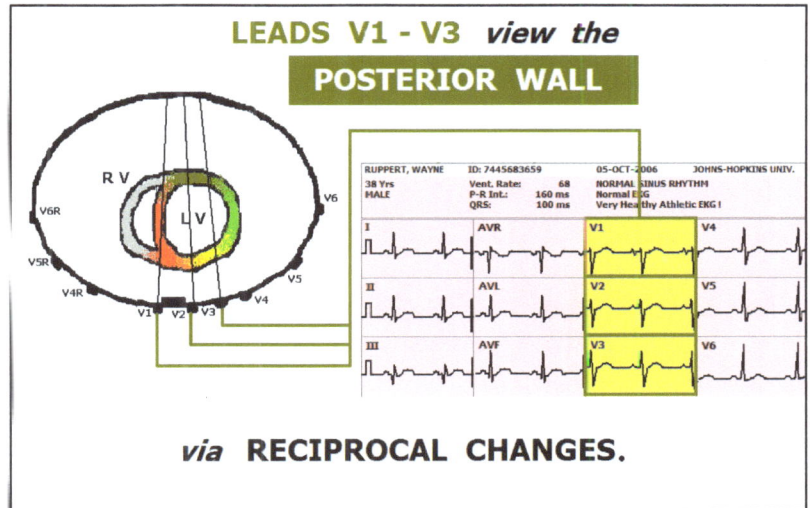

LEADS V1 - V3 *view the* POSTERIOR WALL
via RECIPROCAL CHANGES.

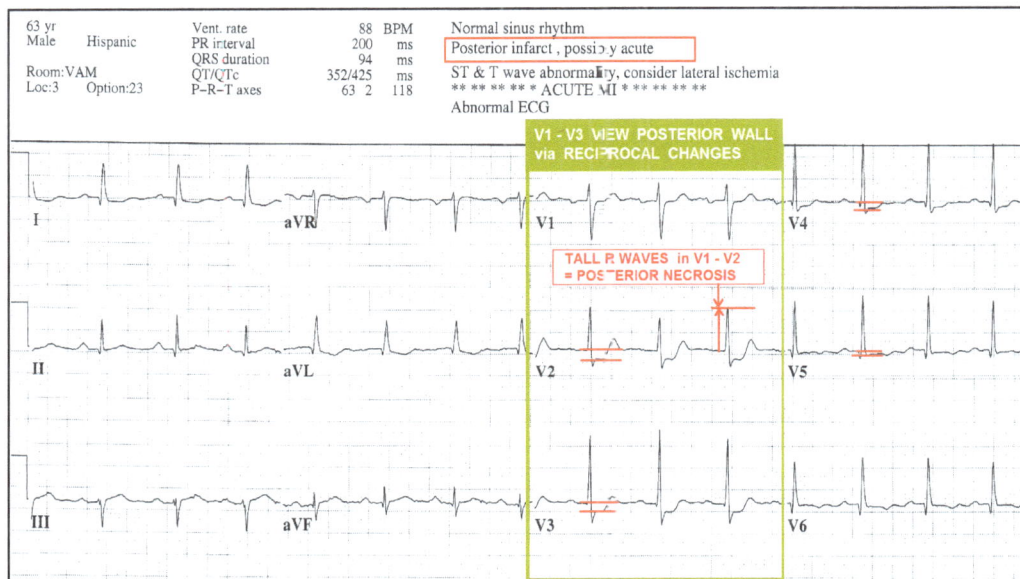

63 yr		Vent. rate	88	BPM
Male	Hispanic	PR interval	200	ms
		QRS duration	94	ms
Room: VAM		QT/QTc	352/425	ms
Loc:3	Option:23	P–R–T axes	63 2 118	

Normal sinus rhythm
Posterior infarct , possibly acute
ST & T wave abnormality, consider lateral ischemia
** ** ** ** ** ACUTE MI ** ** ** ** **
Abnormal ECG

V1 - V3 VIEW POSTERIOR WALL via RECIPROCAL CHANGES

TALL R WAVES in V1 - V2 = POSTERIOR NECROSIS

If we obtained an 18 lead ECG on this patient, it would most likely show ST elevation in leads V7, V8 and V9.

The 18 lead ECG is explained on pages 43 - 46.

Most cases of posterior wall MI also involve inferior and/or inferior-lateral wall infarction. This case study is particularly challenging because it involves the posterior wall exclusively, which is less common.

CASE STUDY SUMMARY

| ST ELEVATION: NONE. | ST DEPRESSION: V1 - V3 |

SUSPECTED DIAGNOSIS: ACUTE NSTEMI - BASED ON SYMPTOMS & ELEVATED MARKERS

SUSPECTED "CULPRIT ARTERY" (if applicable):
POSTERIOR LATERAL VESSEL(S) - originate off of RCA or CIRCUMFLEX

IMMEDIATE CONCERNS FOR ALL ACUTE MI PATIENTS:

- BE PREPARED TO MANAGE SUDDEN CARDIAC ARREST (PRIMARY V - FIB / V- TACH, BRADYCARDIAS / HEART BLOCKS)
- STAT REPERFUSION THERAPY: THROMBOLYTICS vs. CARDIAC CATHETERIZATION and PCI
- CONSIDER NEEDS FOR ANTI-PLATELET and ANTI-COAGULATION THERAPY

| CRITICAL STRUCTURES COMPROMISED: | POTENTIAL COMPLICATIONS: | POSSIBLE CRITICAL INTERVENTIONS: |
| 20 - 30% of LV MUSCLE MASS | POSSIBLE MINOR - MODERATE LV FAILURE. | SMALL FLUID CHALLENGE INOTROPIC AGENTS |

CHIEF COMPLAINT and SIGNIFICANT HISTORY:

67 y/o FEMALE presents to ED with intermittent exertional CHEST PRESSURE x 1 day.   Pt. DENIES shortness of breath, nausea.   CHEST PRESSURE does not radiate.

RISK FACTOR PROFILE:

💣☀ CIGARETTE SMOKER x 40 YEARS
💣☀ HYPERTENSION
💣☀ AGE >65

PHYSICAL EXAM: Pt. CAO x 4 in NAD, SKIN WARM, DRY, COLOR NORMAL. PUPILS PERLA, NO JVD
LUNGS = DECREASED, CRACKLES IN BASES. HEART SOUNDS NORMAL S1, S2, NO ANKLE EDEMA,

VITAL SIGNS: BP: 133/88   P: 68   R: 20   SAO2: 95 % on 2 LPM O2

LABS: TROPONIN: 4.8   CK: 525   CK MB: 29

QUADRAD OF ACS CHECKLIST

☑ **SYMPTOMS of ACS**
- ✔ ◆ TYPICAL ACS - eg:
- ◆ ATYPICAL ACS - eg:

☑ **ECG ABNORMALITIES**
- ◆ ST ELEVATION (J POINT plus 40 ms)
- ◆ HYPERACUTE T WAVES - and/or -
- ◆ NEW or PRESUMABLY NEW LBBB
- ✔ ◆ ST DEPRESSION (>0.5 mm @ J POINT) and/or
- ◆ INVERTED or BIPHASIC T WAVES and/or
- ◆ DYNAMIC ST SEGMENT and/or T WAVE CHANGES IN SERIAL EKGs

☑ **RISK FACTORS - 3 or more**
- ◆ FAMILY HISTORY
- ◆ DIABETES
- ◆ ↑ LDL and/or ↓ HDL
- ✔ ◆ SMOKING
- ✔ ◆ AGE: 65 or MORE
- ✔ ◆ HYPERTENSION

☑ **CARDIAC MARKERS**
- ◆ ELEVATED TROPONIN and/or CK/MB

4 TOTAL

SUSPECTED ACUTE MI:

INITIAL MANAGEMENT

- **VITAL SIGNS**

- **"O.M.I."**
  - Oxygen
  - Monitor (ecg)
  - IV   (plus draw lab samples)

- **12 LEAD ECG**
  Obtain and interpret within 10 minutes of patient's arrival.

- **"M.O.N.A."**
  - Morphine
  - Oxygen (if not already done)
  - Nitroglycerin
  - Aspirin

- **RAPID, FOCUSED ASSESSMENT**

- **HEART / LUNG SOUNDS**

- **SEND LAB SAMPLES:**
  - Cardiac Markers
  - Electrolytes
  - Coagulation Studies

67 yr
Female   Hispanic

Room:S7
Loc:3   Option:23

Vent. rate   67   BPM
PR interval   188   ms
QRS duration   106   ms
QT/QTc   458/483   ms
P–R–T axes   27 –3   –111

POS:

I

aVR

V1

V4

II

aVL

V2

V5

III

aVF

V3

V6

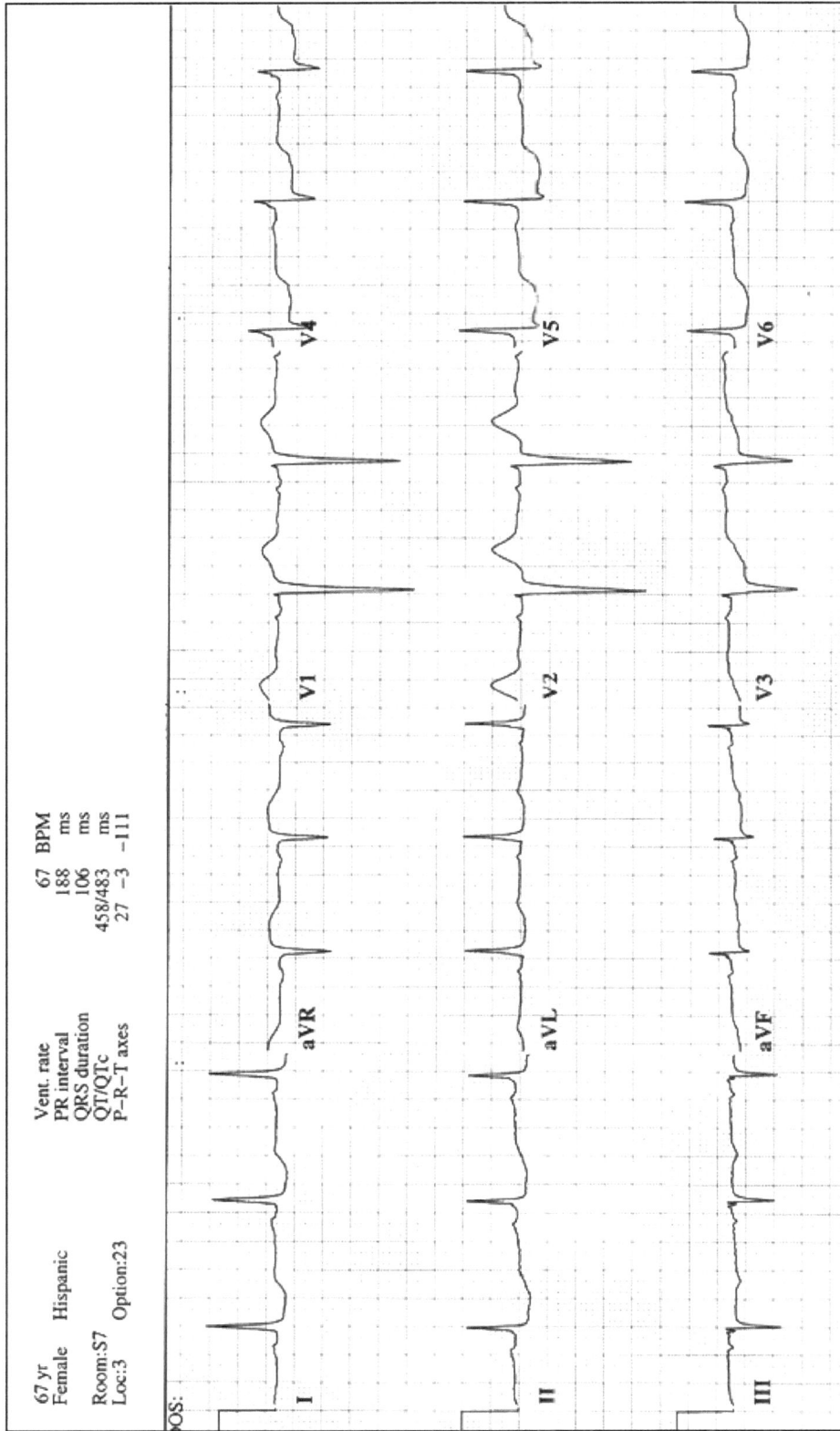

CASE STUDY QUESTIONS:

NOTE LEADS WITH ST ELEVATION:	NOTE LEADS WITH ST DEPRESSION:

WHAT IS THE SUSPECTED DIAGNOSIS ?

WHAT IS THE "CULPRIT ARTERY" -- if applicable ?

LIST ANY CRITICAL STRUCTURES COMPROMISED:	LIST ANY POTENTIAL COMPLICATIONS:

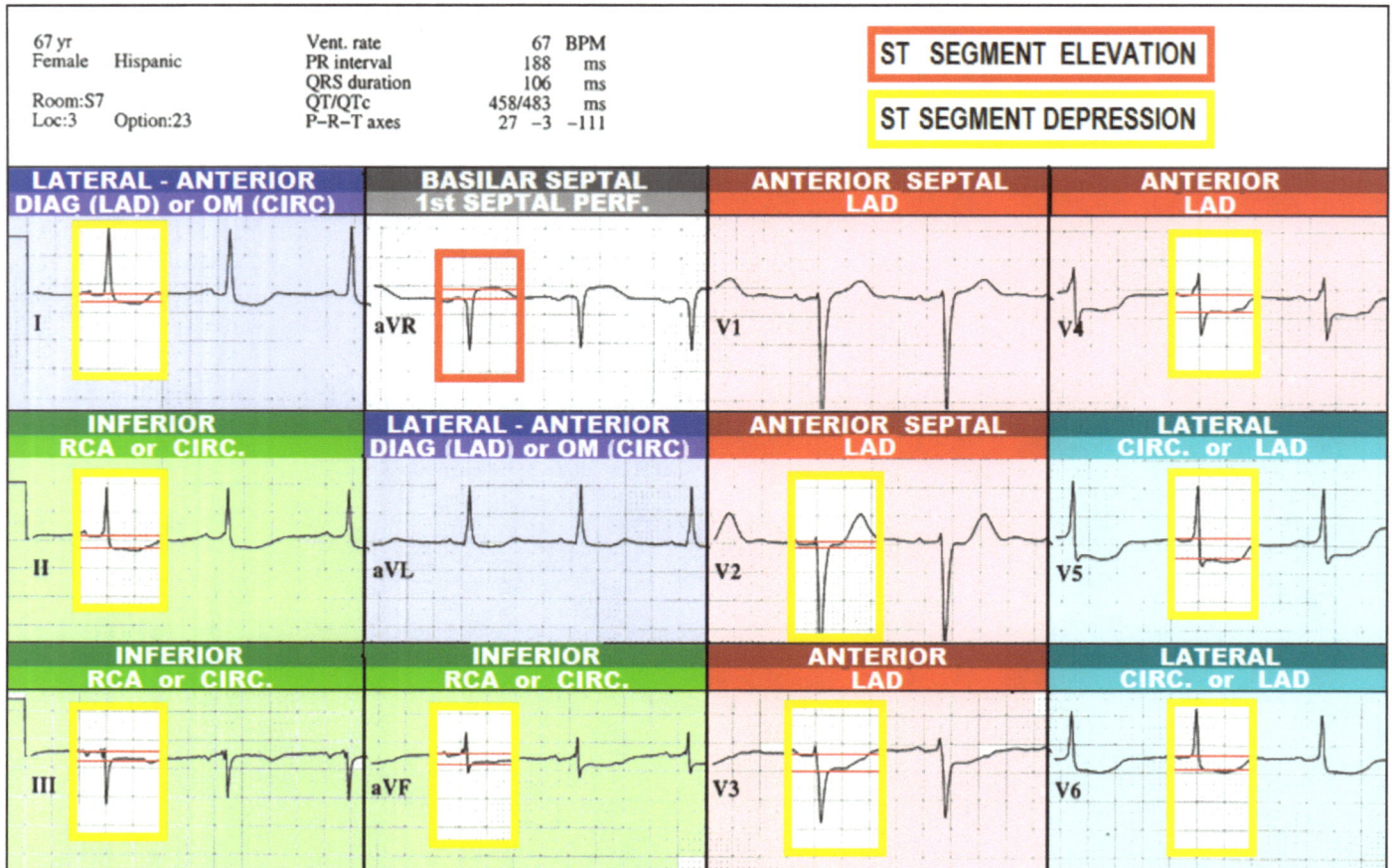

ST SEGMENT ELEVATION

ST SEGMENT DEPRESSION

LATERAL - ANTERIOR DIAG (LAD) or OM (CIRC)	BASILAR SEPTAL 1st SEPTAL PERF.	ANTERIOR SEPTAL LAD	ANTERIOR LAD
I	aVR	V1	V4
INFERIOR RCA or CIRC.	LATERAL - ANTERIOR DIAG (LAD) or OM (CIRC)	ANTERIOR SEPTAL LAD	LATERAL CIRC. or LAD
II	aVL	V2	V5
INFERIOR RCA or CIRC.	INFERIOR RCA or CIRC.	ANTERIOR LAD	LATERAL CIRC. or LAD
III	aVF	V3	V6

The most obvious finding on our patient's ECG is profound ST segment depression in 9 of the 12 leads. As demonstrated by the above color-coded ECG, ST depression is noted in three inferior leads (II, III, aVF), three anterior leads (V2, V3, V4), and two lateral leads (V5, V6). The ST depression in lead I can either be from involvement of the proximal LAD or the proximal circumflex arteries.

☞ **LEAD aVR – sometimes referred to as *"the forgotten 12th lead"* – can be a source of valuable information.** In this case study, lead aVR is the only lead with ST elevation.

- In cases of myocardial ischemia and NSTEMI, ST segment elevation of lead aVR has been associated with a high incidence of triple vessel disease,[61] *which is true in this case study*.
- In cases of anterior wall STEMI, elevation of lead aVR indicates the patient's lesion is proximal to the origin of the first septal perforator.[62]
- When the ST elevation of lead aVR is higher than that of V1, it is considered an indicator that the left main coronary artery is obstructed.[63] Please review Case Study 4 (p 183), STEMI, and involving occlusion of Left Main Coronary Artery.

While reviewing ECGs for inclusion in this curriculum, we noticed the correlation between J point elevation in lead aVR and the incidence of severe multi-vessel disease.

Based on her typical ACS symptoms, positive risk factor profile, elevated cardiac markers, and lack of significant ST segment elevation on her 12 lead ECG, our patient was diagnosed with NSTEMI. Based on her ECG findings, we projected that significant triple vessel disease and/or occlusion of the left main coronary artery would be discovered.

---

[61] Ann Noninvasive Electrocardiol 2010;15(2):175–180
[62] Kurisu, et al, HEART 2004, September: 90 (9):1059-60
[63] Yamaji, et al, JACC 2001, November: 38:1348-54

She was taken to the cardiac catheterization lab, where the following images were obtained:

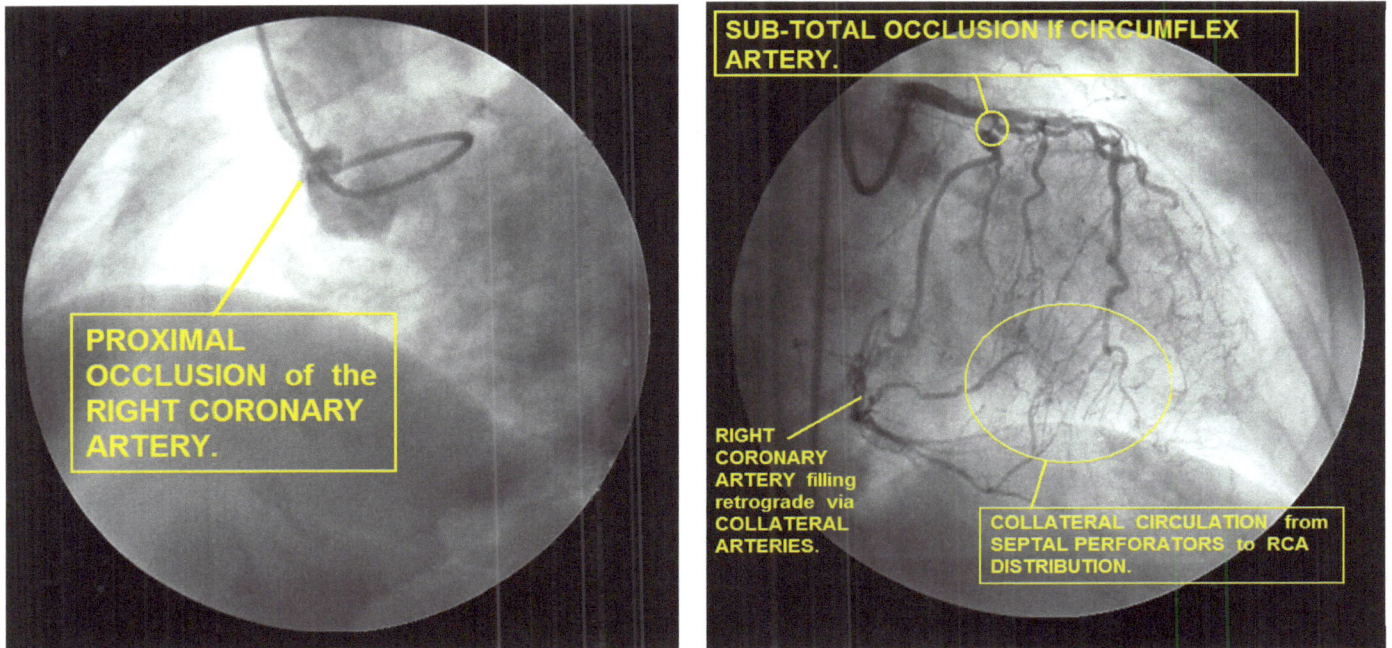

Immediately after her visit to the cardiac cath lab, she was transferred to the cardiac surgical suite where she underwent successful triple vessel coronary artery bypass grafting. She was discharged from the hospital the following week.

There are multiple causes of ST segment depression on the ECG. The images below illustrate how the ECG exemplifies transmural (full-thickness) myocardial infarction, and subendocardial (partial-thickness) myocardial infarction.

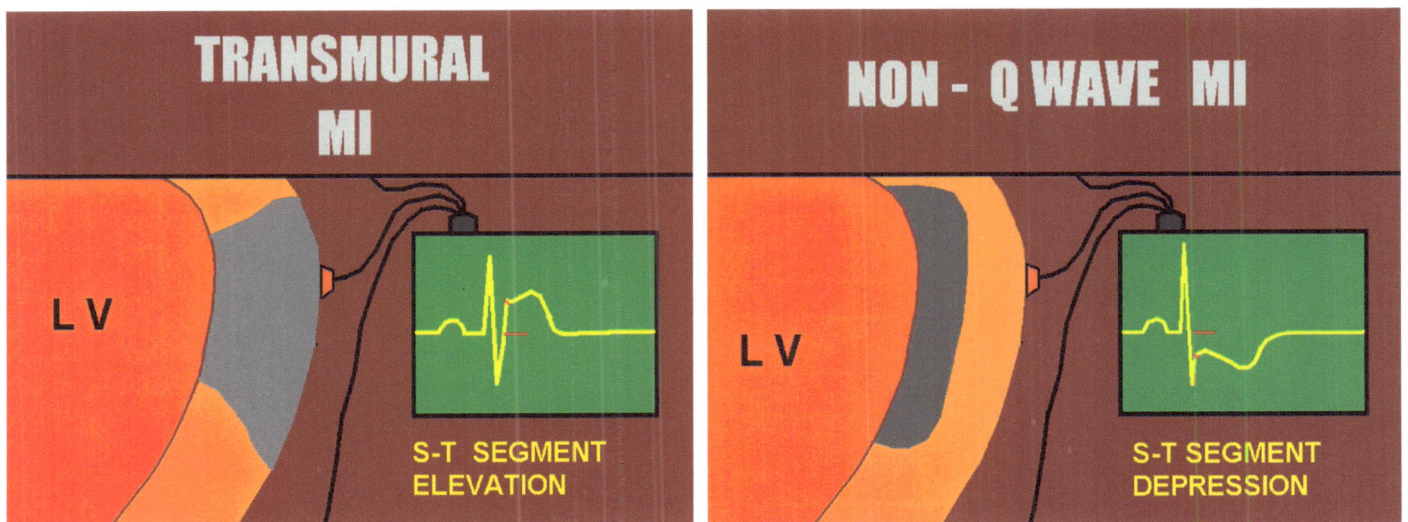

CHIEF COMPLAINT and SIGNIFICANT HISTORY:

45 y/o FEMALE c/o CHEST PAIN, SHORTNESS of BREATH and WEAKNESS x "SEVERAL DAYS." She states she has been under "a great amount of stress" in the past month, and recently started taking diet pills containing EPHEDRA.

RISK FACTOR PROFILE:

FAMILY HISTORY

PHYSICAL EXAM: Pt. CAO X 4, skin warm, dry, color normal.   Lung sounds clear, HS Normal S1, S2.   No JVD, No ankle edema.

VITAL SIGNS: BP: 106/66   P: 80   R: 24   SAO2: 95 % on 2 LPM O2

LABS: TROPONIN: 135

QUADRAD OF ACS CHECKLIST

☑ SYMPTOMS of ACS
- ✔ ◆ TYPICAL ACS - eg:
- ◆ ATYPICAL ACS - eg:

☑ ECG ABNORMALITIES
- ◆ ST ELEVATION (J POINT plus 40 ms)
- ◆ HYPERACUTE T WAVES - and/or -
- ◆ NEW or PRESUMABLY NEW LBBB
- ◆ ST DEPRESSION (>0.5 mm @ J POINT) and/or
- ✔ ◆ INVERTED or BIPHASIC T WAVES and/or
- ◆ DYNAMIC ST SEGMENT and/or T WAVE CHANGES IN SERIAL EKGs

☐ RISK FACTORS - 3 or more
- ✔ ◆ FAMILY HISTORY
- ◆ DIABETES
- ◆ ↑ LDL and/or ↓ HDL
- ◆ SMOKING
- ◆ AGE: 65 or MORE
- ◆ HYPERTENSION

☑ CARDIAC MARKERS
- ✔ ◆ ELEVATED TROPONIN and/or CK/MB

3 TOTAL

This patient presented to the ED after enduring ACS-like symptoms for several days.   What motivated her to go to the ED was the worsening symptoms of fatigue and shortness of breath.

During her initial evaluation in the ED, her ACS-like symptoms and ECG abnormalities gave her two points on the "Quadrad of ACS Checklist" – enough to warrant obtaining cardiac markers.

Another factor which aroused the ED physician's suspicion was the patient's admitted use of diet pills containing ephedra in a medically supervised weight reduction program.   The physician was aware that ephedrine alkaloids have been known to cause coronary vasospasm secondary to potent a-adrenergic stimulation.[64] Furthermore, the patient confided that she has been under "more stress in her life than ever" due to an unresolved problem in her life.   Extreme emotional duress has been linked to incidents of acute stress-induced cardiomyopathy.

After seeing her elevated cardiac marker value, the ED physician consulted with the on-call interventional cardiologist.

---

[64] Weiner, et al, Cathet Cardiovasc Diagn 1990;20:51-3.

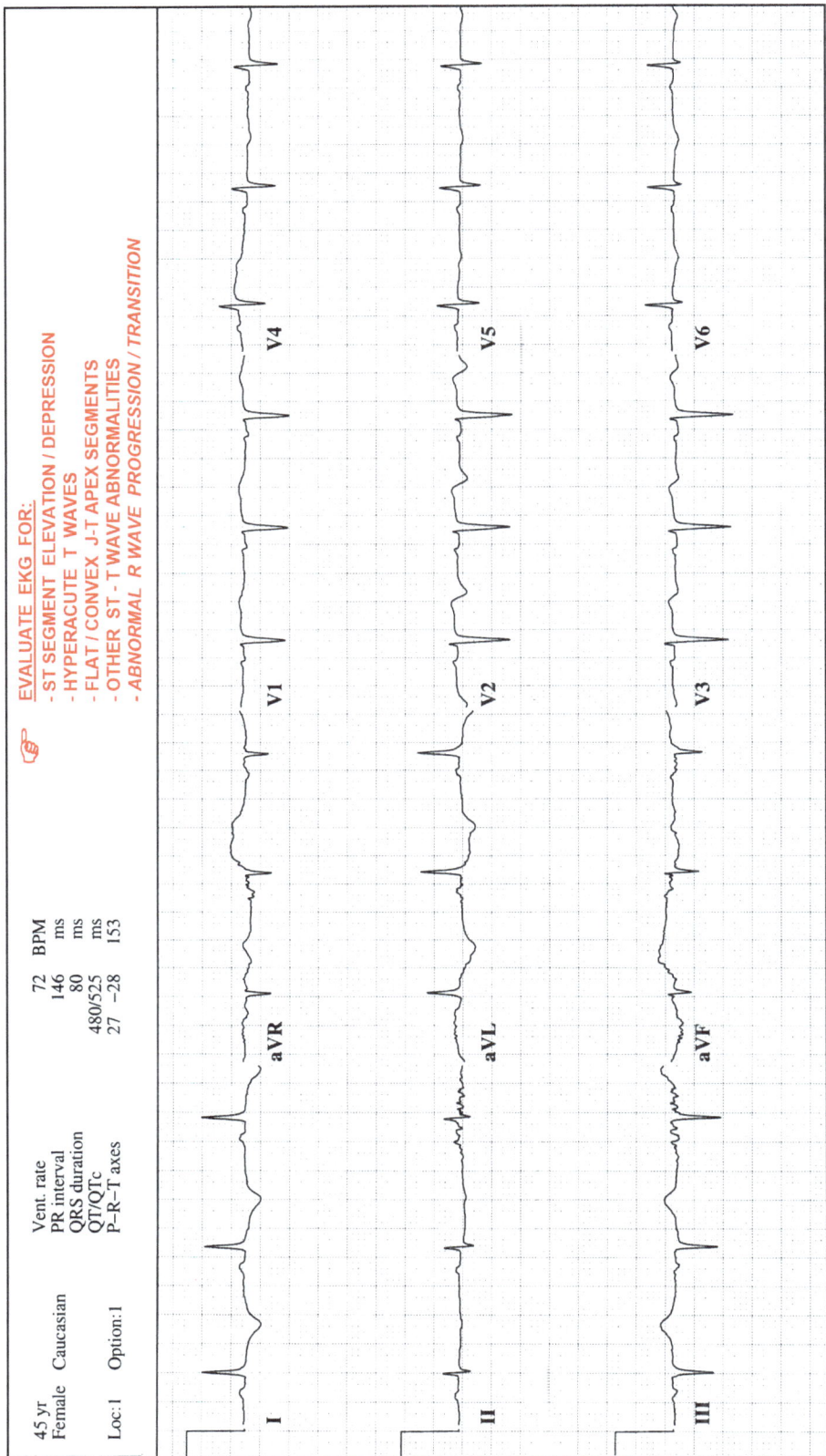

45 yr
Female   Caucasian

Loc:1   Option:1

Vent. rate	72	BPM
PR interval	146	ms
QRS duration	80	ms
QT/QTc	480/525	ms
P–R–T axes	27	–28	153

☞   EVALUATE EKG FOR:
- ST SEGMENT ELEVATION / DEPRESSION
- HYPERACUTE T WAVES
- FLAT / CONVEX J-T APEX SEGMENTS
- OTHER ST - T WAVE ABNORMALITIES
- *ABNORMAL R WAVE PROGRESSION / TRANSITION*

I   aVR   V1   V4

II   aVL   V2   V5

III   aVF   V3   V6

CASE STUDY QUESTIONS:

| NOTE LEADS WITH ST ELEVATION: | NOTE LEADS WITH ST DEPRESSION: |

WHAT IS THE SUSPECTED DIAGNOSIS ?

WHAT IS THE "CULPRIT ARTERY" – if applicable ?

| LIST ANY CRITICAL STRUCTURES COMPROMISED: | LIST ANY POTENTIAL COMPLICATIONS: |

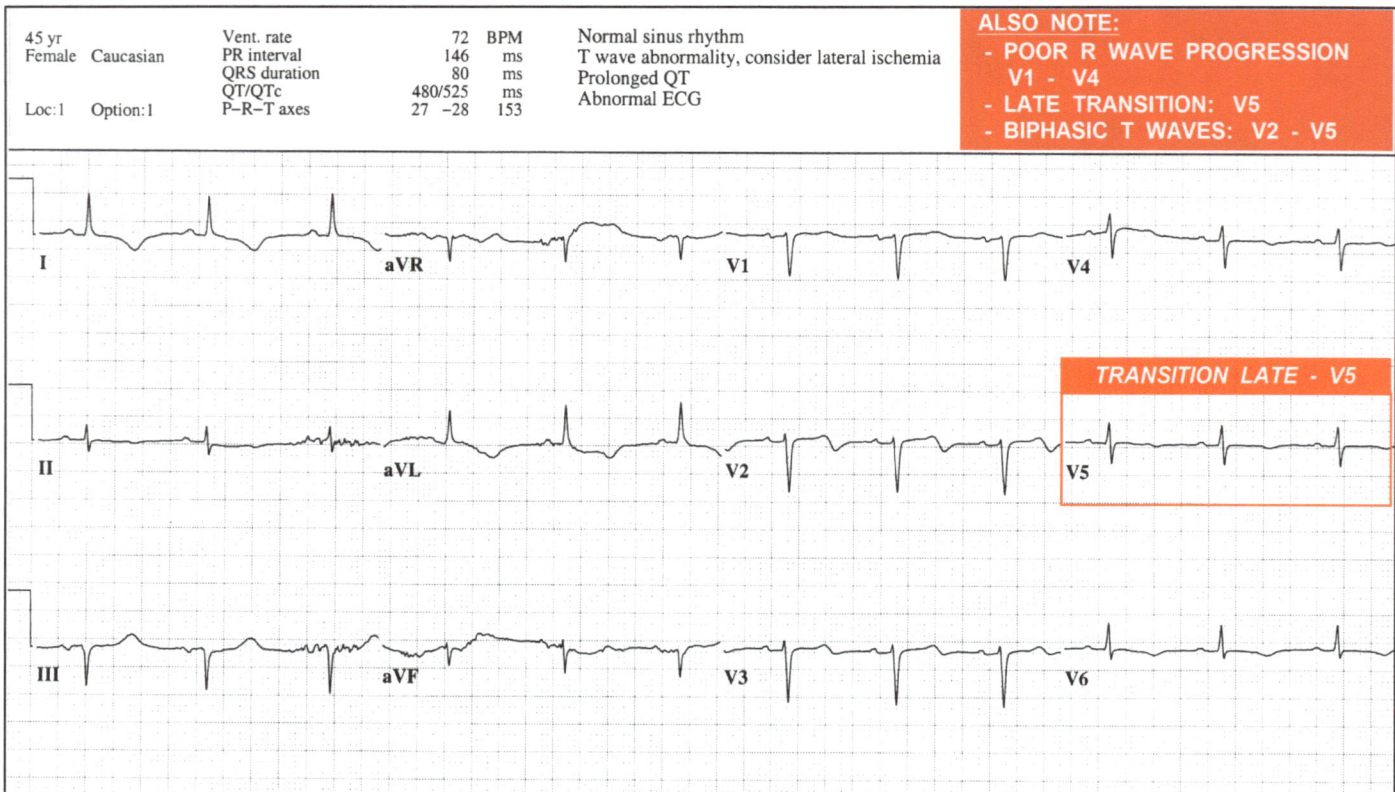

45 yr		Vent. rate	72	BPM	Normal sinus rhythm
Female	Caucasian	PR interval	146	ms	T wave abnormality, consider lateral ischemia
		QRS duration	80	ms	Prolonged QT
		QT/QTc	480/525	ms	Abnormal ECG
Loc:1	Option:1	P–R–T axes	27 –28	153	

ALSO NOTE:
- POOR R WAVE PROGRESSION
  V1 - V4
- LATE TRANSITION: V5
- BIPHASIC T WAVES: V2 - V5

TRANSITION LATE - V5

After evaluating the patient in the emergency department, taking the above ECG and cardiac marker elevation into consideration, he elected to proceed immediately to the cardiac catheterization lab, where the following images were obtained:

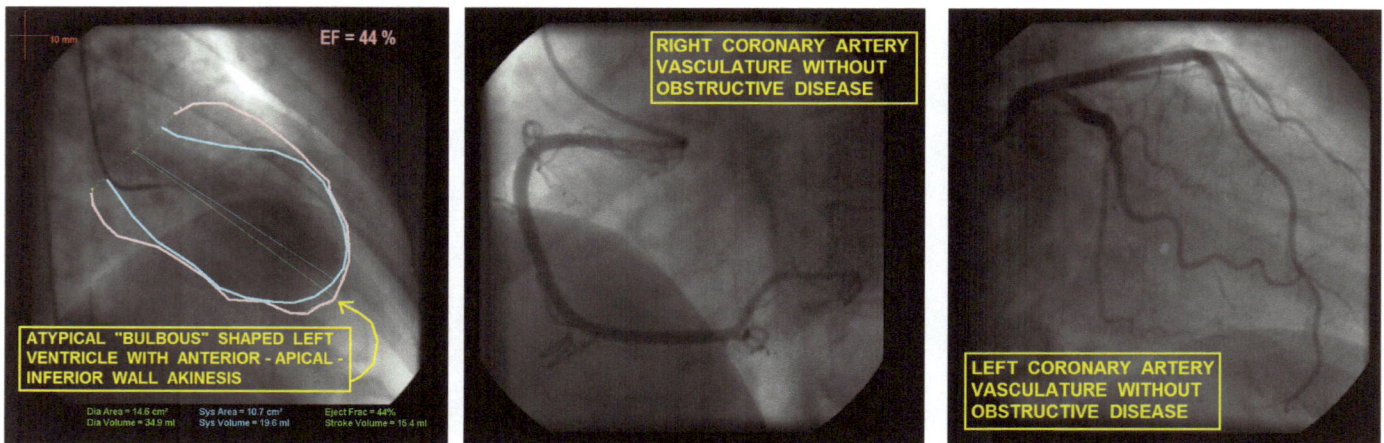

EF = 44 %

ATYPICAL "BULBOUS" SHAPED LEFT VENTRICLE WITH ANTERIOR - APICAL - INFERIOR WALL AKINESIS

Dia Area = 14.6 cm² Sys Area = 10.7 cm² Eject Frac = 44%
Dia Volume = 34.9 ml Sys Volume = 19.6 ml Stroke Volume = 15.4 ml

RIGHT CORONARY ARTERY VASCULATURE WITHOUT OBSTRUCTIVE DISEASE

LEFT CORONARY ARTERY VASCULATURE WITHOUT OBSTRUCTIVE DISEASE

As you can see in the above images, the patient is free of obstructive cardiovascular disease. The patient's left ventricular angiogram identified severe anterior-apical wall akinesis. The cardiologist also noted that the atypical shape of her left ventricle is consistent with that of patients afflicted with "tako-tsubo" (Japanese for octopus trap) cardiomyopathy, based on the peculiar appearance of a rounded bottom and narrow neck on the end-systolic left ventriculogram.[65]

---

[65] G. William Dec MD, *Circulation.* 2005;111:388-390.)

Based on the patient's disease-free cardiovascular status, the classic "tako-tsubo" shape of her left ventricle, her recent use of ephedrine alkaloids, and elevated personal stress factors in her life, the cardiologist diagnosed her condition as "Apical Ballooning Syndrome."

Apical ballooning syndrome, also known as "broken heart syndrome" and "acute stress induced cardiomyopathy," may account for up to 2% of all incidents of acute myocardial infarction.[66] This condition is uncommon but often life-threatening. ABS can be provoked by extreme emotional distress and a-adrenergic substances (including ephedrine alkaloids).

Apical ballooning syndrome (ABS) is characterized by the sudden onset of angina-like chest pain, ECG changes which include ST-segment elevation in 50-60% of cases, diffuse T-wave inversions, abnormal QS-wave development, and prolongation of the Q-T interval. . Cardiac marker elevation is relative to the extent of ventricular injury. Wall motion abnormalities involving the lower anterior wall and apex on echocardiography or left ventricular angiography is often noted. The patient's clinical presentation mimics acute myocardial infarction but always occurs in patients without evidence for hemodynamically significant coronary arterial stenoses by angiography.

"Clinical presentations of ABS often include ACS-like symptoms, and may include cardiogenic shock and ventricular tachyarrhythmias. Clinicians should also consider ruling out other conditions on the growing list of potentially reversible conditions in the initial differential diagnosis, which include cardiotoxins, such as cocaine and/or alcohol; antiretroviral agents; nutritional deficiencies (e.g. thiamine, selenium, carnitine); endocrine disturbances (hyperthyroidism, hypothyroidism, pheochromocytoma); viral myocarditis; Lyme carditis; hypersensitivity reactions; infiltrative processes, such as hemochromatosis; peripartum disease; and tachycardia-induced cardiomyopathy."[67]

This patient's management was focused on controlling the factors which contributed to her development of ABS: cessation of use of ephedrine alkaloids, and measures to limit her perceived stress due to her personal situation. In addition, beta blockers were used to control adrenergic stimulation. Her clinical course was typical of most patients afflicted with ABS: within 30 days, her LV function had returned to normal.

Case contributed by: Matthew Glover, MD, FACC

---

[66] A. Prasad MD, Circulation 2007;115;e56-e59

[67] G. William Dec MD, *Circulation.* 2005;111:388-390.)

Evaluation of the ECG for changes consistent with NSTEMI and Unstable Angina is achieved by carefully scrutinizing the *J point, ST segment* and *T waves* of each lead for abnormalities.

The table to the right features some of the ECG changes sometimes seen in cases of NSTEMI and unstable angina secondary to obstructive coronary artery disease.

The image below illustrates defines the characteristics of normal J points, ST segments, and T waves. An important concept to remember when evaluating your patient's ECG it *"if it isn't NORMAL, it's ABNORMAL."*

EKG PATTERNS of ISCHEMIA
-- J POINT, ST SEGMENT, and T WAVE ABNORMALITIES --

Pattern		Indication
! DEPRESSED J pt. DOWNSLOPING ST and INVERTED T		- ACUTE (NON-Q WAVE) MI - ACUTE MI - (RECIPROCAL CHANGES) - ISCHEMIA
INVERTED T WAVE		- MYOCARDITIS - ELECTROLYTE IMBAL. - ISCHEMIA
SHARP S-T T ANGLE		- ACUTE MI (NOT COMMON) - ISCHEMIA
BI-PHASIC T WAVE		- SUB-TOTAL LAD LESION - VASOSPASM - HYPERTROPHY
DEPRESSED J POINT with UPSLOPING ST		- ISCHEMIA
DOWNSLOPING S-T SEGMENT		- ISCHEMIA
? FLAT S-T SEGMENT > 120 ms		- ISCHEMIA
? LOW VOLTAGE T WAVE WITH NORMAL QRS		- ISCHEMIA
? U WAVE POLARITY OPPOSITE THAT OF T WAVE		- ISCHEMIA

NORMAL ST - T WAVES

- WHEN QRS WIDTH IS NORMAL (< 120 ms)

ASSESS: V5

- J POINT: ISOELECTRIC (or < 1 mm dev.)
- ST SEG: SLIGHT, POSITIVE INCLINATION
- T WAVE: UPRIGHT, POSITIVE

☞ in EVERY LEAD EXCEPT aVR !!

Recall that NSTEMI and UA patients can present with remarkably normal appearing ECGs. Although such events are atypical, we must remember the ECGs inherent lack of sensitivity, and to consider all findings in the "Quadrad of ACS" – *symptoms, risk factors, ECG findings, and cardiac markers* – into the clinical decision making process.

UNSTABLE ANGINA CASE STUDIES:

Unstable angina is defined as "a new onset of ACS-like chest pain, or changes in previously stable patterns of angina," without elevation of cardiac markers.

The initial assessment priority of patients presenting with ACS-like symptoms is to rule out imminently life-threatening conditions, including STEMI and NSTEMI.

The STAT 12 Lead ECG initially rules out STEMI. If cardiac markers are within normal limits, we initiate serial ECGs and repeat cardiac markers at predetermined intervals.

If ACS-like symptoms persist, and repeated ECGs and cardiac markers remain normal, we must work to rule out obstructive cardiovascular disease as well as other conditions which can mimic ACS such as dissecting thoracic/aortic arch aneurysm, pulmonary embolus, and others.

The priorities of patient evaluation in cases of suspected unstable angina are to definitively rule out obstructive cardiovascular disease. This often necessitates admission to the hospital for additional diagnostic procedures, such as CT scans, stress testing, echocardiograms and cardiac catheterization.

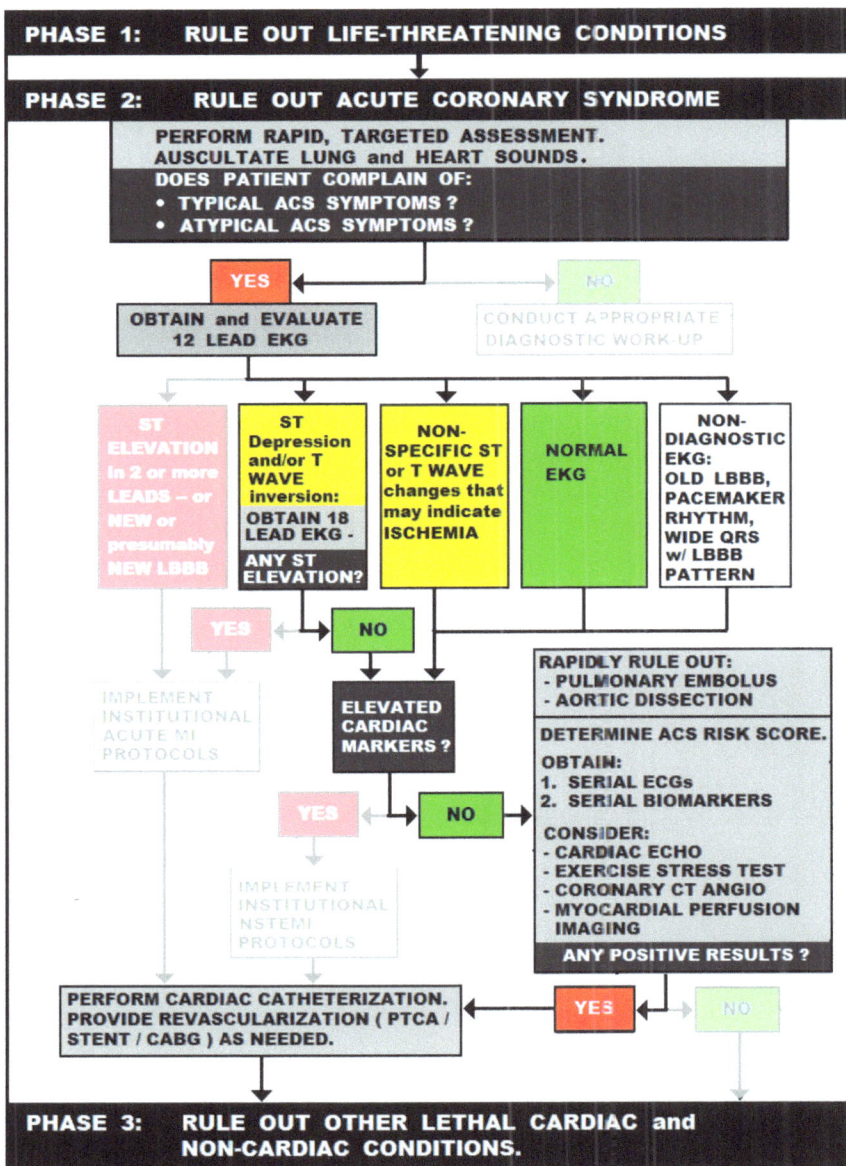

PHASE 1: RULE OUT LIFE-THREATENING CONDITIONS

PHASE 2: RULE OUT ACUTE CORONARY SYNDROME

PERFORM RAPID, TARGETED ASSESSMENT. AUSCULTATE LUNG and HEART SOUNDS. DOES PATIENT COMPLAIN OF:
- TYPICAL ACS SYMPTOMS ?
- ATYPICAL ACS SYMPTOMS ?

YES → OBTAIN and EVALUATE 12 LEAD EKG

NO → CONDUCT APPROPRIATE DIAGNOSTIC WORK-UP

- ST ELEVATION in 2 or more LEADS – or NEW or presumably NEW LBBB
- ST Depression and/or T WAVE inversion: OBTAIN 18 LEAD EKG - ANY ST ELEVATION?
- NON-SPECIFIC ST or T WAVE changes that may indicate ISCHEMIA
- NORMAL EKG
- NON-DIAGNOSTIC EKG: OLD LBBB, PACEMAKER RHYTHM, WIDE QRS w/ LBBB PATTERN

YES → IMPLEMENT INSTITUTIONAL ACUTE MI PROTOCOLS

NO → ELEVATED CARDIAC MARKERS ?

YES → IMPLEMENT INSTITUTIONAL NSTEMI PROTOCOLS

NO → RAPIDLY RULE OUT:
- PULMONARY EMBOLUS
- AORTIC DISSECTION

DETERMINE ACS RISK SCORE.

OBTAIN:
1. SERIAL ECGs
2. SERIAL BIOMARKERS

CONSIDER:
- CARDIAC ECHO
- EXERCISE STRESS TEST
- CORONARY CT ANGIO
- MYOCARDIAL PERFUSION IMAGING

ANY POSITIVE RESULTS ?

PERFORM CARDIAC CATHETERIZATION. PROVIDE REVASCULARIZATION (PTCA / STENT / CABG) AS NEEDED. ← YES ← NO

PHASE 3: RULE OUT OTHER LETHAL CARDIAC and NON-CARDIAC CONDITIONS.

CHIEF COMPLAINT and SIGNIFICANT HISTORY:

42 y/o FEMALE c/o INTERMITTENT CHEST PRESSURE which has been WORSENING during the past week. Also c/o mild DIB. Symptoms previously provoked by exertion, now comes on at rest.

RISK FACTOR PROFILE:

💣 HYPERTENSION
💣 CIGARETTE SMOKER x 15 YEARS
💣 FAMILY HISTORY - FATHER Dx WITH CAD, HAD CABG AT 52

PHYSICAL EXAM: Pt. ASYMPTOMATIC at time of exam. SKIN WARM, DRY, COLOR NORMAL, PERLA, LUNGS= CLEAR, HS NORMAL S1, S2, NO ANKLE EDEMA.

VITAL SIGNS: BP: 148/92   P: 64   R: 20   SAO2: 97 % on 2 LPM O2

LABS: TROPONIN: < .04

QUADRAD OF ACS CHECKLIST

☑ **SYMPTOMS of ACS**
- ✔◆ TYPICAL ACS - eg:
- ◆ ATYPICAL ACS - eg:

☑ **ECG ABNORMALITIES**
- ◆ ST ELEVATION (J POINT plus 40 ms)
- ◆ HYPERACUTE T WAVES - and/or -
- ◆ NEW or PRESUMABLY NEW LBBB
- ✔◆ ST DEPRESSION (>0.5 mm @ J POINT) and/or
- ◆ INVERTED or BIPHASIC T WAVES and/or
- ◆ DYNAMIC ST SEGMENT and/or T WAVE CHANGES IN SERIAL EKGs

☑ **RISK FACTORS - 3 or more**
- ✔◆ FAMILY HISTORY
- ◆ DIABETES
- ◆ ↑ LDL and/or ↓ HDL
- ✔◆ SMOKING
- ◆ AGE: 65 or MORE
- ✔◆ HYPERTENSION

☐ **CARDIAC MARKERS**
- ◆ ELEVATED TROPONIN and/or CK/MB

3 **TOTAL**

This patient presented to the Emergency Department via EMS with intermittent but progressively worsening ACS symptoms. Treatment given by EMS included O2 2 liters per minute via nasal canula, aspirin 325mg, IV NS at KVO rate, and NTG x 2 with relief of symptoms. At the time of ER exam, she was asymptomatic. Cardiac markers were obtained and found to be within normal limits. Her 12 lead ECG is shown on the opposite page.

Based on her ACS symptoms, ECG findings and risk factor profile, the decision was made to admit her to the hospital with a diagnosis of unstable angina. Beta blocker therapy with metoprolol and anticoagulation with low molecular weight heparin was initiated.

Admission orders included continuous telemetry monitoring, O2 prn, IV heplock, aspirin 325 mg once daily, initiation of plavix 75mg once daily, and low molecular weight heparin.

Serial ECGs and cardiac markers were obtained for a twenty-four hour period, and remained unchanged.

Leads selected for telemetry monitoring should include continuous monitoring of the region(s) of suspected myocardial ischemia. In this case, lead II was selected to observe for inferior wall changes.

The following day, she was taken to the cardiac catheterization lab, where the images on page 248 were obtained.

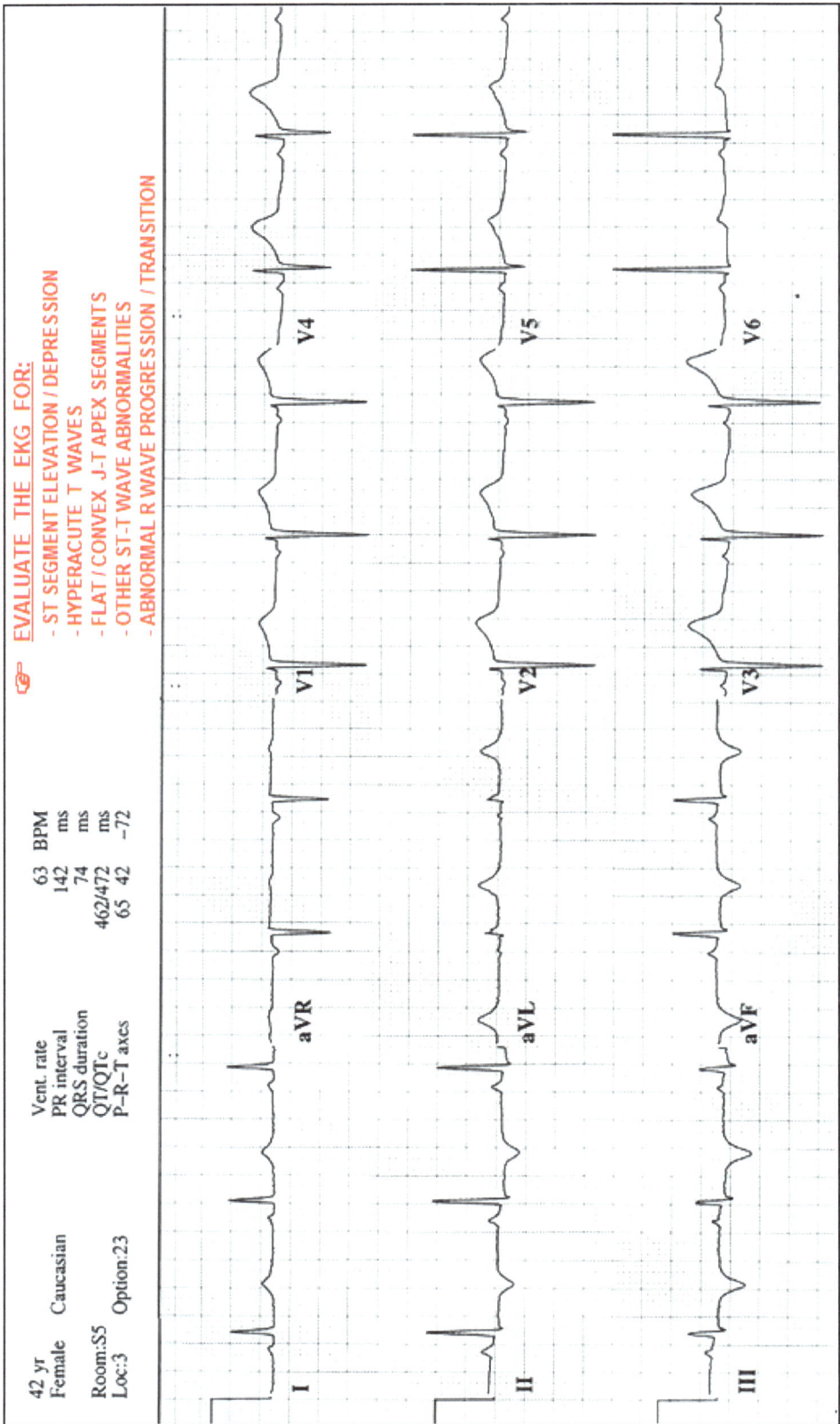

42 yr
Female Caucasian

Room:S5
Loc:3 Option:23

Vent. rate	63	BPM
PR interval	142	ms
QRS duration	74	ms
QT/QTc	462/472	ms
P–R–T axes	65 42	–72

☞ EVALUATE THE EKG FOR:
- ST SEGMENT ELEVATION / DEPRESSION
- HYPERACUTE T WAVES
- FLAT / CONVEX J-T APEX SEGMENTS
- OTHER ST-T WAVE ABNORMALITIES
- ABNORMAL R WAVE PROGRESSION / TRANSITION

I   aVR   V1   V4

II   aVL   V2   V5

III   aVF   V3   V6

CASE STUDY QUESTIONS:

NOTE LEADS WITH ST ELEVATION:	NOTE LEADS WITH ST DEPRESSION:

WHAT IS THE SUSPECTED DIAGNOSIS ?

WHAT IS THE "CULPRIT ARTERY" — if applicable ?

LIST ANY CRITICAL STRUCTURES COMPROMISED: LIST ANY POTENTIAL COMPLICATIONS:

261

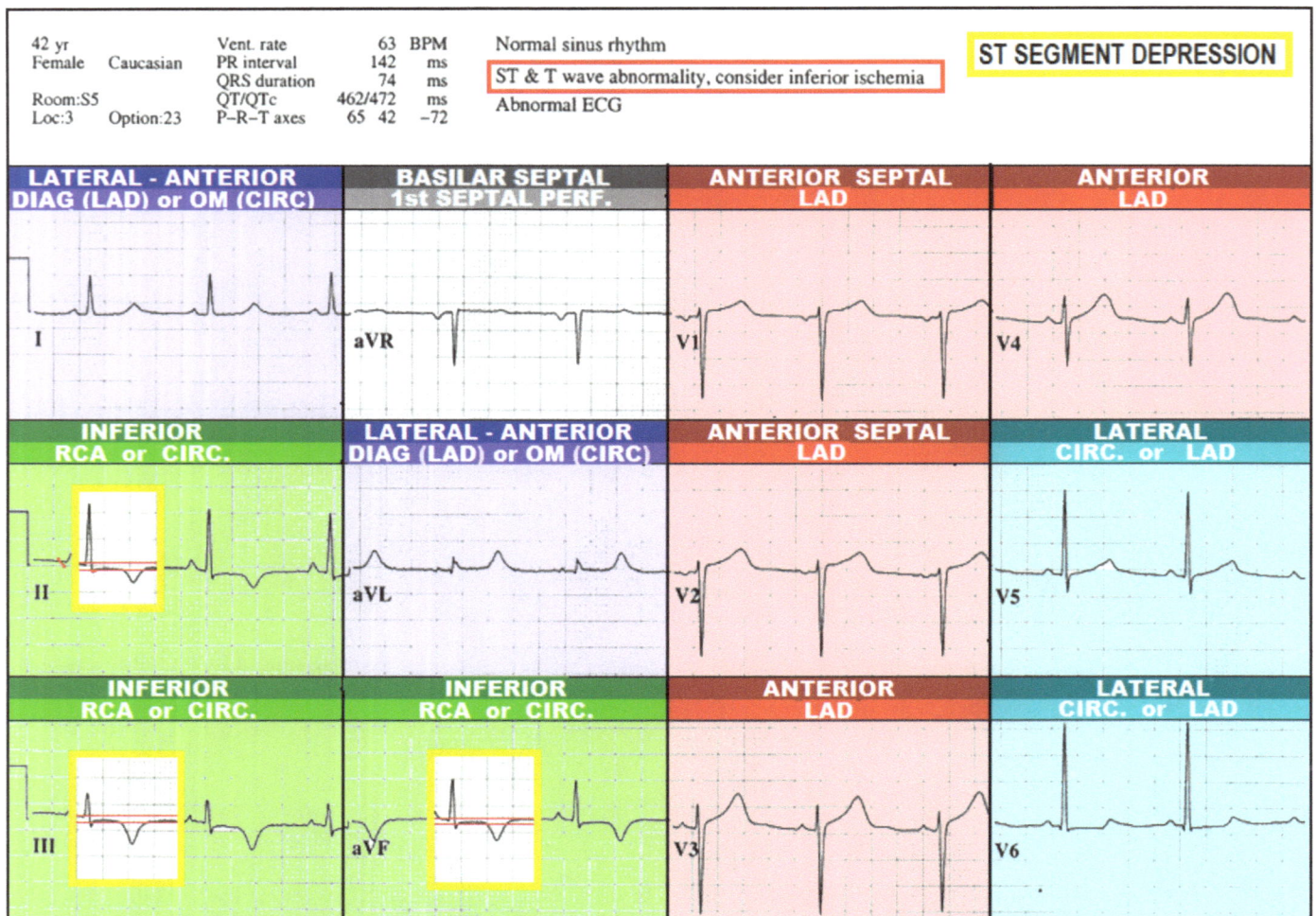

42 yr		Vent. rate	63	BPM	Normal sinus rhythm	**ST SEGMENT DEPRESSION**
Female	Caucasian	PR interval	142	ms		
		QRS duration	74	ms	ST & T wave abnormality, consider inferior ischemia	
Room:S5		QT/QTc	462/472	ms	Abnormal ECG	
Loc:3	Option:23	P–R–T axes	65 42 –72			

LATERAL - ANTERIOR DIAG (LAD) or OM (CIRC)	BASILAR SEPTAL 1st SEPTAL PERF.	ANTERIOR SEPTAL LAD	ANTERIOR LAD
I	aVR	V1	V4
INFERIOR RCA or CIRC.	LATERAL - ANTERIOR DIAG (LAD) or OM (CIRC)	ANTERIOR SEPTAL LAD	LATERAL CIRC. or LAD
II	aVL	V2	V5
INFERIOR RCA or CIRC.	INFERIOR RCA or CIRC.	ANTERIOR LAD	LATERAL CIRC. or LAD
III	aVF	V3	V6

The ECG computer diagnosis correctly identifies the patient's diagnosis as inferior wall ischemia, based on ST depression
in inferior leads II, III, and aVF.   A flat ST segment is noted in lead V6, which could result from ischemia secondary to decreased blood flow in the posterior lateral vessels in the distal RCA distribution.   An expected finding during coronary arterial angiography is obstructive lesions in the right coronary artery, which supply blood to the inferior wall in 75-80% of the population.

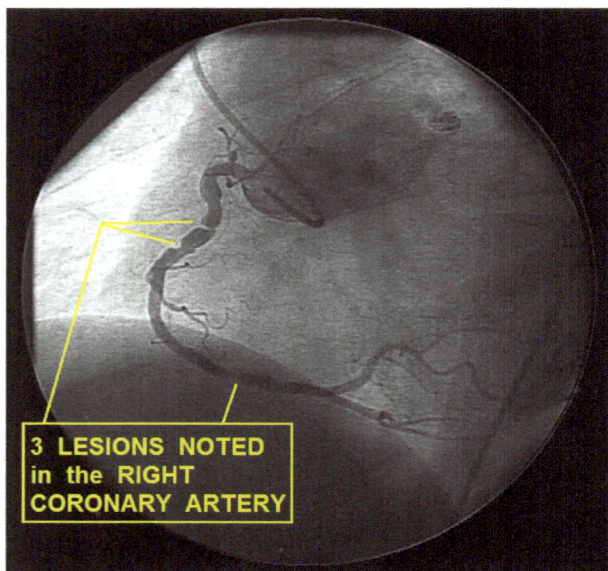

3 LESIONS NOTED in the RIGHT CORONARY ARTERY

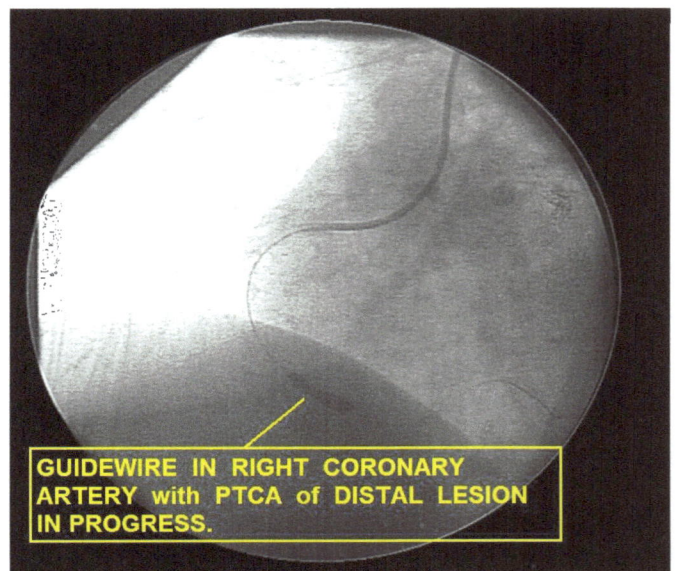

GUIDEWIRE IN RIGHT CORONARY ARTERY with PTCA of DISTAL LESION IN PROGRESS.

POST PTCA / STENTS
(x 2) TO RCA

LEFT CORONARY ARTERY
SYSTEM = DIFFUSE
PLAQUING, NO FOCAL
OBSTRUCTIVE LESIONS

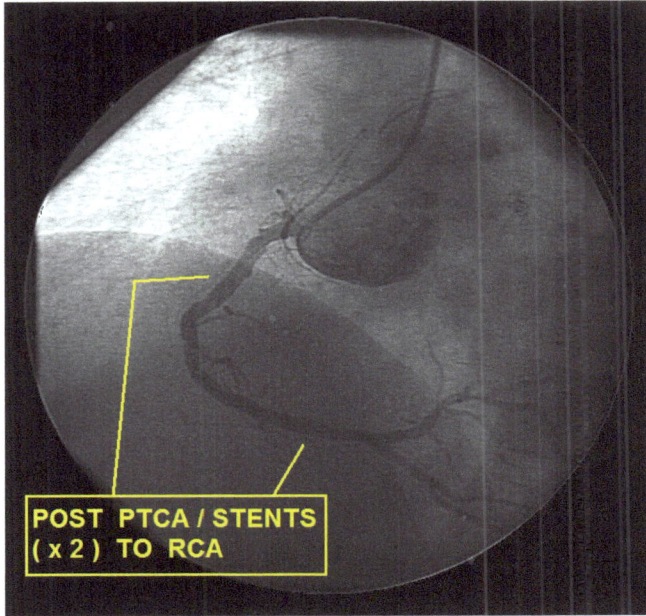

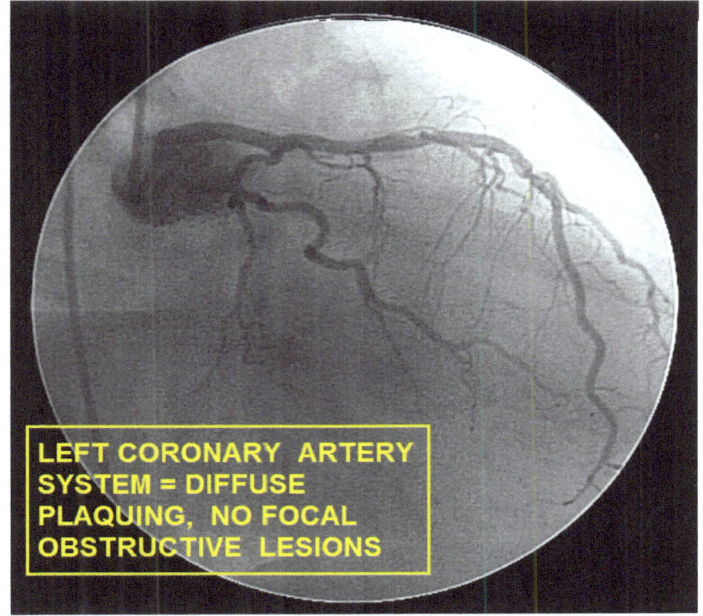

This patient underwent PCTA and Stenting in two locations in her right coronary artery. Her left sided coronary artery anatomy was found to have diffuse plaque formations, but no focal obstructions requiring intervention.

Her post-procedural ECG is shown below. Note that the ST depression and inverted T waves in leads II, III, and aVF have resolved just hours after successful intervention. Also note the ST segment in lead V6 is no longer flat; an indication that the ischemia previously noted there most likely resulted from decreased blood flow to the posterior lateral vessels in the distal RCA distribution.

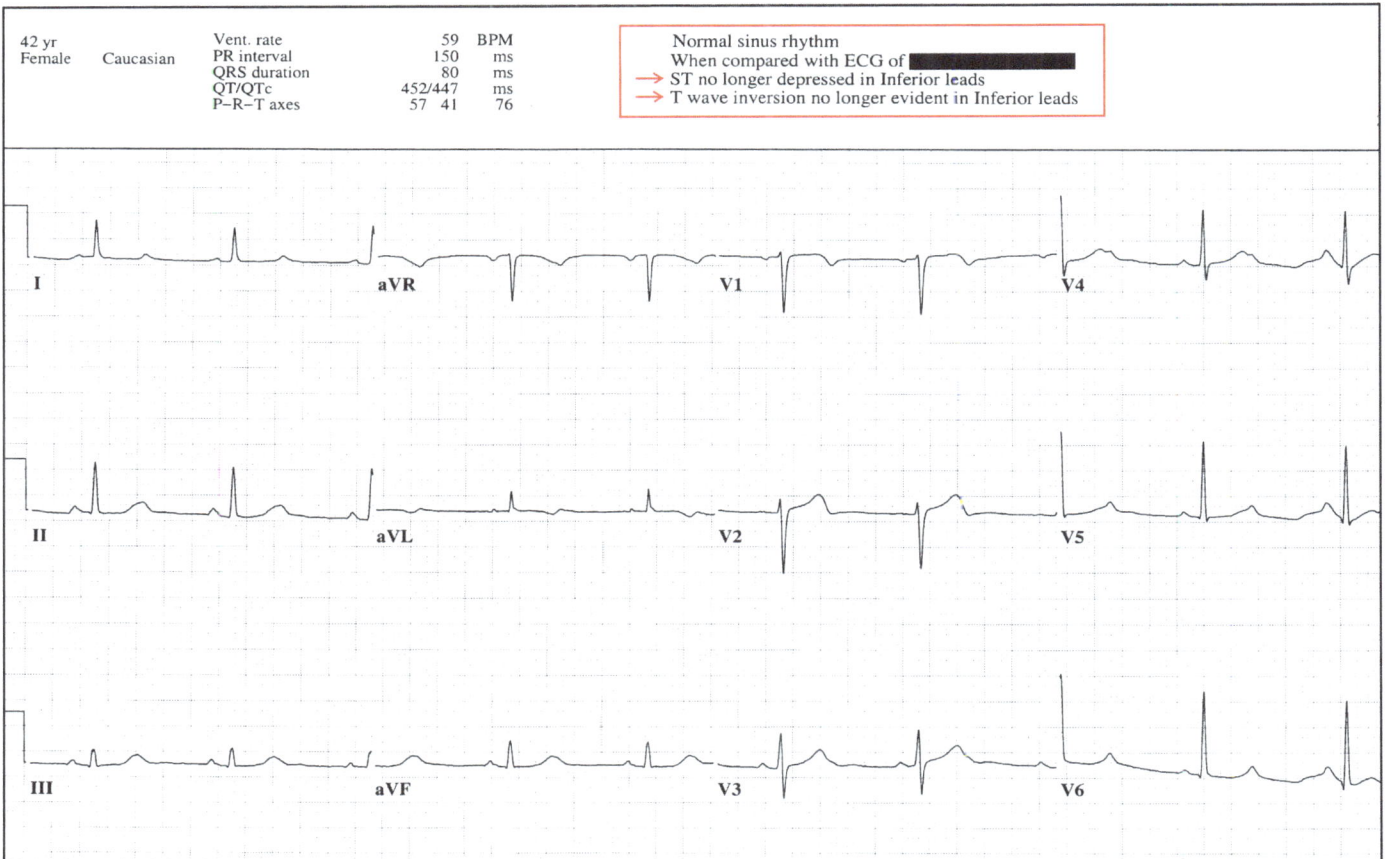

42 yr			Vent. rate	59	BPM
Female	Caucasian		PR interval	150	ms
			QRS duration	80	ms
			QT/QTc	452/447	ms
			P–R–T axes	57 41 76	

Normal sinus rhythm
When compared with ECG of ████████
→ ST no longer depressed in Inferior leads
→ T wave inversion no longer evident in Inferior leads

CHIEF COMPLAINT and SIGNIFICANT HISTORY:

38 y/o MALE presents with sensation of exertional CHEST and NECK PAIN, described as "burning." Patient states symptoms also occur when he is under emotional duress. Symptoms have been occurring intermittently for approx. 2-3 weeks.

RISK FACTOR PROFILE:

💣 HYPERTENSION
💣 DIABETES x 5 YEARS

PHYSICAL EXAM: Pt. ASYMPTOMATIC at time of exam. SKIN WARM, DRY, COLOR NORMAL, PERLA, LUNGS= CLEAR, HS NORMAL S1, S2, NO ANKLE EDEMA.

VITAL SIGNS: BP: 144/92   P: 78   R: 16   SAO2: 100% on room air

LABS: TROPONIN: < .04

QUADRAD OF ACS CHECKLIST

☑ **SYMPTOMS of ACS**
- ✔ ◆ TYPICAL ACS - eg:
- ◆ ATYPICAL ACS - eg:

☐ **ECG ABNORMALITIES**
- ◆ ST ELEVATION (J POINT plus 40 ms)
- ◆ HYPERACUTE T WAVES - and/or -
- ◆ NEW or PRESUMABLY NEW LBBB
- ◆ ST DEPRESSION (>0.5 mm @ J POINT) and/or
- ◆ INVERTED or BIPHASIC T WAVES and/or
- ◆ DYNAMIC ST SEGMENT and/or T WAVE CHANGES IN SERIAL EKGs

☐ **RISK FACTORS - 3 or more**
- ◆ FAMILY HISTORY
- ✔ ◆ DIABETES
- ◆ ↑ LDL and/or ↓ HDL
- ◆ SMOKING
- ◆ AGE: 65 or MORE
- ✔ ◆ HYPERTENSION

☐ **CARDIAC MARKERS**
- ◆ ELEVATED TROPONIN and/or CK/MB

☐ **TOTAL**

This patient complained of exertional chest and neck pain, which he described as a "burning sensation," which did not radiate to shoulders, jaw or arms. His first episode was approximately three weeks ago, and occurred during physical exertion. In the ensuing weeks, episodes have become more frequent, and have been provoked by emotional distress. For the past week, he states the chest pain has come on at rest, and has awakened him in the morning on two occasions.

Since his past medical history included hypertension and insulin-controlled diabetes mellitus, he feared his new onset of chest discomfort may be heart-related.

During exercise stress testing, ST segment elevation in leads II, III, and aVF were noted, along with the onset of his symptoms. At this point, the stress test was aborted, with resolution of ST elevation and symptoms.

He subsequently was referred for an urgent cardiac catheterization, with a diagnosis of "unstable angina."

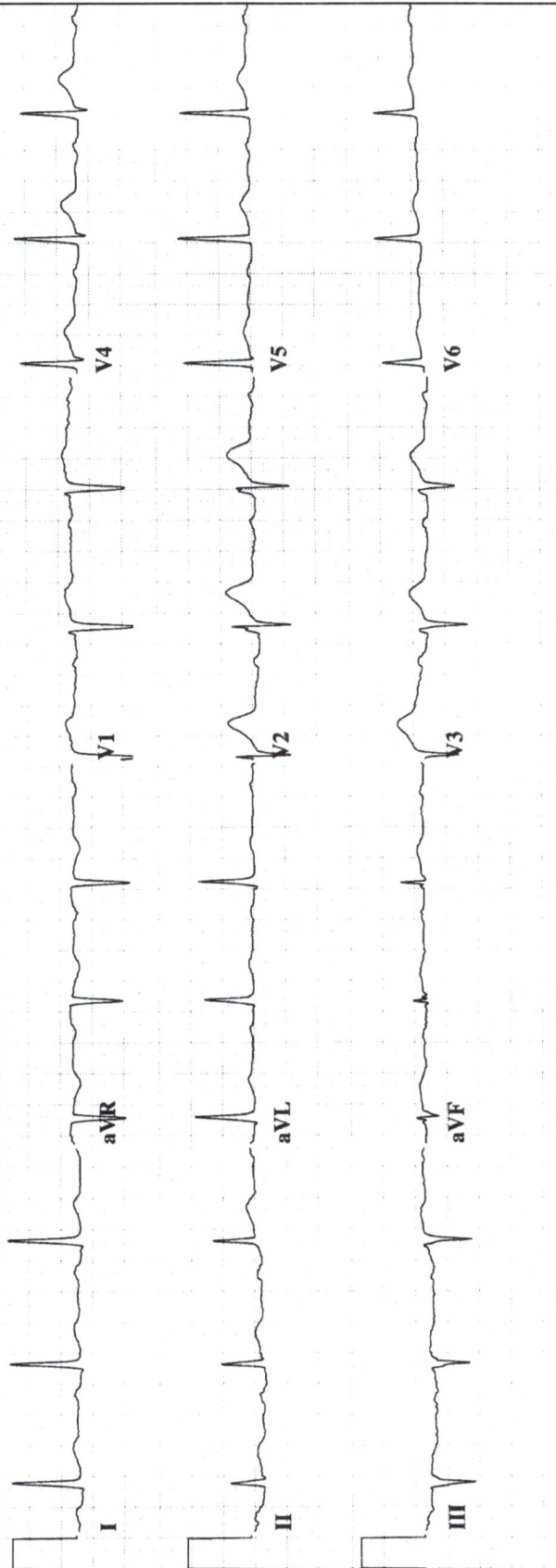

38 yr
Male

Hispanic

Vent. rate	74	BPM
PR interval	212	ms
QRS duration	86	ms
QT/QTc	364/404	ms
P–R–T axes	28 2	27

☞ EVALUATE EKG FOR:
- ST SEGMENT ELEVATION / DEPRESSION
- HYPERACUTE T WAVES
- FLAT / CONVEX J-T APEX SEGMENTS
- OTHER ST - T WAVE ABNORMALITIES
- *ABNORMAL R WAVE PROGRESSION / TRANSITION*

I   aVR   V1   V4

II   aVL   V2   V5

III   aVF   V3   V6

CASE STUDY QUESTIONS:

NOTE LEADS WITH ST ELEVATION:

NOTE LEADS WITH ST DEPRESSION:

WHAT IS THE SUSPECTED DIAGNOSIS ?

WHAT IS THE "CULPRIT ARTERY" – if applicable ?

LIST ANY CRITICAL STRUCTURES COMPROMISED:

LIST ANY POTENTIAL COMPLICATIONS:

38 yr		Vent. rate	74	BPM	Sinus rhythm with 1st degree A–V block
Male	Hispanic	PR interval	212	ms	Abnormal ECG
		QRS duration	86	ms	No previous ECGs available
		QT/QTc	364/404	ms	
Loc:7	Option:35	P–R–T axes	28 2	27	

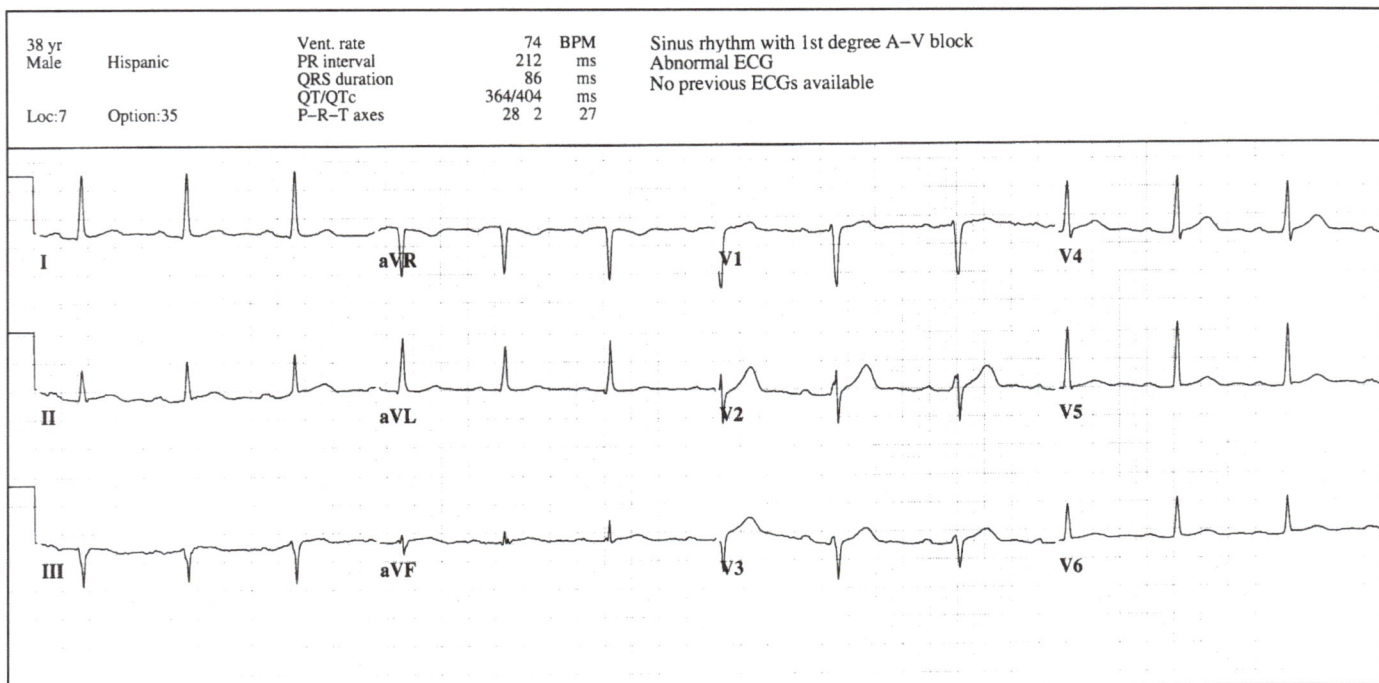

As noted by the ECG computer diagnosis, first degree heart block is present, with a P-R interval of 212ms. Other than a slight R wave progression abnormality in lead V3, no other abnormalities are noted.

He was taken to the cardiac cath lab, where the following images were obtained:

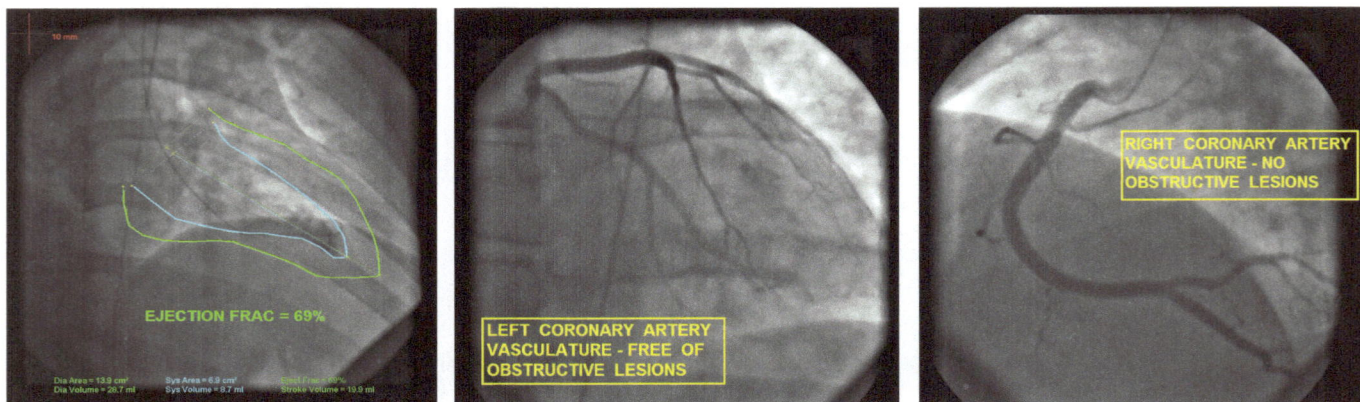

His left ventricular angiogram, seen to the above left, is normal, and shows no sign of injury. His ejection fraction is measured at 69%. Reference for normal range is 55 – 70%.

His left coronary artery system (above middle) shows diffuse, non-obstructive LAD disease in the mid to distal segment. The right coronary artery (above right) is remarkably free of obstructive coronary artery disease.

Within seconds after the above right image was obtained, the patient began complaining of a severe "burning" pain in his chest and neck.   The 6 lead ECG tracing at the top of the next page was recorded during the patient's episode of chest pain. ST segment elevation is noted in leads II, III, and aVF, which is consistent with occlusion of a dominant right coronary artery.   Repeat angiography of the right coronary artery revealed severe mid-segment vasospasm, as seen in top right image on the next page.

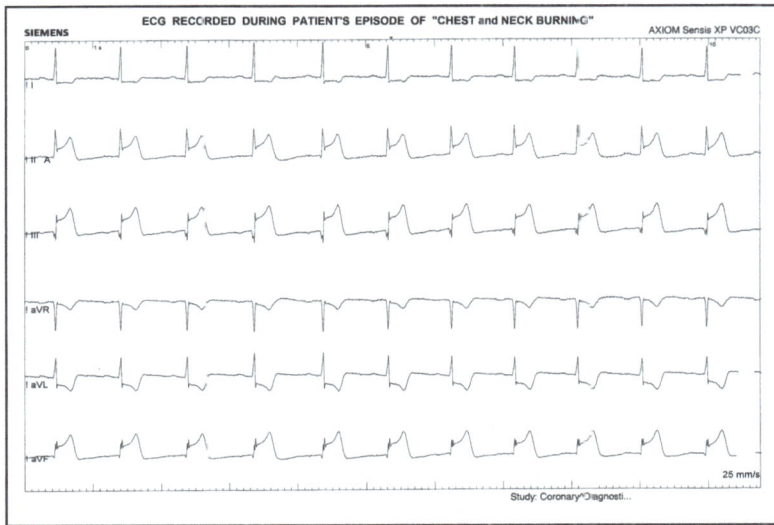

ECG RECORDED DURING PATIENT'S EPISODE OF "CHEST and NECK BURNING"

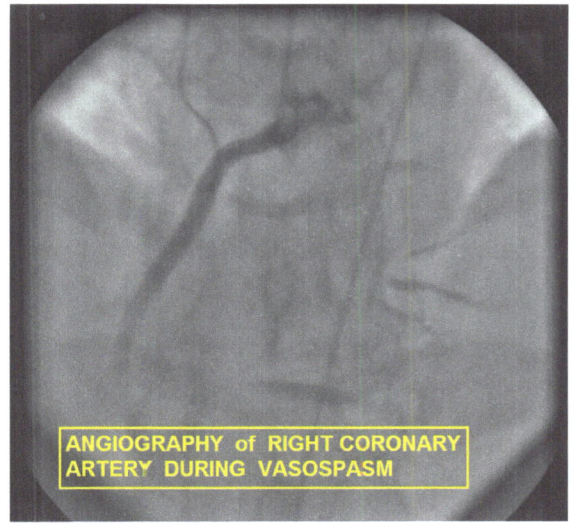

ANGIOGRAPHY of RIGHT CORONARY ARTERY DURING VASOSPASM

Next, 400 micrograms of intra-coronary nitroglycerine was administered, which effectively resolved the arterial vasospasm. The ECG and angiography below were taken just after abatement of the patient's symptoms:

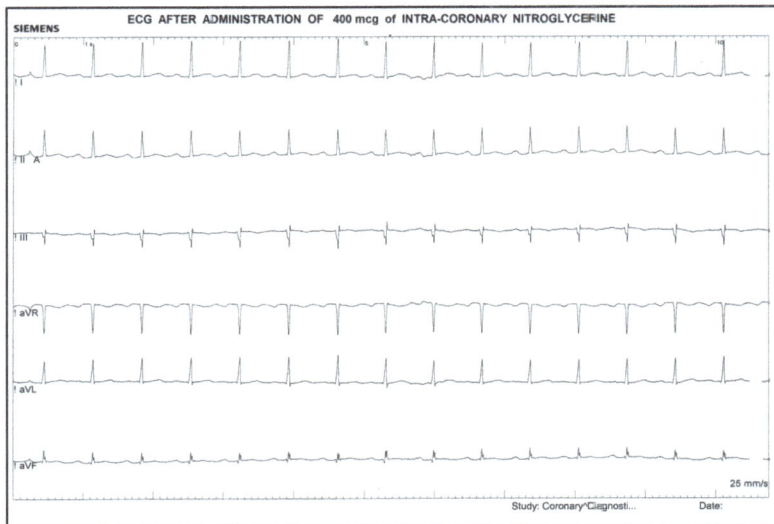

ECG AFTER ADMINISTRATION OF 400 mcg of INTRA-CORONARY NITROGLYCERINE

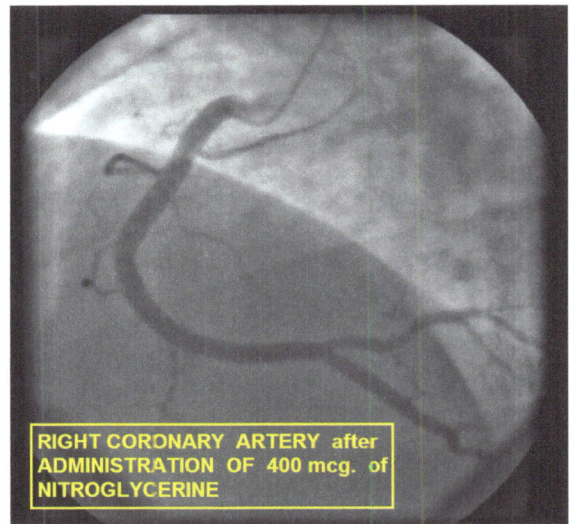

RIGHT CORONARY ARTERY after ADMINISTRATION OF 400 mcg. of NITROGLYCERINE

The patient was diagnosed with "Prinzmetal's Variant Angina" secondary to coronary artery vasospasm, and was placed on calcium channel blocker and nitrate therapy.

Prinzmetal or variant angina is caused by focal coronary artery vasospasm, and was first described by Myron Prinzmetal in 1959 as a syndrome of episodic chest pain that comes on at rest with ST segment elevation.[68] Prinzmetal angina is classified as unstable angina due to its unpredictability[69], and has been associated with myocardial infarction, ventricular dysrhythmias and cardiac arrest. The primary mechanism of vasospasm is hypercontraction of vascular smooth muscle cells. Variant angina is not an indicator of CAD; many patients are free of atherosclerotic plaque. Some factors known to provoke coronary artery vasospasm include: vasoconstrictor medications, stimulants such as cocaine, ephedrine and amphetamines, emotional duress, exposure to cold and alcohol withdraw.

Typical Prinzmetal's variant angina occurs at rest, in the early hours of the morning. The pain is often described as severe chest tightness or pressure. Variant angina is usually treated with and responds well to calcium channel blockers and nitrates.[70]

---

[68] Prinzmetal et al, *Am J Med*. 1959;27:375-388.

[69] National Institutes of Health, Library of Medicine, www.NIH.gov

[70] National Institutes of Health, Library of Medicine, www.NIH.gov

CHIEF COMPLAINT and SIGNIFICANT HISTORY:

45 y/o MALE c/o EXERTIONAL CHEST PRESSURE x past 2 months, getting worse. In last week, CHEST PRESSURE has come on at rest. DYSPNEA sometimes present. Pain is relieved when patient rests, however now takes longer than 20 minutes to subside.

RISK FACTOR PROFILE:

- FAMILY HISTORY: father died of AMI age 50, brother had CABG age 44
- CIGARETTE SMOKER x 20 YEARS
- HYPERTENSION
- ELEVATED LDL, TRIGLYCERIDES, LOW HDL CHOLESTEROL

PHYSICAL EXAM:
Pt. asymptomatic at time of exam, skin warm, dry, color normal, pupils PERLA, no JVD, lungs = clear, heart sounds normal S1, S2. Abd. soft, non-tender, No ankle edema

VITAL SIGNS:
BP: 177/96   P: 64   R: 16   SAO2: 99 % on room air

LABS:
TROPONIN: < .04

QUADRAD OF ACS CHECKLIST

☑ **SYMPTOMS of ACS**
- ✔ TYPICAL ACS - eg:
- ◆ ATYPICAL ACS - eg:

☐ **ECG ABNORMALITIES**
- ◆ ST ELEVATION (J POINT plus 40 ms)
- ◆ HYPERACUTE T WAVES - and/or -
- ◆ NEW or PRESUMABLY NEW LBBB
- ◆ ST DEPRESSION (>0.5 mm @ J POINT) and/or
- ◆ INVERTED or BIPHASIC T WAVES and/or
- ◆ DYNAMIC ST SEGMENT and/or T WAVE CHANGES IN SERIAL EKGs

☑ **RISK FACTORS - 3 or more**
- ✔ FAMILY HISTORY
- ◆ DIABETES
- ✔ ↑ LDL and/or ↓ HDL
- ✔ SMOKING
- ◆ AGE: 65 or MORE
- ✔ HYPERTENSION

☐ **CARDIAC MARKERS**
- ◆ ELEVATED TROPONIN and/or CK/MB

2 **TOTAL**

This patient presented with typical unstable angina symptoms, and an impressive risk factor profile, with respect to family history.

Note the progressive worsening and intensity of his symptoms, specifically the change from "exertional chest pressure" to "chest pressure comes on at rest" – a key factor which differentiates stable angina from unstable angina.

stable angina	VS.	unstable angina
1. SYMPTOMS START DURING PHYSICAL EXERTION.		1. SYMPTOMS MAY START AT ANY TIME, EVEN DURING REST
2. SYMPTOMS ARE "PREDICTABLE"		2. SYMPTOMS ARE *NEW*, *DIFFERENT*, or *WORSE* THAN PREVIOUS EPISODES

He was initially evaluated in the emergency department, and was admitted with the diagnosis of unstable angina.

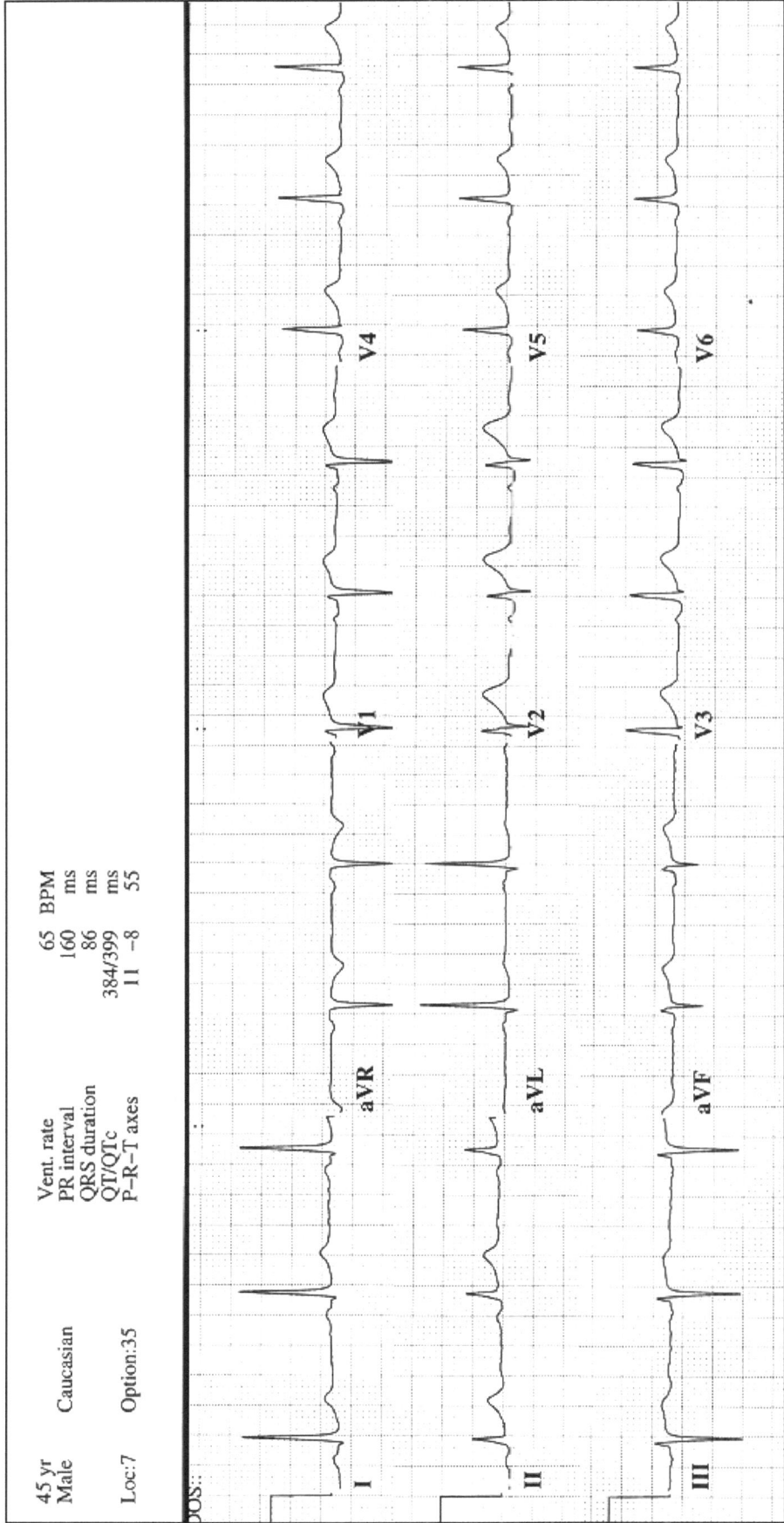

45 yr
Male
Caucasian

Loc:7   Option:35

Vent. rate	65	BPM
PR interval	160	ms
QRS duration	86	ms
QT/QTc	384/399	ms
P–R–T axes	11 –8	55

I   aVR   V1   V4

II   aVL   V2   V5

III   aVF   V3   V6

CASE STUDY QUESTIONS:

NOTE LEADS WITH ST ELEVATION:

NOTE LEADS WITH ST DEPRESSION:

WHAT IS THE SUSPECTED DIAGNOSIS ?

WHAT IS THE "CULPRIT ARTERY" – if applicable ?

LIST ANY CRITICAL STRUCTURES COMPROMISED:

LIST ANY POTENTIAL COMPLICATIONS:

269

His resting ECG demonstrates very subtle ST segment changes in leads III and aVL. Since lead III views the inferior wall, and aVL views the anterior-lateral region (one lead of two different regions), this is not enough "change" to define an abnormality. (Remember that traditional ECG interpretation guidelines define that ECG changes must be evident in "two or more contiguous leads.")

After his stress test revealed ST segment depression in leads I, II, III, aVL, aVF, V1 – V6, and ST elevation in lead aVR, he was sent to the cardiac cath lab, where the following angiographic images were obtained:

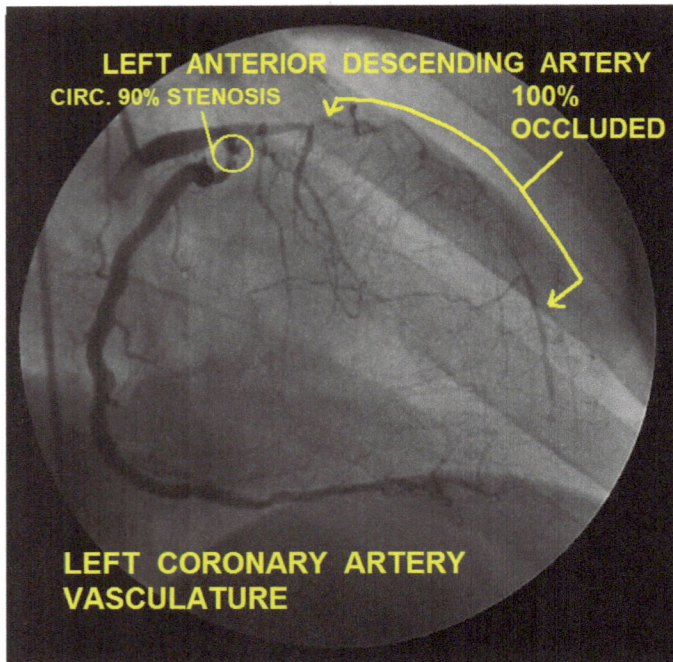

LEFT ANTERIOR DESCENDING ARTERY
CIRC. 90% STENOSIS 100% OCCLUDED
LEFT CORONARY ARTERY VASCULATURE

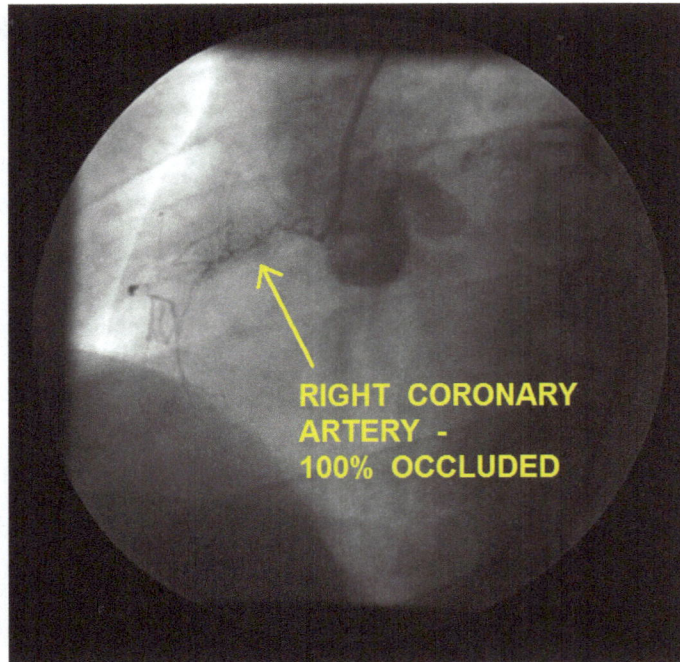

RIGHT CORONARY ARTERY - 100% OCCLUDED

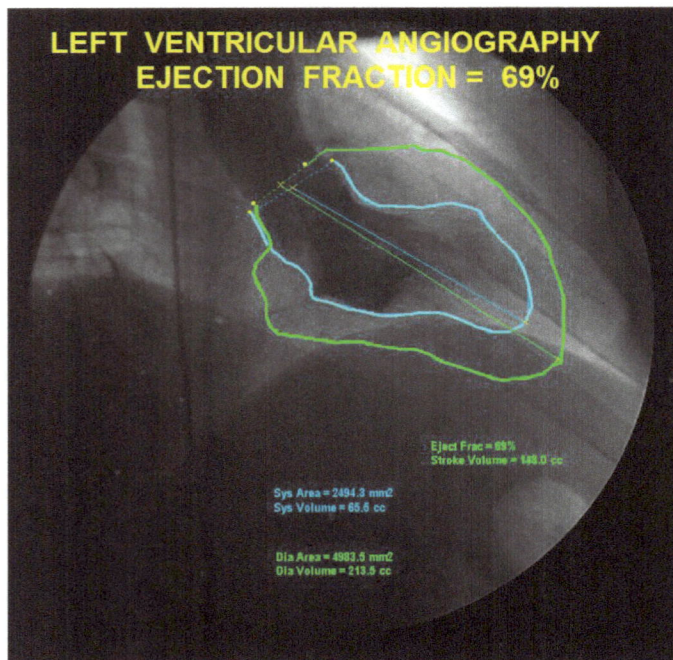

LEFT VENTRICULAR ANGIOGRAPHY
EJECTION FRACTION = 69%

Eject Frac = 69%
Stroke Volume = 148.0 cc
Sys Area = 2494.3 mm2
Sys Volume = 65.6 cc
Dia Area = 4983.5 mm2
Dia Volume = 213.5 cc

When coronary angiography was performed in the cardiac cath lab, the resulting images left the cardiologist and staff (myself included) astonished. The fact that his left ventricular ejection fraction is 69% defies explanation, especially when one considers that the normal range is 55 – 70%. Due to the advanced degree of diffuse disease, his vessels are not suitable for bypass grafting (there is no place to attach a bypass graft to). His options were: cardiac transplant or laser revascularization. He opted for laser revascularization, and one year after these images were obtained, he remained symptom-free, with no measurable myocardial damage.

This case study underscores the importance of not relying on the ECG – which can be NORMAL -- to rule out obstructive cardiovascular disease. In this case study, the clinician took the patient's *ACS symptoms* and *risk factor profile* – two factors of the Quadrad of ACS – into consideration as he engaged in the clinical decision making process.

BRUGADA SYNDROME *and Other Infarction Mimics:*

Brugada Syndrome is a genetically determined disorder affecting the cardiac electrical system and causes paroxysmal episodes of polymorphic ventricular tachycardia. When the polymorphic VT terminates spontaneously, patients may experience palpitations, lightheadedness and syncope. In sustained episodes, VT degenerates into ventricular fibrillation, resulting in mortality. Current studies indicate that Brugada Syndrome is responsible for up to 12% of all unexpected sudden deaths, and up to 50% of all sudden deaths in patients with a structurally normal heart. This disease usually afflicts individuals in their 30s; however patients ranging in ages from 6 months to 74 years have been diagnosed with the disorder. Brugada syndrome is statistically more prevalent in males of Southeast Asian descent.

Although Brugada Syndrome has no relationship with coronary artery disease and ACS, this recently discovered and lesser-known condition warrants inclusion in this curriculum because patients may present for medical help after suffering from Brugada Syndrome induced syncope, with ACS being suspected as a primary diagnosis, especially when ST segment elevation – a common finding – is noted on the 12 Lead ECG. If clinicians are familiar with patient profiles and the typical clinical presentation associated with Brugada Syndrome, accurate diagnosis will most likely occur; patients will be treated appropriately, and mortality will be prevented. It is unknown how many patients suffering from Brugada Syndrome-mediated syncope have sought medical help, been evaluated for ACS, and have been "medically cleared" without being correctly diagnosed with Brugada Syndrome.

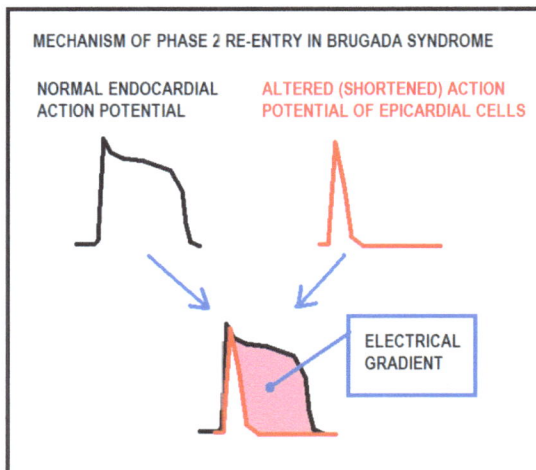

MECHANISM OF PHASE 2 RE-ENTRY IN BRUGADA SYNDROME

NORMAL ENDOCARDIAL ACTION POTENTIAL

ALTERED (SHORTENED) ACTION POTENTIAL OF EPICARDIAL CELLS

ELECTRICAL GRADIENT

Brugada Syndrome has been linked to a mutation of gene SCN5A, which encodes for the cardiac sodium channel. This mutation alters repolarization of epicardial cells, predominantly of the right ventricle, significantly shortening their refractory period. The resulting electrical gradient between abnormal epicardial cells and normal endocardial cells provides the ideal substrate for arrhythmias based on phase 2 re-entry. (See diagram to left).

The degree of repolarization aberrancy fluctuates, and is affected by changes in the body's *autonomic system, temperature, electrolytes,* and the *presence of antiarrhythmic medications*. The result is that the characteristic ECG markers of Brugada Syndrome are known to present ***intermittently,*** with periods where the patient's ECG is normal. Also, there are patients with "concealed" versions of Brugada Syndrome, whose ECGs always present as normal. It should also be noted that while antiarrhythmic drugs such as beta blockers and Amiodarone may mask the ECG markers of Brugada Syndrome, most do not protect against sudden cardiac death; the most effective treatment currently is the implantation of a cardio-defibrillator (ICD). Recent studies indicate Quinidine, a class Ia sodium channel blocker, may effectively prevent VF in patients with Brugada Syndrome.[71]

HISTORY: The first known case of Brugada Syndrome occurred in 1986, involving a three year old boy from Poland. The patient presented after experiencing several episodes of unconsciousness, and had been resuscitated by his father. The boy's older sister had died suddenly at the age of two. At the time of her death, she was receiving Amiodarone, and had a ventricular pacemaker implanted. The ECGs of both siblings featured the ECG abnormalities which have become known as the "typical patterns" of Brugada Syndrome. The identification of two more patients resulted in presentation of these cases at the North American Society of Pacing and Electrophysiology (NASPE) conference in 1991.

CLINICAL PRESENTATION: Formal components of the Brugada Syndrome include: ***right bundle branch block, ST segment elevation in leads V1, V2 and sometimes V3***, and ***sudden death***. Patient presentations range from those who are asymptomatic, to those with sudden death. Asymptomatic patients may be discovered by presentation of the "typical Brugada pattern ECG" during a routine examination. Others are discovered during ECG evaluation after the sudden death of a family member is found to have the disease. Typical complaints of symptomatic Brugada

---

[71] B. Belhassen, MD et al, Circulation, 2004;110:1731-1737

Syndrome patients who present to emergency departments and physician's offices are of episodic "lightheadedness, dizziness, palpitations," and/or "fainting," secondary to runs of polymorphic ventricular tachycardia.

According to recommendations published on www.brugada.org, the website maintained by the Ramon Brugada, Senior Foundation, *Brugada Syndrome* should be ruled out in patients who present with:

1. syncopal episodes of unknown cause or vaso-vagal origin or have a diagnosis of idiopathic ventricular fibrillation and/or
2. incidence of sudden, unexpected death of genetically (blood) related family member(s),   and/or
3. ECG findings characteristic of Brugada Syndrome (see the examples on page 275).

DIAGNOSIS can be easily made in cases where patients present with characteristic ECG markers for Brugada Syndrome. (See examples on pages 273-274). In cases of where the ECG is normal, a Drug Study Protocol should be administered, using Ajmaline, Flecainide, or Procainamide infusions; either of these agents will "unmask" the ECG markers of Brugada Syndrome.   Genetic testing for Brugada Syndrome is conducted by the Ramon Brugada, Senior Foundation.   For information about the Drug Study Protocol and/or genetic testing for Brugada Syndrome, visit www.brugada.org.

PROGNOSIS: An online PubMed search for "Mortality from Brugada Syndrome" nets 108 published scientific papers on this subject. The summary of what I have extrapolated from this material is:
1. There is a clear relationship between patients with Brugada Syndrome and Sudden Death.
2. The highest degree of risk of sudden death (10.2 – 38% annual fatal arrhythmic events)[72],[73] correlates with patients whom are symptomatic (syncope) with ECG presence of a Brugada ECG pattern, or test positive in the Brugada drug study (see "DIAGNOSIS," above).
3. The lowest degree of sudden death risk, according to two studies, is in the subgroup of patients whom are asymptomatic. In one study, 2 previously asymptomatic patients out of 105 suffered sudden death at night during a 5.6 year follow-up.[74]   In the second study, conducted by Probst et al, the event rate for sudden death in asymptomatic patients was 0.5% per year.[75]

According to information posted by the Brugada Foundation, prognosis for individuals not treated for Brugada Syndrome is poor: one third of all patients who suffered from syncopal episodes or were resuscitated from a near-death experience presented with new episodes of polymorphic VT within two years.   Incidentally, one-third of all asymptomatic patients discovered to have characteristic Brugada Syndrome markers on their ECG experienced polymorphic VT within the two year follow-up period.

The Brugada Foundation (www.brugada.org) recommends that patients who present with *family histories of sudden, unexpected death* and/or those who present with complaints of *syncope of unknown etiology* should be screened for Brugada Syndrome. The screening process should include:
1. ECG studies
2. Brugada Drug Study Protocol
3. EP Study for inducible VT/VF
4. Genetic testing for the SCN5A mutation.

TREATMENT: At present, ICD implantation has proven to be 100% effective.   Current literature suggests that Quinidine may be an effective therapy for VF prevention in asymptomatic Brugada Syndrome patients. A clinical study (NIH Study #NCT00789165) is in progress for the use of Quinidine in asymptomatic Brugada Syndrome patients.[76]

In patients who underwent ICD implantation, there was a 0% mortality during a mean 5.6 year follow-up period,[77] and a 0% mortality rate at up to 10 years, as reported by Brugada et al.

---

[72] Y. Miyasaka, MD et al, J Am Coll Cardiol, 2001; 38:771-774

[73] S. Kamakura et al, Circ Arrhythm Electrophysiol. 2009 Oct;2(5):495-503

[74] G. Veerakul et al, Circulation. 2008;118:S_982

[75] V Probst, et al; Circulation 2010 Feb 9;121(5):635-43

[76] Sami Viskin, MD & C. Antzelevitch, www.clinicaltrials.gov (Study Identifier: NCT00789165)

[77] G. Veerakul et al,

CHIEF COMPLAINT and SIGNIFICANT HISTORY:

37 y/o FEMALE patient arrives via EMS after being involved in a low speed motor vehicle accident. Per EMS crew, patient was the driver and sole occupant of a car that struck a tree. Patient does not recall accident. Upon further questioning, patient admits to other episodes of syncope and near-syncope. Patient denies feeling any chest pain / pressure or shortness of breath. She states she "felt great" today, until just before the the accident, when she "suddenly felt lightheaded and must have blacked-out."

RISK FACTOR PROFILE:

💣☀️**FAMILY HISTORY:** MATERNAL AUNT DIED AT AGE 31, UNEXPECTEDLY. WAS RULED AS A "HEART ATTACK." THERE WAS NO PRIOR KNOWN HISTORY OF CAD.

PHYSICAL EXAM: Pt. CAO x 3, skin warm, dry, color normal. Abrasions /contusions on face (airbag deployment). Patient appears to be in excellent physical condition, states she exercises several times per week (aerobics, weight training, swimming).

VITAL SIGNS: BP: 112/66, P: , R: 20, SAO2: 100% on room air.

LABS: TROPONIN: < .04 BMP and CBC: all values within normal limits.

37 yr		Vent. rate	62	BPM
Female	Caucasian	PR interval	180	ms
		QRS duration	88	ms
		QT/QTc	418/424	ms
		P-R-T axes	37 22	47

Normal sinus rhythm
Normal ECG
No previous ECGs available

← **NOTE COMPUTER INTERPRETATION !**

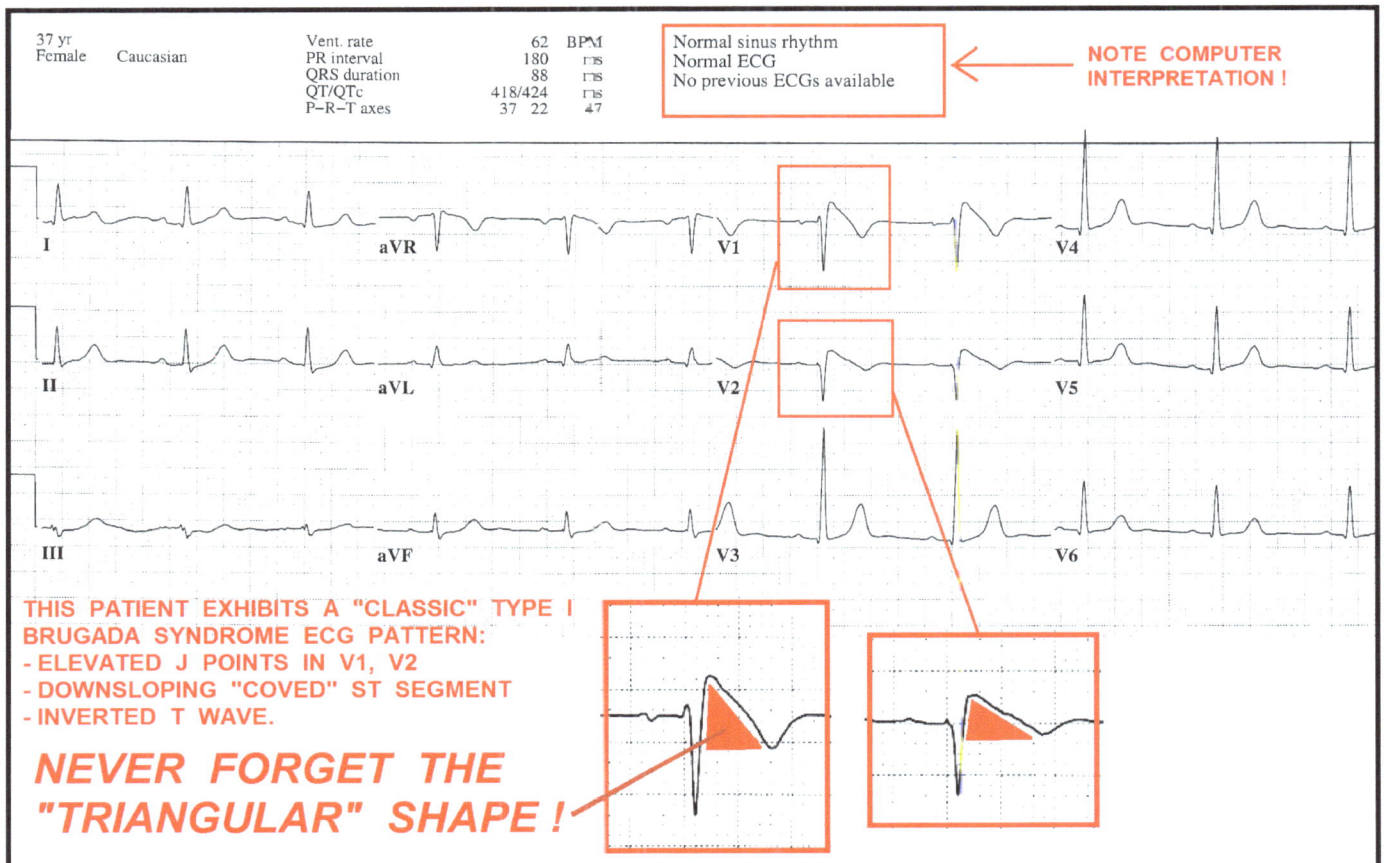

I aVR V1 V4

II aVL V2 V5

III aVF V3 V6

THIS PATIENT EXHIBITS A "CLASSIC" TYPE I
BRUGADA SYNDROME ECG PATTERN:
- ELEVATED J POINTS IN V1, V2
- DOWNSLOPING "COVED" ST SEGMENT
- INVERTED T WAVE.

NEVER FORGET THE "TRIANGULAR" SHAPE !

Patient was admitted to the hospital and received implantable cardio-defibrillator (ICD) prior to hospital discharge.

33 y/o FEMALE

Vent. rate	129	BPM
PR interval	*	ms
QRS duration	112	ms
QT/QTc	398/583	ms
P–R–T axes	* 121	−2

Undetermined rhythm
Incomplete right bundle branch block
Right ventricular hypertrophy
ST elevation consider anterior injury or acute infarct
** ** ** ** ** ACUTE MI * ** ** ** **
Abnormal ECG
No previous ECGs available

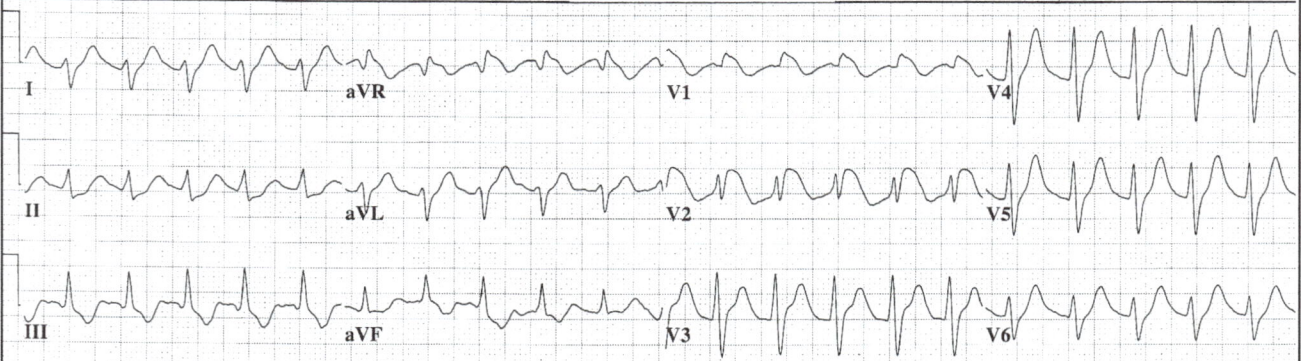

(Leads: I, aVR, V1, V4 / II, aVL, V2, V5 / III, aVF, V3, V6)

PT. BROUGHT TO EMERGENCY DEPARTMENT BY EMS AFTER SUFFERING SPONTANEOUS CARDIAC ARREST.   PATIENT DID NOT EXPERIENCE ANY SYMPTOMS PRIOR TO COLLAPSE.   HAD SEVERAL EPISODES OF NEAR-SYNCOPE IN THE PAST 10 YEARS. CARDIAC CATHETERIZATION REVEALED NO EVIDENCE OF CARDIOVASCULAR DISEASE. NORMAL LV FUNCTION.
DIAGNOSIS: BRUGADA SYNDROME.   PT. RECEIVED ICD PRIOR TO HOSPITAL DISCHARGE.
VISIT: www.BRUGADA.org FOR MORE INFORMATION.

---

42 y/o FEMALE

Vent. rate	86	BPM
PR interval	200	ms
QRS duration	148	ms
QT/QTc	414/495	ms
P–R–T axes	64 114	17

Normal sinus rhythm with sinus arrhythmia
Right bundle branch block
ST elevation consider anterior injury or acute infarct
** ** ** ** ** ACUTE MI * ** ** ** **
Abnormal ECG
No previous ECGs available

Confirmed By:

D.O.S.:

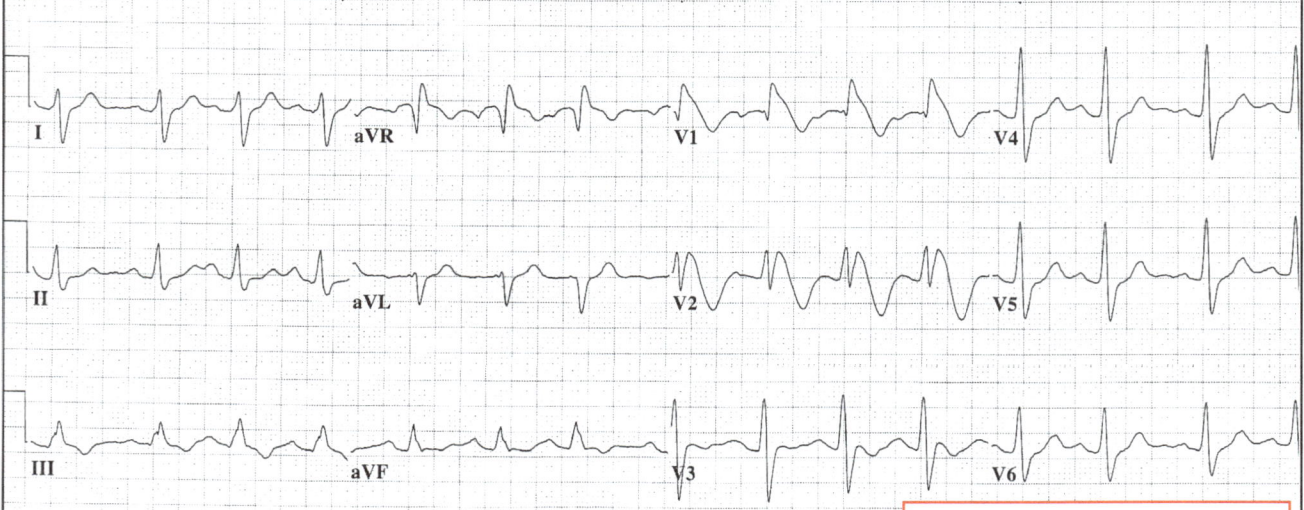

(Leads: I, aVR, V1, V4 / II, aVL, V2, V5 / III, aVF, V3, V6)

BRUGADA SYNDROME.
PATIENT HAD HISTORY of SYNCOPE of UNKNOWN ETIOLOGY.
FAMILY HISTORY of SUDDEN DEATH of YOUNG, HEALTHY ADULTS.
VISIT: www.BRUGADA.org FOR MORE INFORMATION !

THE ONLY KNOWN TREATMENT FOR BRUGADA SYNDROME is IMPLANTATION of an ICD. THIS PATIENT HAD ICD IMPLANTED PRIOR TO HOSPITAL DISCHARGE.

ADDITIONAL 12 LEAD ECGs OF "STEMI – MIMICS:"

The following ECGs are those of conditions which can result in ST segment elevation on the 12 lead ECG. The conditions we feature here are: *Acute Myocarditis, Acute Pericarditis* (2 ECGs), *Early Repolarization* (2 ECGs) and *Hyperkalemia.* Our presentation in this section is not complete: there are several other conditions known to result in ECGs with ST segment elevation: Acute Cor Pulmonale, Myocardial Metastases, Acute Cholecystitis, Intercranial Hemorrhage, Acute Pancreatitis, and Hypoglycemia, and more.

We present these ECGs to you to demonstrate how these other conditions can result in ECGs which look convincingly like STEMI. We have learned that in most cases, if a thorough history and physical exam are obtained, along with serial cardiac markers, ECGs, and ACS Risk Factor Profiles are generated, the diagnosis of STEMI can often safely be excluded. In many cases, such as early repolarization, if old ECGs are available, diagnosis of STEMI can be excluded (see ECG, top of page 278). Note that all of these ECGs feature computer-printed diagnoses proclaiming: "Acute Myocardial Infarction."

Of final note, it must be said that when it comes to patient safety, STEMI must be aggressively ruled out when patients present with ECGs like the ones on the next several pages. Again, this is more easily achieved in some cases than in others. Once STEMI is ruled out, we must be careful to rule out other potentially serious conditions.

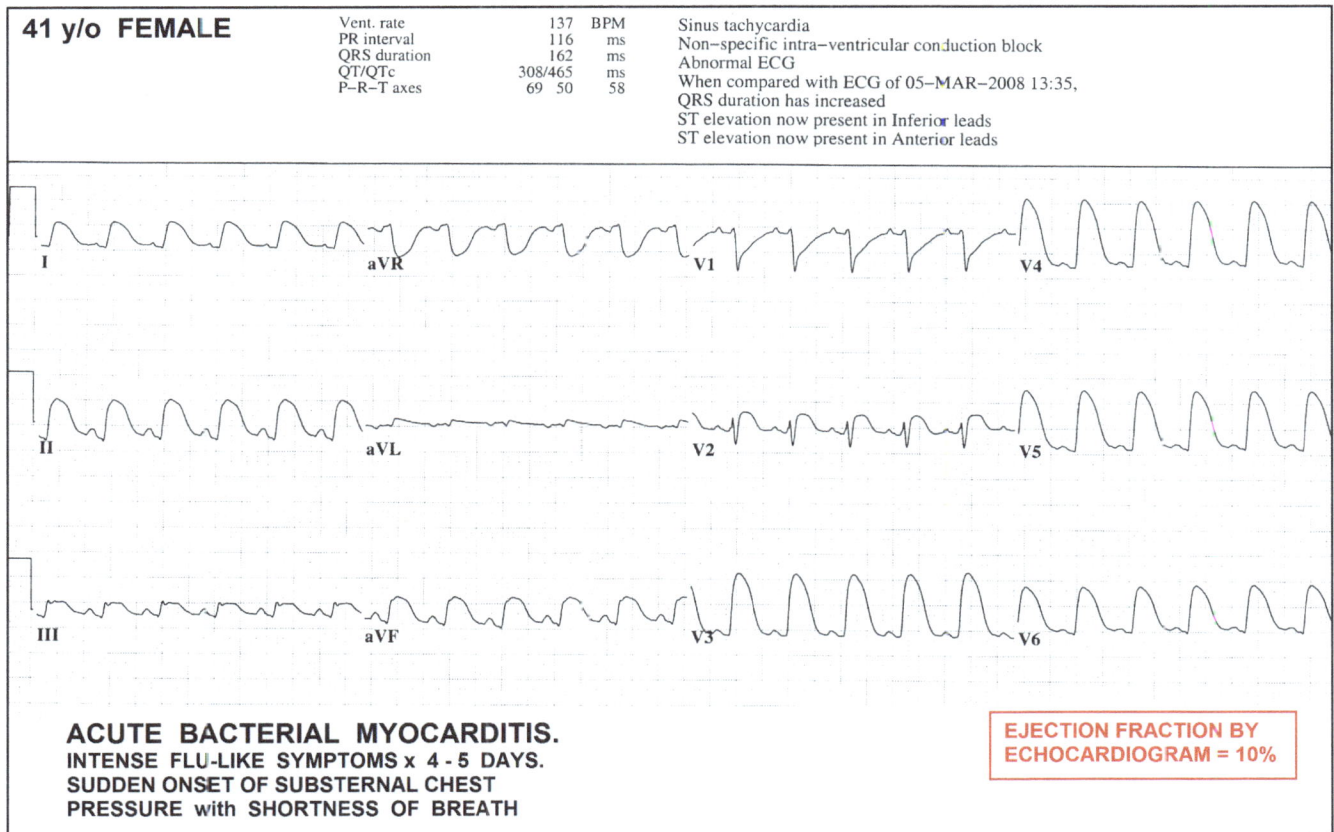

41 y/o FEMALE				
Vent. rate	137	BPM	Sinus tachycardia	
PR interval	116	ms	Non–specific intra–ventricular conduction block	
QRS duration	162	ms	Abnormal ECG	
QT/QTc	308/465	ms	When compared with ECG of 05–MAR–2008 13:35,	
P–R–T axes	69 50	58	QRS duration has increased	

Sinus tachycardia
Non–specific intra–ventricular conduction block
Abnormal ECG
When compared with ECG of 05–MAR–2008 13:35,
QRS duration has increased
ST elevation now present in Inferior leads
ST elevation now present in Anterior leads

ACUTE BACTERIAL MYOCARDITIS.
INTENSE FLU-LIKE SYMPTOMS x 4 - 5 DAYS.
SUDDEN ONSET OF SUBSTERNAL CHEST
PRESSURE with SHORTNESS OF BREATH

EJECTION FRACTION BY
ECHOCARDIOGRAM = 10%

23 y/o MALE:

Vent. rate	56	BPM
PR interval	128	ms
QRS duration	96	ms
QT/QTc	410/395	ms
P–R–T axes	23 66	47

**UNEDITED COPY – REPORT IS COMPUTER GENERATED ONLY, WITHOUT PHYSICIAN INTERPRETATION
Sinus bradycardia with sinus arrhythmia
ST elevation consider inferolateral injury or acute infarct
** ** ** ** * ACUTE MI * ** ** ** **
Abnormal ECG
No previous ECGs available

Confirmed By: UNEDITED   ER

ACUTE PERICARDITIS.
SHARP SUBSTERNAL CHEST PAIN x 1 DAY, HAD VIRAL SYMPTOMS with MOUTH ULCERS x 3 DAYS.   CHEST PAIN INCREASES WITH DEEP INSPIRATION.

TESTED POSITIVE FOR COXSACKIE A and B VIRUS

---

37 y/o MALE:

Vent. rate	97	BPM
PR interval	152	ms
QRS duration	92	ms
QT/QTc	364/462	ms
P–R–T axes	66 34	30

**UNEDITED COPY – REPORT IS COMPUTER GENERATED ONLY, WITHOUT PHYSICIAN INTERPRETATION
Sinus rhythm with Premature supraventricular complexes
ST elevation consider anterolateral injury or acute infarct
ST elevation consider inferior injury or acute infarct
** ** ** ** * ACUTE MI * ** ** ** **
Abnormal ECG

ACUTE PERICARDITIS.
SHARP CHEST PAIN x 1 DAY, PROGRESSIVELY INCREASED PAIN, INCREASES WITH DEEP INSPIRATION. RECENT HISTORY OF VIRAL SYMPTOMS.

NOTE: THIS PATIENT EXPERIENCED SUDDEN VENTRICULAR FIBRILLATION in the EMERGENCY DEPARTMENT, WAS DEFIBRILLATED x 1 WITH RETURN OF SINUS RHYTHM. RECOVERED FULLY.

Note: The above patient was taken immediately to the cardiac catheterization suite after the episode of VF, and was found to have clean arteries.   Endomyocardial biopsy was performed, which confirmed an additional diagnosis of *myocarditis*. *Spontaneous ventricular fibrillation has been reported in cases of myocarditis, and in one study, was found to occur in 20% of myocarditis cases.* [78]   This case study demonstrates the importance of obtaining a thorough diagnosis in cases of suspected pericarditis, and keeping patients in a monitored, ACLS capable unit until myocarditis is ruled out, and sufficient recovery has occurred.

---

[78] A. Ristic el al, Herz. 2000 Dec;25(8):729-33

64 y/o MALE

Vent. rate	65	BPM	Sinus rhythm with 1st degree A–V block
PR interval	232	ms	ST elevation consider anterolateral injury or acute infarct
QRS duration	86	ms	*** ** ** ** * ACUTE MI ** ** ** **
QT/QTc	400/416	ms	Abnormal ECG
P–R–T axes	53 43 –46		

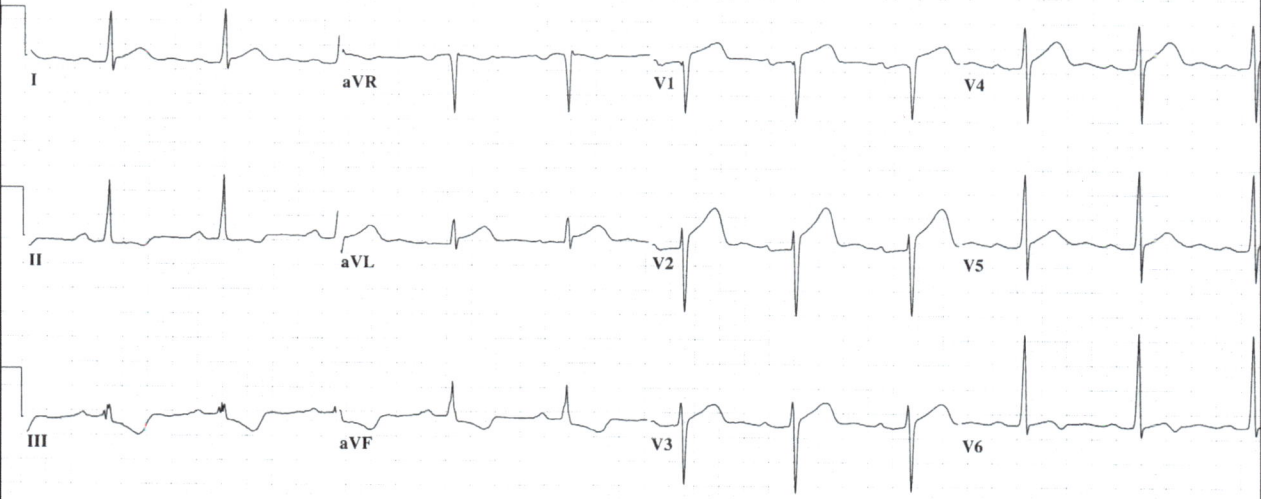

I aVR V1 V4
II aVL V2 V5
III aVF V3 V6

Dx: EARLY REPOLARIZATION. PT. ASYMPTOMATIC HAD 7 EKGs SPANNING 11 YEARS WITH IDENTICAL FINDINGS. NOTE U WAVES V3 - V5.

---

54 y/o FEMALE

Vent. rate	82	BPM	*** AGE AND GENDER SPECIFIC ECG ANALYSIS ***
PR interval	*	ms	Unusual P axis, possible ectopic atrial rhythm with complete heart block and
QRS duration	132	ms	Wide QRS rhythm
QT/QTc	360/420	ms	Non–specific intra–ventricular conduction block
P–R–T axes	159 31 21		ST elevation consider inferior injury or acute infarct
			ST elevation consider anterior injury or acute infarct
			*** ** ** ** * ACUTE MI ** ** ** ** ...

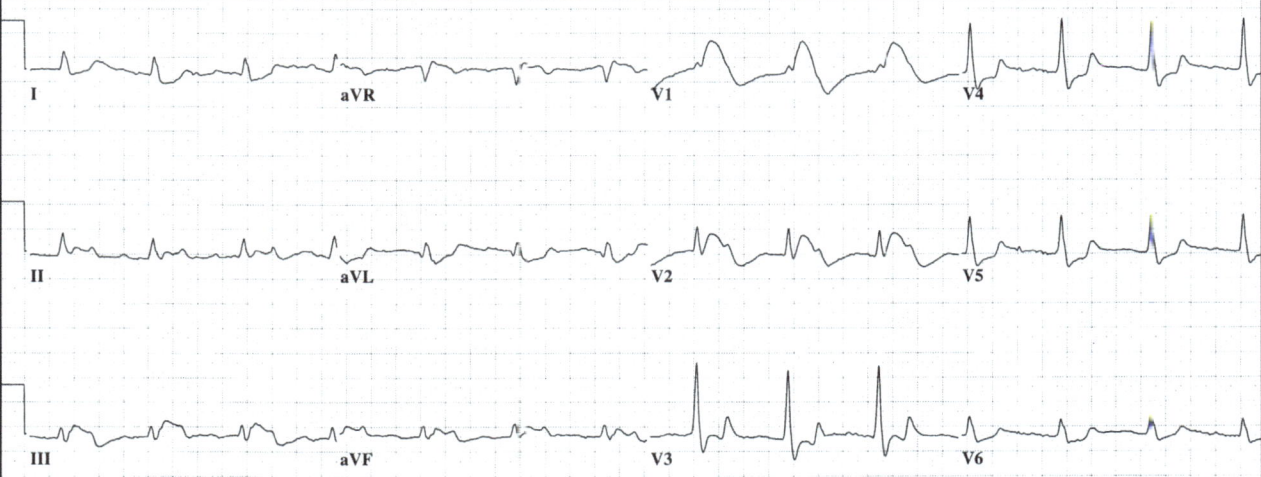

I aVR V1 V4
II aVL V2 V5
III aVF V3 V6

HYPERKALEMIA - K+ 8.6

PT. FOUND UNRESPONSIVE BY FRIENDS. NO PRECIPITATING COMPLAINTS. Dx: ACUTE RENAL FAILURE.

Pt. EXPERIENCED CARDIAC ARREST, SUCCESSFUL RESUSCITATION with NaHCO3 100 mEq, CALCIUM CHLORIDE 1.0 gram, INSULIN 10 units, and DEXTROSE 25 gm. IV. DISCHARGED 11 DAYS LATER.

NSTEMI and Unstable Angina:

58. (p. 241) Patients diagnosed with NSTEMI are having an MI, but there is no qualifying ST segment elevation on the 12 Lead ECG.
    a. true
    b. false

59. (p. 241) Which of the following ECG findings may be seen on a patient suffering from NSTEMI?
    a. ST segment depression
    b. inverted T waves
    c. a normal ECG
    d. all of the above

60. (p. 241) Where are the two "blind spots" of the 12 Lead ECG?
    a. septal wall
    b. right ventricle
    c. posterior wall
    d. b and c

61. (p. 241) According to the algorithm on page 241, what one thing do all NSTEMI patients have in common?
    a. elevated cardiac markers
    b. morbid obesity
    c. elevated cholesterol
    d. ST segment depression in the leads viewing the effected region of myocardium

62. (p. 241) Acute right ventricular MI and posterior wall MI are two examples of transmural (full-thickness MI) that don't have ST segment elevation on the ECG, and are therefore diagnosed as "NSTEMI."
    a. true
    b. false

63. (p. 245) Patients can experience acute transmural (full muscle thickness) MI and have no ST segment elevation or depression on their 12 Lead ECG.
    a. true
    b. false

64. (p. 249) If a patient has isolated posterior wall MI (with no other regions of the heart involved in the MI), their primary ECG abnormality will be:
    a. ST segment elevation in leads V5 and V6
    b. ST elevation in leads II, III, and aVF
    c. ST elevation in leads V1 – V3
    d. ST segment depression along with development of tall R waves in leads V1 – V3.

65. (p. 252) In cases of NSTEMI or Unstable Angina, Elevation of the ST segment in lead aVR is associated with a high incidence of:
    a. significant triple vessel disease
    b. acute cor pulmonale
    c. pulmonary edema
    d. mitral valve regurgitation

66. (p. 257) It is possible to experience Acute MI from emotional duress.
    a. true
    b. false

67. (p. 257) Apical Ballooning Syndrome (ABS) accounts for an estimated 2% of all cases of AMI. There is often NO cardiovascular disease noted during cardiac catheterization. Causes of ABS include:
    a. severe emotional duress
    b. elevated LDL cholesterol
    c. a-adrenergic substances
    d. a and c

68. (p. 258) Your NSTEMI patient may have which of the following symptoms:
    a. typical ACS symptoms
    b. atypical ACS symptoms
    c. no symptoms
    d. all of the above

69. (p. 259) The definition of unstable angina is: *a new onset of ACS-like chest pain, or changes in a previously stable pattern of angina, without* _____.*"*
    a. shortness of breath
    b. elevation of cardiac markers
    c. congestive heart failure
    d. ST segment depression on the ECG

70. (p. 258) While there are numerous "patterns of ischemia" one can memorize, the most important thing regarding ECG changes associated with ACS is to remember "if it isn't NORMAL, it is ABNORMAL." What defines NORMAL in all leads on the 12 lead ECG except lead aVR?
    a. J points within 1mm of the isoelectric line
    b. ST segments have a "slight, positive inclination"
    c. T waves are upright
    d. all of the above

71. (p. 260) If you are monitoring the ECG of a patient whose diagnosis is "Unstable Angina," what ECG lead is best to monitor?"
    a. Lead II
    b. a lead which views the region of suspected ischemia
    c. MCL1
    d. any lead: it really doesn't matter, as long as you can see a good P wave and QRS complex.

72. (p. 267) Prinzmetal's variant angina has been known to:
    a. frequently come on in the morning, and while the patient is at rest
    b. cause myocardial infarction, ventricular dysrhythmias and cardiac arrest
    c. often cause ST segment elevation on the ECG
    d. all of the above

73. (p. 270) The ECGs of patients with unstable angina secondary to severe underlying CAD will always demonstrate some form of *J point, ST segment*, and/or *T wave abnormality*.
    a. True
    b. False

ANSWERS TO REVIEW QUESTIONS:

1.	B	53.	A	105.	A
2.	A	54.	C	106.	C
3.	B	55.	A	107.	D
4.	B	56.	B	108.	C
5.	D	57.	D	109.	D
6.	A	58.	C	110.	C
7.	A	59.	B	111.	A
8.	A	60.	A	112.	A
9.	D	61.	B	113.	A
10.	B	62.	D	114.	B
11.	B	63.	B	115.	B
12.	A	64.	B	116.	D
13.	D	65.	D	117.	A
14.	A	66.	A	118.	B
15.	A	67.	D	119.	D
16.	D	68.	D	120.	A
17.	A	69.	C	121.	D
18.	A	70.	D	122.	D
19.	B	71.	A	123.	A
20.	C	72.	C	124.	A
21.	A	73.	B	125.	A
22.	C	74.	C	126.	D
23.	A	75.	B	127.	A
24.	B	76.	D	128.	A
25.	D	77.	D	129.	D
26.	A	78.	D	130.	D
27.	B	79.	D	131.	B
28.	A	80.	D	132.	D
29.	D	81.	C	133.	B
30.	A	82.	B	134.	D
31.	B	83.	D	135.	B
32.	D	84.	B		
33.	B	85.	A		
34.	C	86.	B		
35.	A	87.	B		
36.	B	88.	A		
37.	B	89.	A		
38.	B	90.	A		
39.	C	91.	C		
40.	A	92.	D		
41.	B	93.	B		
42.	A	94.	A		
43.	A	95.	D		
44.	B	96.	D		
45.	C	97.	D		
46.	A	98.	D		
47.	B	99.	D		
48.	A	100.	A		
49.	B	101.	D		
50.	A	102.	D		
51.	D	103.	B		
52.	D	104.	A		

INDEX of SUBJECT and REFERENCE SOURCES:

*This project would not have been possible without assistance from my **editorial team**, shown in the photograph to the right, taken during an evening manuscript review session, November 2009*

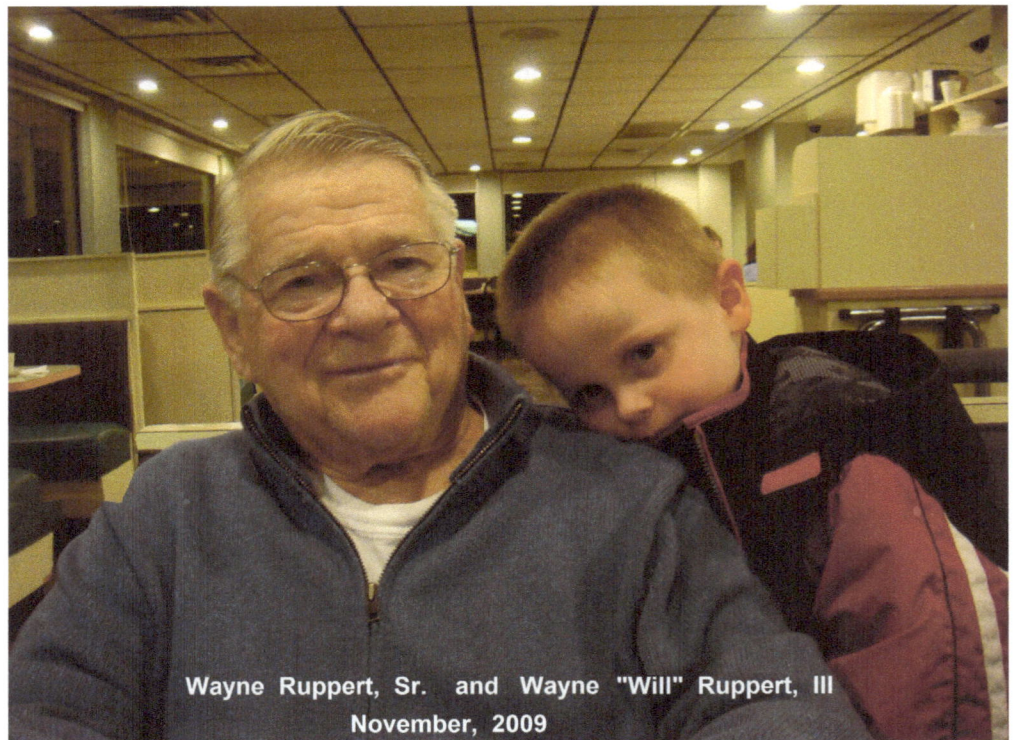

Wayne Ruppert, Sr. and Wayne "Will" Ruppert, III
November, 2009

APPENDIX: ECG EXAMPLES of FASCICULAR BLOCKS:

80 y/o MALE

Vent. rate	101	BPM
PR interval	126	ms
QRS duration	86	ms
QT/QTc	312/404	ms
P-R-T axes	52 -49	163

Sinus tachycardia
Left anterior fascicular block
Minimal voltage criteria for LVH, may be normal variant
ST & T wave abnormality, consider lateral ischemia
Abnormal ECG
No previous ECGs available

LEFT ANTERIOR FASCICULAR BLOCK

see page 71 for more information about LAFB.

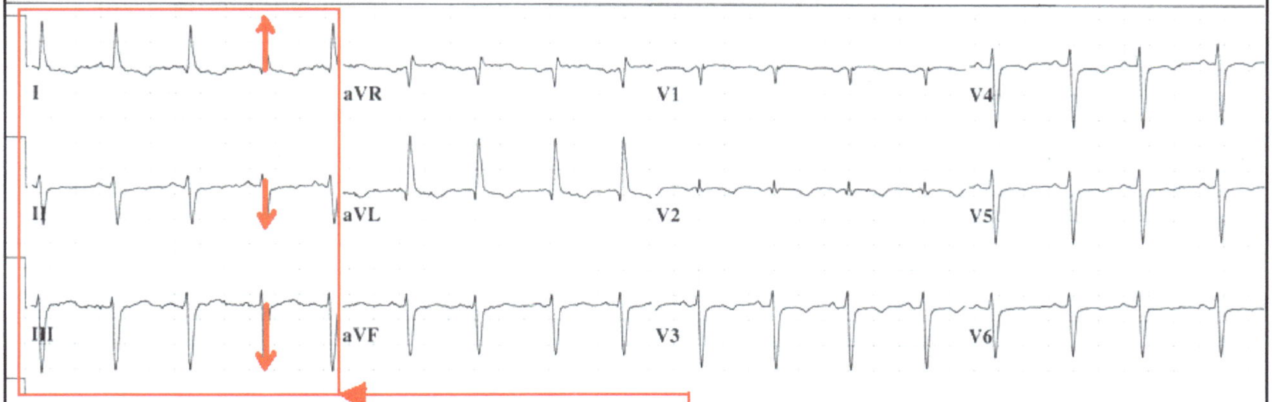

ECG Characteristics of Left Anterior Fascicular Block:

1. "UP-DOWN-DOWN" Pattern in Leads I, II, and III.
2. QRS between 80 - 120 ms.
3. "Q1-S3" pattern (small Q wave Lead I, deep S wave Lead III)
4. Left Axis Deviation.

note the mainly negative deflecting QRS complexes in Leads II and III are NOT caused by old Inferior MI (NO Q waves) - these are " rS " complexes.

76 y/o FEMALE

Vent. rate	82	BPM
PR interval	128	ms
QRS duration	86	ms
QT/QTc	392/457	ms
P-R-T axes	38 112	-142

Sinus rhythm with Possible Premature atrial complexes
Left posterior fascicular block
ST & T wave abnormality, consider anterolateral ischemia
Abnormal ECG

LEFT POSTERIOR FASCICULAR BLOCK

Confirmed By:

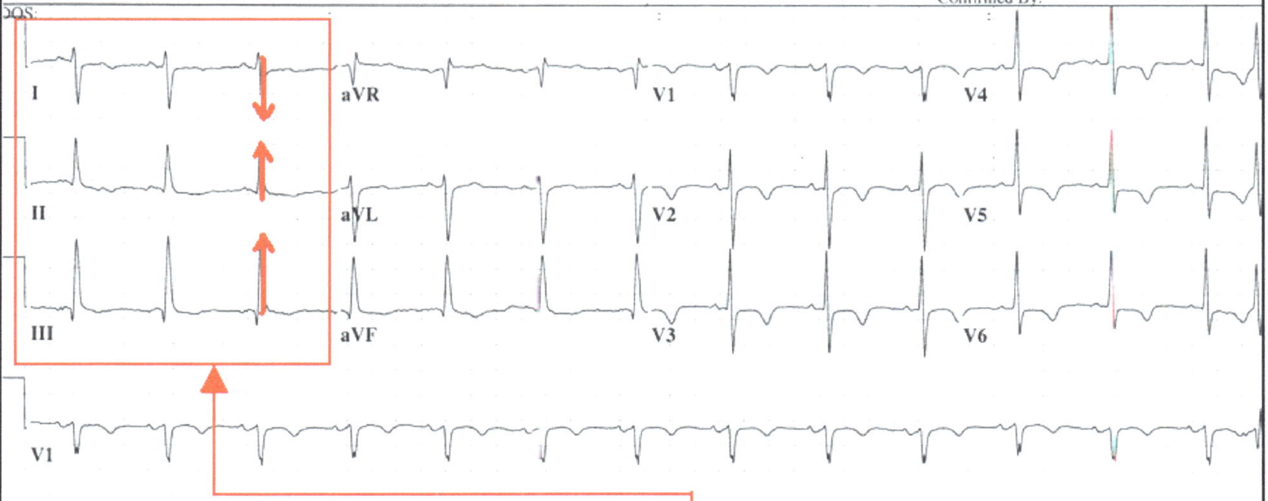

ECG Characteristics of Left Posterior Fascicular Block:

1. "DOWN - UP - UP" PATTERN, Leads I, II, and III.
2. QRS DURATION between 80 - 120 ms.
3. "S1 - Q3 PATTERN" (small Q wave Lead III, deep S wave Lead I).
4. Right Axis Deviation

Note there is NO Q WAVE present in Lead I - QRS complexes are " rS " complexes.
If Q Waves were present, we would have to consider "Lateral Wall Necrosis " (old MI) as a more likely diagnosis over that of LPFB.

62 y/o FEMALE

BIFASCICULAR BLOCK

Vent. rate	66	BPM
PR interval	192	ms
QRS duration	154	ms
QT/QTc	452/473	ms
P–R–T axes	69 –55	22

Normal sinus rhythm
Right bundle branch block
Left anterior fascicular block
*** Bifascicular block ***
Abnormal ECG

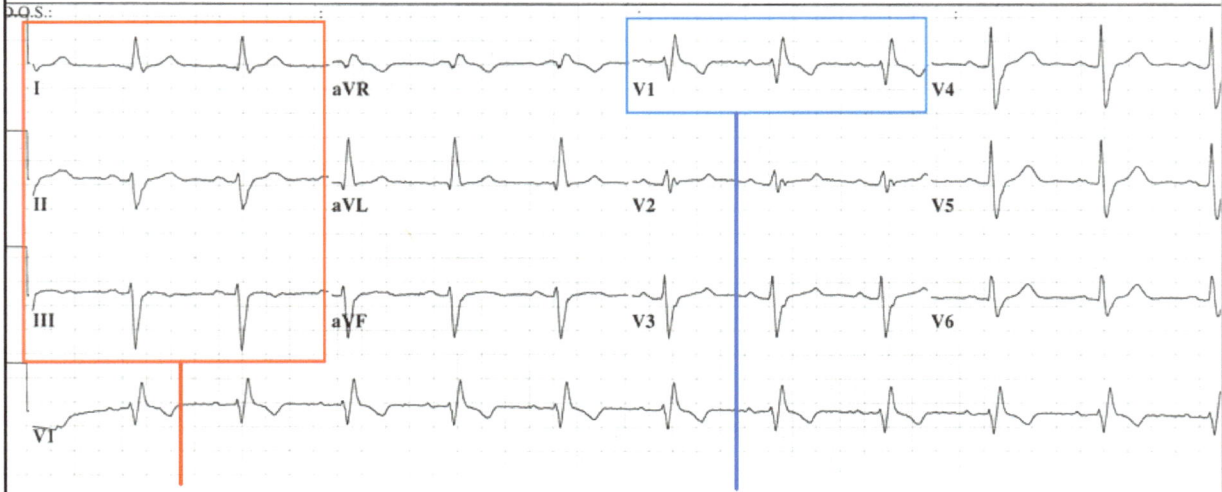

LEFT ANTERIOR FASCICULAR BLOCK
1. "UP-DOWN-DOWN" PATTERN in Lead I
2. Q1 - S3 PATTERN
3. LEFT AXIS DEVIATION

RIGHT BUNDLE BRANCH BLOCK
1. QRS DURATION GREATER THAN 120 ms
2. rSR' PATTERN in LEAD V1

71 y/o MALE

BIFASCICULAR BLOCK

Vent. rate	132	BPM
PR interval	*	ms
QRS duration	124	ms
QT/QTc	328/485	ms
P–R–T axes	* 120	12

Atrial fibrillation with rapid ventricular response
Right bundle branch block
Left posterior fascicular block
*** Bifascicular block ***
Abnormal ECG

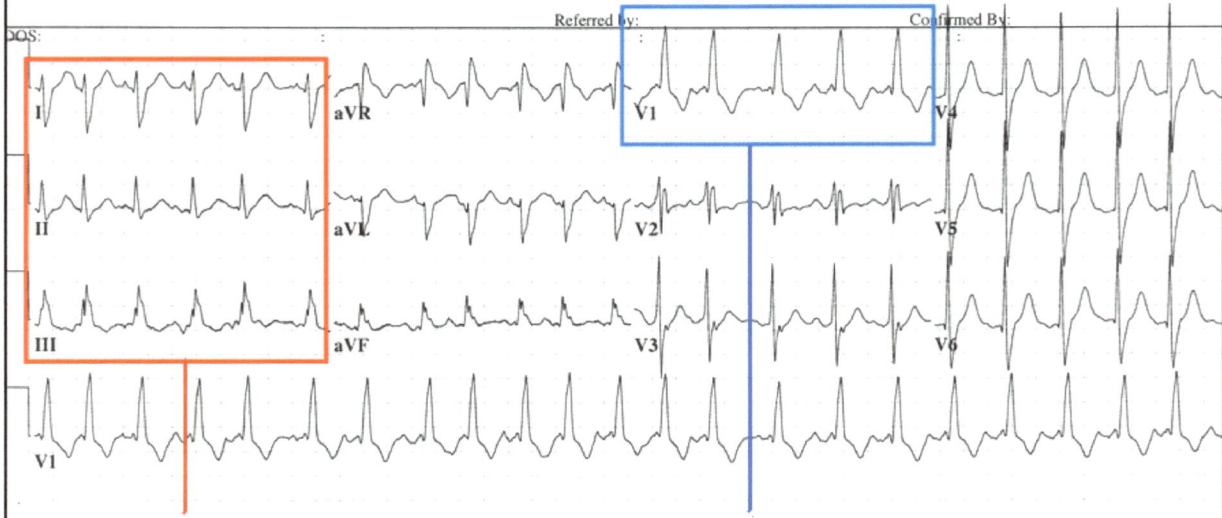

LEFT ANTERIOR FASCICULAR BLOCK
1. "DOWN-UP-UP" PATTERN
2. S1-Q3 (not much Q in Lead III) !
3. RIGHT AXIS DEVIATION

RIGHT BUNDLE BRANCH BLOCK
1. QRS DURATION GREATER THAN 120 ms
2. rSR' PATTERN in LEAD V1

288

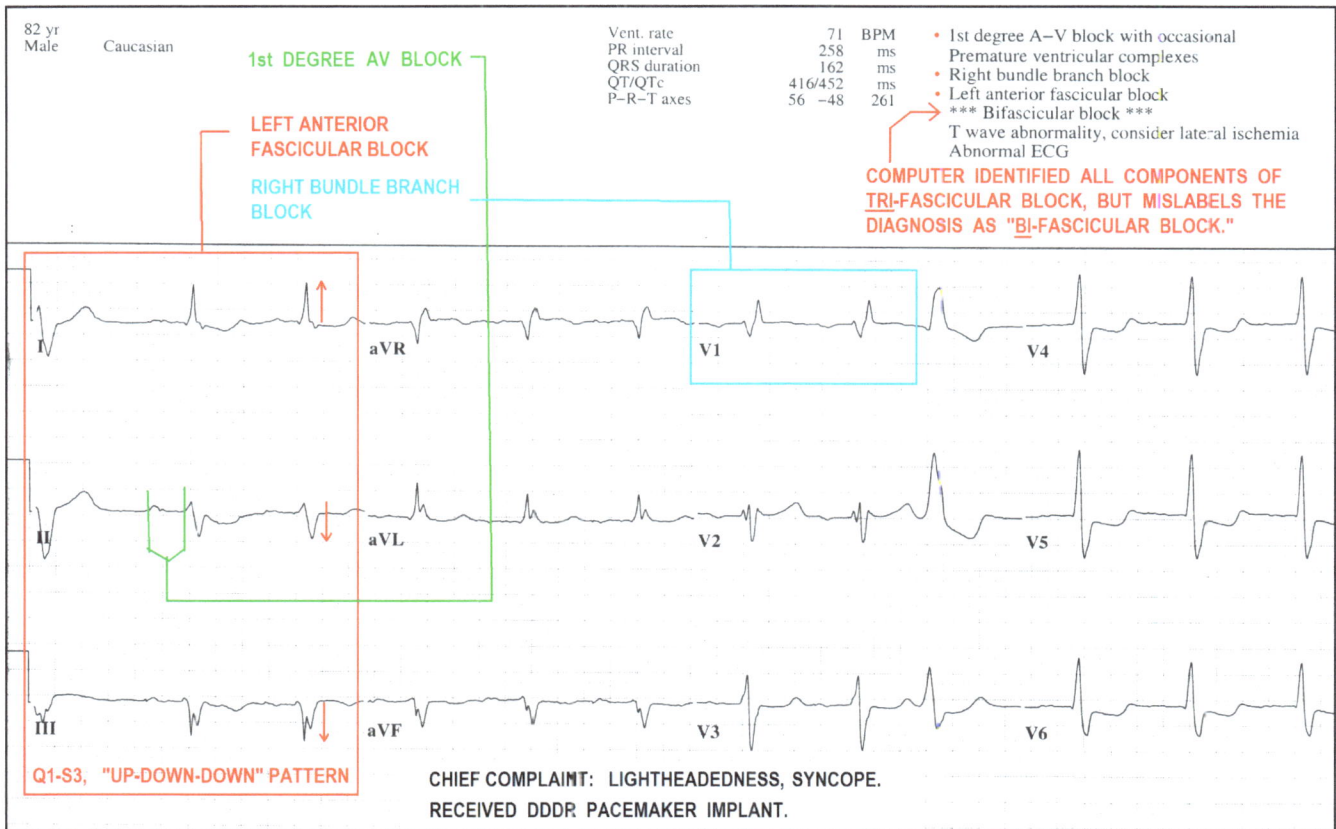

ECG Header Information:

82 yr
Male   Caucasian

1st DEGREE AV BLOCK

LEFT ANTERIOR
FASCICULAR BLOCK

RIGHT BUNDLE BRANCH
BLOCK

Vent. rate	71	BPM
PR interval	258	ms
QRS duration	162	ms
QT/QTc	416/452	ms
P-R-T axes	56 -48	261

- 1st degree A–V block with occasional Premature ventricular complexes
- Right bundle branch block
- Left anterior fascicular block
*** Bifascicular block ***
T wave abnormality, consider lateral ischemia
Abnormal ECG

COMPUTER IDENTIFIED ALL COMPONENTS OF TRI-FASCICULAR BLOCK, BUT MISLABELS THE DIAGNOSIS AS "BI-FASCICULAR BLOCK."

Leads: I, aVR, V1, V4
II, aVL, V2, V5
III, aVF, V3, V6

Q1-S3, "UP-DOWN-DOWN" PATTERN

CHIEF COMPLAINT: LIGHTHEADEDNESS, SYNCOPE.
RECEIVED DDDR PACEMAKER IMPLANT.

The above ECG demonstrates "classic" Tri-Fascicular Block.   Such samples are hard to come by; by the time most patients seek medical care, they're already in complete heart block; they've either bypassed this phase, or they're asymptomatic until they deteriorate into complete heart block.

This gentleman complained of episodes of extreme fatigue, lightheadedness and syncope.   While in the hospital awaiting his appointment in the Electrophysiology Lab, he experienced a run of complete heart block. He responded favorably to 0.5 mg of IV Atropine. He underwent successful pacemaker implantation.

LONG QT SYNDROME CASE STUDY 1:

The ECG below is that of a 22 year old female who was previously diagnosed with "epileptic seizure disorders." She was prescribed several antiseizure medications, none of which were effective in controlling her periodic seizure activity. After visiting several physicians, only one obtained a 12 Lead ECG, which is shown below. Using the "Quick Peek" method (above left), one can rapidly see that the patient's QT duration exceeds that of the R-R Interval!

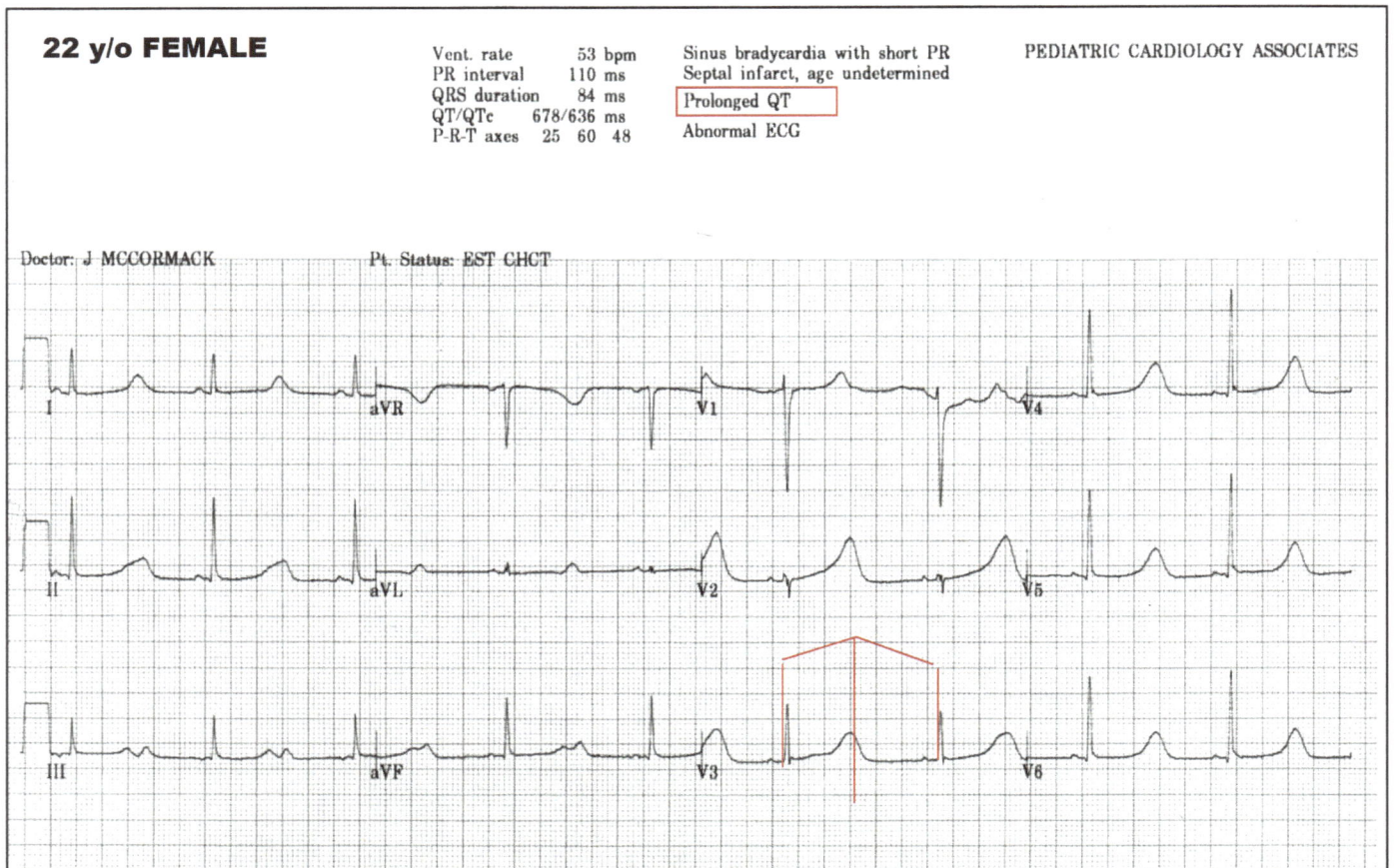

22 y/o FEMALE

Vent. rate	53 bpm
PR interval	110 ms
QRS duration	84 ms
QT/QTc	678/636 ms
P-R-T axes	25 60 48

Sinus bradycardia with short PR
Septal infarct, age undetermined
Prolonged QT
Abnormal ECG

PEDIATRIC CARDIOLOGY ASSOCIATES

Doctor: J MCCORMACK   Pt. Status: EST CHCT

This patient was referred to a local electrophysiologist specializing in the pediatric patient population, and is well known for his expertise in the area of Long QT Syndromes. During exercise stress testing, the patient developed Torsades. At this point, an AICD was implanted.

Subsequent genetic testing confirmed an abnormality of gene KCNQ1, confirming the physician's suspected diagnosis of LQTS Type I. It is significant to note that other members of her family, including a small child, suffered syncopal episodes, tested positive for Type 1 LQTS, and received AICDs. All family members are currently alive and well.

Cardiac events (Torsades, sudden death) in LQTS Type 1 are typically triggered by Exercise and exertional stress. Several incidents have been described as occurring during athletic events and while swimming.[111]

Case contributed by Jorge McCormack, MD, FACC

LONG QT SYNDROME CASE STUDY 2:

ECG of a 15 year old male who suffered sudden cardiac arrest.   Immediate bystander CPR and application of AED resulted in successful resuscitation.   Prior to the event, patient had no known history of any medical problems. There was a familial history of sudden death.

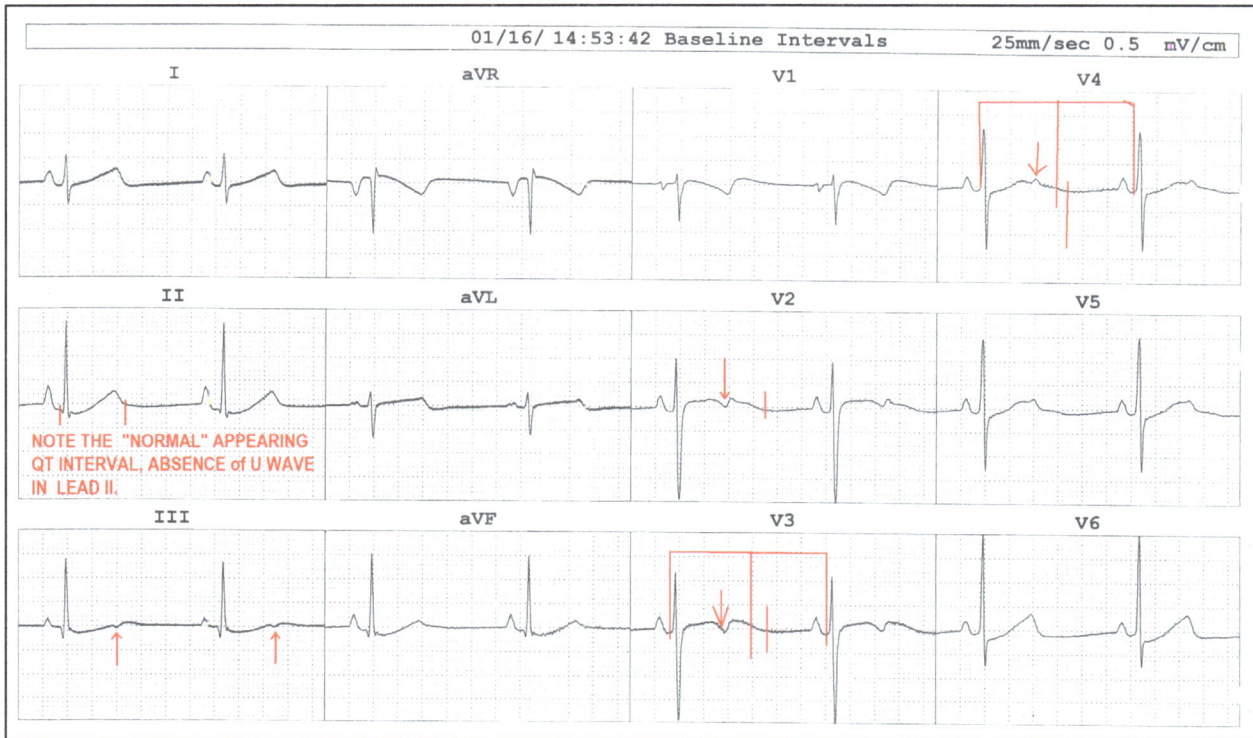

An EP study (shown below) revealed the presence of abnormal electrical signals originating in the ventricles consistent with timing of the U wave (or second half of the "notched" T wave), combined with positive genetic testing for LQTS Type 2 resulted in the patient receiving an AICD.

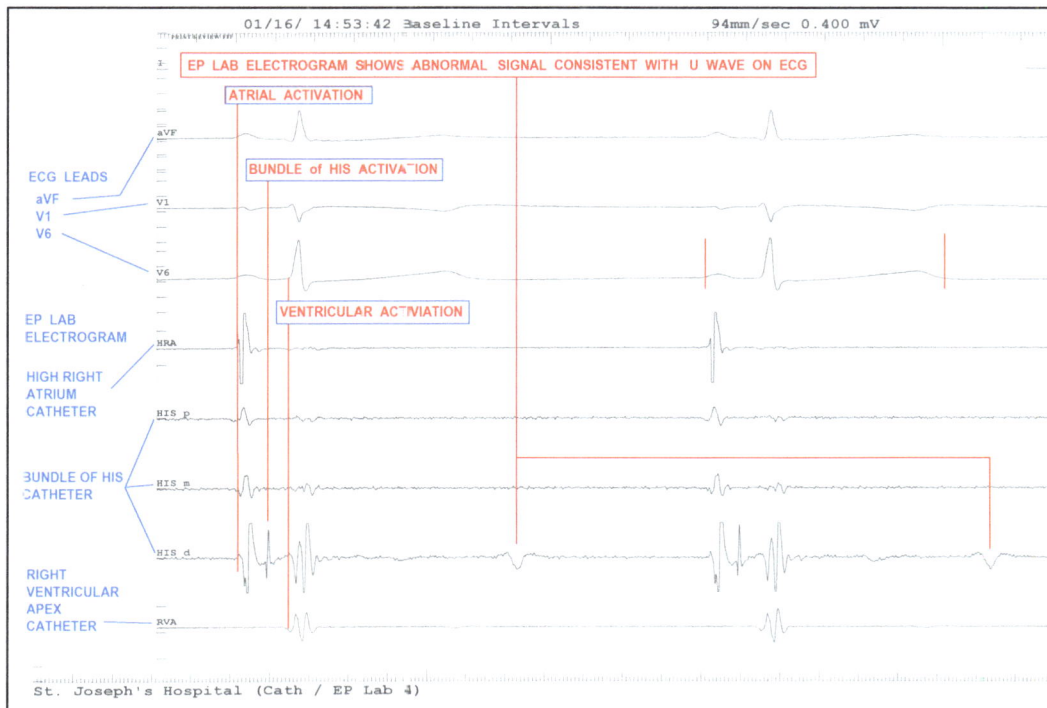

The ECG below is that of a 56 year old man with no previous history of cardiac disorders who suffered from episodes of syncope after being put on Ritalin.   Note the prevalence of U waves in leads aVR, V1, V2 and V3. U waves of opposite polarity (positive T, negative U) are noted in leads V4, V5 and V6.

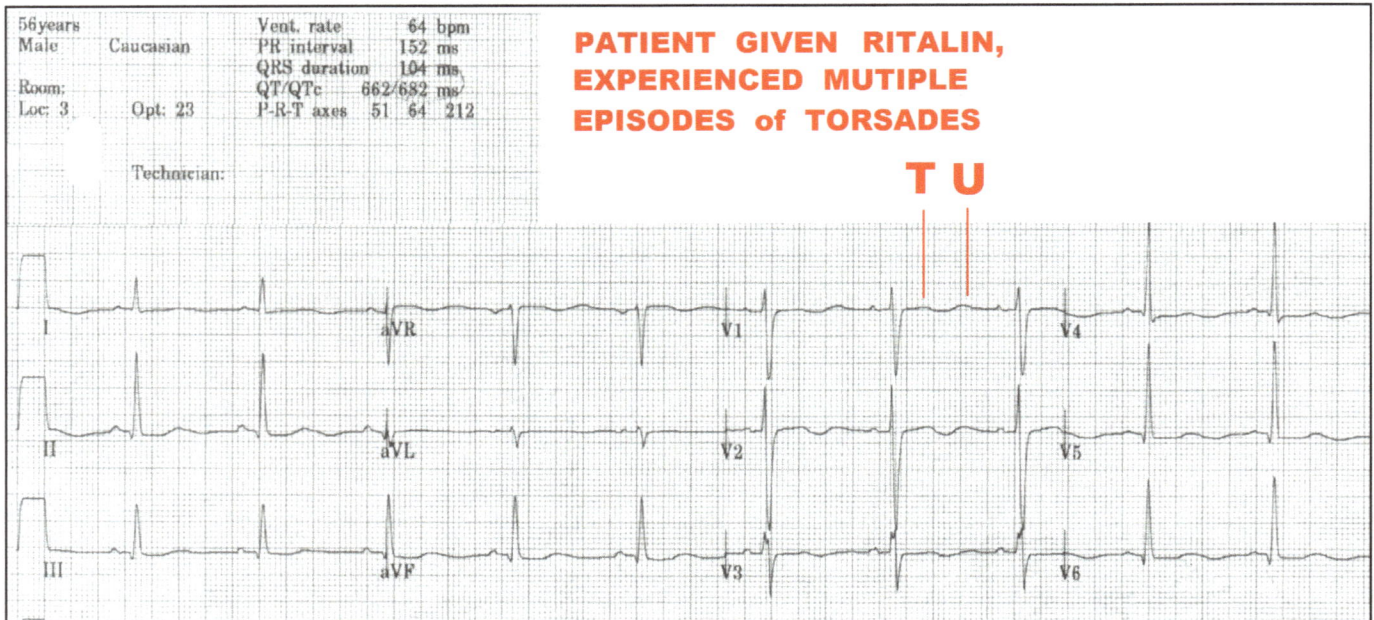

Part of his diagnostic workup included cardiac catheterization to rule out CAD. (U waves of opposite polarity from T waves are considered a sign of ischemia).   During cardiac catheterization, he was found to have no obstructive CAD, however he suffered another episode of syncope – caused by run of Torsades, recorded on the Cath Lab's hemodynamic monitoring system.

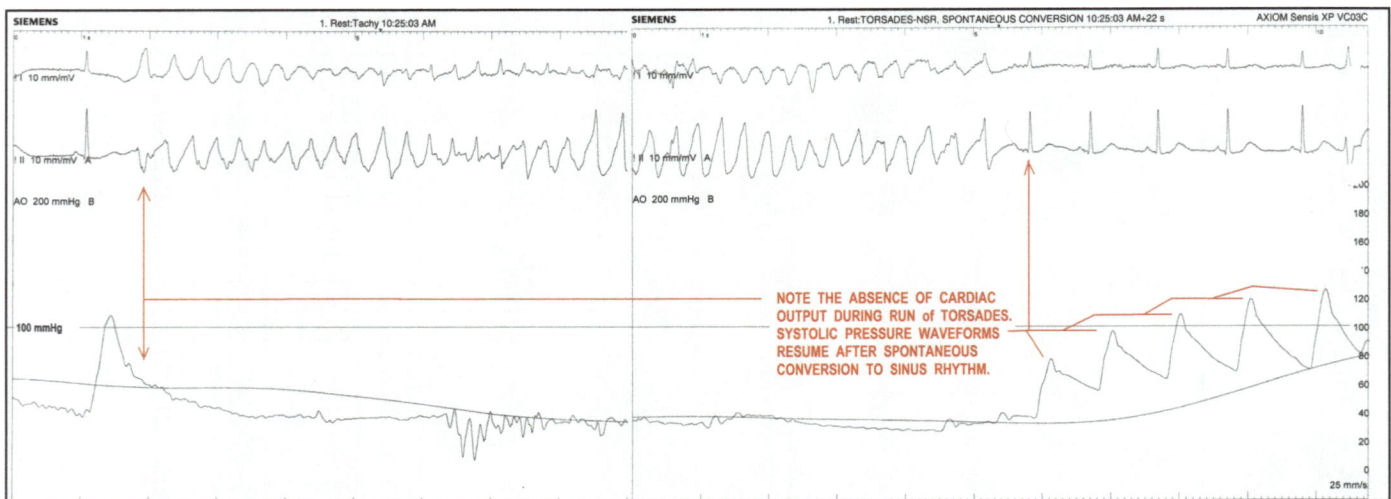

This patient was found to have the Acquired form of Long QT Syndrome, induced by Ritalin, which is one of many medications known to increase QT intervals.